Engineering in Medicine 2

Advances in

Artificial Hip and Knee Joint Technology

Edited by
M. Schaldach and D. Hohmann
in Collaboration with
R. Thull and F. Hein

With 525 Figures

Springer-Verlag Berlin Heidelberg New York 1976

This book is edited by
MAX SCHALDACH, Prof. Dr.
Zentralinstitut für Biomedizinische Technik
der Friedrich Alexander Universität Erlangen / Nürnberg
Turnstr. 5
852 Erlangen (Germany)

DIETRICH HOHMANN, Prof. Dr.
Direktor der Orthopädischen
Universitäts-Klinik Erlangen
852 Erlangen (Germany)

ISBN 3-540-07728-6 Springer-Verlag Berlin Heidelberg New York
ISBN 0-387-07728-6 Springer-Verlag New York Heidelberg Berlin

Library of Congress Cataloging in Publication Data. Main entry under title:
Advances in artificial hip and knee joint technology.
(Engineering in medicine ; v. 2). Bibliography: p. . Includes index. 1. Artificial joints. 2. Biomedical materials. 3. Hip joint – Surgery. 4. Knee – Surgery. I. Schaldach, Max, 1936– II. Hohmann, Dietrich, Dr. med. III. Series. RD686.A38. 617'.582. 76-11760. ISBN 0-387-07728-6

Printed in Germany

Printing and binding: Druck- und Verlagsanstalt K. Triltsch, Würzburg

FOREWORD

Implantable joint prostheses which have been under development for more than 25 years, are today being used with success in the rehabilitation of many cases, including patients with extremely severe joint pathology. However, artificial joint designs still pose problems with respect to their function, anchoring, materials employed and the interaction of the prosthesis with the surrounding biological tissues. Some of these problems are associated with considerable therapeutic complications.

Further improvement in the artificial joint requires the application of all the modern experimental and research techniques and the close cooperation of medical doctors, engineers and scientists. The International Symposium on Advances in Artificial Hip and Knee Joint Technology held at Erlangen on October 30 and 31, 1975 under the auspices of the Societas Physica Medica Erlangensis, had as its aim the promotion of just this interdisciplinary cooperation. One of the traditional objectives of the Societas has been the advancement of diagnosis and therapy by the adaptation of medical skill to modern technology and scientific engineering concepts.

The major objective of this volume is to present, in expanded form, the lectures given by internationally recognized scientists and clinical researchers in the field of artificial joints in the locomotor system, and to make that information available to a wider public. The experience discussed covers the principles and primary methods of joint replacement. Particular emphasis is on problems of pressing importance at the present time, such as improvement of the general design, the fixation systems and implantable materials for hip and knee joints, as well as the postoperative management of a steadily increasing number of patients.

Erlangen 1976

D. Hohmann

M. Schaldach

CONTENTS

CHAPTER 4

TRENDS IN HIP AND KNEE PROSTHESES DEVELOPMENT

LIST OF LECTURERS

BECK, H.
Friedrich-Alexander-Universität,
Chirurgische Klinik
Krankenhausstrasse 12
D-8520 Erlangen
(Federal Republic of Germany)

BLAUTH, W.
Orthopädische Universitätsklinik und
Poliklinik
Klaus-Groth-Platz 4
D-2300 Kiel
(Federal Republic of Germany)

DEBRUNNER, H.U.
Universität Bern
Orthopadische Klinik und Poliklinik
Inselspital
CH-3010 Bern
(Switzerland)

FREEMAN, M.A.R.
Imperial College of Science and Technology
Exhibition Road
London SW 7
(United Kingdom)

FRIEDEBOLD, G.
Freie Universität Berlin,
Orthopädische Klinik und Poliklinik im
Oskar-Helene-Heim
Clayallee 229
D-1000 Berlin 33
(Federal Republic of Germany)

GSCHWEND, N.
Klinik Wilhelm Schulthess
Neumünsterallee 3/10
CH-8032 Zürich
(Switzerland)

HENCHE, H.R.
Orthopädische Universitätsklinik
Felix-Platter-Spital
CH-4055 Basel
(Switzerland)

HOHMANN, D.
Universität Erlangen-Nürnberg
Orthopädische Klinik und Poliklinik
Rathsbergerstrasse 57
D-8520 Erlangen
(Federal Republic of Germany)

HUGGLER, A.H.
Kantonsspital Chur
Orthopädische Abteilung
CH-7000 Chur
(Switzerland)

HULBERT, S.F.
Tulane University
Biomaterials Laboratory
New Orleans, LA. 70118
(USA)

KLAWITTER, J.J.
Tulane University
Biomaterials Laboratory
New Orleans, LA. 70118
(USA)

KNAPPEN, F.-J.
Winterthur-Versicherungsgruppe
Obere Laube 44
D-7750 Konstanz
(Federal Republic of Germany)

KUMMER, B.
Universität Köln
Anatomisches Institut
Lindenburg
D-5000 Köln 41
(Federal Republic of Germany)

MITTELMEIER, H.
Orthopädische Universitätsklinik und Poliklinik
D-6650 Homburg (Saar)
(Federal Republic of Germany)

MÜLLER, M.E.
Universität Bern
Orthopädische Klinik und Poliklinik
Inselspital
CH-3012 Bern
(Switzerland)

PAUL, J.P.
University of Strathclyde
Bioengineering Unit
106 Rottenrow
Glasgow 64 ONW
(United Kingdom)

SAUER, B.W.
Clemson University
Clemson, SC. 29631
(USA)

SCHALDACH, M.
Universität Erlangen-Nürnberg
Zentralinstitut für Biomedizinische
Technik
Turnstrasse 5
D-8520 Erlangen
(Federal Republic of Germany)

SCHREIBER, A.
Orthopädische Universitätsklinik Balgrist
Forchstrasse 340
CH-8008 Zürich
(Switzerland)

SCHULITZ, K.P.
Universität Heidelberg
Orthopädische Klinik und Poliklinik
Schlierbacher Landstrasse 200 a
D-6900 Heidelberg-Schlierbach
(Federal Republic of Germany)

THULL, R.
Universität Erlangen-Nürnberg
Zentralinstitut für Biomedizinische
Technik
Turnstrasse 5
D-8520 Erlangen
(Federal Republic of Germany)

UNGETHÜM, M.
Orthopädische Klinik München
Harlachinger Strasse 51
D-8000 München 90
(Federal Republic of Germany)

VERNON–ROBERTS, B.
The London Hospital Medical College
Turner Street
London E1 2AD
(United Kingdom)

WEBER, B.G.
Kantonsspital
Klinik für Orthopädische Chirurgie
CH-9006 St. Gallen
(Switzerland)

WEIGHTMAN, B.
Imperial College of Science and Technology
Exhibition Road
London SW7
(United Kingdom)

WILLERT, H.-G.
Orthopädische Universitätsklinik
Friedrichsheim
Marienburgstrasse 2
D-6000 Frankfurt/Main – Niederrad 71
(Federal Republic of Germany)

ZITTER, H.
Montanuniversität
Institut für Allgemeine und Analytische
Chemie
Franz-Josef-Strasse 18
A-8700 Leoben
(Austria)

ZWICKER, H.U.
Universität Erlangen-Nürnberg
Institut für Werkstoffwissenschaften II
Martensstrasse 5
D-8520 Erlangen
(Federal Republic of Germany)

Chapter 1
Principles and Techniques of Hip and Knee Joint Replacement

STATE OF THE ART OF HIP AND KNEE JOINT REPLACEMENT

G. Friedebold and R. Kölbel

A dream seemed to come true when George McKee's first patient with an artificial hip joint took his first steps, was able to move, sit and walk painlessly and unobtrusively. Payr, one of the fathers of joint surgery had hoped to realize this dream conceived 150 years ago: Restoration of the ruin of a joint with its pain, contracture or instability. The optismism of this great surgeon, expressed in 1934 was based on the results of conventional interposition arthroplasties improved by Lexer himself and are followed up and reported sporadically (4). It was not until 30 years later that the resolution of some of the problems by positive fixation of artificial joint components by Charnley (5) opened up a new epoch of joint surgery.

Ten years have since passed; partial arthroplasties were introduced or interposition arthroplasties with a metal cup (21,27,40,48). Articulations of one artificial articular component on its biological counterpart is basically different from total joint replacement in that a body of low compliance is pressed against cartilage and bone, and in that the interaction of cartilage surfaces and synovia is disturbed both in static and dynamic loading and shearing relative movements. For a method whose objective it is to obtain lasting and normal function of an artificial organ, 10 years is not a very long period of time for assessment. Even for patients over 65 years, 10 years experience does not permit us to promise lifelong service since life expectancy may be well over 75 years.

Excellent early results have contributed to an optimism among patients and surgeons that is unprecedented for an operation which is not life-saving.

In the meantime complications and failures have been reported – only occasionally at first, but subsequently in ever increasing numbers. Thrombosis and early infection are mentioned because of their general surgical importance and due to the fact that, in contrast to some other surgical procedures, infection is fatal for the outcome of the arthroplasty.

The incidence of periarticular calcifications, an occasional finding, may be influenced by operative technique. Attempts at local or systemic drug application to prevent calcifications have not been satisfactory. Their clinical significance is doubtful as they are not always associated with compromised motion (16).

Loosening with or without infection is the most important cause of failure. In patients with artificial joints which may have been functional for years, walking and movement become painful due to loosening, at a time when the results in these patients have long been listed as sucesses. Increasing incidence of failure within the ten-year-limit raises the question as to whether we can truly speak of a victory over the problems of arthroplasty, or, has the problem of arthroplasty really been solved in the spirit of our great teacher Payr?

Osteoarthritis, a chronic degenerative lesion of the joints caused by a number of etiologic factors arises as a consequence of a disturbed balance of the biological potential of the joint and the mechanical stress and strain. These are of paramount importance in the case of the lower limb; hence the large proportion of degenerative lesions of hip and knee joint. Endoprostheses have been designed for most of the peripheral joints. However, experience has not yet led to unequivocal conclusions. To sum up the results of arthroplasty of the last decade and the present state of the art one will have to look at the hip and knee, the replacement of which is of eminent practical significance.

There is a time lag in the development of implants: When Walldius (51), later Young (53), Shiers (45) and a few others reported on initial results after knee joint replacement, hip replacement had already spread like wildfire. While attempts to modify or improve McKee's and Charnley's models were in full swing, the followers of Walldius, Young and Shiers were still using their original designs – gaining experience and analysing it. Meanwhile, knee joint replacement has been advanced and today we are in a position to evaluate, not only a vast number of design models, but also an appropriate variety of such failures as loosening and late infection. There may still be a time lag as regards their appearance in statistics.

Before reviewing the problems as they present themselves, we shall first deal with some aspects of joint replacement in general and of hip and knee replacement in particular. Present-day solutions, as regards engineering and biological aspects, appear as powerful therapeutic media. Nevertheless the application should occur carefully, taking into account the conditions in the individual patient. Hence we shall finally dwell upon indications.

GENERAL ASPECTS OF JOINT REPLACEMENT AT THE HIP AND KNEE

In the lower extremity, both great joints are subjected to high static and dynamic loads. The general aspects we have to deal with apply equally and basically to both the hip and knee joints.

IMPLANT MATERIALS

Starting with the original designs of McKee and Farrar and Charnley the combinations of metal on metal and of metal on plastic have gained in popularity. With modified designs, these models are currently in use. Although the range of application is quite restricted for hemiarthroplasties, we still have to deal with the combination metal on cartilage. The recent application of ceramics seems to have opened up new perspectives. The application of materials of this type is now at the stage of clinical trial and will not be included in this review.

MATERIAL PROPERTIES

In contrast to temporary implants, higher mechanical strength is required of permanent implants, which are subjected to a greater number of load cycles (14). A combination of required properties in a single material will be achieved by alloying certain basic metals, however, the optimization of one specific property may mean less than optimal values for others. As yet, there is not ideal alloy and experimental research is still going on (42). At present, alloys of three basic metals are being used. Their properties are listed in Table 1.

Improvements will certainly be possible through cooperation between metallurgists and bioengineers familiar with mechanical loads on permanent implants, with the severe environment to which they are exposed in the body, and with the requirements of body compatibility of solid materials and their wear and corrosion products (11,13). After initial experience with Teflon and other polymers, high density polyethylene has been found to be the plastic material which meets most practical requirements. As a paraffin derivative it is chemically inert, even its wear particles produce little tissue reaction. No carcinogenic effect has been proven in man. Its tensile and bending strength properties exclude it as a sole material for use as fixation parts or to bridge defects. Since Charnley (8) demonstrated its properties as a bearing material in combination with metal surfaces of defined radii, the metal on plastic combination has become universal in a vast number of joint replacement implants for the hip and knee.

In the early stages, total joint replacements were designed for direct fixation to bone. Today we are witnessing a swing back of interest to this idea. But ever since the introduction of polymethylmethacrylate as a means of fixation, the majority of surgeons have used it. In the polymerized state this material has adequate compressive and shear strength, it is inert and non toxic. Hypersensitivities have been reported in surgeons but not in patients.

Table 1 Comparison of requirements and properties for the employment of metallic materials for artificial joints

	Steel	CoCrMo-Alloy Cast - Forged	Titanium TiAlV-Alloy
1. High static strength, low modulus of elasticity	+	++	++
2. High fatigue strength	++	+ +++	+++
3. Max. corrosion resistance under intracorporeal conditions	+	++	+++
4. Body compatibility for implant and wear particles	+	+++	+++
5. Workability	+++	+	++
6. Low cost	++	+	+

CHARACTERISTICS OF MATERIALS AS ARTICULATING SURFACES

Loading and articulation at normal joints are fairly slow dynamic actions. Biologic materials and designs are perfectly adapted to them. The changes we impose on this balance by different types of alloarthroplasties have to be considered:

In hemialloarthroplasty a metallic body articulates with hyaline cartilage. We realize today the importance of the change in the lubricating mechanism and the stress distribution which this means and which may over different periods of use lead to replacement by fibrocartilage or removal of hyaline cartilage and erosion of the underlying bone (Fig. 1). In the case of optimal matching of the surfaces, moderate loading and solid subchondral bone cobalt-chrome-molybdenum femoral head replacements of the Moore (29), Thompson (50) or Eicher (12) types may well serve their purpose. Their use, however, is restricted to subcapital fractures of the femur and their sequelae in the very old.

In the knee McIntosh's (25) replacement of the tibial plateaus is still in use in certain (posttraumatic) conditions (Fig. 2). Surface replacement of the femoral condyles has had some good results as regards mobility, but load-bearing may be painful.

Apparently the tibial articular surfaces are softer than the femoral condyles which seem well able to support the friction and pressure by a McIntosh plateau made of a cobalt-chrome-alloy. Again, good matching of the surfaces is a prerequisite of success.

METAL ON METAL JOINTS

The classical metal on metal joint, made of cast cobalt-chrome molybdenum-alloy, has been followed by the Stanmore metal-to-metal hip, the Ring prosthesis (41) and Sivash's metal-to-metal hip (47) which was at the time made of titanium. They each have a great number of supporters to this day. For electrochemical reasons, the use of identical metals for the articulating surfaces is obligatory. Their geometry is of critical importance: Maintenance of a passivated surface layer may be of relative importance for the service life of the articulating surfaces. This may be destroyed by excessive pressures i.e. mismatch-

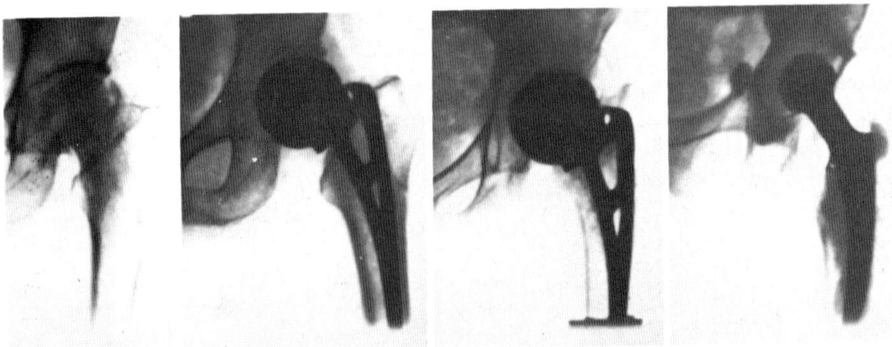

Fig. 1 Erosion of the hyaline cartilage of the hip socket in hemialloarthroplasty. Shifting of the head of a Moore prosthesis towards the small pelvis

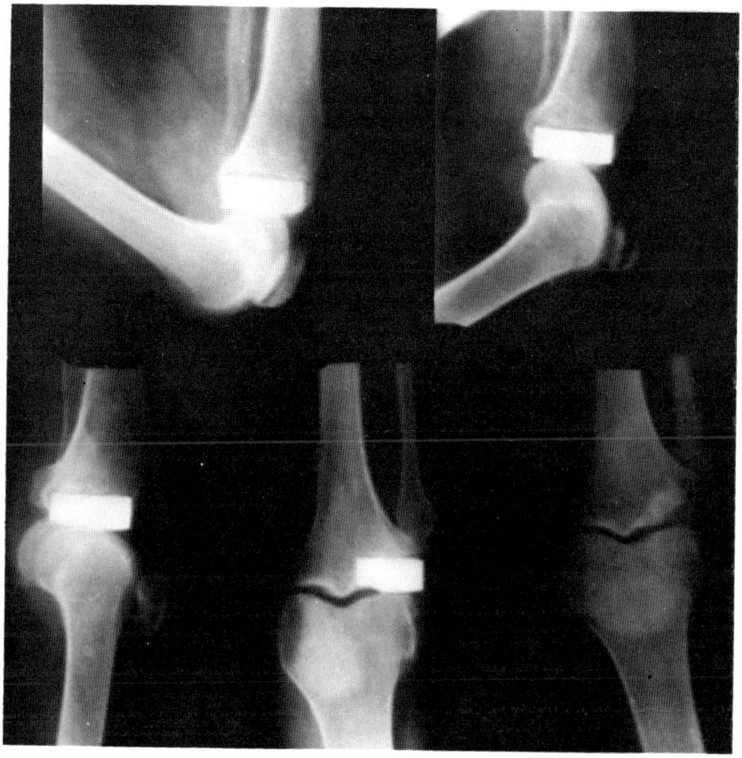

Fig. 2 Employment of McIntosh's plateau for the reconstruction of the lateral articular surfaces of the tibia destroyed by compression fracture

ing of the radii. On the other hand exactly congruent joints tend to seize up, thereby causing considerable torques to be applied to the zone of fixation. Loosening of the acetabular and the femoral part is the result. Oval areas of contact, which lead both to corrosion and blocking, have been demonstrated by means of a staining technique using ink (Fig. 3).

The horseshoe type of bearing developed at Stanmore appears to have been only partially successful. Parsons (36) found that an increase of the radius of the acetabular cup as well as a central recess contributed towards the solution of the problem of friction torque (Fig. 4). A difference of 0.2 mm between the radii of ball and socket seems to be a compromise agreed upon for metal-to-metal joints today. This point may not be of equal relevance for metal-to-metal knee joints, however; too much play of the axis and malalignment of the hinge lead to unequal load distribution and consequently to corrosion and wear on corresponding surfaces (Fig. 5).

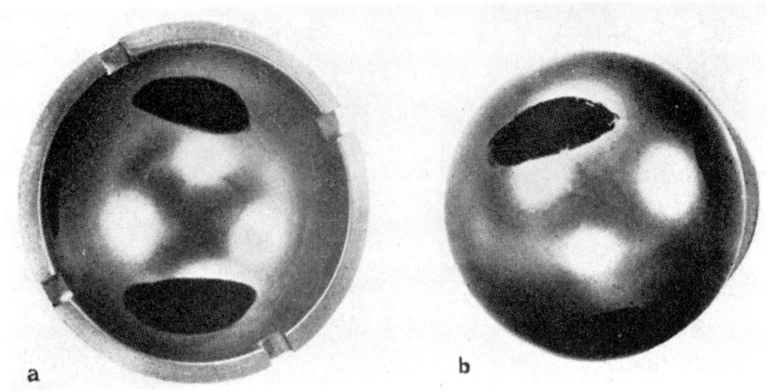

Fig. 3 Staining of the contact surfaces in total hip joint replacement (37)

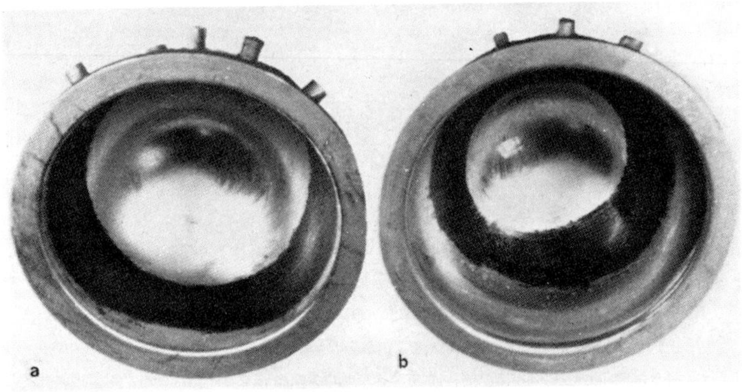

Fig. 4 Joint for the replacement of the hip joint and reduction of the forces of friction by varying radii (37)

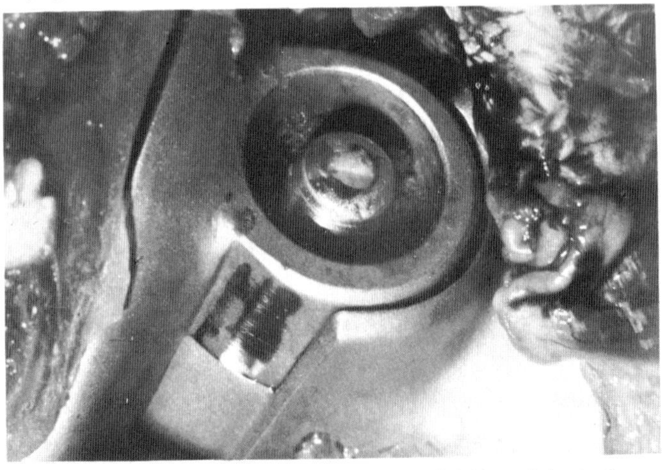

Fig. 5 Corrosion of the metallic joint surface of an artificial knee joint in the presence of too much play of the axis

METAL–TO–PLASTIC JOINTS

High density polyethylene was employed because of its low friction, but only as a second choice to Teflon, which is superior in vitro but did not pass the clinical test. In the dry state, the coefficient of friction for metal on polyethylene is only about half, and lubricated with Ringer's solution only about one tenth, that of contemporary metal-to-metal surfaces. Seizing up has never been a problem with the low friction arthroplasty. Charnley's stainless steel head has a diameter that is 0.127 mm smaller than the plastic acetabulum which can easily adjust to this difference.

Most of the metal-to-plastic modifications of this type of bearing have larger diameters and seem to function equally well. This raises the question as to whether friction is indeed such an important factor as Charnley has always claimed – especially since smaller heads produce greater linear wear. It must not be overlooked, however, that greater friction means greater static and dynamic stressing of a rigid zone of fixation and may contribute to loosening. This may be the real significance of low friction (15).

This aspect has not played an equally important role in the considerations of th original all-metal hinges which are still being widely used. A number of knee replacement implants are now commercially available, in which a metallic femoral component articulates with a polyethylene tibial plateau. This may be cemented to the bone directly or mounted on a metal stem. In some models, plastic is only used as a buffer in full extension. The use of plastic in fixed hinges has so far not been proven essential, since motion occurs in one plane only. Conditions are different for design concepts which allow for relative sliding torsion similar to the natural joint. In such designs the likely danger of higher corrosion and wear exclude the use of metal-to-metal bearing surfaces.

METALLOSIS AND THE EFFECTS OF WEAR PRODUCTS

Friction between metallic parts and metal on plastics under static and dynamic loads necessarily produces wear of the articulating surfaces. Mechanically this is of minor importance as long as wear particles will be eliminated from the joint space by the body fluids. The Stanmore horseshoe bearing was designed with this aspect in mind.

The wear rate is higher in plastic materials than in the harder metals. Here, careful handling of passivated surfaces is as important as careful positioning to avoid mechanical contact between the neck of the femoral component and the rim of the metallic acetabulum (Fig. 6). Present designs allow a larger range of movement than earlier ones.

Consequently, problems from wear are less likely to result from mechanical causes than from possible chemical and toxic effects. The laws of relations between large metal parts and the body have their complements on the microscopical or biochemical level. Here we have to look at the reactions caused by the contact of pure metallic and polymer particles of very small dimensions with vital cells and their products (Figs. 7,8).

The toxic effects of stainless steel and cobalt-chrome-molybdenum alloys have been examined by Pappas and Cotten (35) and, with slightly different methods, by Mital and Cotten (28). The former exposed tissue cultures to powders of both materials and counted

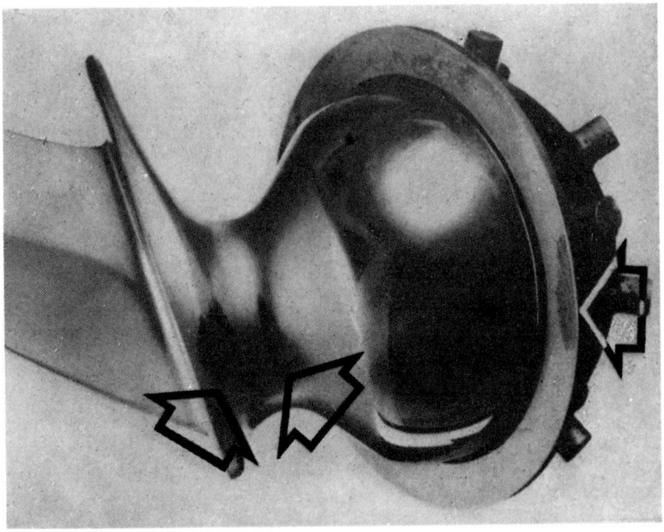

Fig. 6 Representation of the wear corrosion resulting from mechanical contact between the rim of the acetabulum and the neck collar of the femoral shaft (37)

their populations in the replication phase; the latter used suspensions of metal particles in solutions simulating body fluids for the same type of investigation, counting populations in the lag-phase. The tissue cultures showed metallic inclusions in mitotic cells and in cells after 15 subcultures. The toxicity indicated by these experiments, more so for cobalt-chrome-molybdenum than for stainless steel, which is certainly not negligible, has as yet not shown any correlation with clinical experience. Both materials are well tolerated. Prompted by the high variance of the experiments mentioned, Gerber et al. (17) developed standardized organ cultures of growing bones in order to obtain sensitive and reproducible tests of toxicity. In fact their results led to dose-effect curves which could be utilized in testing the effects of soluble substances on tissues. Metallic inclusions were also found in lymphatic tissues. The question as to whether in fact, a period of 10 years is sufficient to judge this negative side of endoprosthetics exhaustirely and finally remains unanswered.

Fig. 9 shows a Young's knee in situ three years afters implantation. Its femoral component had come loose, it was painful and required replacement. Changes in the zone of contact between cobalt-chrome-molybdenum and vital bone are more impressive than those at the bone cement border where mechanical stresses must have been considerably higher, especially after loosening (Figs. 10,11). It would be hard to believe that such masses of necrotic tissue, together with cement fragments of various sizes should be biologically inert (Fig. 12). Undoubtedly, in the case shown, mechanical loosening has promoted the effect of metallosis (Fig. 13).

It still remains uncertain whether this is due to a basic difference or to an acceleration of the natural course of events, and – again – whether 10 years is really an adequate period of time to evaluate knee replacement.

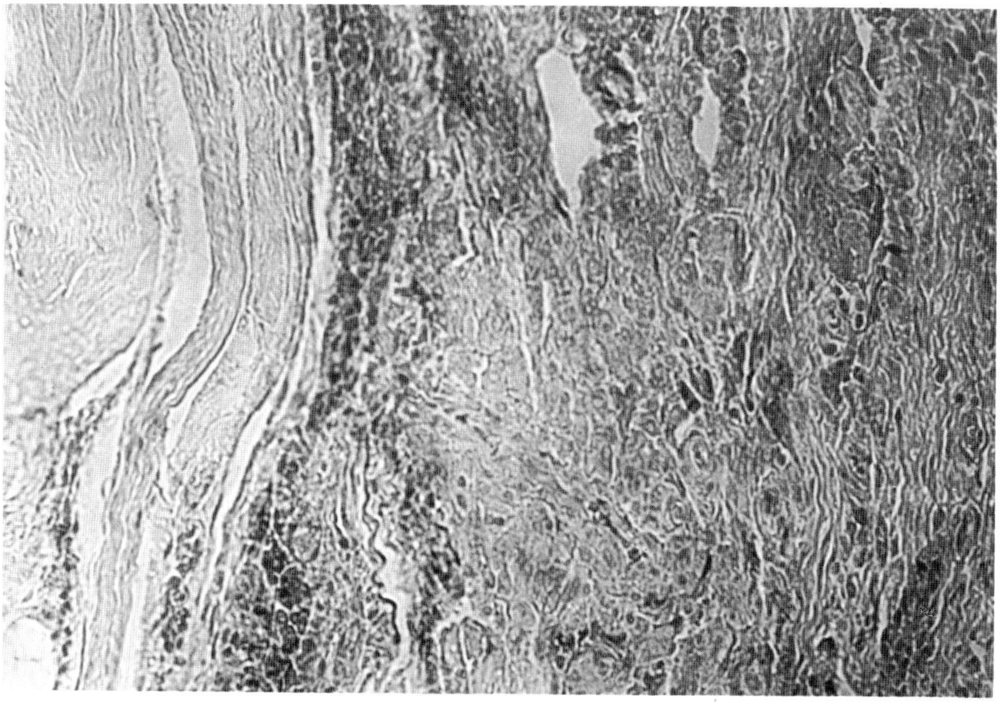

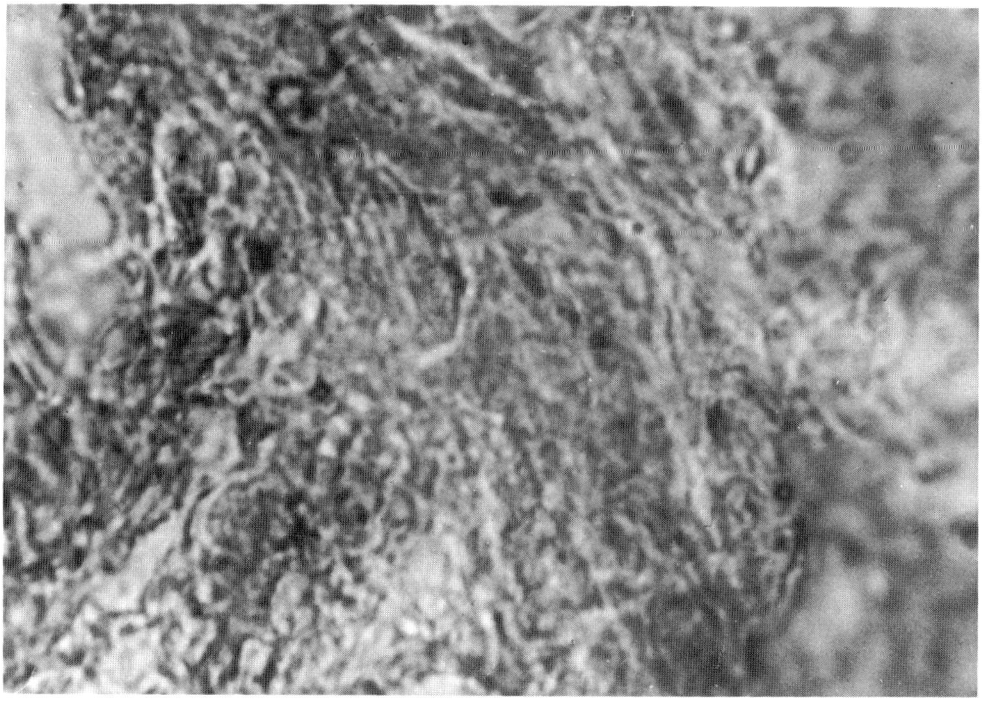

Figs. 7,8 Histological sections through tissue with metallic inclusions (particles) from the neighbourhood of the artificial joint

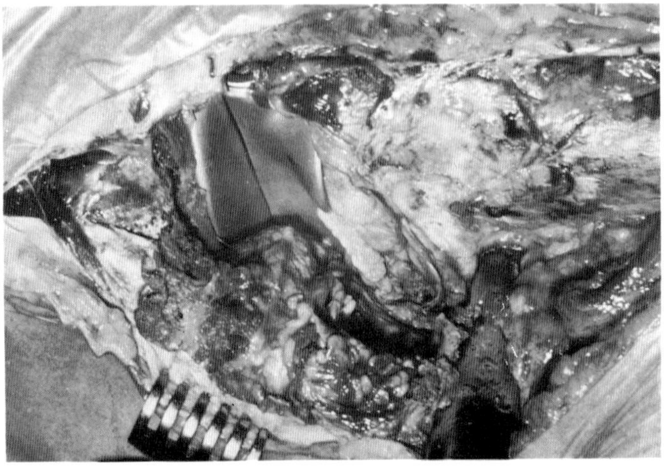

Fig. 9 Young's knee in situ, three years after the initial implantation

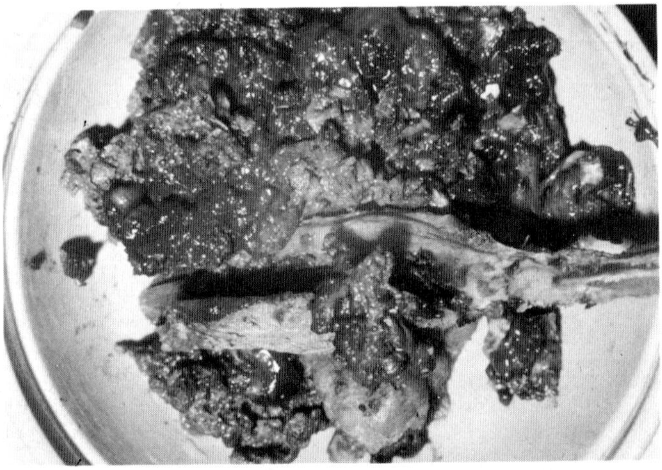

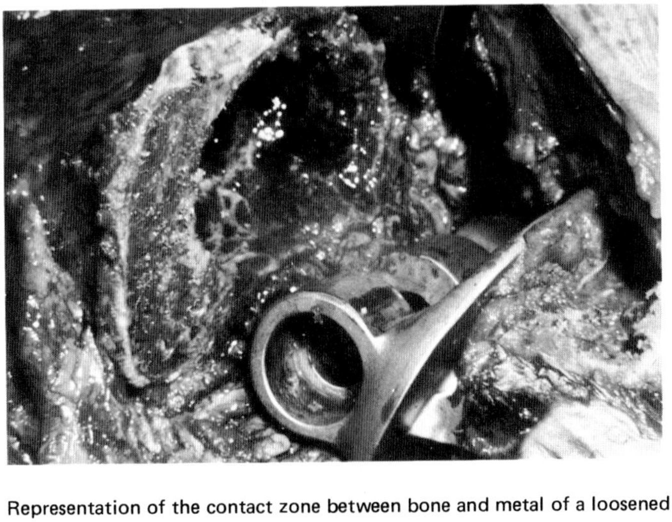

Figs. 10,11 Representation of the contact zone between bone and metal of a loosened Young's knee

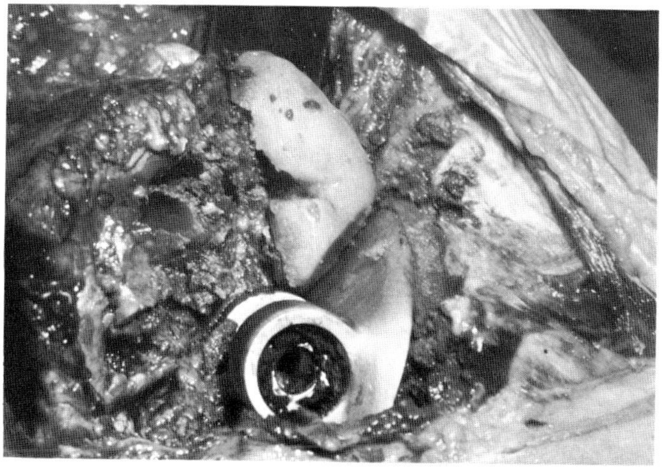

Fig. 12 Tissue mass and loosened cement removed on the occasion of a surgical revision of the case in Fig. 9

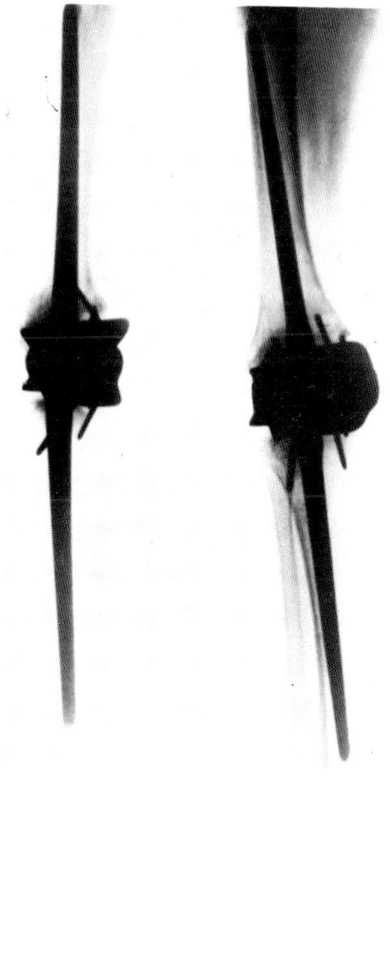

Fig. 13
X-ray picture of the loosened Young's prosthesis

The question of the individual response of connective tissues, as is known in the context of scar formation, also remains unanswered. There was no infection in the joint shown here. It seems to be merely a matter of time for the metallotic changes of the surrounding tissues to arrive at the most superficial covering layer.

In metal-to-plastic joints, the linear wear rate – 0.2 mm per year for the Charnley hip – may not impair mechanical function of the joint. However, volumetric wear may amount to as much as one ml per year, depending on the dimensions of the joint. This represents a quantitative problem for the surrounding tissues in that their capacity for storage is limited. If wear volume is overwhelming, the resulting granulation tissue may erode the bone in the zone of fixation and cause loosening. For HDP no specific effect of the particles has been reported so far.

FIXATION

Before the introduction of acrylic cement the construction of joint implants required special features in order to achieve an anchorage adequate for mechanical stability, which is a prerequisite for bone healing and adaptation. At the same time, a certain amount of elasticity was required to allow for equal load distribution at the interface between the stems of hip and knee replacements and the inner surface of the medullary cavities. Such a design meant absolute reliability of the seating at the points of load transfer to bone, at the base of the neck of the femur as well as at the femoral and tibial condyles for hinge knee replacements which were additionally fastened with screws.

The principle of fixation without cement (41,47) has been given renewed attention recently. This is due to the fact that the shortcomings of acrylic cement have so far largely excluded younger patients from the benefits of joint replacement, and to the advent of ceramics in endoprosthetics. The application of acrylic cement creates a large area of intimate bonding of implant and bone. This area is fairly rigid, it loses its natural mechanical properties, its compliance and hence some of its properties essential to load transfer.

The implant itself does not replace the mechanical properties of the joint components which it doubles for. Biological reactions will therefore be concentrated on the vital side of the interface only. This is the weak link in the chain of load transfer: Bone – cement – prosthesis – prosthesis – cement – bone. Whereas problems at the prosthesis/cement interface can be avoided by an appropriate geometry of the implant-surface, the cement/bone interface is subjected to great mechanical stresses. Its stability may be jeopardised by any technical error – incorrect choice of implant design, malalignment of stems, errors in the position of cups or the anteversion of the femoral head, inappropriate preparation of bone or use of cement – or by other conditions such as – excessive body weight, pronounced reactions of juvenile connective tissues, and excessive physical activity. All these factors may considerably increase the stresses at the cement/bone interface (1). Deepening of the acetabulum, necessary to completely accomodate the load-bearing part of the artificial acetabulum, may be a problem. Chiari (10) recommends preliminary pelvic osteotomy for hypoplastic acetabula.

The critical role attributed to this interface has led to considerable activity in experimental and basic research. Oest, Müller and Hopfauer (33) have just recently given an excellent review of the scope of application of current types of acrylic cements in implant fixation. They also show the limitations. In our institution the mechanical properties of the cement/ bone bond under static and cyclic loading as well as the significance of the dimensions of cement plugs at the acetabulum were investigated (22).

The cementing of an implant is associated with four problems. They have been over-estimated and are probably of lesser practical importance:

1. The stability of the cement depends largely on its homogeneity which may be disturbed by inclusion of blood and fat during the setting stage. This may compromise the ultimate strength of the fixation. Careful aspiration and employment of clotting agents have proven useful. Curettage of the medullary cavity, avoided by some surgeons for reasons of mechanical disadvantages, does not cause more than the usual amount of bleeding.
2. Production of heat during polymerization is certainly associated with necrosis of a layer of tissue. This neither influences the stability immediately – since there are no defects – nor does it produce any lasting effects on the capacity to form connective tissue. Consequently this is not of practical importance (23,32,34,39). Charnley and Crawford (6) did not answer the question as to whether necrosis found in the surrounding tissue 3 to 8 years after implantation is due to the initial thermal effect.
3. The rapid packing of cement into the medullary cavity may be regarded as a cause of intraoperative complications, with symptoms similar to those of fat embolism (Fig. 14). This is rare. Insertion of a catheter into the depth of the medullary cavity in order to facilitate the escape of air, blood and detritus is a useful precaution (43).

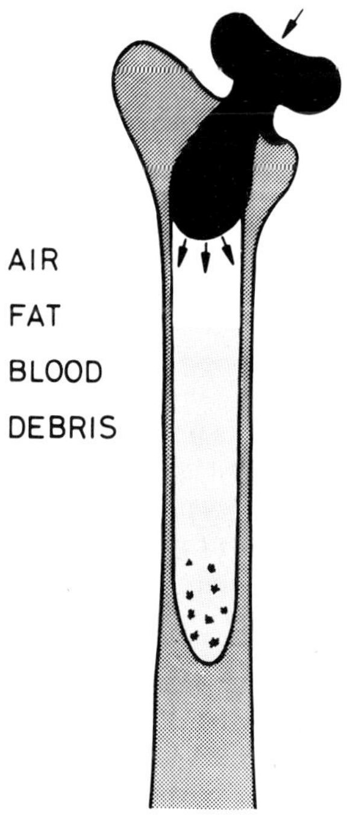

Fig. 14
Schematic representation of the possibility of pressing the contents of the medullary cavity of a long bone (air, fat, blood, debris) into opened veins during the introduction of the cement (37)

4. A sudden drop in blood pressure at the time of application of acrylic cement has been ascribed to toxic effects of free monomers of methylmethacrylic acid. Two precautionary procedures should be observed: Cement should not be introduced as long as it sticks to the surgeon's gloves. This sticky stage is indicative of free monomer at the surface of the cement in the plastic stage. Blood volume deficits ought to be compensated or slightly overcompensated, which require close cooperation with the anesthetist.

PARTICULAR PROBLEMS OF THE HIP AND KNEE

A review of this kind shows that the majority of problems in endoprosthetics are of a common nature. Differences result from different functional-anatomical conditions. With regard to relevant complications such as mechanical loosening and infection they raise particular questions which will now be dealt with.

TOTAL HIP REPLACEMENT

The number of different implants for total hip replacement can scarcely be determined. Known models might now exceed a hundred; not counting the ideas which never leave the designer's desk. The reasons for continuing efforts to produce new types of prosthesis cannot merely be dissatisfaction with current ones, since a large number meet most requirements. Clinical failures must be ascribed, less to shortcomings of design, material and manufacture, than to a much greater extent, to inadequate use and inappropriate indications.

Is there such a thing as an ideal model? Let me first deal with the two kinds of complication that signify complete failure of an arthroplasty.

Loosening of a hip replacement

This always occurs at the bone/cement interface of either the acetabular or the femoral component, or both. Factors favouring loosening have already been mentioned. Pain is the preeminent symptom, occurring initially on loadbearing, later even at rest. Occasionally some sudden occurrence, not necessarily a traumatic one, may be the triggering event. Gradual onset is, however, more common. Indicative of loosening is the painfree interval which may have lasted for years after implantation. A stable functional joint may be associated with occasional pain in the inguinal region. This will usually occur a short time after the operation and is of no pathognomonic significance.

A diagnosis of loosening is easy enough to establish if complete instability precludes load-bearing, or relative movements of bone and implant can be felt or even heard. Frequently, however, it is difficult to prove. Table 2 shows a number of clinical signs indicative of loosening. Persistent pain makes surgical revision a necessity (2,31,52).

Table 2 Signs of loss of fixation

X-ray:	extended zone around the prosthesis
X-ray image-intensifier:	mobility between prosthesis and bone
Arthrography during traction:	radiopaque fluid between cement and bone
Scintigraphy:	"hot" zones around the joint
BSR:	slightly increased

In the occasional rare case replacement of only one of the components of the joint will be considered. This does not apply to metal-to-metal joints. Even for so-called interchangeable components, matching may not be exact after a period of use of one part. Should there be any doubt both parts must be replaced. Provided a reasonable fit is obtained, replacement of one part is less objectionable in metal-to-plastic joints.

Late infection

Whereas in cases of aseptic loosening function will be restored by an exchange operation, this approach is an exception in late infection. The concept of a haematogeneous bacterial infection at a locus minoris resistentiae has been disputed (3). It may be true for a proportion of the cases. For the rest, late reactivation of a local postoperative focus of infection cannot be denied. Occasionally persistent minor complaints may "bridge the gap" between infection and clinical manifestation. Abscesses and fistulae make the diagnosis clear enough. As a rule, however, we are dealing with deep, more or less active chronic infection localized at the bone/cement interface. They may lead not only to loosening, but finally to widespread osteomyelitis of the acetabular fossa and the femoral medullary cavity. Diagnosis may remain uncertain at any stage. Some clinical findings are listed in Table 3.

Severe pain is the predominant symptom, necessitating surgical action although proof of deep infection is lacking before the operation. Even during surgery, the findings may leave doubts as to whether loosening has been caused by infection or not. These are the cases in which the attempt at salvage by replacement of the prosthesis may be successful. The employment of bone cement with an antimicrobial action appears useful through controlled release of the drug. However, the implantation of foreign bodies in the presence of necrotic and putrefying tissue appears opposed to general surgical practice. At a round table discussion three years ago this was confirmed by the participating experts. Prevention of infection, i.e. aseptic precautions in the operating room, will not be discussed here.

Table 3 Signs of deep infection

BSR:	much increased
Leukocytosis	
X-ray:	extended zone around the prosthesis and erosion of bone
Scintigraphy:	very "hot" zones around the joint

Problems will be multiplied with each repeat replacement, especially that of infection. The decision as to what measures to take rests entirely with the personal experience and to the best of the individual surgeon's belief. Removal of an implant creates a Girdlestone-type condition which provides more stability if done as a primary procedure (18,37). The attempt to manage without bracing is always justified and successful in most instances.

The incidence of infection will probably never be zero. Endeavors to perfect hip replacement in the face of an already impressive success rate will necessarily be aimed at adapting implant mechanics to those of the skeleton in order to avoid loosening. So called iso-elastic implants, an objective pursued by Morscher and Mathys (30), seem to promise more flexibility of the zone of fixation. There will be better modifications of current acrylic cement and even ceramics and polyethylene have been shown to have some prospects as regards fixation. All these experimental results indicate solutions to our current problems, if not ways to achieve the ideal hip joint replacement.

THE KNEE JOINT

Motion of the transverse axis in flexion is the particular anatomical-functional feature of the knee joint. It causes a combined sliding and rolling relative movement, allowing also for rotatory movements and dissipation of rotatory moments. In contrast to the hip joint the knee joint is stabilized mainly by ligaments. The early implant designs eliminated all but simple hinge type movements. Their practical value is apparent even after ten years as in the case of a patient (Fig. 15) in whom a Young's knee prosthesis has been functional for ten years. Use of such simple hinges is still justified. Young's knee joint had to be blocked at 90 ^{o} of flexion to protect popliteal soft tissues. In more recent designs this problem has been solved by a posterior position of the axis (Fig. 16). Meanwhile practical realization of more physiological design concepts seems to be within reach. This may or may not mean the ideal knee joint.

Here, loosening and infection represent preeminent complications. Loosening in particular is a criterion for the long-term practical value of a knee joint replacement.

Loosening

In hinge joints, loosening occurs also at the highly stressed zone of fixation between bone and cement. If axial loads act at right angles to the axis of the hinge, stresses will be evenly distributed at the interface. A normal range of loading, as in daily activities of elderly patients, will be tolerated. Higher loads and mechanical moments such as result from the physical activities of younger patients, may be expected to provoke loosening even in well aligned implants of the current types. Rotatory moments as occur in walking are thought to contribute to excessive stressing of the fixation. In hinge type joints, these moments cannot be dissipated by muscular action in knee flexion or terminal rotation but will be transferred to, and act on, the zone of fixation.

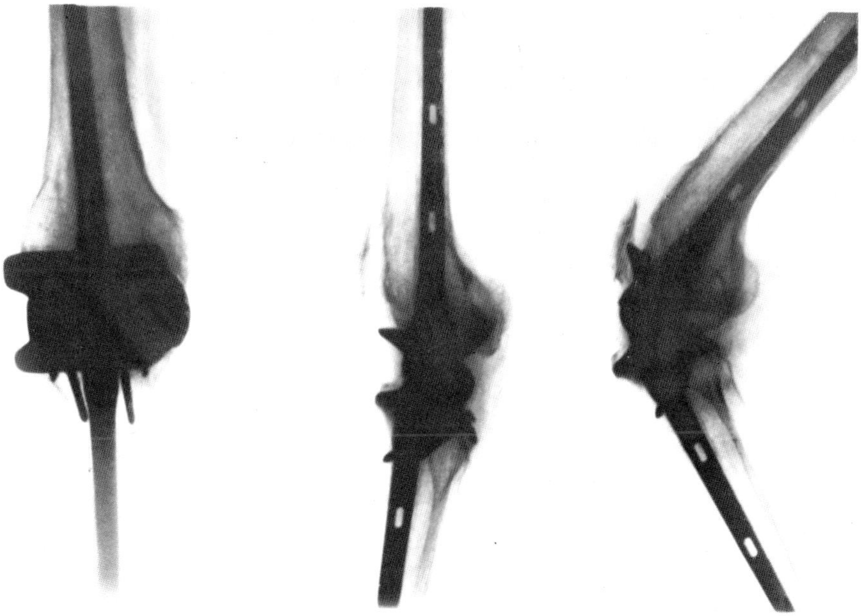

Fig. 15 Young's knee prosthesis with good function after ten years' implantation

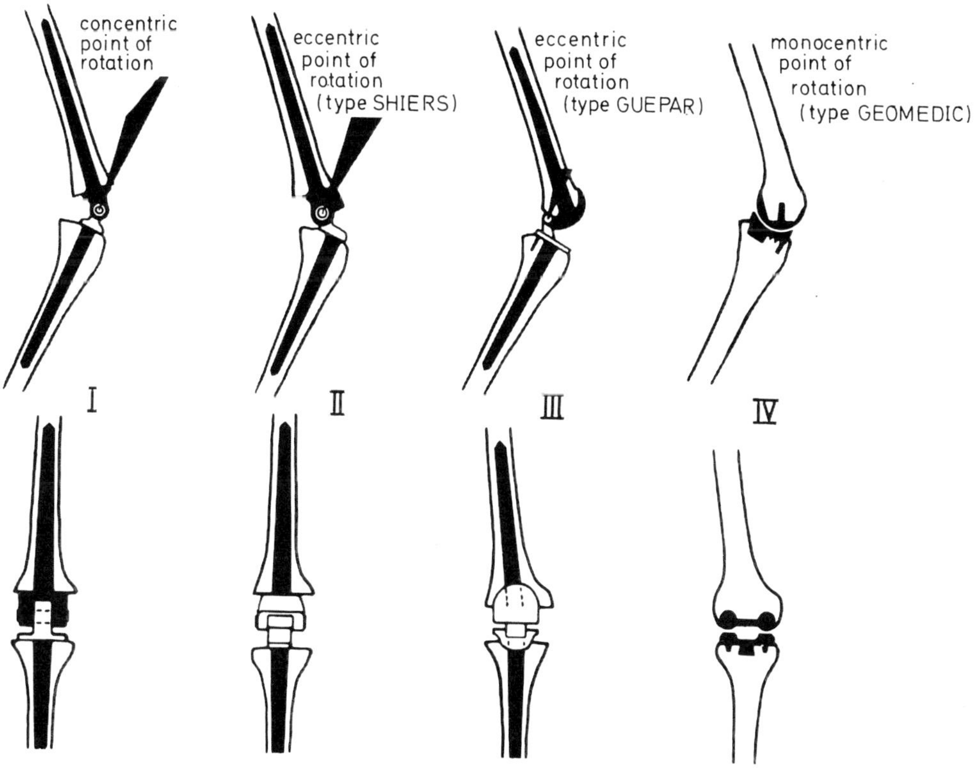

Fig. 16 Repositioning the axis of an artificial knee joint more posteriorly to avoid pressure damage in the popliteal fossa when flexion is too great

The diagnosis of loosening presents fewer problems than in the case of the hip. Exchange of prosthetic components is associated with higher risks than in the hip. It is a good deal more difficult to remove cement from two long bones (Table 2)

Infection

Infection usually appears to start in the soft tissues surrounding the implant. This may be due to the kind of tissue, skin, fat and fibrous tissue which represent rather a thin cover. Long-term chronic inflammation may precede eventual break-down of the skin. The risks of replacing the implant in a such knee joint are such as to forbid the attempt. In overt osteomyelitis of the femur and tibia all implants have to be removed before a reversion to arthrodesis can have any chance of success. It is on account of this possibility of preserving a "second line of defense" that we favor models requiring only a limited degree of bone resection (Table 3).

Is there an "ideal" knee endoprosthesis? The urge to live actively means significantly higher loads in younger patients. To satisfy such demands in patients with knee replacements requires adaptation of knee design concepts to the natural knee as regards range of movement. Development and clinical trials of models meeting this demand are presently being carried out.

Moreover, since the introduction of polyethylene to knee arthroplasty by Gunston in Charnley's laboratory (19), the low friction idea has been realized for the knee, too. 10-year results have not as yet been presented. The criteria of loosening and infection have not been applied to the evaluation in a convincing fashion. At last year's meeting of the DGOT (Saarbrücken 1974), nearly all current models were presented, however, the follow-up periods were almost all below three years. Excellent individual results in elderly patients do, however, justify the use of simple hinges.

INDICATIONS

At the present stage of development of hip and knee endoprosthetics, we are in a position to establish standard indications, which are generally accepted and which need not be listed here.

The individual surgeon may extend the range of indications based on his experience with certain implant types. This approach, however, ought to be reserved to those familiar with the complete range of joint operations short of arthroplasty and for whom the indications of high tibial osteotomy are not identical with those for knee replacement.

As long as the employment of alloarthroplasty is restricted to the elderly, most current implants will meet the demands as to materials, design and type of fixation.

The more generously the age limit is lowered, the more relevant will be the problems listed, and the more critically one ought to judge the situation. Still's disease, ankylosing spondylitis and severe bilateral early osteoarthritis of the hip in women may force a decision in favor of alloarthroplasty. In a patient who is fully aware of possible consequences such as second and third interventions, and is willing to accept these possibilities one will be hard put to reject such an argument as: "I would prefer to have a good joint as long as I am young". We are all familiar with the task of advocating arthrodesis when the success story of arthroplasty is being emphasized by the lay press. Arthrodesis has become a suspicious word and the well-meaning surgeon who mentions it may lose his patient's confidence.

This review was not meant to damp an optimistic approach to endoprosthetics in the hip and knee – great progress has undoubtedly been made – but, was meant to show the limitations, to show the necessity, and direction, of further developments and to suggest where critical restriction of indications should be employed.

REFERENCES

1. Andersson, G.B.J., Freeman, M.A.R., Swanson, S.A.V.: Loosening of the cemented acetabular cup in total hip replacement. Journal of Bone and Joint Surgery 54-B, 590 (1972)
2. Böhler, J.: Expertengespräch Alloarthroplastiken, DGOT-Kongress Berlin 1972, Zeitschrift für Orthopädie III, 552 (1973)
3. Buchholz, H.W.: Die tiefe Infektion bei der totalen Endoprothese. In: Cotta-Schulitz, edit., Der totale Hüftgelenkersatz, Stuttgart: G. Thieme-Verlag 1973
4. Bürkle de la Camp, H.: Die Untersuchungsbefunde von zwei homioplastisch verpflanzten Kniegelenken. Deutsche Zeitschrift für Chirurgie 217, 109 (1929)
5. Charnley, J.: Arthroplasty of the hip. A new operation. Lancet I, 1129 (1961)
6. Charnley, J., Crawford, W.J.: Histology of bone in contact with self-curing acrylic cement. Journal of Bone and Joint Surgery 50-B, 228 (1968)
7. Charnley, J.: Total prosthetic replacement of the hip. Reconstr. Surg. Traumat. II, 9 (1969)
8. Charnley, J.: Long-term results of low-friction arthroplasty of the hip. Paper read at British Orthopaedic Association Meating, 1970
9. Charnley, J.: Acrylic cement in Orthopaedic Surgery, Edinburgh – London: Livingstone, 1970
10. Chiary, K.: A contribution to the surgical technique of total arthroplasty of the hip in extreme dysplasia. In: G. Chapchal, edit., Arthroplasty of the Hip, Stuttgart: G. Thieme Verlag 1973
11. Contzen, H., Straumann, F., Paschke, E.: Grundlagen der Alloplastik mit Metallen und Kunststoffen, Stuttgart: G. Thieme Verlag 1967
12. Eicher, P.: Use of a prosthesis in the fresh intracapsular fracture of the hip. Am.Acad.orthop. Surg. 16, 287 (1959)
13. Evans, E.M., Freeman, M.A.R., Miller, A.J., Vernon-Roberts, B.: Metal sensitivity as a cause of bone necrosis and loosening of the prosthesis in total joint replacement. Journal of Bone and Joint Surgery 56-B, 626 (1974)
14. Frank, E., Zitter, H.: Metallische Implantate in der Knochenchirurgie. Heidelberg-Berlin-New York: Springer-Verlag 1971
15. Freeman, M.A.R.: Observations on the fixation of the femoral component of total hip prostheses using acrylic cement (discussion). Journal of Bone and Joint Surgery 52-B, 177 (1970)

16. Friedebold, G., Hanslik, L., Radloff, H., Weigert, M., Gerbia, W.: Ergebnisse der totalen Alloarthroplastik der Hüfte. In: Cotta-Schulitz, edit., Der totale Hüftgelenkersatz, Stuttgart: G. Thieme Verlag 1973

17. Gerber, H., Bürge, M., Cordey, J., Ziegler, W., Perren, S.M.: Quantitative Bestimmung der Gewebsverträglichkeit von Korrosionsprodukten in der Organkultur. In: Chirurgisches Forum 75 für experimentelle u. klinische Forschung, Berlin-Heidelberg-New York: Springer Verlag 1975

18. Girdlestone, G.R.: Pseudarthrosis. In: Discussion on treatment of unilateral Osteoarthritis of the hip joint. Proceedings of the Royal Society Med. 38, 363 (1945)

19. Gunston, F.H.: Polycentric knee arthroplasty. Journal of Bone and Joint Surgery 53-B, 272 (1971)

20. Jones, G.B.: Arthroplasty of the knee. In: A.G. Apley, edit., Modern Trends in Arthroplastics, London: Butterworths 1972

21. Judet, R.: Experience of hip arthroplasties by acrylic prostheses since 1946. Journal of Bone and Joint Surgery 36-B, 691 (1954)

22. Kölbel, R.: Problems of mechanical strength of the interface PMMA – cancellous bone in implant fixation. In: Biopolymere und Biomechanik von Bindegewebssystemen, Berlin-Heidelberg-New York: Springer Verlag 1974

23. Kuner, E.H.: Verhandlungen der Deutschen Gesellschaft für Orthopädie und Traumatologie Kiel 1970

24. Lexer, E.: Wiederherstellungschirurgie, Leipzig: J.A. Barth-Verlag 1920

25. McIntosh, D.L.: Arthroplasty of the knee in rheumatic arthritis using the hemiarthroplasty prosthesis. In: G. Chapchal, edit., Synovectomy and Arthroplasty in Rheumatic Arthritis. Stuttgart: G. Thieme Verlag 1967

26. McKee, G.K., Watson-Farrar, J.: Replacement of arthritic hips by the McKee-Farrar prosthesis. Journal of Bone and Joint Surgery 48-B, 245 (1966)

27. Merle d'Aubigne, R., Maurer, P.: Resultats des arthroplasties cervico-cephaliques dans la chirurgie de la hanche. Revue de Chirurgie Orthopedique 42, 19 (1956)

28. Mital, M., Cotten, J.: Toxicity of metal particles in tissue culture. Journal of Bone and Joint Surgery 50-A, 535 (1968)

29. Moore, A.: Metal hip joint. A new self-locking metallic prosthesis. Sth.med. J. (Bgham, Ala) 45, 10.15 (1952)

30. Morscher, E., Mathys, R.: Erste Erfahrungen mit einer zementlosen isoelastischen Totalprothese der Hüfte. Zeitschrift für Orthopädie 113, 745 (1975)

31. Müller, M.E.: Expertengespräch Alloarthroplastiken DGOT-Kongress Berlin 1972. Zeitschrift für Orthopädie III, 552 (1973)

32. Münzenberg, K.J.: Submikroskopische Veränderungen des Knochens durch Hitze und Palacos. Verhandlungen der Deutschen Gesellschaft für Orthopädie und Traumatologie Kiel 1970

33. Oest, O., Müller, K., Hopfauer, W.: Die Knochenzemente, Stuttgart: Ferdinand Enke Verlag 1975

34. Ohnsorge, T.: Untersuchungen von Knochenzement mit dem Rasterelektronenmikroskop. Verhandlungen der Deutschen Gesellschaft für Orthopädie und Traumatologie Kiel 1970

35. Pappas, A.M., Cotten, J.: Toxicity of metal particles in tissue culture. Journal of Bone and Joint Surgery 50-A, 535 (1968)

36. Parsons, D.W., Goddard, D., Ansell, R.H.: Observations on the fixation of the femoral component of total hip prostheses using acrylic cement. Journal of Bone and Joint Surgery 52-B, 177 (1970)

37. Parsons, D.W.: Total hip replacement. In: A.G. Apley, edit., Modern Trends in Orthopaedics – 6, London: Butterwortsh 1972

38. Payr, E.: Gelenksteifen und Gelenkplastik, Berlin: J. Springer Verlag 1934

39. Peters, G.: Verhandlungen der Deutschen Gesellschaft für Orthopädie und Traumatologie Kiel 1970

40. Rettig, H.: Die Hüftarthroplastik mit Spezialendoprothese. Zeitschrift für Orthopädie 82, 290 (1952)

41. Ring, P.A.: Operative treatment of osteoarthritis of the hip. British Medical Journal 1, 827 (1960)

42. Ruedi, Th.P.: Titan und Stahl in der Knochenchirurgie Handbuch der Unfallheilkunde 123. Berlin-Heidelberg-New York: Springer Verlag 1975

43. Schulitz, K.P., Dustmann, H.O., Koch, H.: Fettembolie beim Einsetzen von Totalendoprothesen mit Acrylzement. In: Cotta-Schulitz, edit., Der totale Hüftgelenkersatz, Stuttgart: G. Thieme Verlag 1973

44. Semlitsch, M.: Oberflächenuntersuchungen an Metallen und Kunststoffen für künstliche Hüftgelenke mit dem Rasterelektronenmikroskop. In: Der totale Hüftgelenkersatz, Stuttgart: G. Thieme Verlag 1973

45. Shiers, L.G.P.: Hinge arthroplasty for arthritis. Rheumatism 17, 3 (1961)

46. Shikita, T., Oonishi, H.: Abnutzung und Sanierung der Totalendoprothesen des Hüftgelenkes. In: Der totale Hüftgelenkersatz, Stuttgart: G. Thieme Verlag 1973

47. Sivash, K.M.: The development of a total metal prosthesis for the hip joint from a partial joint replacement. Reconstruction Surgery and Traumatology II, 53 (1969)

48. Smith-Petersen, M.N.: Arthroplasty of the hip. A new method. Journal of Bone and Joint Surgery 21, 269 (1939)

49. Swanson, S.A.V., Freeman, M.A.R., Heath, J.C.: Laboratory tests on total joint replacement prostheses. Journal of Bone and Joint Surgery 55-B, 759 (1973)

50. Thompson, F.R.: Two and a half years experience with vitallium intramedullary hip prosthesis. Journal of Bone and Joint Surgery 36-A, 489 (1954)

51. Walldius, B.: Arthroplasty of the knee using an endoprosthesis. 8 Years experience. Acta Orthopaedica Scandinavica 30, 137 (1960)

52. Witt, A.N.: Expertengespräch Alloarthroplastiken DGOT-Kongress Berlin 1972. Zeitschrift für Orthopädie III, 552 (1973)

53. Young, H.H.: Use of a hinged vitallium prosthesis for arthroplasty of the knee. Journal of Bone and Joint Surgery 45-A, 1627 (1963)

BIOMECHANICS OF THE HIP AND KNEE JOINT

B. Kummer

The hip joint is an almost ideal spherical joint. It is in equilibrium when the resultant of all the forces acting on it passes through its geometrical centre. The stress on the surface of the joint is then determined by the magnitude of the resultant force (vectorial sum of muscle forces and body weight) and of the area of support on which the force is acting. Furthermore, the stress distribution is given by the position of the force within the area of support.

In contrast to the hip joint, the knee is undetermined in the statical sense, that means that in a given position many different combinations of stressing forces are possible without disturbing the equilibrium. Consequently, different positions of the resultant force may occur, even those with extreme disproportionate stress distributions.

The movement in the knee joint is governed by the ligaments. The cruciate ligaments play the most important role. If the tibial surface is accepted as given, then the contour of the femoral condyles may be regarded as the curve, depicted by the ligament-governed tibia.

SOME REMARKS ON THE GENERAL MECHANICS OF THE LOWER EXTREMITY

The mechanics of extremity joints can only be understood from a knowledge of the mechanical conditions of the entire body, or at least of the extremity in question. This concerns statics as well as dynamics.

STATICS OF THE LOWER EXTREMITY

The most important requirement of statics is that the centre of gravity of a body must be on a vertical line passing through its area of support (Fig. 1). This means that for a standing man the gravity vertical line falls within an area between the points of support.

Bipedal stance

The supporting area in bipedal stance is delimited by the tangents to the convexities of the standing surfaces (Fig. 2). The foot of the gravity vertical line within this area may vary in relation to the actual posture of the whole body. If a symmetrical stance is presumed, the body weight is distributed on both legs equally.

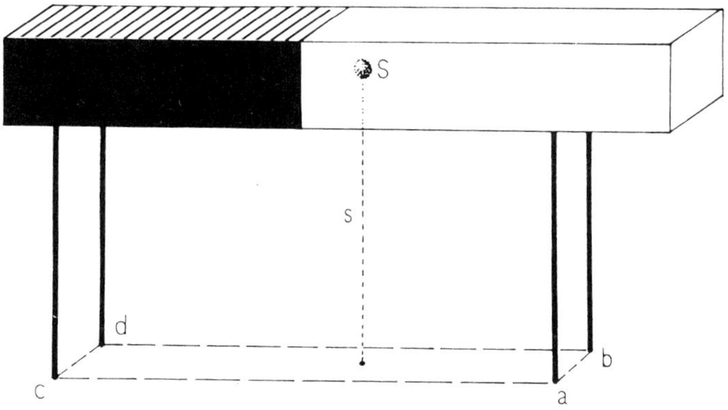

Fig. 1 Heavy bar, supported by four legs (a to d). The vertical, s, from the centre of gravity, S, must fall within the area of support

What is meant by the term "body weight" will depend on the part of the leg to be considered.

With regard to the level of the hip joints the weight to be considered is the sum of the masses of trunk, head, and both arms. Pauwels (23) calls this part of the total body mass G_4, because it is composed of four partial masses (Fig. 3). Thus, the primary loading of each hip joint is $G_4/2$.

At the level of the knee joints, the weight G_4 is augmented by the weights of both thighs etc.

The important fact in the statics of bipedal stance is the absence of any tilting moment in the frontal plane, since the gravity vertical line of the mass borne lies between the two supporting extremities. Although in the sagittal plane the gravity vertical line generally falls in front of or behind the hip or knee axis (Fig. 4), thus tending to bend or extend these joints, the contraction of antagonistic muscles is necessary to prevent those movements.

Monopodal stance

When the body is supported on only one leg, its centre of gravity, S_6, has to be balanced vertically above the bearing area of the foot (Fig. 5). This fact determines the posture as a whole including the posture of the leg, joint positions etc.

With regard to the hip joint of the supporting leg, the centre of gravity, S_5, has to be considered, and the moment of the mass G_5 must be balanced in the joint by means of the abductor muscles. Magnitude and direction of the joint resultant then depend on the

- direction and tension of the hip-abductors,
- posture of the pelvis, and
- length and posture of the leg.

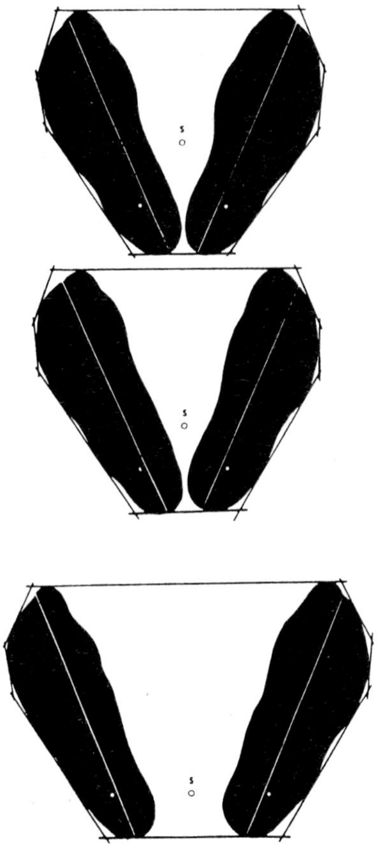

Fig. 2
Area of support at various postures of a standing man. S = position of the gravity vertical (11)
Top: "military bearing"
Centre: "easy bearing"
Bottom: "normal posture" (H.v.Meyer)

Moreover, direction and tension of the abductor muscles are related to the lever arm of the load (depending, among other things, on the width of the pelvis), to the length of the femoral neck and trochanter, and to the angle between neck and shaft (1) (Fig. 6). Furthermore, it must be remembered that the posture of the leg is strictly determined by the position of S_6, on account of the equilibrium conditions.

DYNAMICS OF THE LOWER EXTREMITY

The dynamic stressing of the skeleton is, in principle, similar to the static stressing. Differences between the two may concern magnitudes and directions of the forces, but the equilibrium conditions at the joints are still valid.

Slow motion

When the change of speed is so slow that the inertial forces involved are negligible, the subsequent stages of the movement may be considered as static.

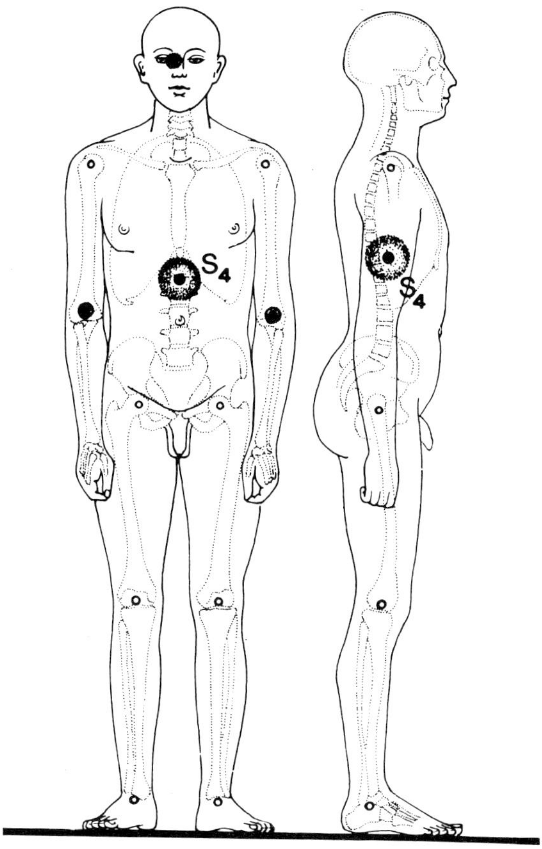

Fig. 3
Position of the partial mass G_4 of the human body

High speed and acceleration

Only higher speeds require considerable accelerations or decelerations. Consequently, inertial forces arise from the accelerated masses. The total "load" acting on the parts of the extremity is then the resultant of the weight of the body (or some of its parts), and the force of inertia. In further considerations, this resultant force takes the place of the load and must be balanced at the levels of the joints by muscular forces. It goes without saying, that the line of action of the total load passes through the area of support (Fig. 7).

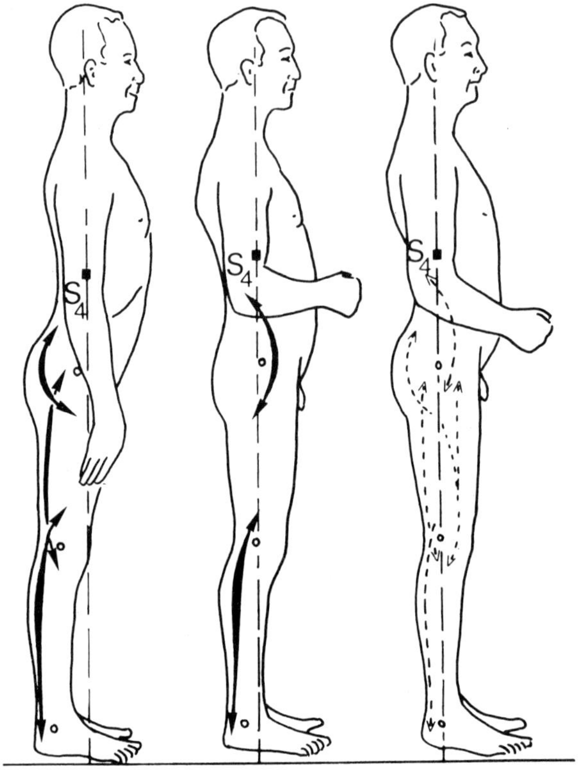

Fig. 4
Position of the centre of gravity, S_4, relative to the main joints of the lower extremity.
A: military bearing
B: easy bearing
C: normal posture
In A and B the principal muscles for the balance of the hip and knee joint are indicated by black arrows. In C "ready-for-action" muscles are indicated

MECHANICS OF THE HIP JOINT

To a first approximation, the hip joint may be considered as an ideal spherical joint. This implies three degrees of freedom for rotation and consequently three main axes for abduction-adduction, extension-flexion, and internal-external rotation movements. There is virtually no degree of freedom for translation.

EQUILIBRIUM CONDITIONS

The equilibrium conditions of a spherical joint are relatively easy to determine on account of its practically unlimited rotational ability: since the sum of all rotational moments must be zero, the resultant of all forces must pass through the geometrical centre of the joint.

Equilibrium in bipedal stance

Theoretically, instable equilibrium without any muscle action should be possible in bipedal stance. In every case, the resultant of the stressing forces is directed vertically in the projection on a frontal plane.

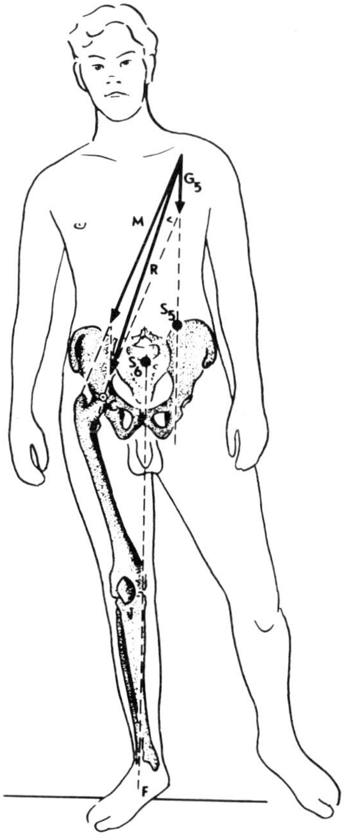

Fig. 5
Man standing on his right leg. The gravity vertical line from S_6 falls in the supporting area of the right foot. The weight G_5 is to be balanced in the right hip joint. M: abductor muscles of the right hip, R : hip resultant, S_5 : centre of gravity of the body mass to be borne in the right hip joint (14)

In a sagittal plane, the gravity vertical line of S_4 can pass through the articular centre, or behind the joint, or in front of it, depending on the posture of the individual (cf. Fig. 2). Thus, either the flexors of the hip (Mm. iliopsoas et rectus femoris) or the extensors (M. gluteus maximus, ischiocrural muscles) are responsible for the maintenance of equilibrium.

Monopodal stance

As has been mentioned above, in monopodal support the weight G_5 has to be balanced in the hip joint. This is effected by the abductor muscles.

The resultant of the forces can be determined from the known vector of the load G_5 and the position and direction of the muscular force M (22,23). The position of the latter is given by the fact that the equilibrium conditions require the forces G_5 and M to be in the same plane as the articular centre C (Fig. 5). This "plane of stressing" deviates from the sagittal plane through the joint by a very small angle, which can be neglected.

The exact direction of the muscular force M is not so easy to determine (3). It is commonly believed that the force exerted by the abductors (Mm. glutei medius et minimus) is directed from the apex of the trochanter to the centre of the surface of origin of these muscles.

In addition to this difficulty, the magnitude and inclination of the hip resultant, R, depend on virtually all the morphological parameters of the skeleton of the lower extremity including the pelvis (1). A computer program has been developed to permit the magnitude and inclination of R to be determined individually (Figs. 8,9). In the meantime, similar calculations have been made by Hamacher and Roesler (6,7,24), Brinckmann et al. (2), and Debrunner (3).

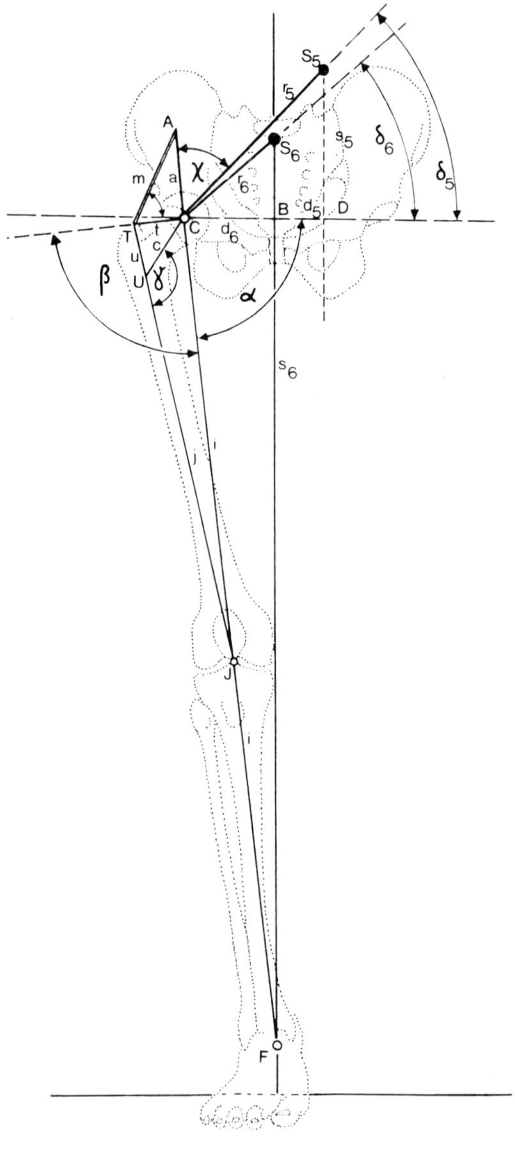

Fig. 6
Some distances and angles in the human pelvis and leg skeleton.
A : insertion of abductors at the pelvis, a : distance AC, B : intersection of s_6 with a horizontal through C, C : centre of the hip joint, c: length of the femoral neck (distance CU), D : intersection of s_5 with the horizontal through C, d_5 : distance DC, d_6 : distance BC, F : centre of the ankle joint, i : distance CF, J : centre of the knee joint, j : distance JU, k : distance CS, m : line of action of the abductors, r_5: distance CS_5, r_6 : distance CS_6, S_5 : gravity centre of the body mass minus the mass of the supporting leg, S_6 : gravity centre of the body mass, s_5 : vertical from S_5, s_6 : vertical from S_6, T : apex of the greater trochanter, t : distance CT, U : intersection of the line through J and T with the neck-axis, u : distance TU, α: angle between i and the horizontal, β : angle between i and t, γ : angle between j and c (projection of angle between neck and shaft), δ_5 : angle between r_5 and the horizontal, δ_6 : angle between r_6 and the horizontal, χ: angle between a and r_5 (1)

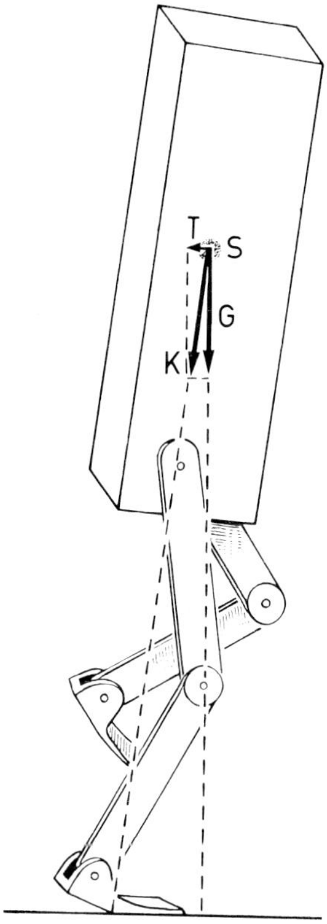

Fig. 7
"Total load" of an accelerated body. G : weight of the body, K : "total load" (resultant of G and T), S : centre of gravity, T : force of inertia

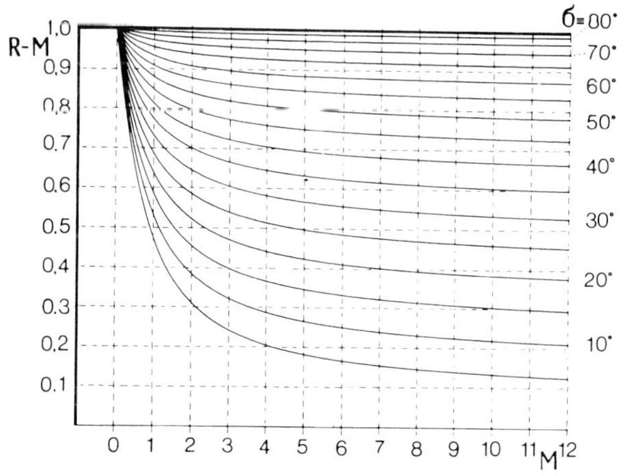

Fig. 8 Determination of the hip resultant R of the muscle force M and its inclination σ (1)

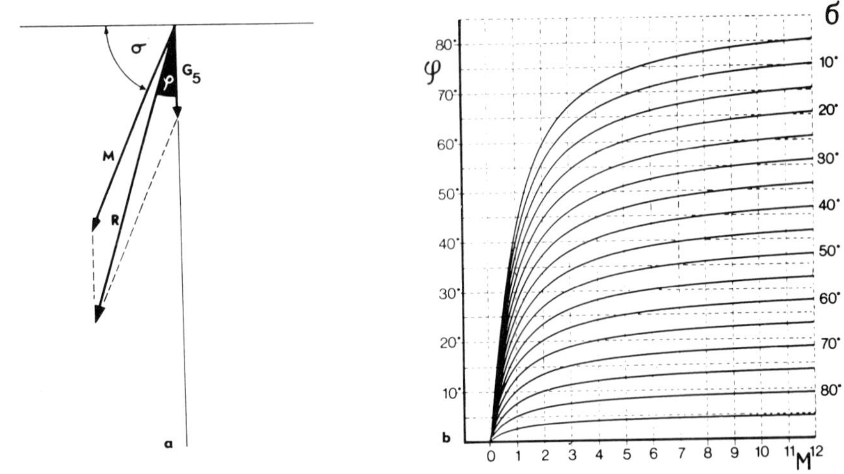

Fig. 9 Determination of the angle of inclination φ of the hip resultant, depending on the muscle force M and its inclination σ.

a. Scheme for explanation of the geometry. G_5 : weight to be balanced in the hip joint, M : force of abductors, R : hip resultant, φ : inclination of R to the vertical, σ : inclination of M to the horizontal (1)

STRESSING OF THE HIP JOINT

In the following considerations it shall be presumed that in synovial joints friction is negligible, and the pressure is not hydrostatic. Under these conditions, the stresses on the articular surface are normal stresses and are proportional to the normal forces transmitted from one articulating element to the other.

Stress distribution in the articular surfaces

Since there is no reason to assume that stress distributions in the acetabulum and femoral head should be different in any particular position of the joint, the stresses in but one component, the acetabulum, may be considered. Furthermore, attention will be paid only to monopodal stance or the supporting phase of the gait, because this represents the situation of maximal articular stress.

As is demonstrated in Fig. 10, in a spherical joint, the area of support need not be identical with the area of contact nor with the anatomical articular surface. The supporting area is delimited either by the borders of the anatomical articular surface or by a principal circle on the sphere, comparable to the equator on the globe if the point of penetration of the stressing force R (the hip resultant) is taken as the "pole".

With this assumption we may say that below the equator no normal forces can be transmitted from the socket to the articular head and that where the border of the socket lies above the equator, it delineates the area of force transmission. It goes without saying that for reasons of equilibrium, the pole cannot go outside the borders of the area of contact.

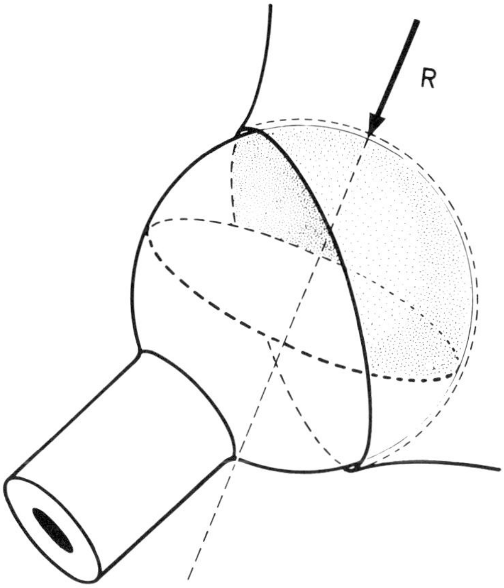

Fig. 10
The supporting area of a spherical joint as a "spherical biangle". The spherical head may be covered by cartilage : anatomical surface, its contact with the socket comprises the area of contact, shadowed biangle : area of support.
R : hip resultant, penetrating the joint at the "pole"

For theoretical calculation of the stresses, the hip resultant is divided into partial forces distributed in such a way that the sums of rotational moments of opposite sides everywhere are equal to zero (Fig. 11).

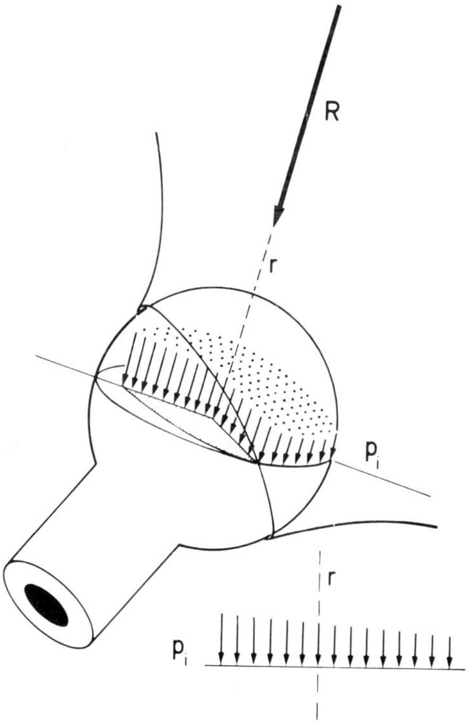

Fig. 11
Division of the hip resultant, R, into partial forces p_i. The distribution of the p_i takes place in a plane, perpendicular to the line of action r of R (15)

If p_i are the partial forces, then

$$R = \Sigma p_i, \qquad (1)$$

and, assuming an elastic, but not visibly deformable material, the principal stresses in the articular surface are proportional to the normal components of p_i:

$$\sigma_i = -p_i \sin \alpha_i \qquad (2)$$

where α_i is the angle between p_i and the equator (angle of latitude).

If the principal circle through the pole and the apex of the border of the socket is taken as the "zero meridian" and the angle of inclination of the acetabular border to the equatorial plane may be ρ, the smallest angle α on the zero meridian will be

$$\alpha_o = \rho \qquad (3)$$

(Fig. 12). This angle increases as the resultant, R approaches the acetabular border. Because of the fact that the sum of all moments have to be equal to zero, the stresses must increase in the area between R and the border of the surface of contact. Consequently, increasing angle ρ means increasing stresses at the articular border (Fig. 12).

Since the magnitudes of the transmitted normal forces, and consequently the normal stresses, depend on the angle α, the stresses will be greatest and equal to the partial force p_i at the pole, and will decrease to zero at the equator (Figs. 13-15).

Theoretically, an elastic layer like the articular cartilage should be able to distribute the stresses over a great part of the supporting surface to an almost uniform magnitude. This is particularly so when the articulating head is a little bit wider than the socket and touches first the border of the acetabulum and relieves the roof of the socket (5).

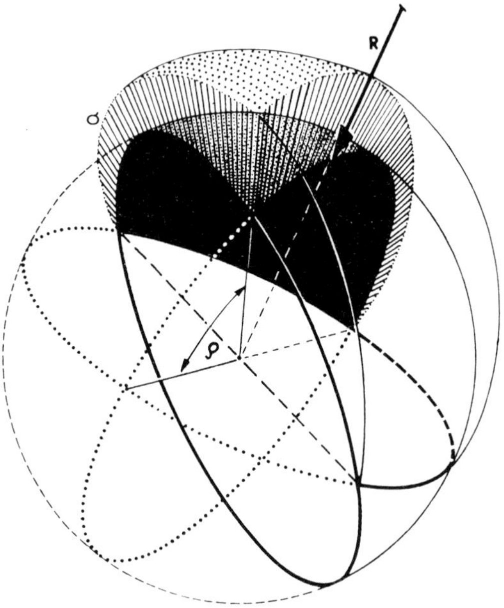

Fig. 12
Stress distribution in a spherical joint. R : hip resultant, ρ : angle between the plane of the border of the socket and the equatorial plane (15)

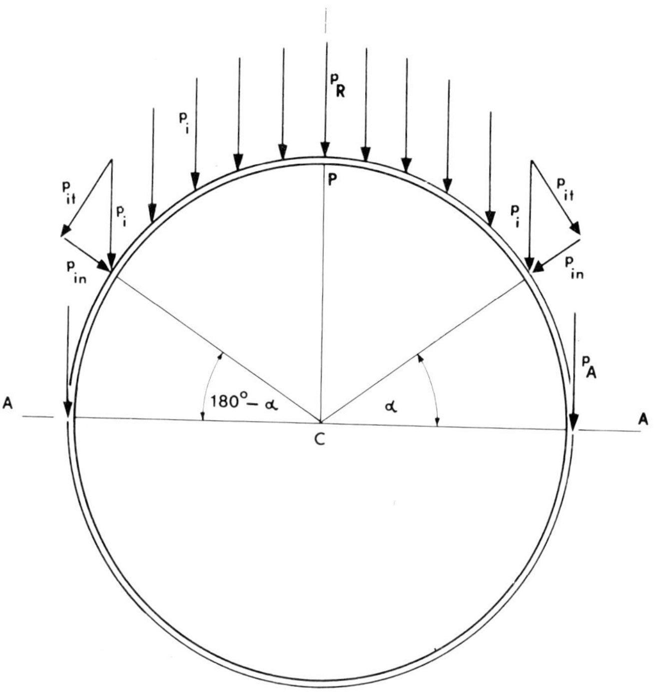

Fig. 13 Determination of the normal forces p_{in} from the partial forces p_i. Each force p_i can be divided into the normal component p_{in} add the tangential component p_{it}. The relation of p_{in} to p_{it} depends on the "latitude" (14)

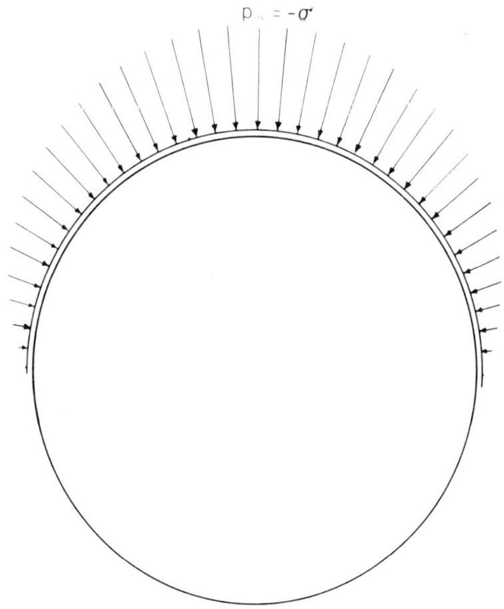

Fig. 14
Distribution of the normal forces p_{in} in a spherical joint. The maximum $p_{in} = p_i$ lies on the pole, on the equator $p_{in} = o$ (14)

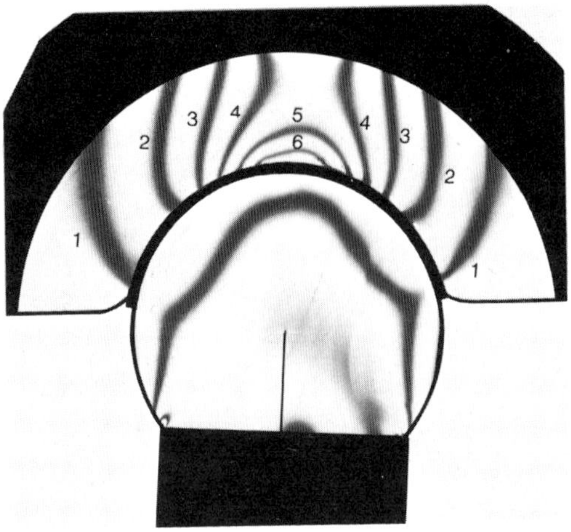

Fig. 15
Stress distribution in a spherical joint as determined by a photoelastic experiment. The numbers indicate orders of interference fringes. They are proportional to the local stresses

It may be presumed that the radius of the head is somewhat greater than the radius of the socket, but that the double layer of compressible cartilage is able to compensate the incongruity (Fig. 16). Furthermore, the stresses arising from the compression of the cartilage at the border of the socket may be exactly as great as the maximal stress at the pole (Fig. 17). The superposition of the two diagrams (1. from compression of the cartilage, due to incongruity, and 2. from the loading of the joint) then gives a uniform stress over the entire area of support.

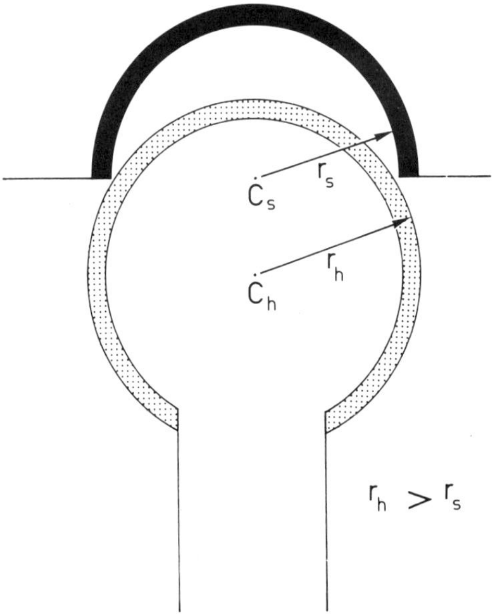

Fig. 16
Incongruent ball-and-socket joint. Both articular surfaces are covered by an elastic layer. c_h and c_s : centres of head and socket respectively, r_h and r_s : radii of head and socket (15)

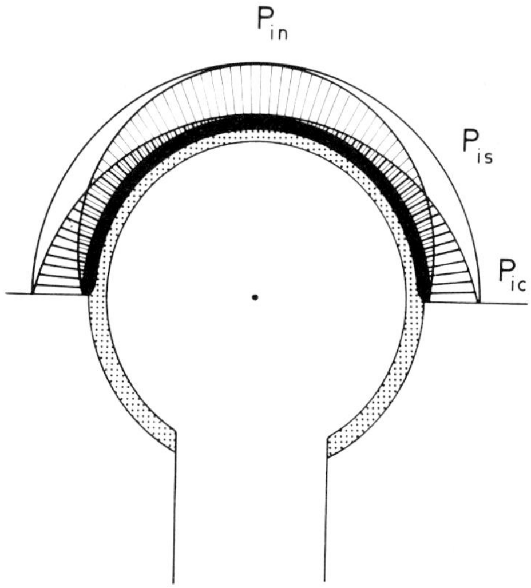

Fig. 17
Stress distribution in an incongruent ball-and-socket joint with elastic layer on both surfaces. p_{ic} : normal stresses due to compression of the cover, p_{in} : normal stresses due to loading, p_{is} : sum of p_{in} and p_{ic} (uniform over the whole area of support) (15)

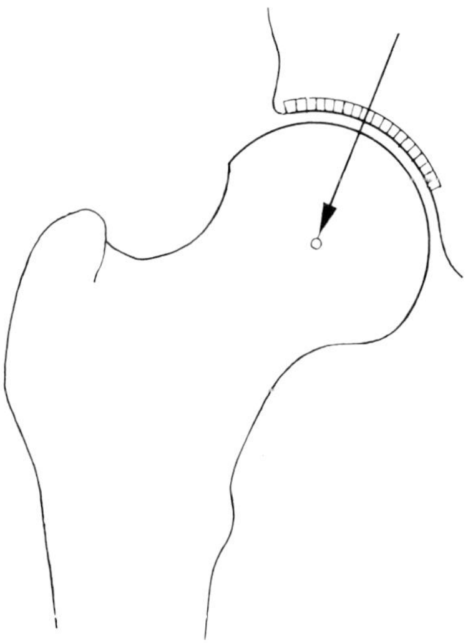

Fig. 18
Stress distribution in the normal human hip joint (23)

Pauwels (22,23) has maintained that the densification in the subchondral bone exactly reflects the stress distribution in the joint, assuming that bone formation and calcification are everywhere proportional to the actual stresses. In a normal hip joint the roof of the socket has a very compact bone structure (Figs. 18,19). Its uniform height indicates that the stresses must be distributed uniformly, probably due to the articular cartilage. If the hip resultant is shifted towards the acetabular border, the stress diagram becomes triangular in shape (Fig. 20) and the densification in the acetabulum shows the same contour (Fig. 21). This stress distribution can also be demonstrated in the photoelastic experiment (Fig. 22).

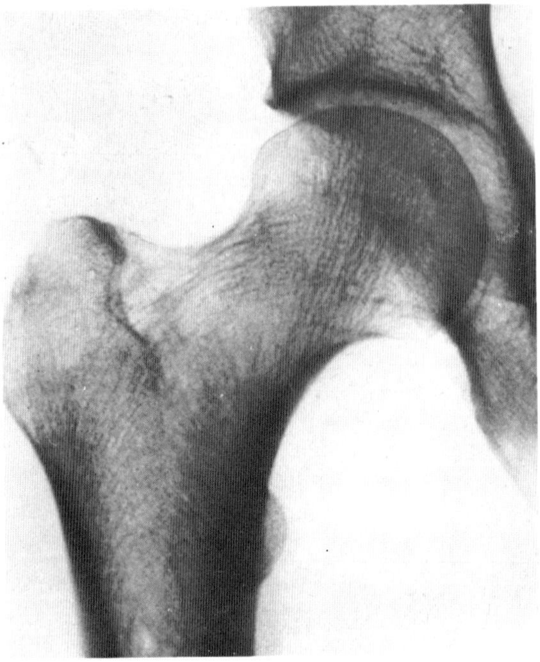

Fig. 19
Bony condensation in the acetabular roof (23)

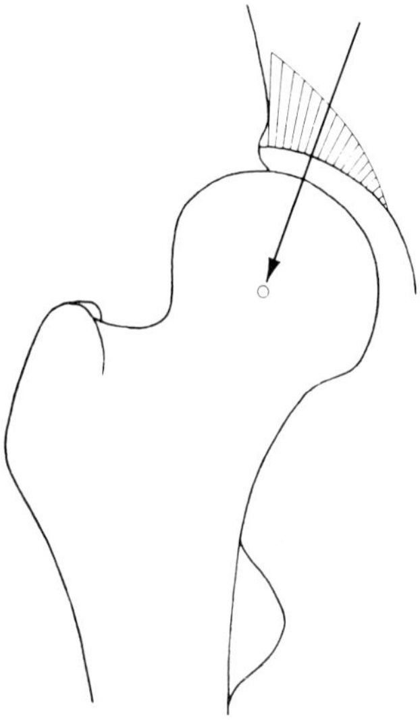

Fig. 20
Triangular stress diagram in a hip joint with laterally shifted force R (23)

Such an unequal stress distribution may influence the development of the articular cartilage. This problem has been discussed by Pauwels (22,23), Kummer (12-14) and Tillmann (26). There are many arguments in favour of the assumption that cartilage can exist only if the mechanical stresses do not exceed certain limits (Fig. 23). Beyond the upper limit, σ_o, cartilage degenerates with the symptoms of arthritis; below the minimal stress, σ_u, it undergoes involution and, generally, is replaced by bone tissue.

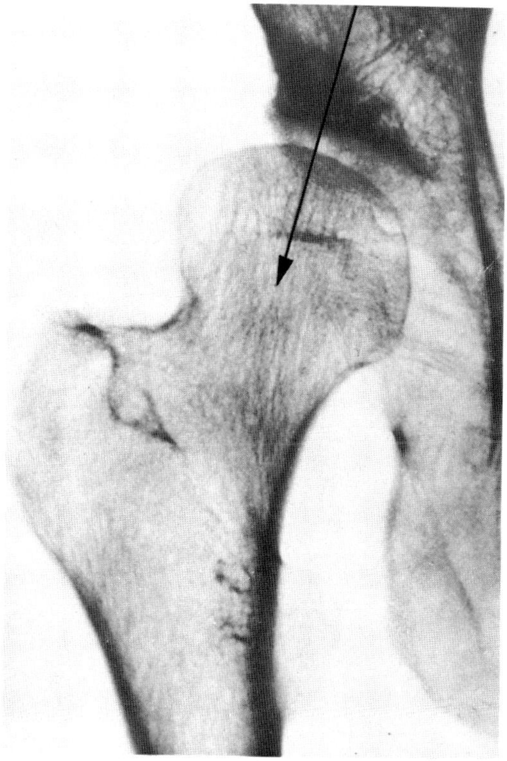

Fig. 21
Triangular condensation in the acetabular roof of a hip joint with subluxation of the head (23)

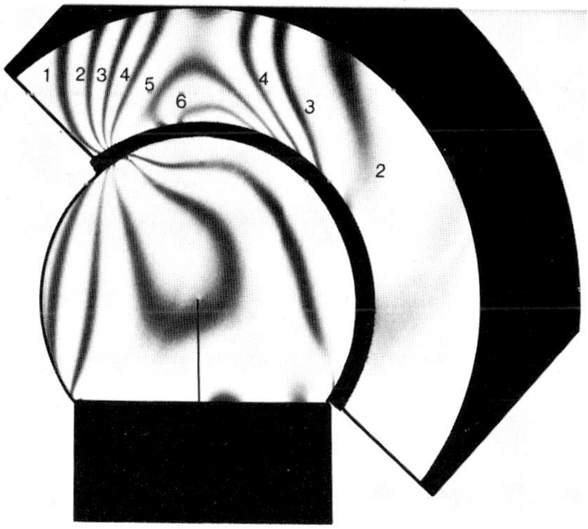

Fig. 22
Interference pattern in a model with subluxation of the head. The stresses are concentrated towards the border of the socket

This reaction of cartilage determines the shape of articular surfaces, so that it may be said that all areas of support in every position of the joint must be covered with cartilage in case the stresses stay between σ_u and σ_o.

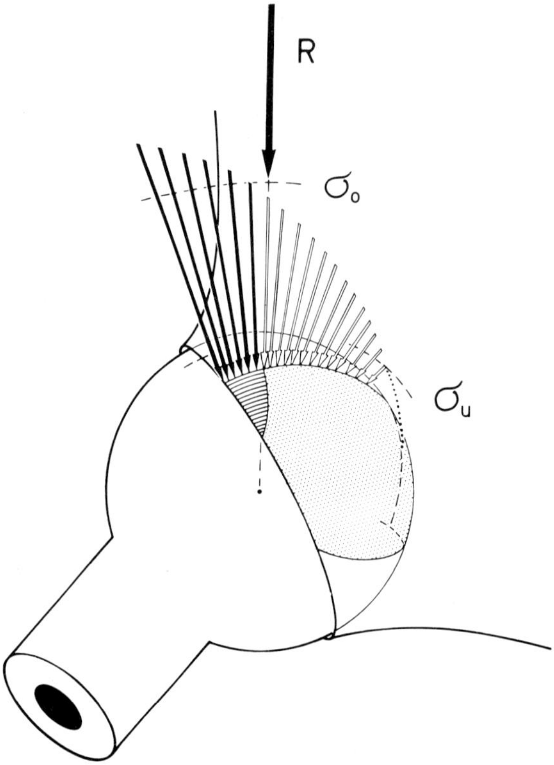

Fig. 23
Reaction of the articular cartilage to the magnitude of stresses. Cartilage develops and is preserved in the area between the lower limit σ_u and the upper limit σ_o. Beyond σ_o cartilage is destroyed, below σ_u it disappears due to ossification (15)

Following this theory, artificial surfaces of joints can be constructed. Presumed is an area of support, shaped as a spherical biangle, delimited by the acetabular border and part of the equator (cf. Fig. 10). When the joint resultant, R, shifts on the articular surface, the supporting area changes its position in the same way. The summation of several overlapping supporting areas can be made visible by photographing a globe with a coloured biangle on its surface at different angles. Superposition of the photographs depicts a surface representing the sum of all of the individual areas of support. Rotation of the articular resultant (and of the biangle of support) through about 180° caused by overlapping a surface with the contour of the facies lunata (Fig. 24). A three-dimensional diagram of the stress distribution in this "acetabular cartilage" is shown in Fig. 25, demonstrating that the stress does not decrease to zero at the border of the acetabular incision, but stays at a minimum value, identical to the lower limit σ_u of the cartilage-stimulating stresses.

Rotation of the hip resultant through more than 270° – as is most probable for the femoral head during movement of the hip – furnishes a total surface similar to the articular surface of the head with the uncovered "fovea capitis" (Fig. 26).

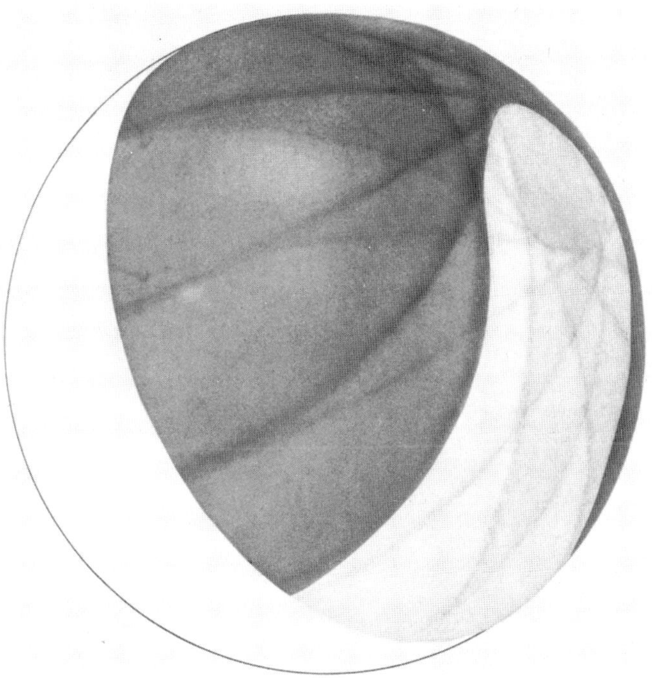

Fig. 24 Photographic reproduction of a "facies lunata" (projected on the surface of a globe) by superposition of spherical biangles in different positions. Range of displacement of the force R : about 180° (14)

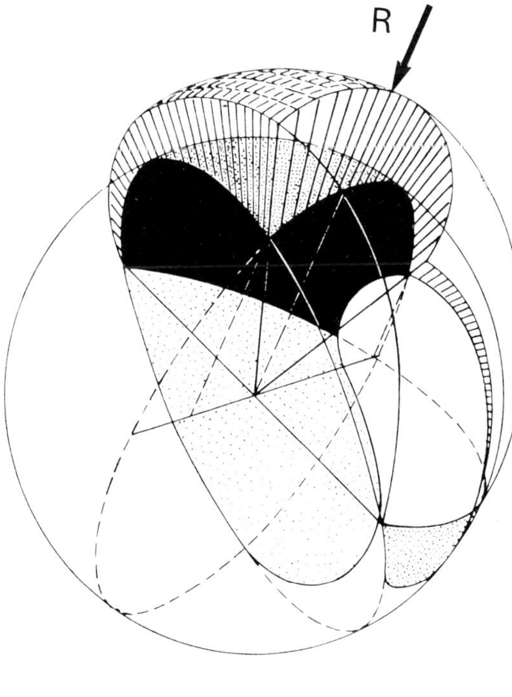

Fig. 25
Three-dimensional distribution of stresses in the facies lunata. For reasons of perspective only half of the diagram is represented

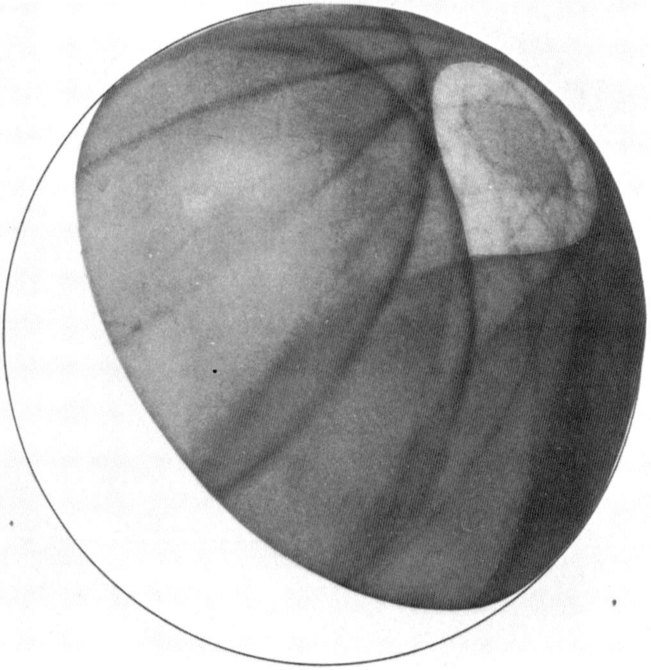

Fig. 26 Photographic reproduction of an "articular surface" of the femoral head by displacing the biangular area for more than 270°. Note the appearance of a "fovea capitis"! (14)

Stress distribution in the femoral neck

The femoral neck is stressed by the same hip resultant, R, that stresses the articular surfaces (Fig. 27a). Since the line of action of the force passes oblique to its axis, the femoral neck is stressed by bending. In a femur with normal angle between neck and shaft, the eccentricity of the stressing force is so great that, at the middle of the neck relatively high compressive stresses arise in the medial wall and somewhat lower tensile stresses in the lateral wall (Fig. 27b). The distribution of stresses can be demonstrated clearly in the photoelastic fringe pattern of a femur model and is reflected in the distribution of bone density as it appears in radiographs.

In coxa vara, the bending moment for the femoral neck increases (Fig. 28a) and consequently the tension bearing parts of the cancellous bone at the lateral side is reinforced (Fig. 28b).

A certain erection of the neck can lead to a position where the line of action of the hip resultant intersects with the border of the marrow space at the middle of the neck (Fig. 29). Under these conditions, the no-loaded line falls within the lateral contour.

This can be demonstrated in photoelastic fringe patterns where the stress in the lateral wall of the neck is near zero.

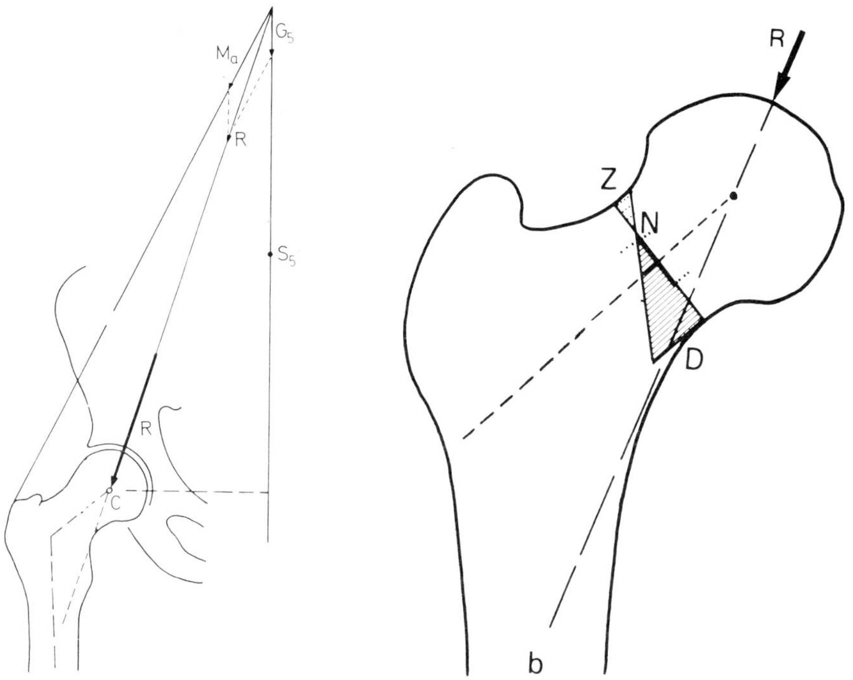

Fig. 27 Stressing of the femoral neck with normal angle between neck and shaft.
a. Determination of the hip resultant, R, from G_5 and M_a.
b. Distribution of stresses in a cross-section at the middle of the neck. D : compressive stresses, R : stressing force, N : no-loaded line, Z : tensile stresses

Extreme erection of the neck as in coxa valga can reduce the bending moment almost to zero (Fig. 30a). If the line of action of the stressing force passes through the neck axis, the cross-section is stressed by pure compression of uniform magnitude (Fig. 30b).

MECHANICS OF THE KNEE JOINT

From the theoretical viewpoint, the knee joint is more difficult to analyse than the hip because the freedom of motion is definitely restricted and in consequence some problems of equilibrium allow a rather large number of equivalent solutions.

GENERAL STATICS OF THE KNEE JOINT

It is characteristic for the knee joint that most of the muscles crossing it go still farther over neighbouring joints and therefore may be contracted for reasons that primarily do not concern the knee joint itself. In this way they can develop an effect synergistic to the load to be borne instead of antagonistic.

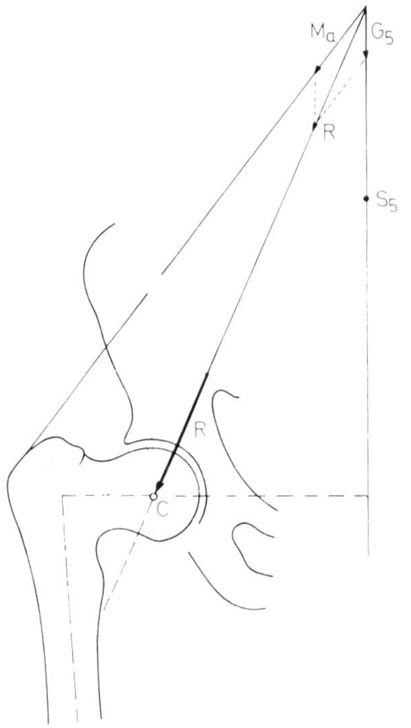

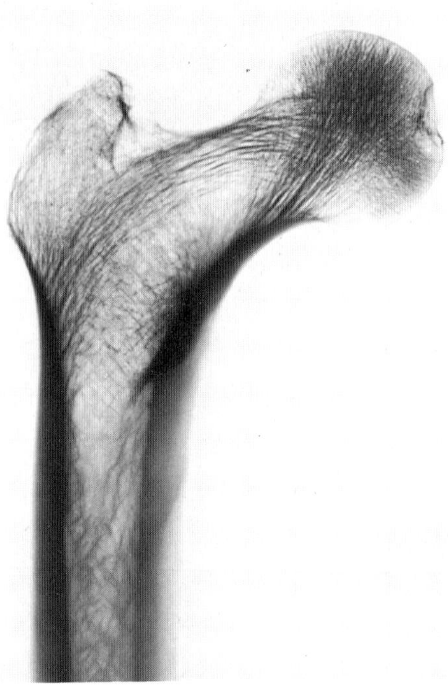

Fig. 28 Increased bending stress in coxa vara.

a. Determination of the hip resultant, R, from G_5 and M_a.

b. Radiograph of a coxa vara (Note the reinforced tension bearing parts at the lateral contour of the neck!)

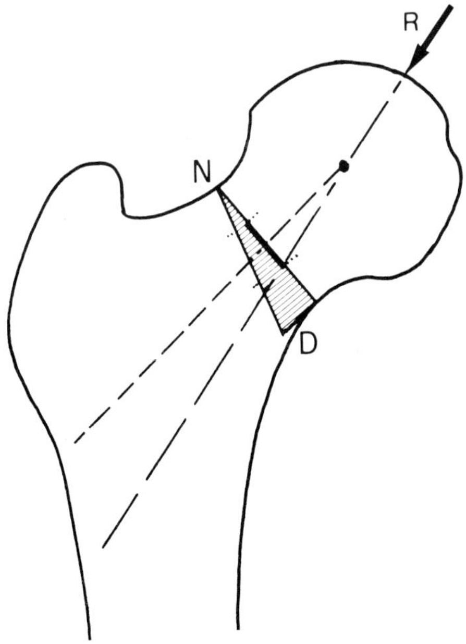

Fig. 29
Stressing of the femoral neck by a force R just at the top of the roof. D : compressive stresses in the medial well of the neck, N : neutral fibre in the lateral wall

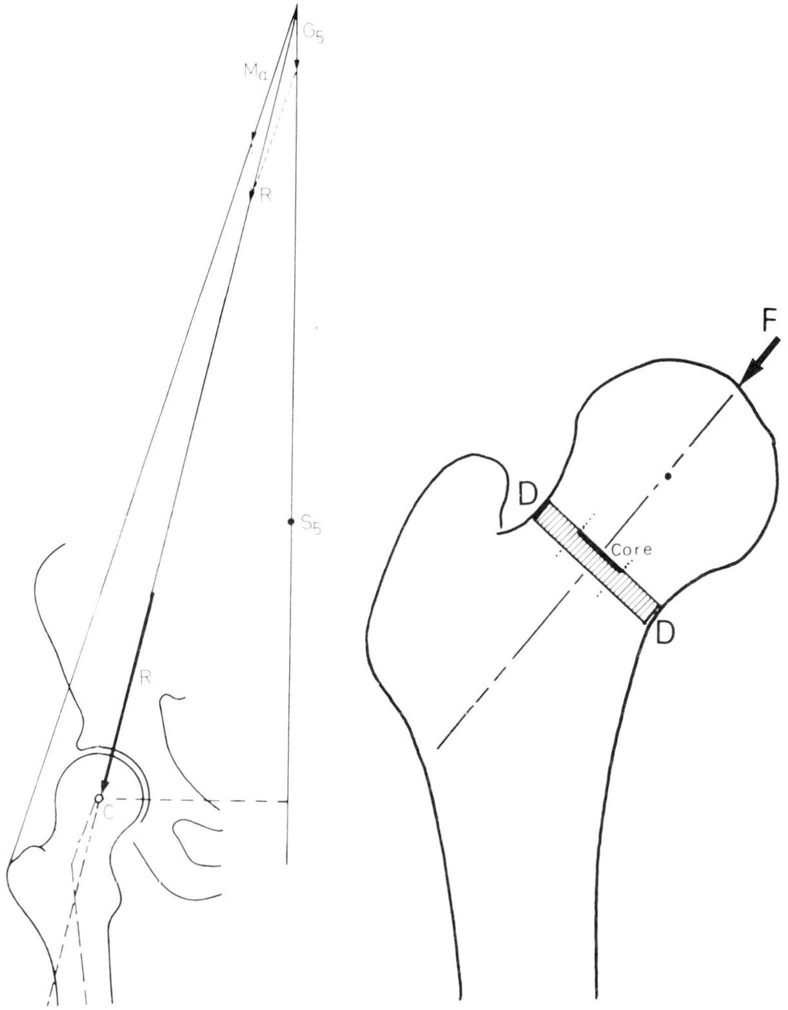

Fig. 30 Stress distribution in the femoral neck of an extreme coxa valga.
a. Determination of the hip resultant, R, from G_5 and M_a.
b. Axial position of the force R and uniform distribution of compressive stresses D

Equilibrium in the sagittal plane

The equilibrium in the sagittal plane is relatively easy to determine because there exists a definite axis of movement. The conditions depend on the fact that part of the equilibrium in the hip joint is maintained by the ischiocrural muscles and, further, that the ankle joints are balanced by the triceps surae. In Fig. 31 the line of action of the weight G to be balanced passes behind the transverse knee axis, consequently the ischiocrural muscles M_i and the triceps surae M_t with the gastrocnemius act as flexors of the joint, being synergists to the body weight.

This explains why the resultant force, R_4, responsible for the loading of the knee in the sagittal plane, is much higher than the ankle- and hip-resultants, R_1 and R_2.

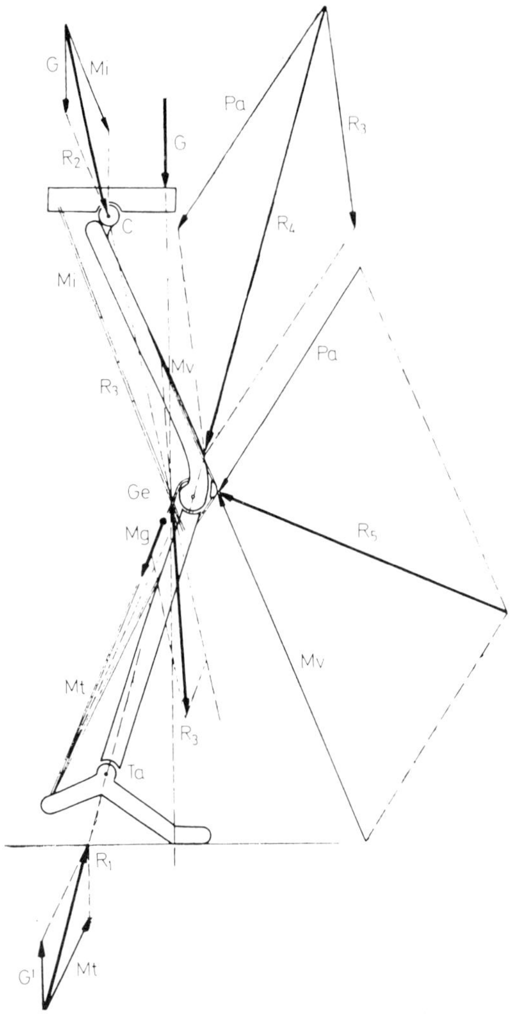

Fig. 31
Stressing of the skeleton of the lower limb in the sagittal plane. C : centre of the hip joint, G : body weight, Ge : centre of the knee joint, Mg : Mm. gastrocnemii, M_i : ischiocrural muscles, M_t : triceps surae, Mv : Mm.vasti, Pa : Lig.patellae R_1 : resultant of G and M_t, R_2 : resultant of G and M_i, R_3 : resultant of R_1 and Mg, R_4 : resultant of R_3 and Pa, R_5 : resultant of M and Pa, Ta : centre of the ankle joint (11)

The balance is effected by the quadriceps femoris in connection with the patella, inserted in its tendon. Even in a slightly flexed knee the patella is pressed against the femur with the considerable force, R_5. This force increases rapidly with further flexion.

Equilibrium in the frontal plane

In the frontal plane, the equilibrium is characterized by the fact that the gravity vertical line falls medially of the knee joint. The resulting tilting moment producing a varus deviation must be compensated by structures on the lateral side of the knee: the lateral collateral ligament and the tractus iliotibialis. The collateral ligament can only be extended passively, but the tractus can be stretched by the tensor fasciae latae and gluteus maximus muscles. Both muscles cross the hip joint and thus can add to the balance in this articulation. Consequently, in monopodal stance or in the supporting phase during walking, the force of the tractus, contributing to the stabilization of the knee joint in the frontal plane, depends on to what extent the lesser glutei, gluteus maximus and tensor fasciae muscles are contributing to the equilibrium of the hip joint.

Furthermore, many positions of the knee resultant in the frontal plane are compatible with equilibrium. It is plausible that as uniform a distribution of stresses as possible represents the minimal stress for the whole articulation. This situation is given when the line of action of the knee resultant falls in the centre of the articulating surface, i.e. in the intercondylar eminence. The more the force R is shifted towards one condyle (internal or external), the higher become the stresses on this side and the more the contralateral condyle is relieved. Thus, equilibrium is garanteed as long as the load R remains between the rotational centres of both condyles. Only if the force R falls outside one of the centres does the femur tend to rotate in the frontal plane (16) and one of the collateral ligaments must come into play.

Maquet (17) shows how the knee resultant, R, can change its position in the frontal plane. This can be caused by a change of the position of the leg, generally related to a shift of the centre of gravity (Fig. 32), or by alteration of the frontal angle of the knee. Varus deformity for example or increased body weight shift the knee resultant medially (Fig. 33 C).

Stress distribution in the articular surface and subchondral bone

It has already been mentioned that the stress distribution in the knee joint depends on the position of the force R (Fig. 34). The more the weight is concentrated on one condyle, the higher are the stresses on this side, as can be seen in the photoelastic experiment carried out by Maquet (16).

The distribution of stresses is again expressed in the condensation of subchondral bone, especially in the tibial condyles. Consequently, the position of the joint resultant can be determined by analysis of the distribution of density in radiographs of the tibial head. Equal density on both sides indicates a central position of the force. Condensation in the medial condyle is characteristic for a medial shift of the force. Lateral condensation for example is observed in genu valgum. This demonstrates also that the medial collateral ligament is elongated by permanent tension, caused by the lateral eccentricity of the stressing force.

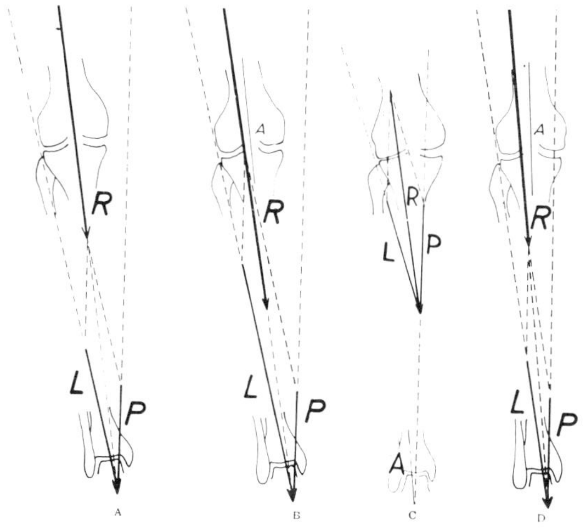

Fig. 32
Possible positions of the resultant force R in the knee joint (17). L : lateral force (tractus), P : body weight.
A. Normal situation
B. Increased tension of L
C. Genu valgum
D. Lateral shifting of P

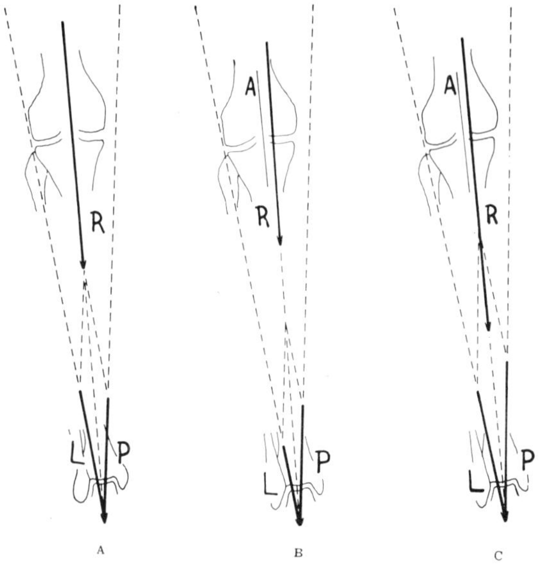

Fig. 33
Possible positions of the resultant force R in the knee joint (17). L : Lateral tensile force (tractus) P : body weight.
A. Normal stressing
B. Relaxation of L
C. Increase in body weight

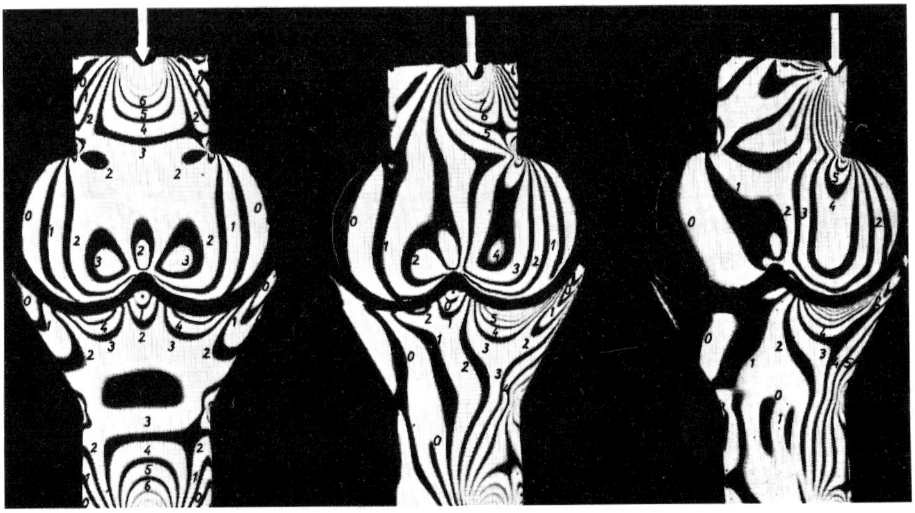

Fig. 34 Interference patterns in photoelastic investigations. The white arrow indicates the position of the load. The numbers represent orders of interference fringes (16)

KINEMATICS OF THE KNEE JOINT

The movements of the knee joint are strictly governed by ligaments. Besides some rotational possibility, they permit, in the first instance flexion and extension of the knee. This is the reason why only the movement in the sagittal plane should be analysed.

The most important structures governing the sagittal movement, are the cruciate ligaments. It has been pointed out by Huson (8-10) that the entire system femur-cruciate ligaments-tibia can be understood as a closed kinematic chain.

Closed kinematic chains

The chain, representing the mechanism of the knee joint consists of four links (Fig. 35):

1. the distal end of the femur, represented by the link A-B,
2. the proximal extremity of the tibia, represented by the link A_1-B_1,
3. the anterior cruciate ligament, link B-B_1 (o), and
4. the posterior cruciate ligament, link A-A_1 (h).

In the four-bar chain of Fig. 35 (19), the links o and h are crossed. When the link p (A_1-B_1) is moved, its pathway will be determined by the crossed links o and h. In every position, p will be the tangent to an ovoid curve.

On the other hand, when an element with the ovoid contour and another straight element are given and connected by two crossed ligaments fastened at A and A_1 or B and B_1 respectively, the two concrete elements can roll on each other in permanent contact.

The ovoid contour described above, is similar to, but not identical with, the contour of a femoral condyle. On the other hand, the straight bar p (A_1-B_1) is not an exact representation of the tibial plateau. If it is replaced by another element adapted to the curved contour of the tibial head (p_1 in Fig. 35), it describes a curve almost identical to the femoral contour.

The knee joint as a closed kinetic chain

The theoretical model explains how the contours of femoral condyles and tibial head determine each other. It explains also that both cruciate ligaments can stay in tension during the whole range of movement. Fig. 36a shows the flexion, a fixed position of the femur assumed. The rolling of the surfaces is evident.

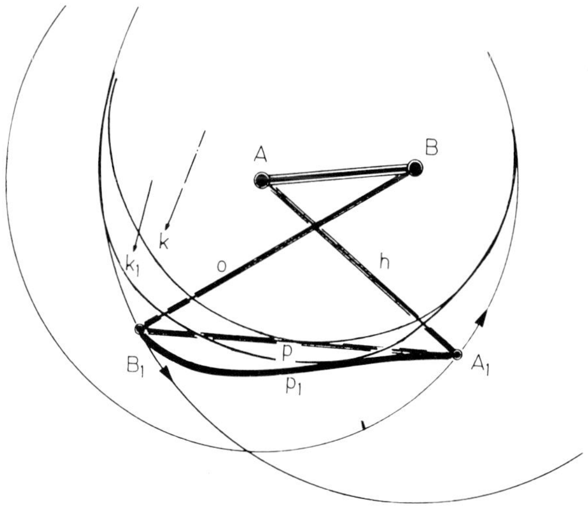

Fig. 35 Closed four-bar chain. A-A_1 : link to be comparable with the posterior cruciate ligament, B-B_1 : link to be comparable with the anterior cruciate ligament. Further explanation in the text (19)

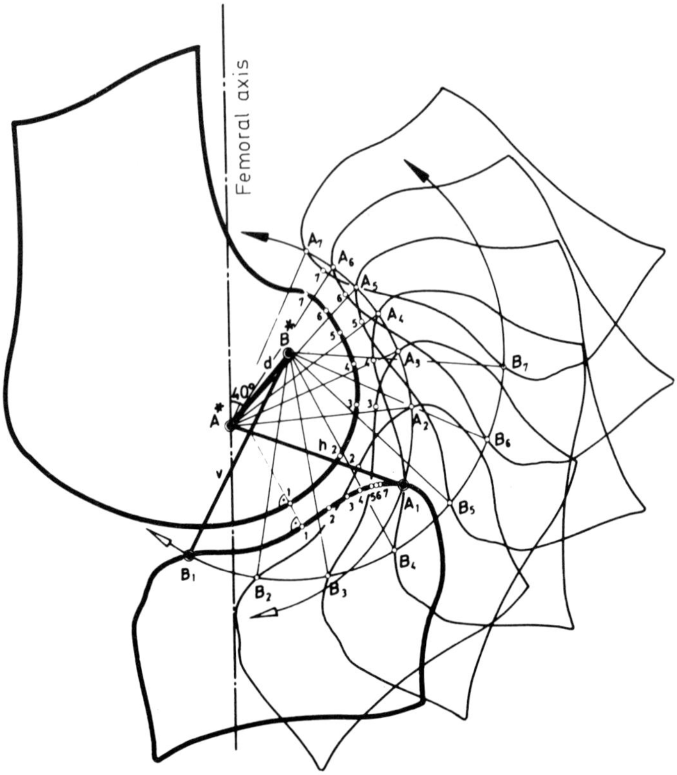

Fig. 36 The knee joint as a closed kinematic chain.
a. Contour of the femoral condyle, produced by movement of the tibial plateau (19)

In Fig. 36b the same movement is shown assuming that the position of the tibia is fixed. The points on both elements, marked with the same numbers demonstrate, that in every position of the knee joint, well defined points of contact exist.

Near the end position of extension, the so-called final rotation is performed. At least one of the causes for it seems to be an inclination of the lateral tibial surface dorsally and distally (10). By the resulting rotation, the joint axis is shifted to a lower position, so that the posterior ligamentous system is stress-relieved (20).

Since the shape and mobility of the joints in general are determined by the influence of biological function, especially the action of muscular forces, even details of the articular surface, it must be doubted whether the complex mechanism of the knee joint can be replaced by a simple hinge.

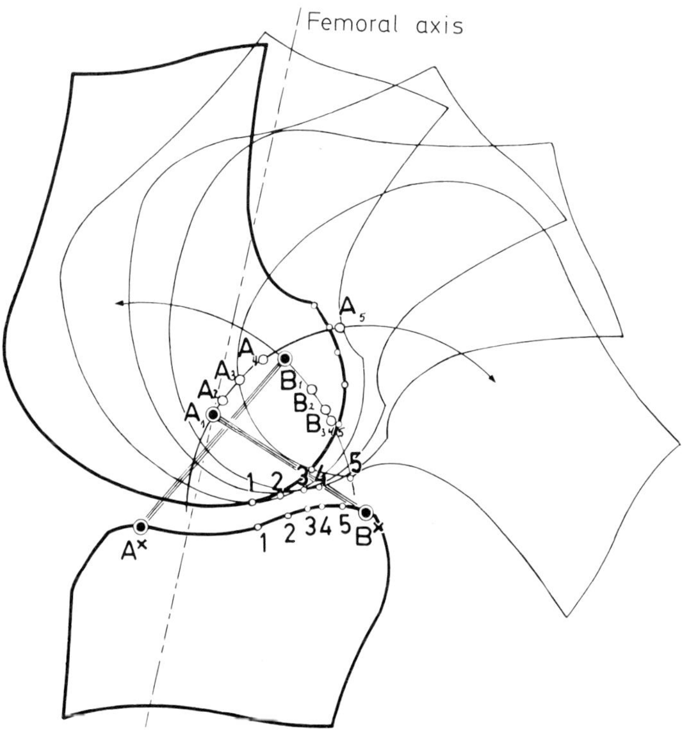

Fig. 36 The knee joint as a closed kinematic chain.
b. Surface of the tibial plateau, produced by movement of the condyle. Further explanation in the text (19)

REFERENCES

1. Amtmann, E., Kummer, B.: Die Beanspruchung des menschlichen Hüftgelenks. 2. Größe und Richtung der Hüftgelenksresultierenden in der Frontalebene. Zeitschrift für Anatomie und Entwicklungsgeschichte 127, 286 (1968)
2. Brinckmann, P., Hoefert, H., Jongen, H.Th., Polster, J.: Die Biomechanik des Hüftgelenks. Der Orthopäde 3, 104 (1974)
3. Debrunner, H.U.: Studien zur Biomechanik des Hüftgelenkes. I. Ein neues Modell für die Berechnung der Hüftbelastung. Zeitschrift für Orthopädie 113, 377 (1975)
4. Frankel, V.H., Burstein, A.H.: Orthopaedic Biomechanics, Philadelphia: Lea u. Febiger 1970
5. Greenwald, A.S., O'Connor, J.J.: The transmission of load through the human hip joint. Journal of Biomechanics 4, 507 (1971)
6. Hamacher, P., Roesler, H.: Die Berechnung von Größe und Richtung der Hüftgelenks-resultierenden im Einzelfall. Archiv für orthopädische und Unfall-Chirurgie 70, 26 (1971)
7. Hamacher, P., Roesler, H.: Ergebnisse der Berechnung von Größe und Richtung der Hüft-gelenksresultierenden im Einzelfall. Archiv für orthopädische und Unfall-Chirurgie 72, 94 (1972)

8. Huson, A.: La chaine cinematique fermee. Bulletin Ass. Anat. 57 (1973)

9. Huson, A.: The functional anatomy of the knee joint: the closed kinematic chain as a model of the knee joint. Proc. Internat. Congr. Ser. 324: The knee joint. Rotterdam 1973, pp. 163-168

10. Huson, A.: Biomechanische Probleme des Kniegelenks. Der Orthopäde 3, 119 (1974)

11. Kummer, B.: Gait and posture under normal conditions, with special reference to the lower limbs. Clinical Orthopaedics and Related Research 25, 32 (1962)

12. Kummer, B.: Die Beanspruchung des menschlichen Hüftgelenks. 1. Allgemeine Problematik. Zeitschrift für Anatomie und Entwicklungsgeschichte 127, 277 (1968)

13. Kummer, B.: General problems in biomechanics of the upright posture and gait (An introduction). VIII. Congr. Internat. Sci. Anthropol. et Ethnol. Tokyo 1968, Sympos. 3: Human posture and locomotion. pp. 316-322

14. Kummer, B.: Die Beanspruchung der Gelenke, dargestellt am Beispiel des menschlichen Hüftgelenks. Verhandlungen der Deutschen Orthopädischen Gesellschaft, 55. Kongr. Kassel 1968, pp. 301-311 (1969)

15. Kummer, B.: Biomechanik der Gelenke (Diarthrosen). Die Beanspruchung des Gelenkknorpels. Biopolymere und Biomechanik von Bindegewebssystemen. 7. Wiss. Konf. Deutscher Naturforscher und Ärzte, 19-28 (1974)

16. Maquet, P.: Biomechanics and osteoarthritis of the knee. 11th Congr. Internat. Chir. Orthop. et Traumatol. Mexico 1969, pp. 317-357

17. Maquet, P.: Biomecanique de la gonarthrose. Acta orthopaedica Belg. 38 Suppl. I, 33 (1972)

18. Maquet, P., Simonet, J., de Marchin, P.: Biomecanique du genou et gonarthrose. Revue de chirurgie orthopedique et reparation de l'appareil moteur 53, 111 (1967)

19. Menschik, A.: Mechanik des Kniegelenkes, 1. Teil. Zeitschrift für Orthopädie 112, 481 (1974)

20. Menschik, A.: Mechanik des Kniegelenkes, 2. Teil: Schlußrotation. Zeitschrift für Orthopädie 113, 388 (1975)

21. Oberländer, W.: Die Beanspruchung des menschlichen Hüftgelenks. 5. Die Verteilung der Knochendichte im Acetabulum. Zeitschrift für Anatomie und Entwicklungsgeschichte 140, 367 (1973)

22. Pauwels, F.: Gesammelte Abhandlungen zur Biomechanik dès Bewegungsapparates, Berlin, Heidelberg, New York: Springer 1965

23. Pauwels, F.: Atlas zur Biomechanik der gesunden und kranken Hüfte, Berlin, Heidelberg, New York: Springer 1973

24. Roesler, H., Hamacher, P.: Die biostatische Analyse der Belastung des Hüftgelenkes. I. Teil. Zeitschrift für Orthopädie 110, 67 (1972); II. Teil. Zeitschrift für Orthopädie 110, 186 (1972)

25. Tillmann, B.: Die Beanspruchung des menschlichen Hüftgelenks. 3. Die Form der Facies lunata. Zeitschrift für Anatomie und Entwicklungsgeschichte 128, 329 (1969)

26. Tillmann, B.: Zur Lokalisation von degenerativen Veränderungen am Femurkopf bei Coxarthrose. Zeitschrift für Orthopädie 111, 23 (1973)

LOADING ON NORMAL HIP AND KNEE JOINTS AND ON JOINT REPLACEMENTS

J.P. Paul

Increasing use is being made of implanted joint replacements in the treatment of patients suffering from degenerative and other joint diseases. The success of these is naturally measured in most cases by the patient himself in his expressed satisfaction with the end result in respect of relief from pain and in restoration of function. The clinician also makes an assessment in terms of the degree of activity which the patient can routinely undertake and the degree of abnormality in the restored pattern of use.

With the rapid development of scientific techniques for the analysis of gait and the associated biomechanical factors, it is natural that these techniques should be applied to this category of patient. In this connection studies have been conducted largely on patients where the lower limb is of greater interest, although tests are underway at the University of Strathclyde to assess the performance of patients with an endoprosthesis at the elbow joint. The functional description of the lower limb includes weight bearing as in stationary standing and in locomotion to alter the position of the individual relative to his surroundings. Both of these are routine situations and frequently repeated during normal daily life. By contrast the arm is used in a wide range of activities and complete assessment of function is necessarily more difficult and wide ranging. The literature therefore shows little on the biomechanical assessment of arm disabilities and it is proposed in this chapter to consider the leg only.

Physiological factors relating to energy expenditure and physical or mental stress can be used in the assessment of a disability. Ralston (23,24), Molbech (15) and James (9) have investigated the use of respired gas analysis to obtain overall body metabolic rate and have compared metabolic rate variation with walking speed for amputees and brace wearers. Fig. 1 shows typical results illustrating the penalty suffered by the amputee in comparison with the corresponding normal individual. Gangula and Datta (4) have investigated the locomotion of patients with similar disabilities but point out that, due to the approximately linear correlation between metabolic rate and cardiac rate elevation, this latter measure can be much more conveniently used for patient assessment. It appears that there is a fruitful technique here which could reasonably be applied to analyse the effectiveness of joint replacement surgery provided the treatment is found to give sufficiently large alterations to the measured parameters to allow their realistic interpretation. This type of measurement however is a gross overall measure of many factors such as mental or psychological stress, respiratory or cardiac deficiencies and, even if it measures only the malfunction of the lower extremity, this may be due to the affected joint or other joints or deficiencies in the muscular or neural systems.

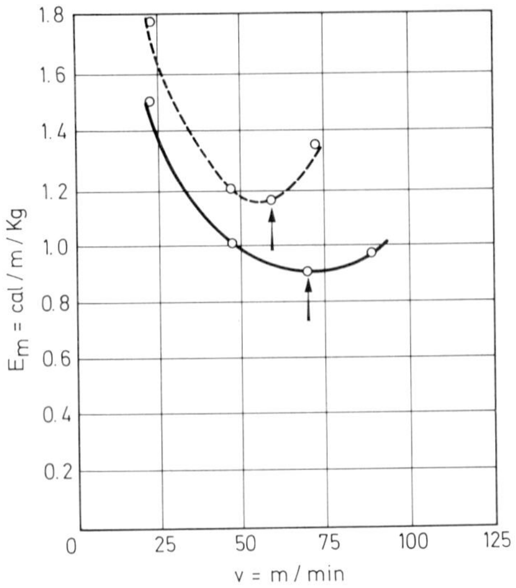

Fig. 1 Variation of metabolic energy consumption E_m with walking speed V. Solid line for above-knee prostheses. Dotted line for same patient using forearm crutches only.

E_m = Energy consumption in calories per metre of distance travelled per kilogram of body mass

V = Mean walking speed – metres per minute (23)

KINEMATIC STUDIES

A study of 30 patients before and after total hip replacement was conducted by Murray et al. (18). This could be said to be the major work reported in which measured body displacements are used as the criterion for walking capability. A similar study was performed by Murray et al. (17) without the advantage of a post-surgical follow up. Fig. 2 taken from (18), illustrates graphically the improvement in gait following surgery and during the post operative period, as measured by:

1. Reduction in lateral leg motion,
2. Increase in range of hip angulation, and to a lesser degree,
3. Increase towards normal range of knee flexion.

This is a useful method of quantifying the complicated phenomena of gait which are normally assessed subjectively by the clinician.

Milner (13) has reported similar studies in which the kinematics of gait were represented by diagrams such as shown in Fig. 3 where the angle of knee flexion is plotted vertically to a base of the angle of hip flexion or extension. This technique was shown by Grieve (5) to be an effective means of assessment of the varying characteristics of locomotion of the normal. Whereas Grieve used a sophisticated data acquisition system involving polarised

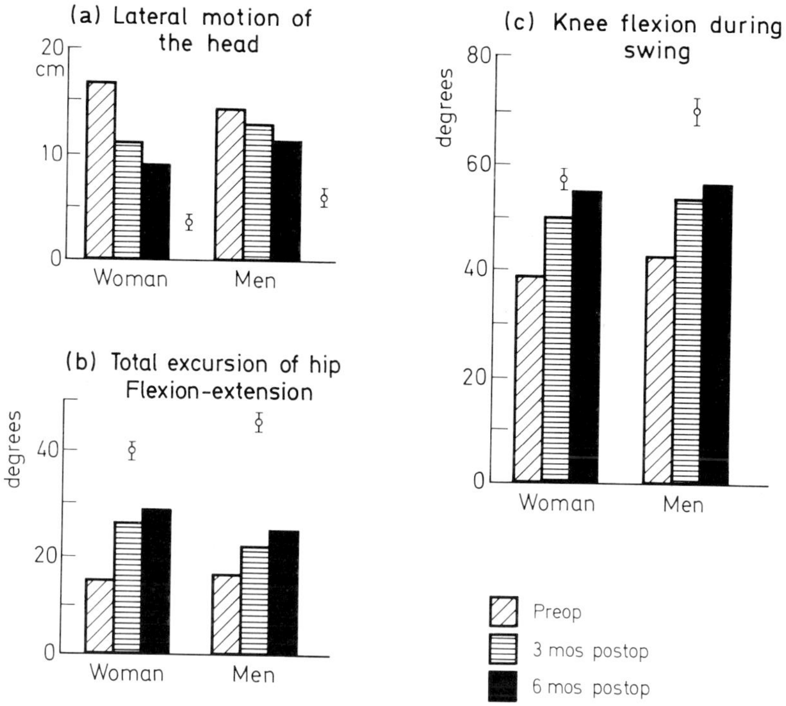

Fig. 2 Changes in patient's gait kinematics following hip joint replacement (18)

light (POLGON), Milner used the more basic method of stroboscopic flash photography. The striking alteration in the characteristics of the joint angulation illustrated in this way is shown in Fig. 4 (14). Since one of the major factors relating to the disability caused by joint disease is the limitation of angulation at the articulations, obviously studies such as these are very good and relevant measures of the change in patient performance corresponding to the surgery and post operative treatment.

GROUND FORCE MEASUREMENT

An effective joint replacement must give a suitable range of angular movement and allow transmission of force between the relevant skeletal segments. If force is taken as the criterion, then it is obviously appropriate to measure some aspect of force and relate this to the assessment of patient performance. Ground to foot force measurement is reported for patients before and after hip surgery (2,8). The authors used measuring devices incorporated in the floor of the clinic (26). This allowed the measurement of the vertical component of force developed between the ground and successive left and right foot contacts with the ground. Separate records were obtained for left and right foot by virtue of having two such devices extending the length of the walking track and separated from each other by a small distance. Fig. 5 shows typical results where the vertical component of force expressed in multiples of body weight is shown varying with time for the left foot and right foot for a patient with hip disease.

Smidt and Wadsworth (27) and Stauffer and Wadsworth (28) reported similar studies in which the three components (vertical, anterior/posterior and medial/lateral) were measured. These are presented in a manner similar to that of (2) and are exemplified by Fig. 6 although their apparatus did not have the facility for registering several successive foot contacts and they report only forces on the affected limb. In the interpretation of the tests reported by these groups two factors are relevant:

1. The loads borne at the extremities are definitely related to the force transmitted at the affected joints. The actual joint forces however depend on the magnitude of the forces transmitted by the muscular and ligamentous connections in the region of the articulation. These are directly related to the external force but involve other factors such as the anatomical disposition and the configuration of the limb at each instant.

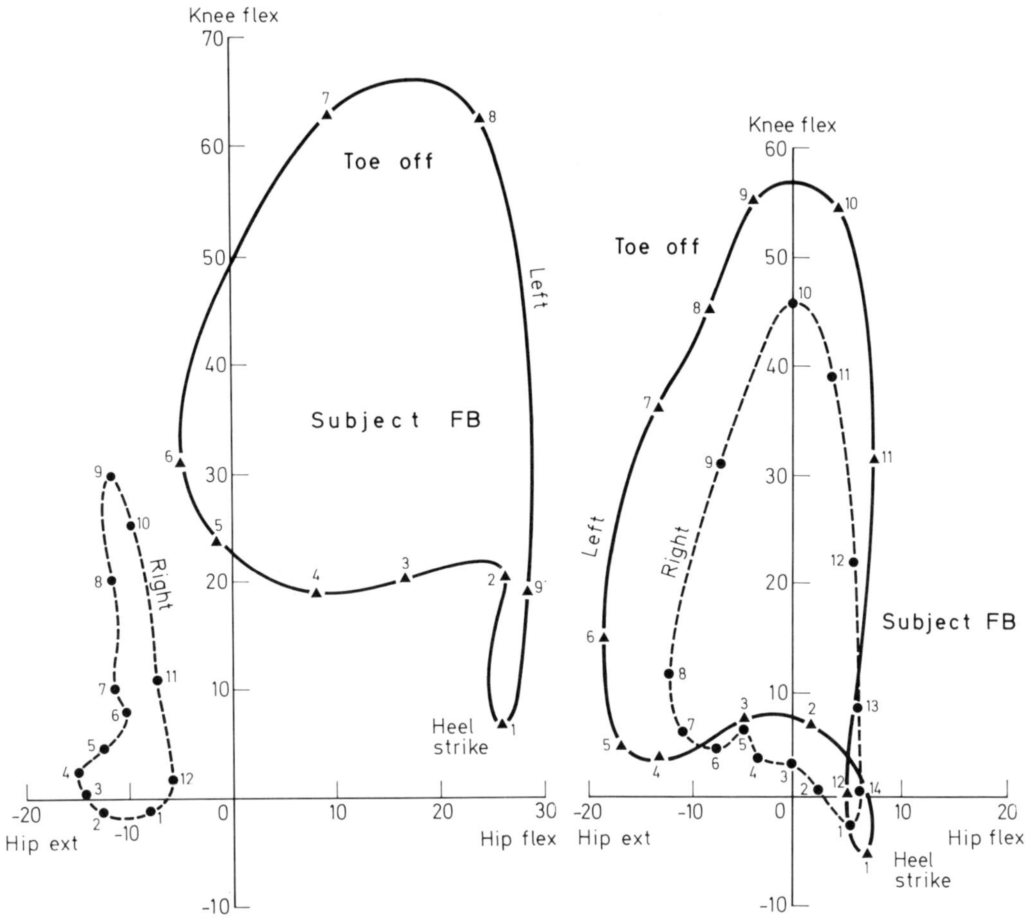

Fig. 3 Angle diagram for patient having osteoarthritis of right hip. Vertical axis knee flexion angle degrees. Horizontal axis, hip flexion angle degrees (14)

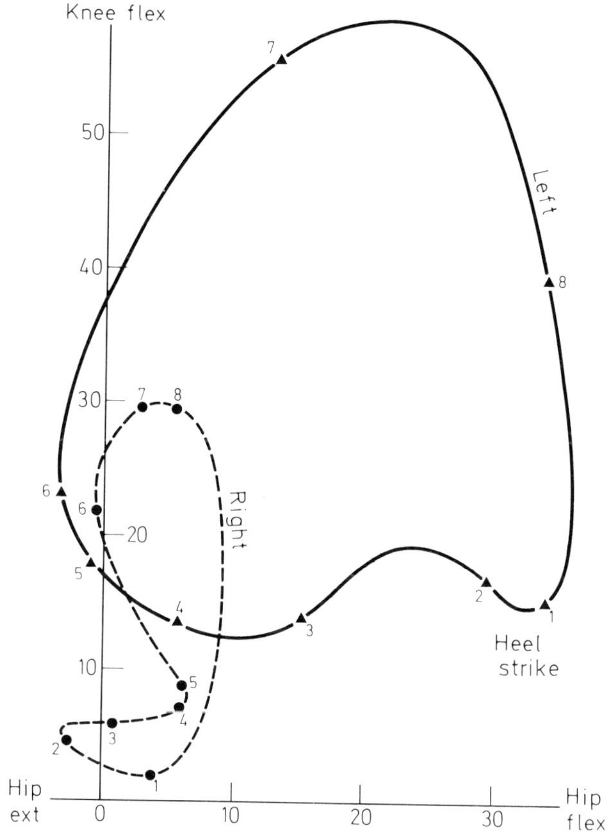

Fig. 4 Angle/angle diagram as in Fig. 3, this time illustrating the improvement in locomotion characteristics of a patient following hip arthroplasty (14)

2. The external force components are however useful in another respect in that the accelerations undergone by the body during locomotion must correspond to the externally applied forces. Thus gait abnormalities which involve abnormal accelerations can be inferred from measurements of the external forces.

ANALYSIS OF FORCES TRANSMITTED BY JOINTS

There have been several studies relating to cadaver specimens or to the analysis of the living subject in conventional standing positions (7,12,22,29,30).

There is only one study known to the writer where an intravital measurement has been made of joint force – this is the classical work of Rydell (25) where data is described collected from two patients in whom a modified prosthesis of the Austen-Moore type was inserted following traumatic fracture of the upper femur. These prostheses had strain gauges fitted to measure the forces transmitted by the device. Six months after surgery they were connected to the appropriate measuring apparatus and some of the results obtained are illustrated in Fig. 7 which shows the variation with time of the components of hip joint force during rapid walking in the female subject. The values of force are expressed as multiples of body weight. This study obviously provides direct and relevant information relating to endoprosthesis design but can only exceptionally be used for patient assessment. Similarly the information acquired pertains only to the affected joint and not the adjacent or contralateral joints.

Basic studies relating to the forces developed between ground and foot and the relative configuration of limb segments were initiated by Saunders et al. (3) and a three-dimensional analysis of the total load actions transmitted between foot and shank, shank and thigh and thigh and pelvis was reported by Bresler and Frankel (1). These authors reported the results of tests on four normal subjects and typical information is shown in Fig. 8.

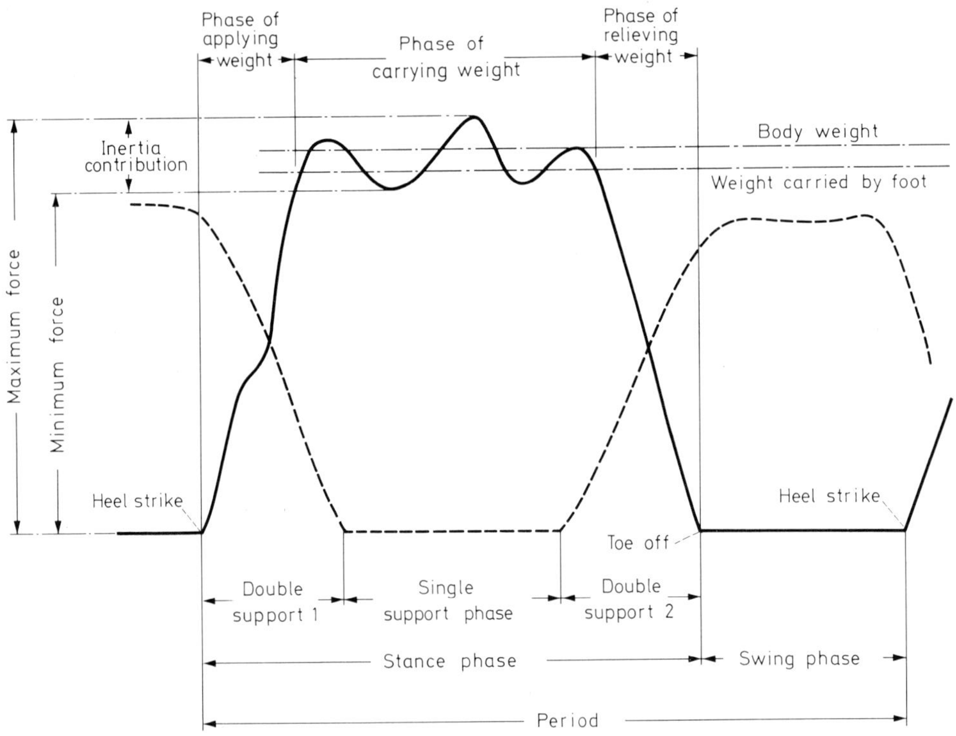

Fig. 5 Variation with time of ground/foot force for left and right foot of a patient with degenerative disease in the hip joint (8)

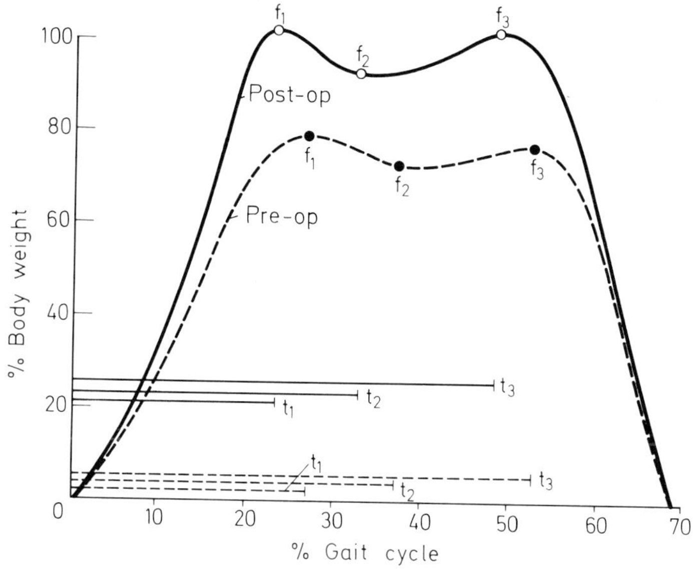

Fig. 6 Graph of vertical component of floor reaction force pre- and post-operatively. f, values represent mean peak loads (in per cent of body weight) while the, t, values represent mean times at which the peak loads occurred during the gait cycle (28)

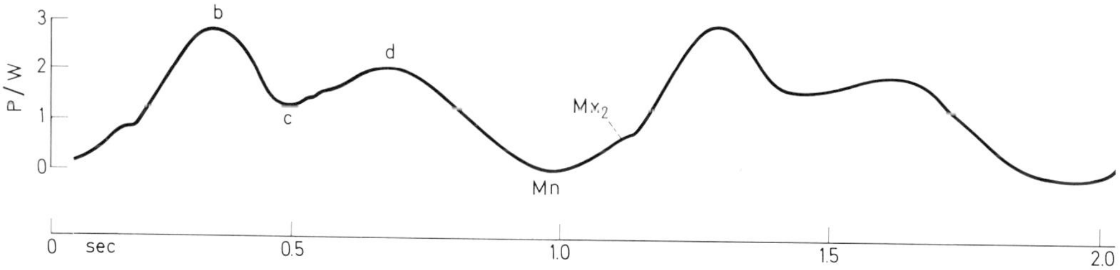

Fig. 7 Variation of resultant hip joint force P with time during the walking cycle for a female subject walking in a straight line on a level surface.W, body weight, = 45 Kg (25)

It should be emphasized however that the force values shown transmitted at the hip, knee and ankle levels are the total resultant forces transmitted between the limb segments. These forces do not relate to the pressures developed at the articulating surfaces. Obviously the pressures at the joint comprise not only the external forces but also the tensions in the tendinous and ligamentous structures passing the joint. For instance, in the knee joint the resultant load transmitted at the tibial/femoral surfaces correspond to the ground to foot force reduced by the effects of the gravity and inertia actions on the shoe, foot and shank together with the tension in the patellar tendon as well as in the tendons of the back of the thigh and the back of the calf muscles (if these are active) and also any force transmitted by the fascia lata or the cruciate or capsular ligaments.

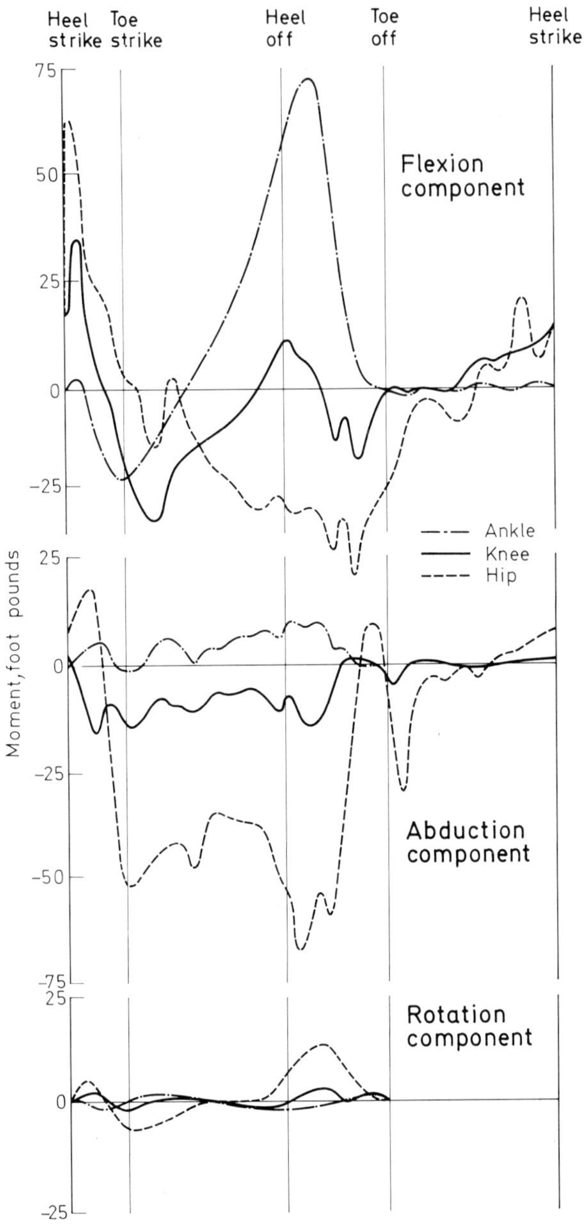

Fig. 8 A Resultant inter-segment moments in the leg during level walking (1)

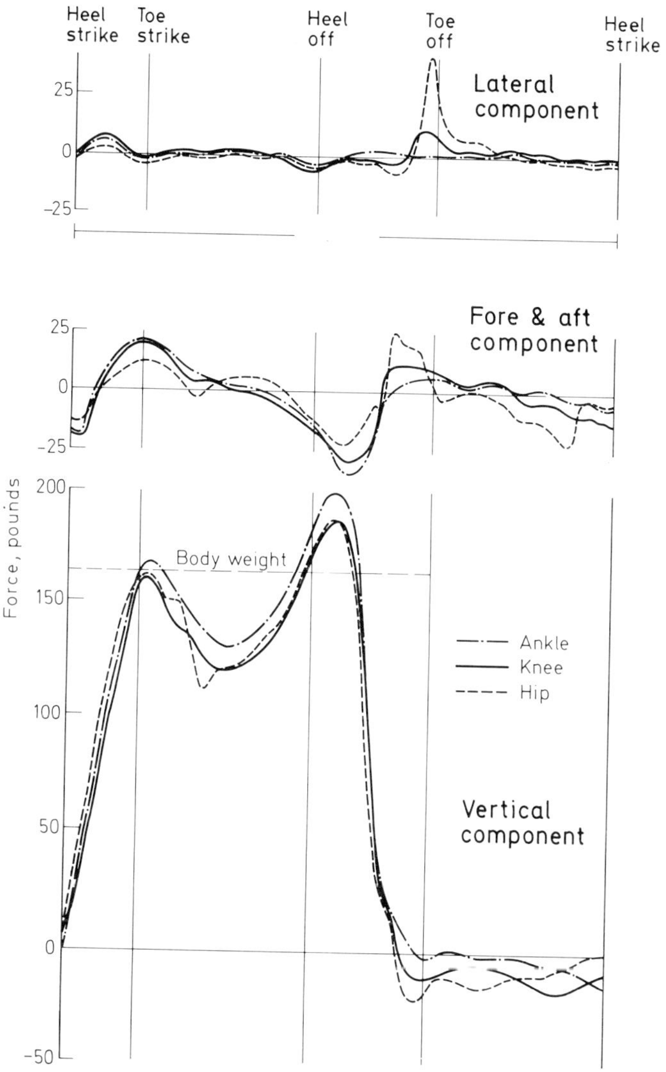

Fig. 8 B Resultant inter-segment forces in the leg during level walking (1)

An exact analysis of all these factors is not possible since the precise load in the relevant muscles cannot be determined nor can the force transmitted by the ligaments at any instant be inferred from external measurements. By making reasonable assumptions for the position of resultant force transmitted by certain groups of muscles and having regard to the phasic pattern of EMG (16,19,20), values were obtained for the knee joint forces transmitted by normal individuals in walking on a level surface and negotiating stairs and ramps. Curves representing averages of 36 tests for the hip joint and 26 tests for the knee joint are shown in Fig. 9. The maximum values of the joint forces during level walking are high in comparison with those of Rydell's patients. It is however instructive to compare these on the basis of body weight, W, and stride length, L, as

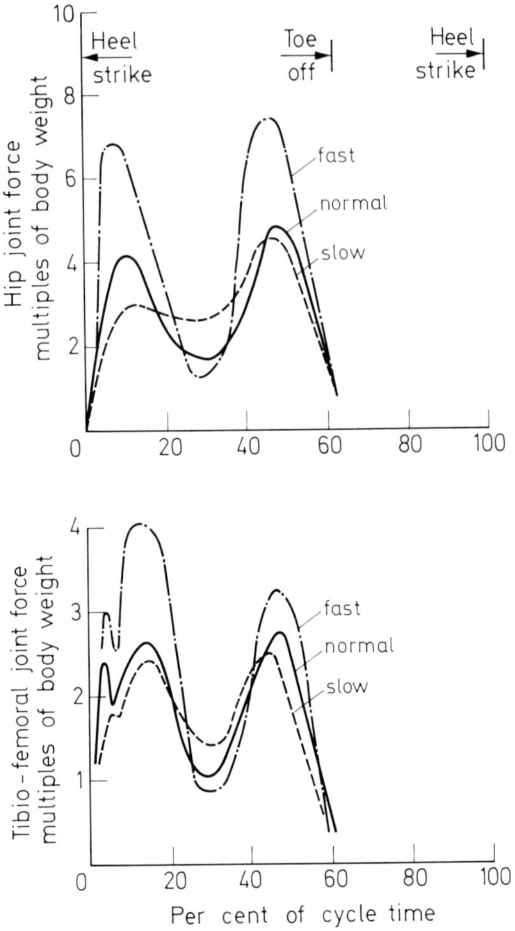

Fig. 9 Variation with time of hip joint and knee joint forces for slow, normal and fast walking (21)

shown in Fig. 10. In Fig. 9 it will be seen that there are two maxima in the hip joint force/time relationship. Some subjects have the greater value in the first peak at approximately toe-off of the contralateral foot whereas others have the maximum in joint force at the heel strike of that foot. Fig. 10 is therefore presented with the ordinate as the mean of the two maximum values and the abscissa as the product of the body mass, M, and stride length, L. Two factors of interest follow from this graph. Firstly, the closeness of the linear regression to the experimental points (t = 6.34) and, secondly, the close correspondence of the results of Rydell with the linear relationship. As mentioned earlier there are as yet no other data relating to direct measurements of joint forces. Until this is available it would be reasonable to assume that the approximate values inferred from external measurements are close to actual. Average values of forces transmitted at the hip and knee joints during other activities are shown in Table 1.

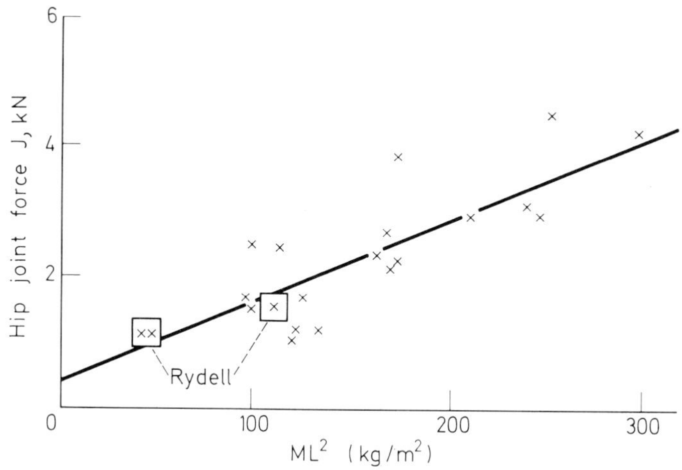

Fig. 10 Relationship between hip joint force J and ML^2 where M, subject body mass, in Kg and L, double stride lenght, in m. The circled points represent the results of Rydell. Joint force is the average of the two maxima shown in the typical curves of Fig. 9 (20)

Table 1 Average maximum values of forces at hip and tibio-femoral joints during a range of activities (10)

Activity	Maximum joint force Multiples of body weight	
	Hip	Knee
Level walking		
slow	4.9	2.7
normal	4.9	2.8
fast	7.6	4.3
Up stairs	7.2	4.4
Down stairs	7.1	4.9
Up ramp	5.9	3.7
Down ramp	5.1	4.4

With these techniques of analysis established for normal individuals, further tests proceeded at the Bioengineering Unit, University of Strathclyde to assess the performance of patients with degenerative joint disease and also with pathological abnormalities. A series of patients with osteoarthritis of clinical significance at one hip joint was assessed by these techniques before and after palliative surgery. The patients analysed were all provided with a Charnley low friction arthroplasty and the results before surgery and six months after are reported (11).

Typical curves representing hip joint loads transmitted in one of these patients are shown in Fig. 11 indicating the pattern of joint force before and after surgery. There is little significant difference between the values of force transmitted. It should be noted however that this phenomenon arises for two distinct reasons. Before surgery the patient had pain in the joint and adopted a gait which was significantly antalgic. With the relief of pain following the arthroplasty the pattern of activity of the abductor muscles much more closely resembled normal, although even six months post operatively they were not developing the maximum value of abductor moment at the hip which might have been expected. The other factor was that before surgery most patients had significant hip flexion deformities. The presence of this deformity required enhanced activity of the extensor muscles which of course produced larger forces at the hip joint. Following surgery this contracture was relieved, the patient walked erect and thus the joint force was correspondingly reduced. It is interesting to look at the results of three patients following surgery in comparison with the spectrum of normal values previously obtained by Paul. This is shown in Fig. 12 and is indicative of the fact that the age of the patients and the surgery they have received has only slightly reduced the values of force they develop at the hip joint in comparison with normal individuals.

A range of tests on patients with pathological knee conditions is reported by Harrington (6). He also conducted some tests on patients who had had knee joint replacements of the Freeman-Swanson and the Waldius type. The knee joint force for these patients is shown to a base of time in Fig. 13 with the corresponding average curve for normal subjects. It will be seen that patients following surgery are developing values of force very similar to the normal individual. Failure of knee joint replacements of the hinge type is frequently reported as being due to rotation of the prosthesis stem relative to the long bone and it is therefore relevant to look, in Fig. 14, at the curves of variation of moment about the long axis of the tibia transmitted during the walking cycle for these patients and the normal. Once again it is seen that the force actions developed by the patients correspond closely to the normal subject values.

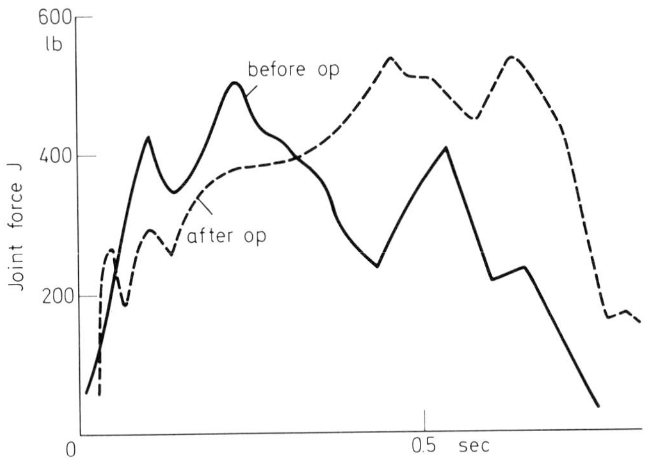

Fig. 11 Hip joint force during level walking for an arthritic patient before and after Charnley low-friction arthroplasty (11)

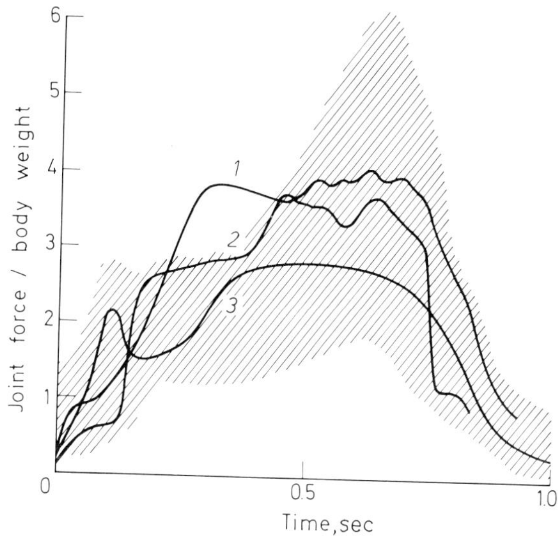

Fig. 12 Hip joint force for three patients after hip arthroplasty compared with the envelope of "normal" values obtained by Paul during level walking (11)

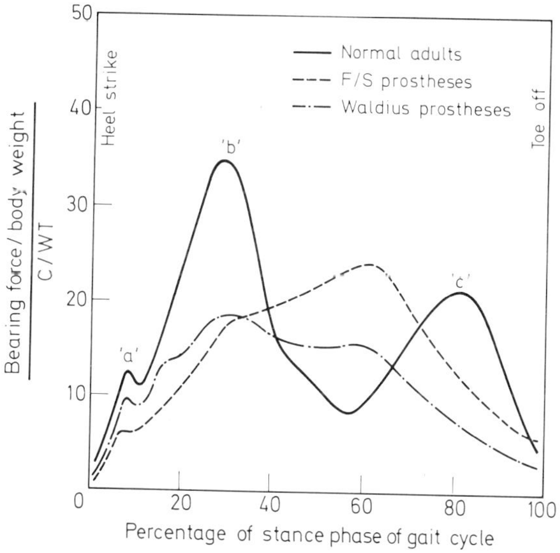

Fig. 13 Forces transmitted at the knee joint for patients with Freeman-Swanson and Waldius type replacements compared with the corresponding curve for normal subjects during level walking (6)

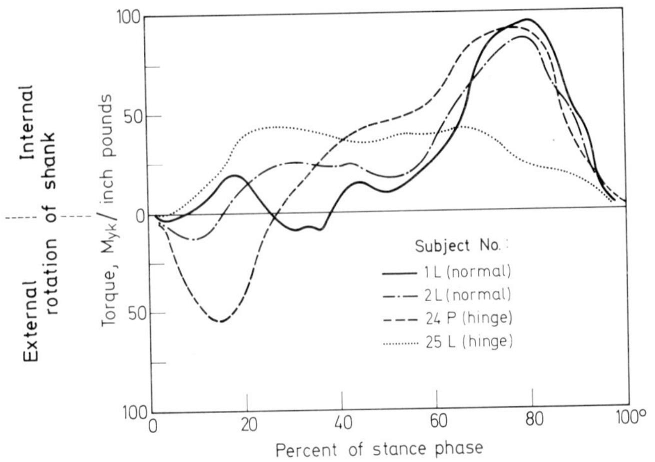

Fig. 14 Moments about the long axis of the tibia for patients with Freeman-Swanson and Waldius type joint replacements compared with values for normal subjects during level walking (6)

Further studies were undertaken by McGrouther relating to the force transmitted at the knee joint of these patients who had required hip surgery. The curves of knee joint force variation with time before and after hip surgery for one patient are shown in Fig. 15 and, as was the case for the hip, there is little major difference between the values. One quantity showing significant difference however is shown in Fig. 16. This is the variation in the position relative to the knee joint of the resultant force transmitted at the tibial/ femoral articulation. In the normal individual this is concentrated almost exclusively in the medial condyle during the stance phase of walking. For the patient whose characteristics are illustrated here it is seen that before surgery the path of this resultant point was on the lateral side of the joint. Following surgery a trajectory is seen which corresponds

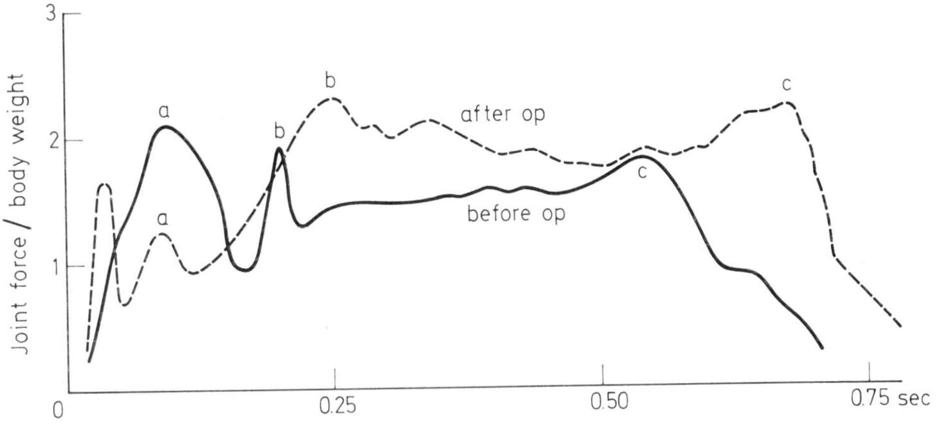

Fig. 15 Forces transmitted during level walking at the knee of a patient before and after hip arthroplasty

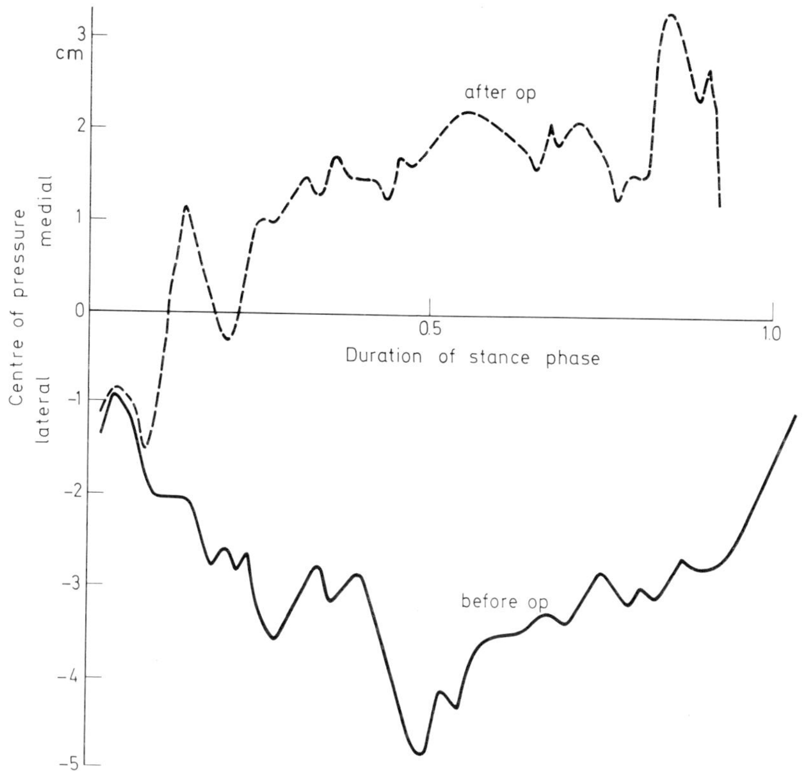

Fig. 16 Level walking data relating to the knee of a patient following hip arthroplasty. Vertical axis represents the medio-lateral offset from the A/P axis of the knee of the line of action of the resultant joint force during the walking cycle (10)

closely to that of the normal. Obviously therefore the hip surgery has had a significant effect on the loading of the knee and analysis of the adjacent and contralateral joints is therefore relevant to studies of this type.

In current clinical practice ankylosing is currently less frequently practiced. It is however of interest to assess the gait of patients in whom this procedure has been undertaken. Fig. 17 represents the results of this type of analysis for a patient who is a "good" walker, some ten years after surgery. The graphs show the variation with time of knee joint force on the affected and contralateral side. For this patient there seems to be no great difference in locomotion pattern, it is unfortunate that techniques of analysis have not yet been extended to analyse the loading at the lumbar and sacral joints where significant changes might be expected.

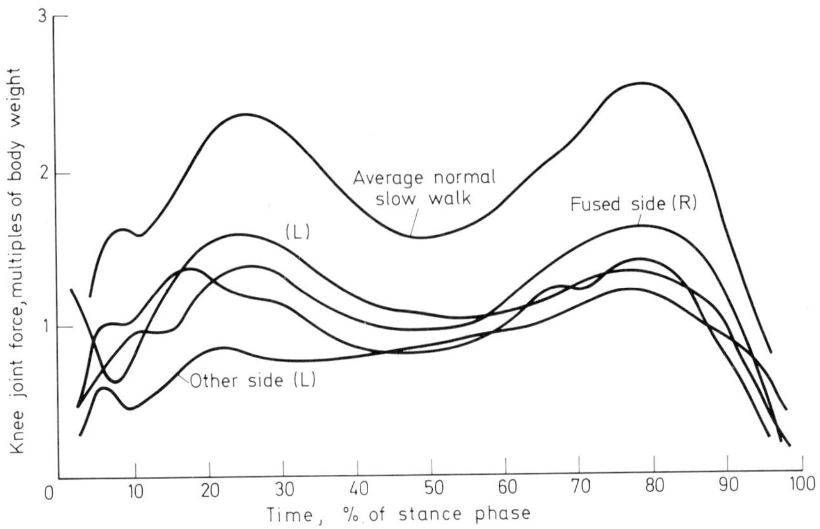

Fig. 17 Knee joint force at right and left knee during walking for a patient with ankylosed right hip

CONCLUSIONS

The practice of orthopaedics involves considerable intuitive knowledge of mechanical principles and it is therefore realistic that patient assessment should increasingly be undertaken on a mechanical basis. The paucity of the results in the professional literature is, however, principally an indication of the experimental difficulties in undertaking this procedure. Fortunately, with the developments of more sophisticated techniques allowing rapid data handling, it will be possible in the future to consider the analysis of locomotion and the associated force actions as possibly being one of the procedures available on a routine basis to the practising clinician.

REFERENCES

1. Bresler, B., Frankel, J.P.: The forces and moments in the leg during level walking. Transaction of the American Society of Mechanical Engineering 72, 27 (1950)
2. Charnley, J., Pusso, R.: The recording and analysis of gait in relation to the surgery of the hip joint. Clinical Orthopaedics and Related Research 58, 153 (1968)
3. Eberhart, H., Inman, V.T., Saunders, J.B.: Fundamental studies of human locomotion and other information relating to artificial limbs. Report of National Research Council on Artificial Limbs, University of California, Berkeley (1947)

4. Ganguli, S., Datta, S.R.: Prediction of energy cost from peak heart rate in lower extremity amputees. Biomedical Engineering 10, 52 (1975)

5. Grieve, D.W.: Gait patterns and the speed of walking. Biomedical Engineering 3, 119 (1968)

6. Harrington, I.J.: The effect of congenital and pathological conditions on the load actions transmitted at the knee joint. In: Total Knee Replacement, Institute of Mechanical Engineering, London: in press.

7. Inman, V.T.: Functional Aspects of the abductor muscles of the hip. Journal of Bone and Joint Surgery 39, 214 (1947)

8. Jacobs, N.A., Skorecki, J., Charnley, J.: Analysis of the vertical component of force in normal and pathological gait. Journal of Biomechanics 5, 11 (1972)

9. James, U.: Oxygen uptake and heart rate during prosthetic walking. Scandinavian Journal of Rehabilitation Medicine 5, 71 (1973)

10. McGrother, D.A.: Load actions transmitted at the knee of arthritic patients. In: Total Knee Replacement, Institute of Mechanical Engineering, London: in press.

11. McGrouther, D.A.: In vivo measurement of joint loading after total hip replacement. Proceedings of the Clemson Conference on Biomaterials (1974)

12. McLeish, R.D., Charnley, J.: Forces in the one-legged stance. Journal of Biomechanics 3, 191 (1970)

13. Milner, M., Dall, D., McConnell, V.A., Brennan, P.K., Hershler, C.: Angle diagrams in the assessment of locomotor functions. S.A.Med.J. 47, 951 (1973)

14. Milner, M., Dall, D., Ruff, A.L., Brennan, P.K.: Pre- and post-operative angle diagram in cases of total hip reconstruction. Digest of the 5th Canadian Medical and Biological Engineering Conference, Montreal (1974)

15. Molbech, S.: Energy cost in level walking in subjects with abnormal gait. In: K.Evang and K.L. Andersen, edit., Physical Activity in Health and Disease, Oslo: Universitatsforlaget 1966

16. Morrison, J.B.: Bioengineering analysis of force actions transmitted by the knee joint. Biomedical Engineering 3, 164 (1968)

17. Murray, M.P., Gore, D.R., Clarkson, B.H.: Walking patterns of patients with unilateral hip. Pain due to osteoarthritis and avascular necrosis. Journal of Bone and Joint Surgery 53-A, 259 (1971)

18. Murray, M.P., Brewer, B.J., Zuege, R.C.: Kinesiological measurements of functional performance before and after McKee Farrar total hip replacement. Journal of Bone and Joint Surgery 54-A, 237 (1972)

19. Paul, J.P.: Forces transmitted by joints in the human body. Proceedings of the Institute of Mechanical Engineering 181, 8 (1967)

20. Paul, J.P.: Forces at the human hip joint. PhD Thesis, University of Glasgow (1967)

21. Paul, J.P.: Force actions transmitted by joints in the human body. Proceedings of the Royal Society-B, in press.

22. Pauwels, F.: Der Schenkelhalsbruch, ein mechanisches Problem, Stuttgart: Ferdinand Enke Verlag 1935

23. Ralston, H.J.: Energy speed relation and optimal speed during level walking. Internationale Zeitschrift für angewandte Physiologie 17, 277 (1958)

24. Ralston, H.J.: Effects of immobilization of the knee on energy expenditure during level walking. Ergonomics, Proc. 2nd I.E.A. Congress, Dortmund (1965)

25. Rydell, N.W.: Forces acting on the femoral head prosthesis. Acta Orthopaedica Scandinavica, Supplement 88 (1966)

26. Skorecki, J.: The design and construction of a new apparatus for measuring the vertical forces in walking. Journal of Strain Analysis 1, 429 (1966)

27. Smidt, G.L., Wadsworth, J.B.: Floor reaction during gait – comparison of patients with hip disease and normal subjects. Phys. Therapy 53, 1056 (1973)

28. Stauffer, R., Smidt, G.L., Wadsworth, J.B.: Clinical and biomechanical analysis of gait following Charnley total hip replacement. Clinical Orthopaedics and Related Research 99, 70 (1974)

29. Stange, F.G.: The hip, London: Heineman 1965

30. Williams, J.F.: A force analysis of the hip joint. Biomedical Engineering 3, 365 (1968)

PRESENT INDICATION FOR HIP JOINT REPLACEMENT AND IMPLANTATION TECHNIQUES

M.E. Müller

Total hip replacement has brought the promise of relief from hip pain, excellent gait and a satisfactory range of hip motion (1). But we have to keep in mind that total hip replacement is a major procedure and local complications such as infection, loosening of the fixation, and migration of the socket into the pelvis may lead to lifelong disability.

Not the very rare primary infection, which can usually be dealt with by early revision, is important, but the low-grade type of infection due to inoculation at the time of surgery or after a post-operative discharge hematoma appearing months or years after surgery.

The indications for total hip replacement involve four different factors:

- technical problems
- the surgeon
- selection of patients
- hip disease

TECHNICAL PROBLEMS

Prior to start operation on hip joints, the operating room conditions have to be improved. The efficiency of a special clean-air operating theatre to reduce air infections has not been proven, but in the greenhouse unnecessary movements are prevented and the enclosure isolates the operating team from circulating personal and "spectators". This is particularly important in teaching hospitals.

Today over 100 different types of total hip implants are on the market, and the choice may be difficult. It now seems that a metal-to-plastic bearing presents some advantages. Net-fitting prostheses appear to lead to more loosenings of the socket compared with components that allow the hip to subluxate in the event of inappropriate movements. The best prosthesis is the one the surgeon is accustomed to. But no one can solve all the total-hip problems with just one prosthesis. Clearly, many different models should be available. In addition, all the necessary instruments such as reamers, special chisels, cold light, etc., must be on hand for total hip replacement and revision operations.

THE SURGEON

When the surgeon performing a total hip replacement is a "super-specialist" for joint replacement and works in a hip center, like Charnley (2), the advantages for teaching purposes or for developing new implants and perfecting new operating techniques are obvious. Furthermore, the overall results of such a hip center should certainly be better than those of a general orthopedic center. Finally, such centers may be needed for the most difficult problems of revision surgery, but most of the time the orthopedic surgeon has to deal with a variety of problems and therefore must be experienced in all aspects of orthopedics. Since the number of patients who need a total hip replacement is very large, there is no doubt that virtually all experienced orthopedic surgeons are confronted with this problem. A good hip surgeon must know the merits and the possibilities of all the other hip procedures with potentially better long term results than total hip replacement. Unfortunately, there are still too many so-called hip surgeons who, for instance, do not know how to cure a slipped femoral epiphysis of more than 50° with a resection osteotomy of the femoral neck. Using this procedure the result is usually a normal hip. In a non-union of the femoral neck with a still living head, an abduction osteotomy re-establishes a normal hip joint. And how many cases of painful coxa valga luxans will become painless and mobile and fully functioning after a shelf operation, a pelvic osteotomy, or a varus osteotomy. Also, double-cup procedures are actually performed more and more frequently in young patients who need an arthrodesis. We must also not forget that after a perfect hip fusion, a patient can ski and work for years without pain (Figs. 1-4).

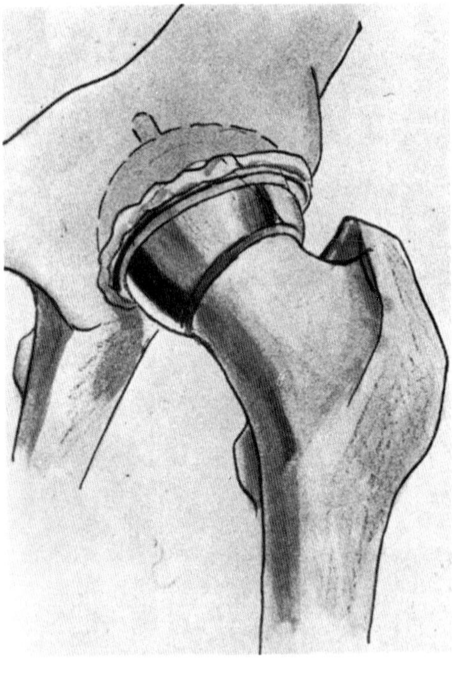

Fig. 1
Double cup prosthesis

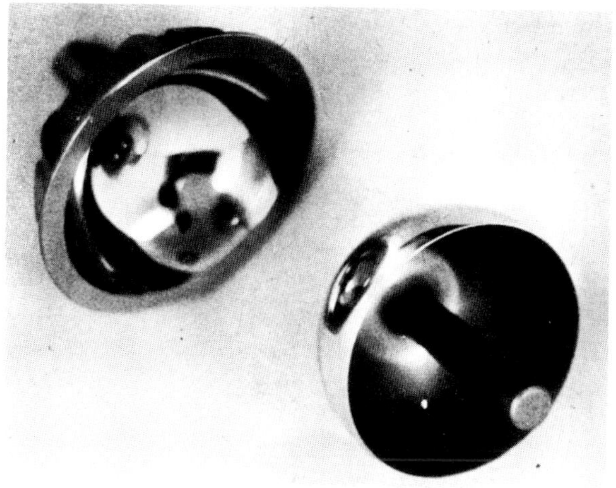

Fig. 2
Joint "body" of the double cup prosthesis

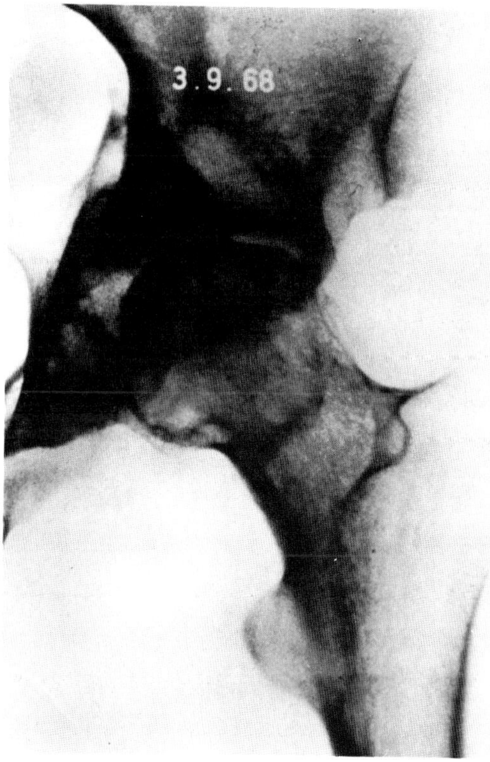

Fig. 3
Arthrosis of the hip joint at an advanced stage. Complete incongruence of the joint

The hip surgeon has to be acquainted with the technical reasons of early failure and the technique of cementing-in a prosthesis. He must be able to employ not only a rigorous aseptic technique, but an atraumatic and precise one.

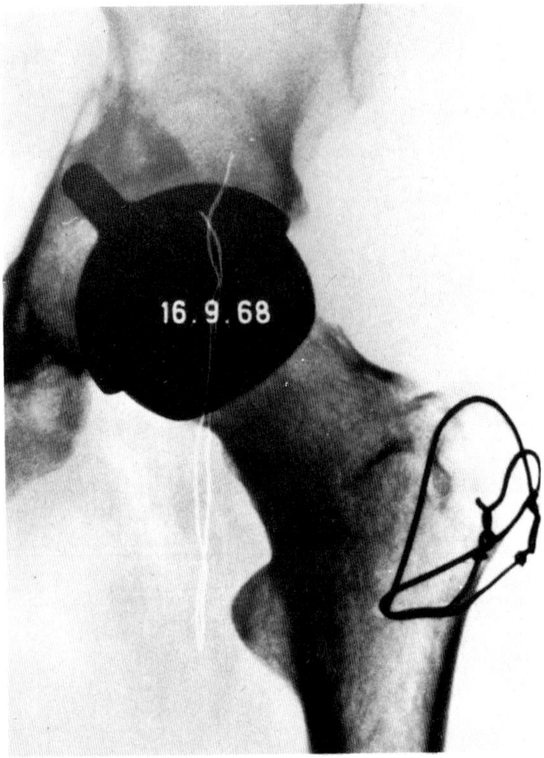

Fig. 4
The case shown in Fig. 3 after provision of a double cup prosthesis

A surgeon who has studied the procedure from books only, who has no interest in mechanical problems, and who does not know how to solve all the complications which may occur during or after surgery, has no place in this field. Especially the revision procedures in case of infection, loosening, and migration of the socket must be known.

The hip surgeon must be constantly involved with the problems of total hip replacement and must be able to check the reliability and efficacy of his total hip replacement for years.

SELECTION OF PATIENTS

Our experience in 15 years of practice in total hip replacement leads us to the conclusion that age as a criterion for selection is best considered restrictively. Thus, we still rarely accept patients below 60 with unilateral disease or below 50 with severe bilateral involvement. We are fully aware that such a strict selection is not practiced by most of the surgeons, but Charnley and many of us still use the same criterion with success.

Younger patients with severely limited mobility due to polyarthritis or ankylosing spondylitis (Figs. 5-6), or those with limited life expectancy, should have the operation

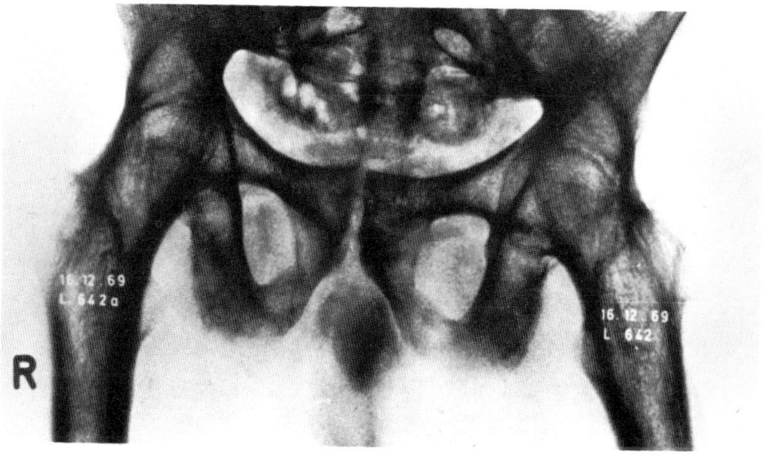

Fig. 5 Indication exception for total hip joint replacement without consideration of the age of the patient; bilateral ankylosis of the hip in Bechterew's disease

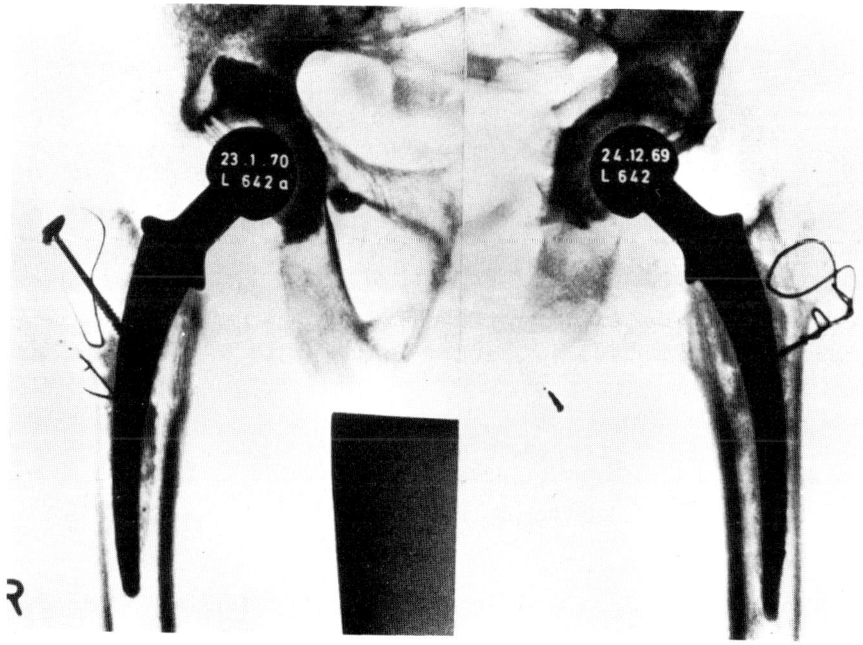

Fig. 6 The case shown in Fig. 5 after surgical treatment

performed. Our youngest patient with total hip replacement was a bedridden 16-year-old boy with polyarthritis who returned to us with a fracture of the femur after a motorcycle accident five years later. As shown previously, most of the patients of the younger age group can be treated very well by means of an intertrochanteric operation, shelf operation, or arthrodesis (Figs. 7-8).

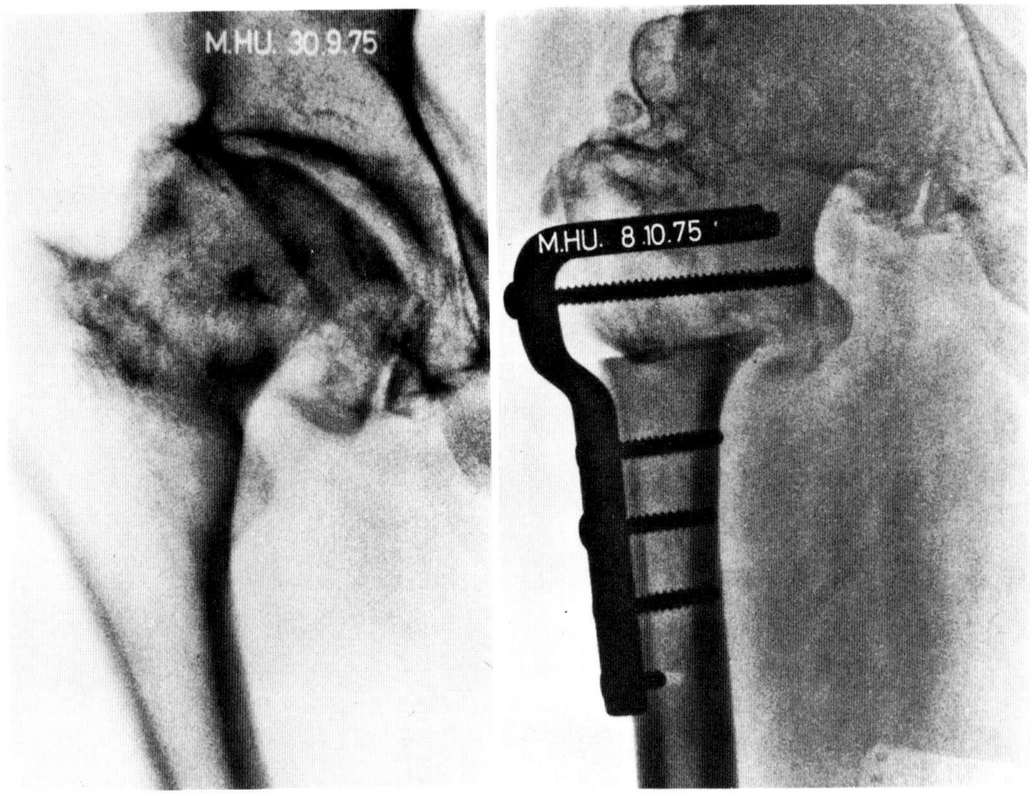

Figs. 7,8 Advanced deformity arthrosis of the hip joint with partially preserved articular space and treatment with high femoral osteotomy as an alternative to total hip replacement

If the disease itself does not limit the activity of the patient, we should always be aware that the patient will rapidly forget his now painless hip, and will try sports and other activities involving great effort, this in spite of all the instructions of his surgeon to restrict the stress put on the artificial joint. A patient, for example, was given a Moore prosthesis at the age of 28 years because of a necrosis of the femoral neck following a neck fracture; she was unable to walk without a stick. After four years, a total hip replacement was carried out and two years later she became dancing champion of Italy in the Shake and Charleston. However, six years after having gone through a total hip replacement, she asked us for a revision of her loose socket.

It should be remembered that a young woman is likely to marry and have children not knowing that loosening problems are often seen after two or three pregnancies. At the age of 27 a patient was subject to a Girdlestone operation after a fracture of the femoral head in an aeroplane accident. Six months after a total hip replacement she married and had two children within 4 years. Loosening problems arose soon after the birth of the second child.

But, as a salvage operation after the failure of other procedures without infection, total hip replacement is preferable at any stage to a Girdlestone procedure and a double-cup arthroplasty is preferable in women before arthrodesis is considered.

In poor-risk, debilitated patients over 80 years of age with aseptic disease and intolerable pain, total hip replacement seems justified. The speed of ambulation and recovery is so spectacular that, if a good anesthesia team is available, age alone is not considered a contraindication. But there may be increased risks in the presence of heart and circulatory disorders, diabetes, kidney diseases, and cerebral sclerosis.

Until recently, there were plenty of patients without much pain or disability demanding the procedure. Such patients should not be considered. In contrast, today we see more and more patients who have friends in whom the procedure has ended with disastrous results and who would now prefer another type of operation for themselves. In such cases the problem can often be solved by means of an intertrochanteric osteotomy, and it is unwise to insist on hip replacement.

HIP DISEASE

After local infection, even without evidence of inflammation at the time of surgery, total hip replacement cannot be recommended. In such cases we have to be very careful to prevent a flare-up of the infection, and we hesitate to follow Buchholz. At the very least we have to reduce the risk to an acceptable level.

We know many diseases that are not suitable for total hip replacement, even if the patient is older than 60. If there is a bilateral highly dislocated hip, we would not touch it. In unilateral cases, the socket must be fixed at its anatomical place and not in a secondary acetabulum (Figs. 9-10). Sometimes a plastic socket of 40 mm or even 36 mm with a femoral head of 22 mm in diameter is used. A narrow stem prosthesis should be available for the very narrow medullary cavities. Finally, in subluxated hips the adjustment and the anchorage of the socket may present some difficulties, particularly when the pelvic wall is very narrow (Fig. 11).

After fresh fracture of the femoral neck without arthritic changes we still prefer the femoral head prosthesis in patients over 70 years. An 80-year-old patient, for example, obtained a prosthesis 15 years ago and is still walking about without any trouble.

Following fracture of the acetabulum, it might be very difficult to adjust the posterior rim of the socket without autogenous bone grafts and a plate.

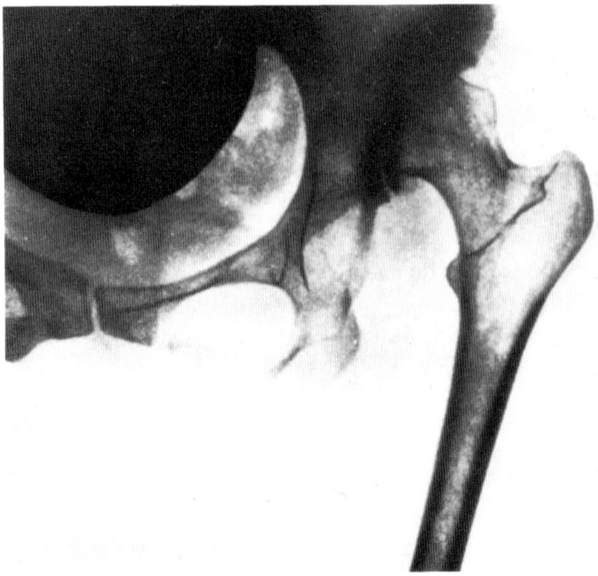

Fig. 9 Subluxation arthrosis with formation of a secondary socket above the acetabulum

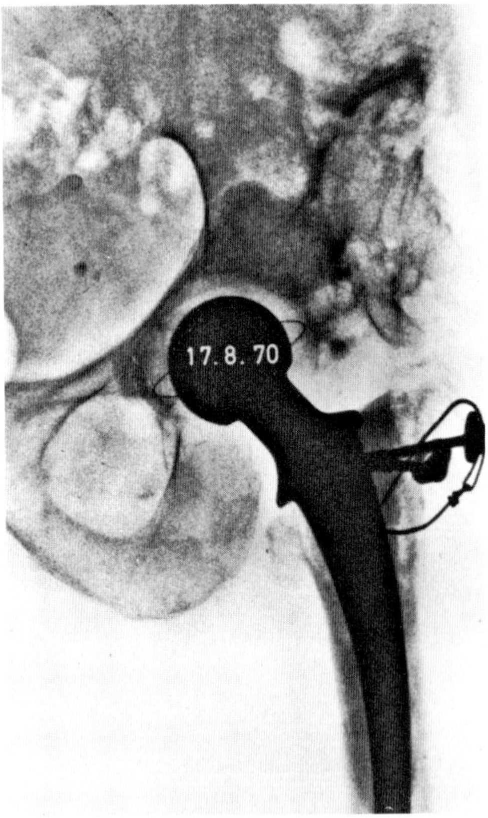

Fig. 10
The case shown in Fig. 9 after surgical treatment: on implantation the socket of the total hip prosthesis is shifted down to the level of the original site

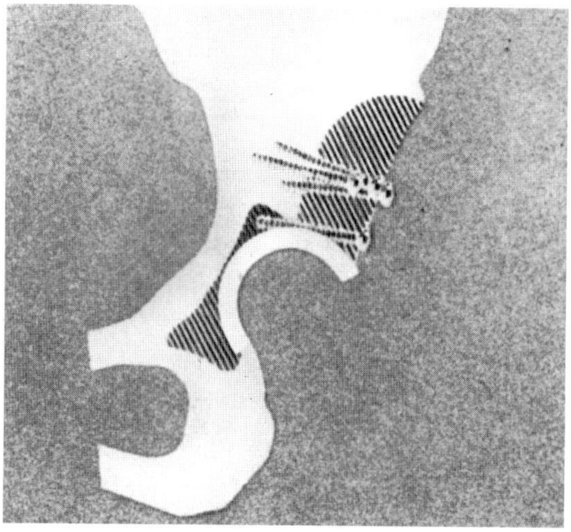

Fig. 11
Schematic representation of the possibility of fixing the socket after shifting it (Figs. 9 and 10)

In bone tumors or tumor-like conditions the en bloc resection of the joint must be followed by the reconstruction of the femur by means of special long stem prostheses. But if pelvis and femoral neck are destroyed by a metastatic process, only a Girdlestone procedure should be considered. In spastic dislocated hips the usually excellent results of the total hip replacement do not last very long. Such a case with migration of the plastic socket into the pelvis 6 years after surgery is demonstrated in Fig. 12.

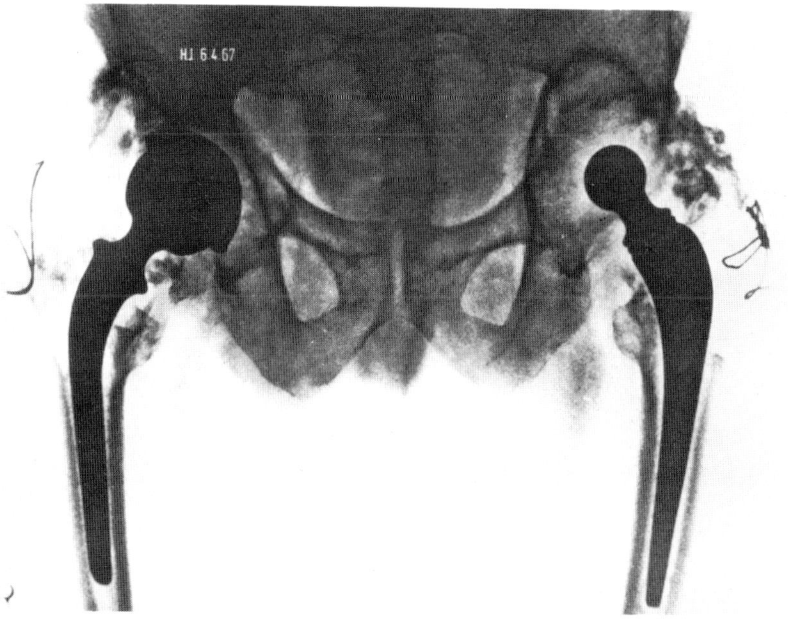

Fig. 12 Representation of a socket migration (left) into the small pelvis after using the total hip replacement in a case with tumorous destruction of the surrounding tissue

In previously operated hip joints, total hip replacement often counts as a salvage operation, but the risks of infection, early loosening, breaking of the femoral shaft, etc., increase. An arthrodesed hip in perfect position should be remobilized if the other hip is stiff or if the patient has constant back pain.

More difficult are the indications for total hip replacement after an unsuccessful total hip operation, especially after infection, migration of the socket and fracture of the pelvis.

CONCLUSION

We are of the opinion that it is difficult for an honest surgeon to give the right advice in every case. I should like to emphasize that the patient should always be informed that, in time, a second or a third operation may become necessary, and that 1 % or 2 % of the operations are followed by an infection within five years after the procedure. I hope that I have made it clear why we restrict the indication for total hip replacement to patients over 50, and why we always give consideration to other procedures such as intertrochanteric osteotomy, shelf operation, arthrodesis, etc., in younger patients.

REFERENCES

1. Stinchfield, F.W., Henry, J.H., Eftekhar, N.S., White, E.S.: Total hip replacement. Current practice in orthopaedic Surgery
2. Charnley, J.: Acrylic cement in orthopaedic surgery, Edinburgh and London: The Williams and Wilkins Co. 1970

HIP JOINT REPLACEMENT IN TRAUMA THERAPY

H. Beck

In trauma therapy, total hip joint replacement should be done more often in secondary arthroses than in acute trauma, and more often in injuries of the femur and their sequelae rather than in trauma involving the acetabulum (Table 1).

In acute trauma a clear indication is given in medial fractures of the femoral neck (type Pauwels II and III). In old patients an uncomplicated healing cannot confidently be expected and for immediate remobilization of old patients a prosthesis is more reliable than nailing. In patients with a life expectancy of less than 3 years, a hemiprosthesis would do the job; but this judgement of the shocked patient in the immediate post-traumatic period can be difficult, sometimes 5 to 8 years later the acetabular cartilage has been worn away and, in the presence of concurrent disease, the situation for changing the prosthesis can be much worse, as, for example, in a patient (Figs. 1a-1c) with an incipient central luxation and breakthrough of the acetabular floor. The 84-year-old patient was first operated on in 1968. Replacement of the prosthesis became necessary at the age of 90.

With increased life expectancy we recommend in the case of steep fracture in patients older than 70, a total replacement. Thus an immediate mobilization and full weight bearing ability are guaranteed. In contrast, in younger patients a joint-conserving osteosynthesis should always be performed.

In laterally located fractures the criteria are similar. The indications for joint replacement should be even more restricted. Delayed healing fractures or pseudarthrosis of the femoral neck in patients above the age of 60 should be treated by arthroplasty, it a valgus-type osteotomy holds out no promise of improvement.

In acute pertrochanteric fracture an indication for hip joint replacement is hardly ever given today; a correctly done arthroplasty gives a full-weight-bearing hip, but the joint replacement with especially designed prostheses after resection of the centrally located fragment carries higher risks – mainly because of higher blood loss – for the elderly

Table 1 Possible indications

A. Femurside injuries	B. Acetabularside injuries
1. femurneck fractures	1. fractures of acetabular rim
2. pertrochanteric fractures	2. fractures of acetabular ground
3. pathologic fractures	3. instability of pelvic girdle
4. femurhead necrosis	

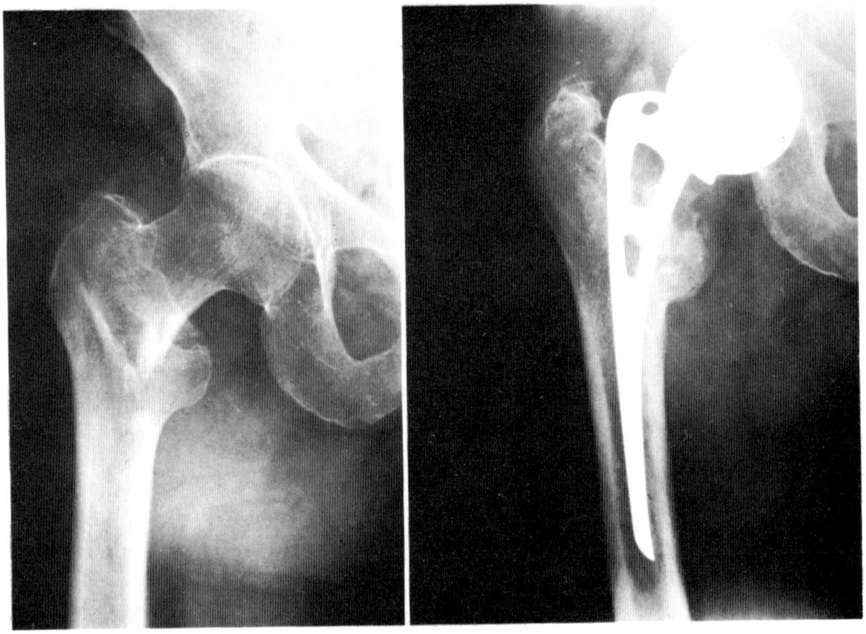

Fig. 1a Pertrochanteric fracture in an 84-year-old woman; poor cardiovascular condition necessitated the implantation of a hemiprosthesis

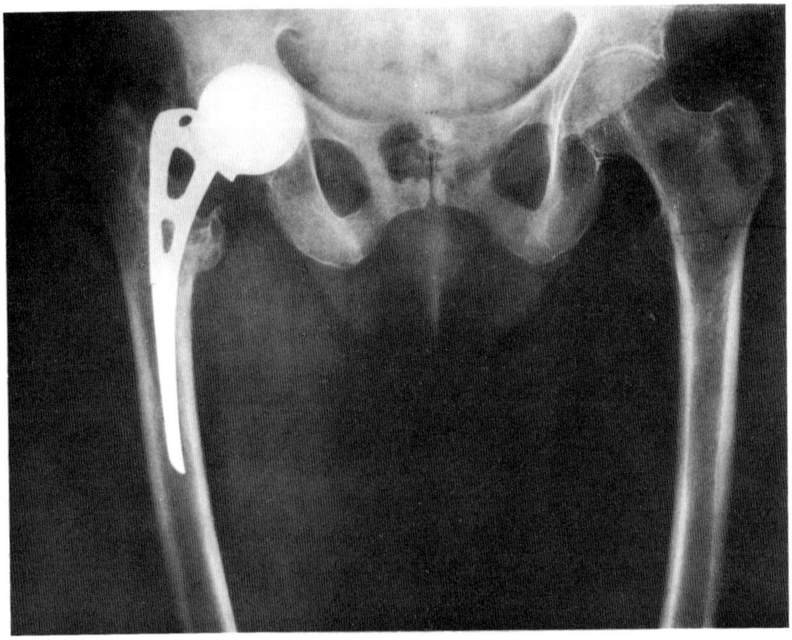

Fig. 1b Incipient perforation of acetabular floor 6 years after implantation

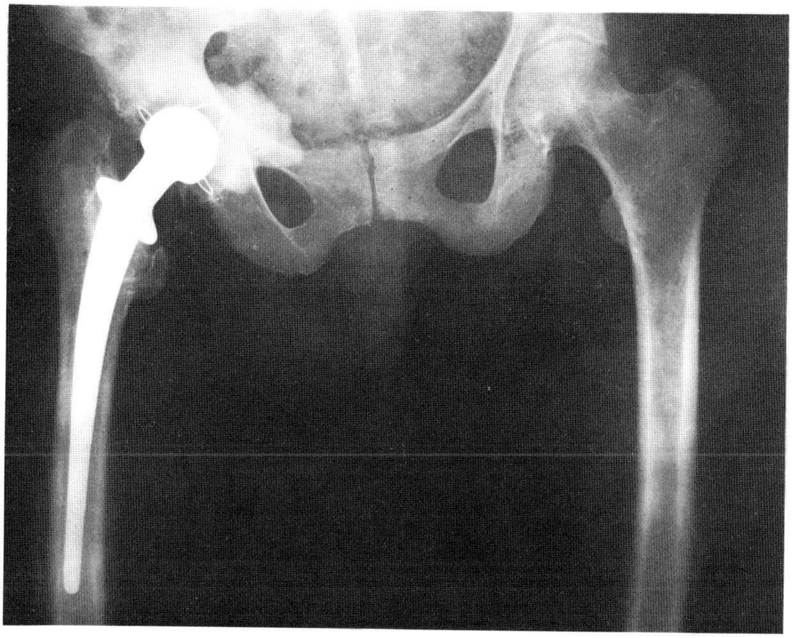

Fig. 1c Change of prosthesis to total hip at age of 90

patients than does cemented osteosynthesis or ascending nailing, methods that easily provide a primary or early weight-bearing ability. If an arthroplasty is performed, an adequate prosthesis with a long stem should be used. Figs. 2a-2c show an inadequate treatment. The prosthesis was replaced at another hospital – again the stem was not long enough to stabilize the defective marrow cavity. 4 years ago the third attempt was successful.

An ascending transtrochanteric nailing would have led to success more quickly and with less risk, in this 80-year-old patient.

In pathologic fractures of palliative operated primary malignant or metastatic tumor with good and sometimes long lasting results an arthroplasty should be performed at all ages. Generous bone resection and implantation of specially designed prostheses are justified, depending on disease and life expectancy. Here (Fig. 3) a Paget-sarcoma with pathologic fracture was treated with a Francobal prosthesis.

Posttraumatic femur head necroses are a relatively frequent indication for total endoprosthesis above the age of 60. Joint conserving methods are usually not possible and an arthrodesis is poorly tolerated by elder patients. These operations should be performed in younger patients.

I think it is essential to speak out against arthroplasties in younger patients. Young people expect more durability of their artificial hips than the joints are able to fill. Furthermore these patients need the arthroplasties for much longer periods than elderly patients; this leads very often to complications so that the operation is a scarcely tolerable risk.

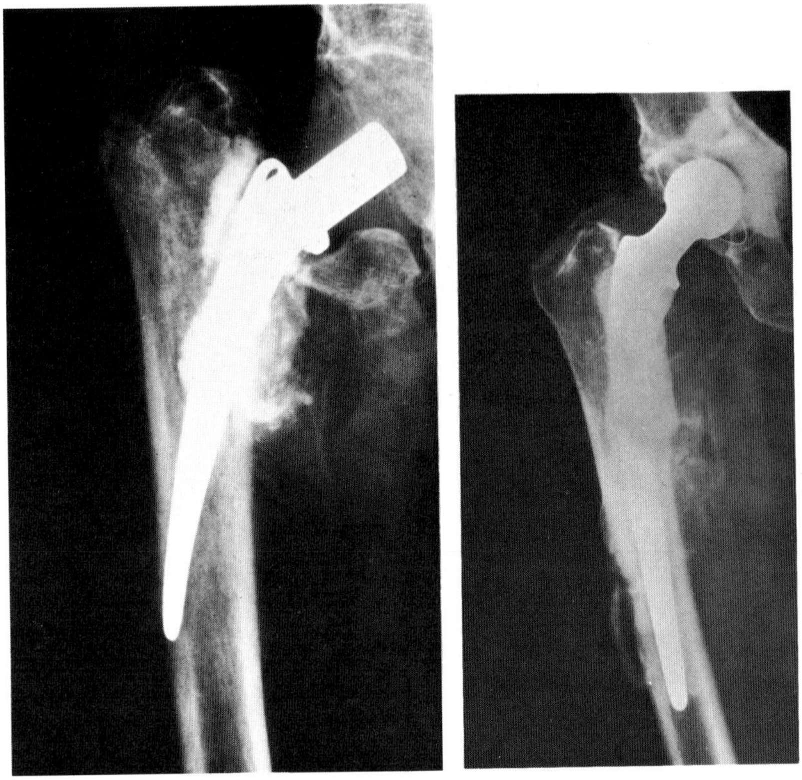

Fig. 2a Wrong position of hemiprosthesis with perforation of the lateral corticalis in a pertrochanteric fracture

Fig. 2b Implantation of a total hip with an inadequately long stem

The situation is different in older patients, who as a rule can be freed from intractable pain for the rest of their lives.

I would like to present a rare case of hip joint replacement (Figs. 4a, 4b): Three years postoperatively a patient was involved in a traffic accident in which he suffered a subtrochanteric fracture and a bending of the prosthesis stem caused by a sudden great force. After 8 months ineffective conservative treatment a replacement of the original arthroplasty by a long stem model was carried out.

In acute trauma of the femur side, the arthroplasty is indicated primarily sometimes and slightly more frequent as a secondary operation. The indication is further limited by age-dependent or posttraumatic or postoperative stability loss of the bones, in which the joint has to be anchored safely for a long period. Be reluctant, if the case history reveals evidence of postoperative infectious complications, as after hip joint replacement a twenty-fold rate of infections has to be put into account.

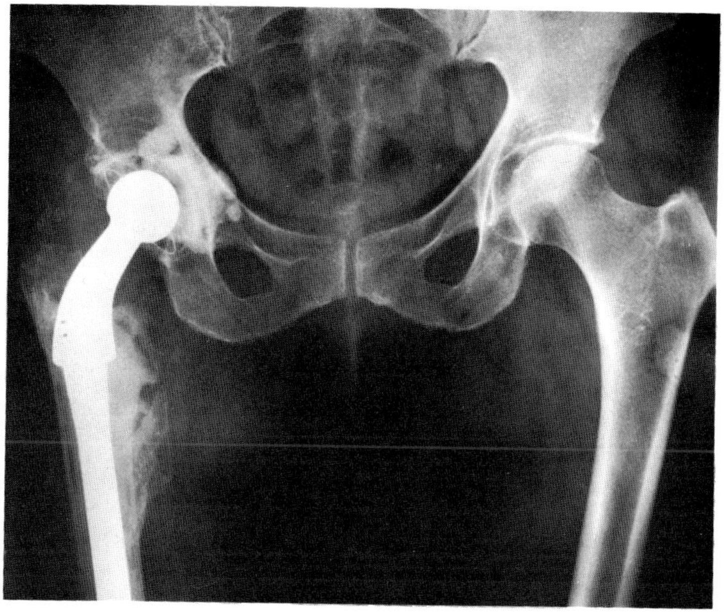

Fig. 2c Second change with efficient long stem 3 years ago brought good weight bearing capacity

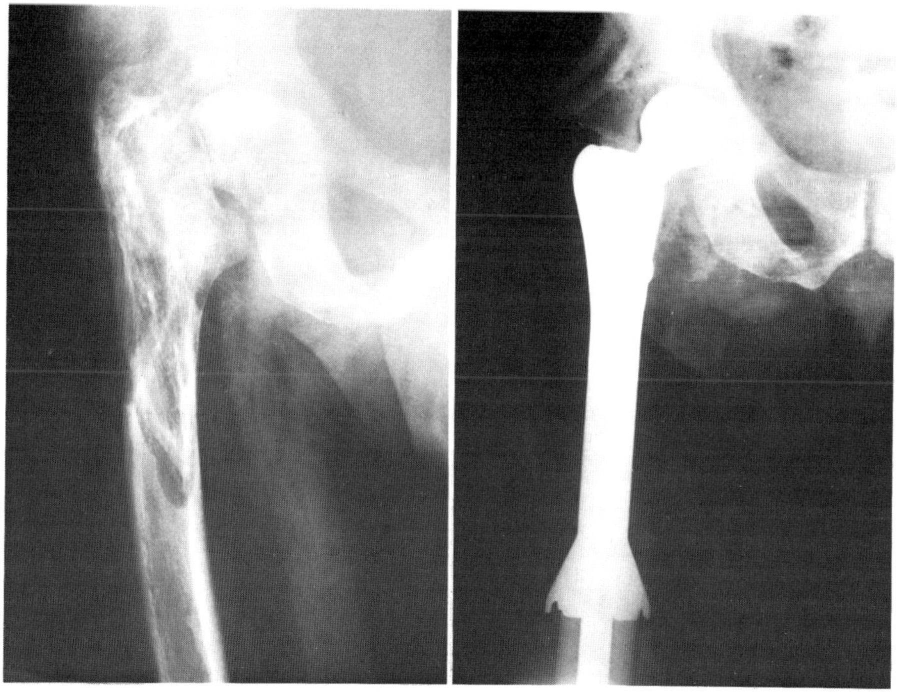

Fig. 3 Pathologic fracture in a Pagets sarcoma treated by resection of proximal femur and substitution of defect by special designed "Francobal" total hip

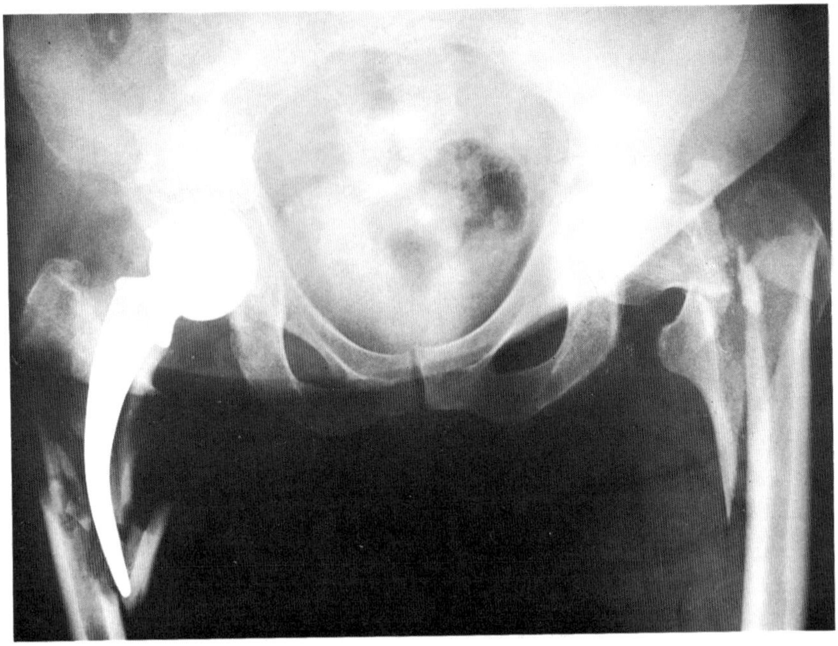

Fig. 4a Stem bending and loosening after a traffic accident 3 years after total hip replacement

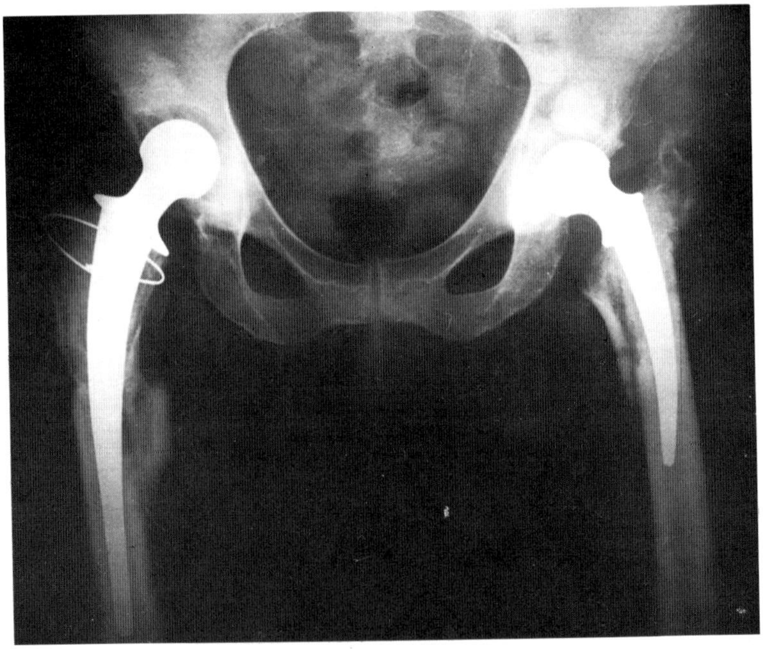

Fig. 4b 10 months after accident pseudoarthrosis necessitated the replacing of the artificial hip on the right side and implantation of a total hip on the left side

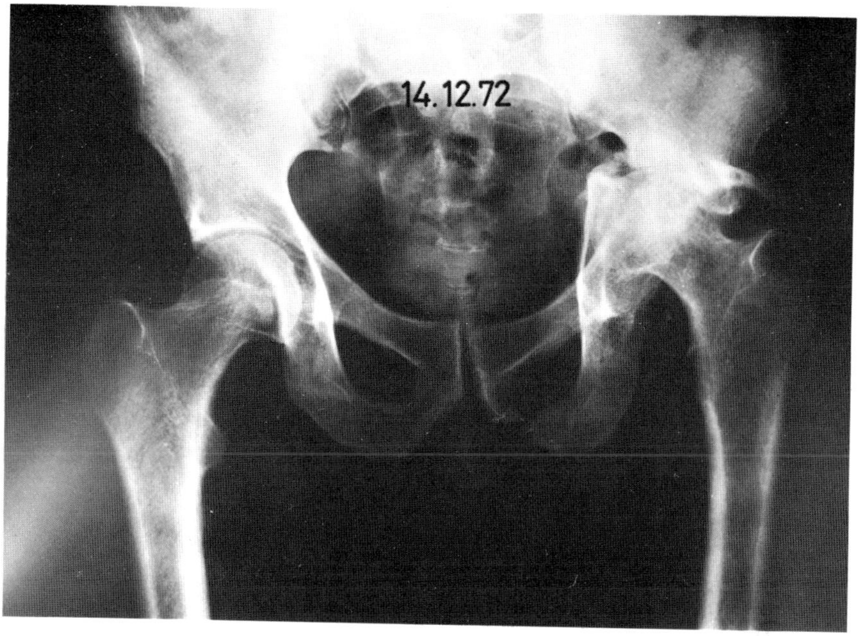

Fig. 5a 17 months after acetabular fracture questionable stability of acetabular floor

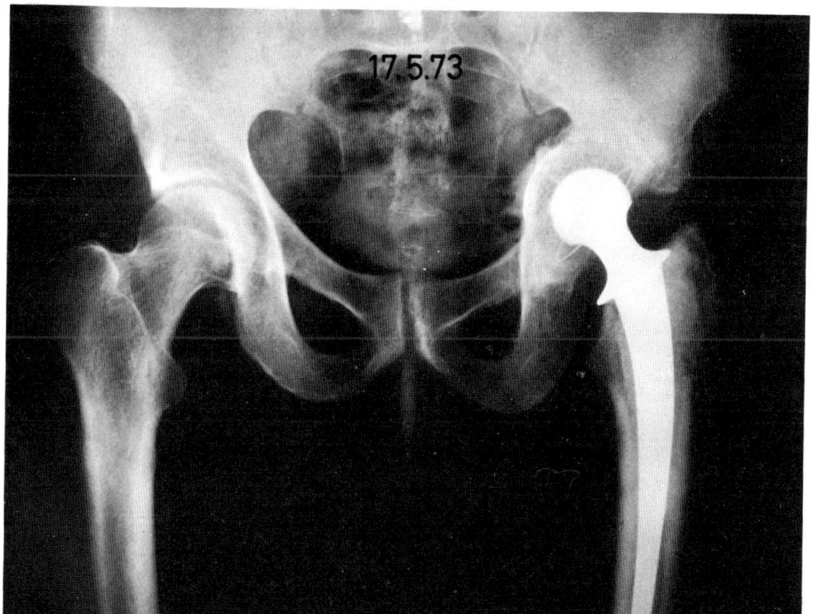

Fig. 5b Safe implantation of total hip 22 months after injury

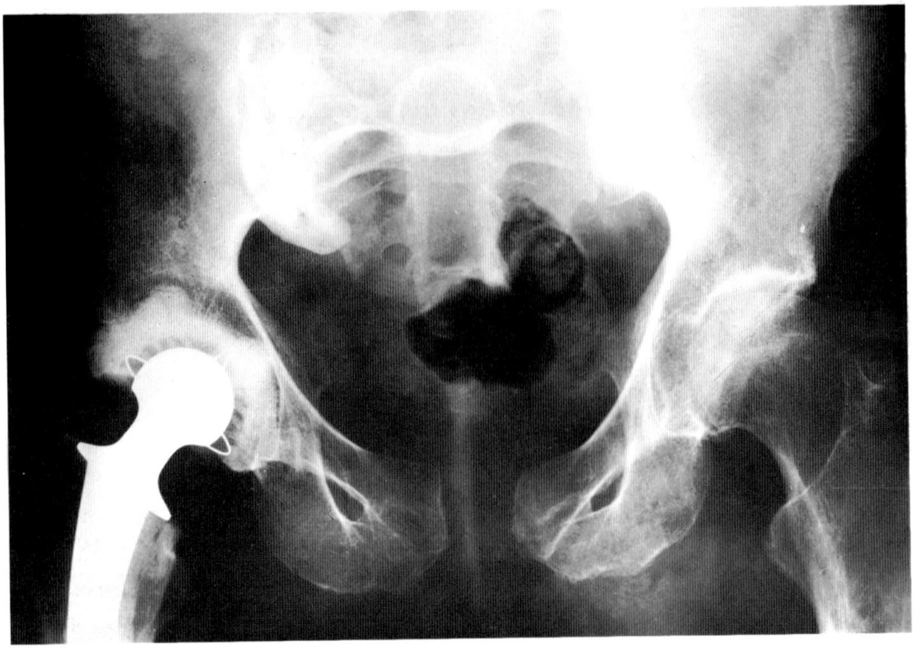

Fig. 6a Acetabular luxation-fracture combined with rupture (instability) of pelvic girdle leads to loosening of cement layer

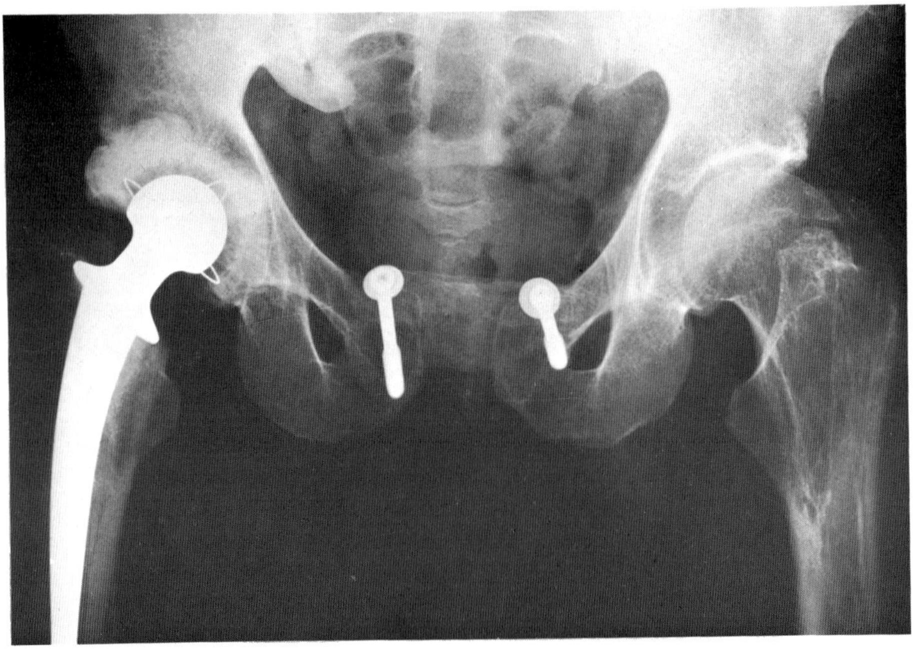

Fig. 6b Stabilization of pelvic girdle by T-shaped bone-graft

Less frequent than after femur side trauma, a hip joint replacement is indicated after acetabular side lesions. In acute trauma such an operation never should be done. It is impossible to achieve a stable and durable fixation of the artificial cup in correct position in these cases. An additional screw-osteosynthesis cannot prevent loosening, and even by additional strengthening of the posterior rim merely questionable stability could be gained.

In defects of the posterior wall, the cement basement has to be supported by huge dowel holes in correct direction. Insufficient anchoring leads to weight-bearing pain, caused by loosening and makes changing of the prosthesis necessary.

The choice of the acetabular model is of great importance. It should be as flat as possible, so it does not overtop the damaged posterior rim. Enclosing instead of open cup allows to spare anteversion, without danger of luxation. Most suitable is the acetabular part of the Le Grange Letournelle-type. In order to allow a hip replacement after fracture of the acetabular rim, it is useful to achieve primarily a reconstruction of the acetabulum; when secondary arthrosis has developed, then the conditions for implantation of a total hip are better and the fixation is as save as in degenerative arthrosis.

Especially in fractures of the acetabular bottom a primary fixation is not possible. Weight depending movements always lead to loosening of the cement layer. In cases when a primary osteosynthesis cannot be performed for good reasons, under conservative treatment a solid healing must be expected patiently like in this man (Figs. 5a, 5b), when 22 months had to forego after the trauma, before an operation could be performed.

Ruptures of the pelvic ring in addition to hip joint trauma are clearly a contraindication for arthroplasty. We had two pitfalls. When the patient puts weight on a pelvis with loosened symphysis or sacroiliacal joint, the diseased semipelvis makes elastic movements.

These movements inevitably lead to loosening of the cup basement. So it is useful to achieve a stabilization of the pelvic ring prior to or simultaneously with the arthroplasty (Figs. 6a, 6b), by bolting the symphysis with a T-shaped bone graft taken of the pelvic rim.

The premises for arthroplasty of the hip joint in trauma therapy are, caused by age, general condition and stability of the bed-building bone parts, usually less favorable than for degenerative arthrosis.

Summarizing, the decision for operation should fall reluctantly, and in younger patients never be considered, before long term results of new material and implantation-techniques are available.

DESIGN CRITERIA, PRESENT INDICATION AND IMPLANTATION TECHNIQUES FOR ARTIFICIAL KNEE JOINTS

N. Gschwend

When comparing the development of the alloarthroplasty of the hip joint with that of the knee joint, the following two essential differences become apparent:

1. The success rate, measured by the number of cases that exhibit postoperatively normal or almost normal articular function, is greater in the case of the total replacements of the hip joint than in the case of the knee joint.

2. The number of existing models for alloarthroplasty of the hip is smaller by far. They differ primarily in the mode of anchoring the individual prosthetic components: with or without cement (Shivas), supporting fin principle (Mittelmeier, Tragrippenprinzip), isoelastic prosthesis (Mathys), shorter stem with three-point support or longer stem, — and, closely connected with this, the materials used: metal/metal, metal/polyethylene, metal/ceramic, porometal, isoelastic materials, etc. On the other hand, apart from minor differences (such as head-cup radius relation, safeguard against dislocation) the mechanics of the joint are the same.

Things are, however, different with the knee joint, for which more than 100 different models are currently available. These show in part considerable design differences that primarily affect the mechanics of the joint itself.

THE PHYSIOLOGY OF THE KNEE JOINT

The complexity of the normal human knee joint can be easily understood from the extremely exacting and varying demands that are imposed on it during walking erect and — in connection with this — its position in the movement chain of the lower extremity. As the intermediate joint of the lower limb, the knee is located between the longest lever arms and is consequently subjected to extremely severe mechanical stresses. In this respect, it resembles the elbow joint, which has the most complicated structure of all the joints of the upper extremity. Both the arm and the leg demonstrate that the construction of the joints becomes ever more simple, the nearer we approach to the periphery.

The knee exhibits an extremely ingenious combination of stability and mobility, each of which — depending on the position of the knee joint — can be either increased or reduced at the expense of the other. Especially marked is the pronounced asymmetry of the medial and lateral articular surfaces (Fig. 1), which corresponds to the total asymmetry of the ligaments. Huson (12) and Menschik (16), who — independently of each other — analyzed these relationships from the standpoint of descriptive geometry, established a direct relationship between the changing radii of curvature of the femoral

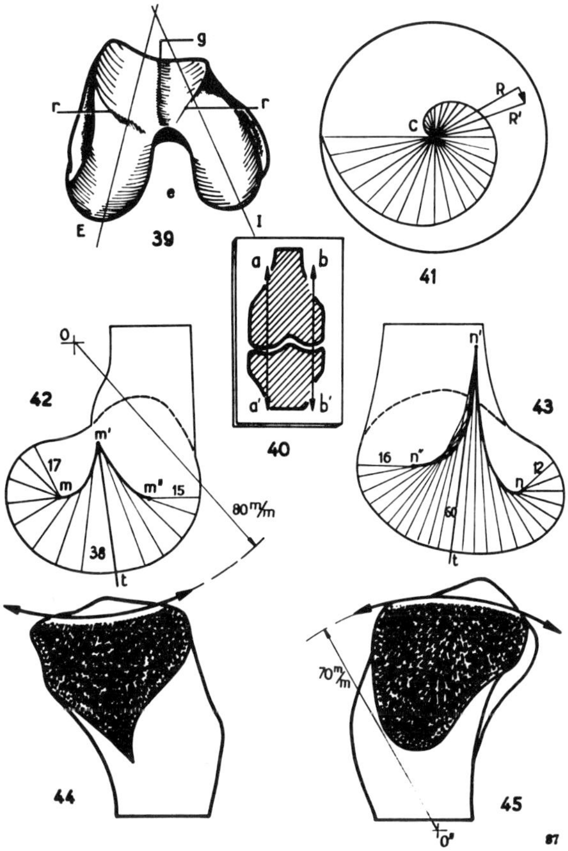

Fig. 1
Complete asymmetry of the joint components of the knee joint, great differences between medial and lateral (13)

condyles and the arrangement and length relation of the cruciate ligaments (Fig. 2). But also the different length and course of the medial and the lateral collateral ligaments, which form – together with the cruciate ligaments – a radial bracing system protecting the knee from forces acting from various directions, are directly related to the rolling-sliding motion sequence of the knee joint. This is characterized by a simultaneous rolling-sliding movement with a continually migrating axis, the relation between the rolling and sliding mechanism of the femoral condyle on the tibial plateau varying during the different phases of flexion. Comparable to an infinitely variable gear, this system on the one hand permits transition to the different flexion and extension positions within the smallest possible space with a minimum expenditure of force, and on the other hand allows the foot to adapt itself to a variable floor through the changing rotation of the lower leg. In this connection, mention should be made of terminal rotation, which is to be regarded as a passive locking mechanism. It is also closely associated with the arrangement of the cruciate ligaments, which is anatomically reflected not only in the configuration of the intercondylar eminences and the dorsal divergence of the femoral condyles, but also in the different length and curvature of the medial and lateral femoral condyles. These extremely complicated correlations, demonstrated in a most convincing manner by Menschik, reveal the great difficulties with which the designer of artificial joints is confronted in his task. Since the individual variability of the anatomical conditions can

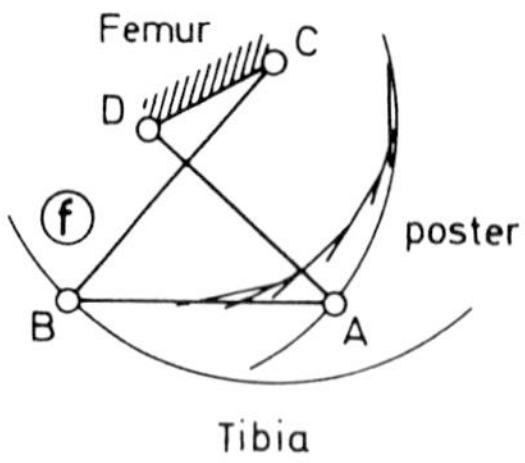

Fig. 2
Determination of the shape of the femoral condyles by the arrangement and relationship of the points of insertion and lengths of the cruciate ligaments

hardly be determined in advance, and the degree of damage to the articular surface, the joint capsule, the ligaments and the muscles is no less difficult to estimate, all attempts at devising a completely perfect replacement of the knee joint appear to be, for the time being, more or less futile. Far from facilitating a normal sequence of motions, they subject the system designed to promote mobility and stability (artificial articular surfaces, their points of anchorage, the ligament apparatus) to abnormal stresses, which must – sooner or later – result in the failure of the former or the latter. Considering the problems involved from this aspect, it is still rather premature to pose the question as to the best artificial joint and to demand clear, model-related indications, since the current prosthesis designs that imitate the natural movement process as nearly as possible, have by no means passed the test of time yet.

CLASSIFICATION OF TYPES OF ARTIFICIAL JOINTS

The different prosthesis designs can be classified and critically analyzed as follows:

CONDYLAR PROSTHESES

The design is based on the assumption of more or less normal ligaments, and a linking between the femoral and the tibial prosthetic component is completely dispensed with (Figs. 3-10).

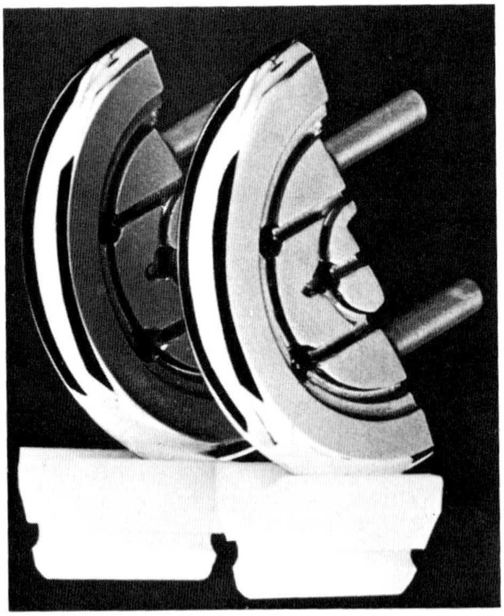

Fig. 3
Polycentric condylar prosthesis, type Gunston

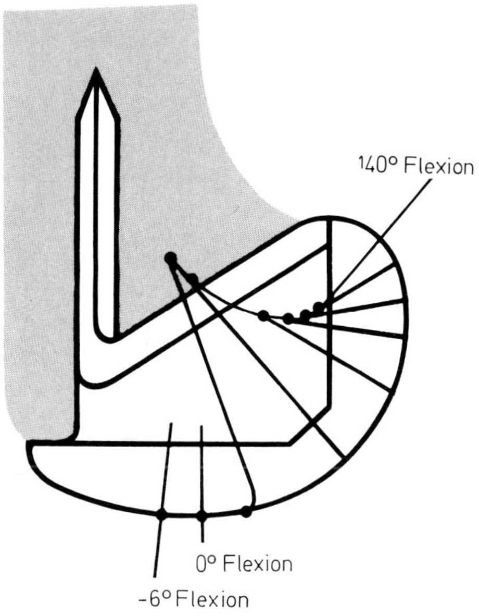

Fig. 4
Polycentric condylar prosthesis, type UCI

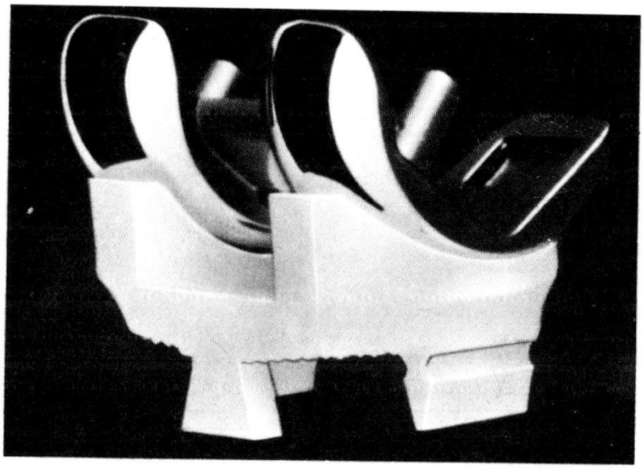

Fig. 5
Unicentric condylar prosthesis, type Geomedic

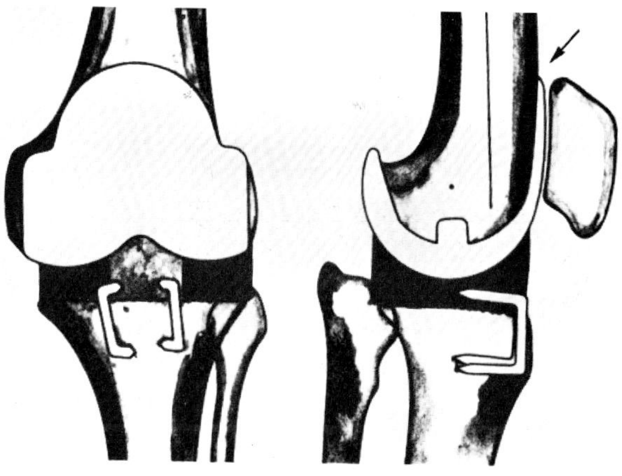

Fig. 6
Unicentric condylar prosthesis, type Kodama

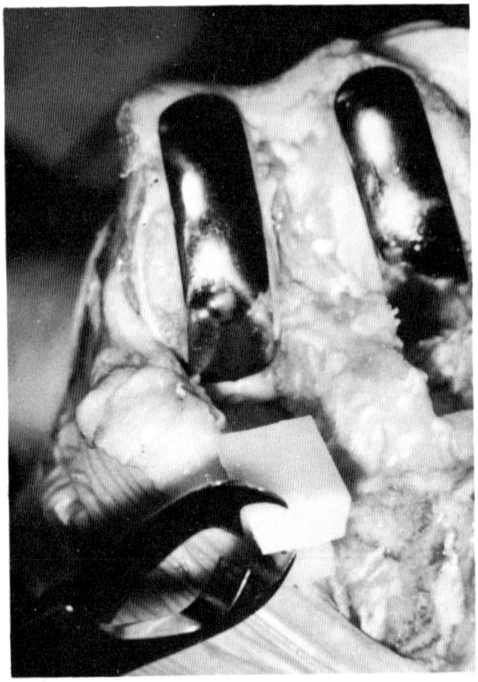

Fig. 7
St. Georg sledge prosthesis: Tibial plateau flat

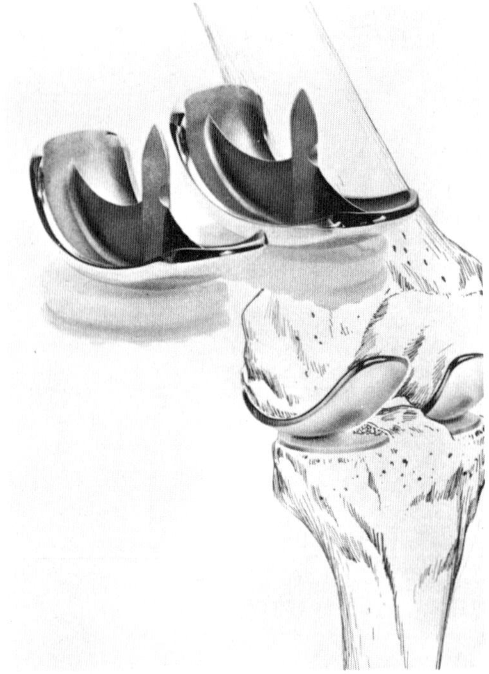

Fig. 8
Marmor modular prosthesis: Larger and slightly concave tibial component

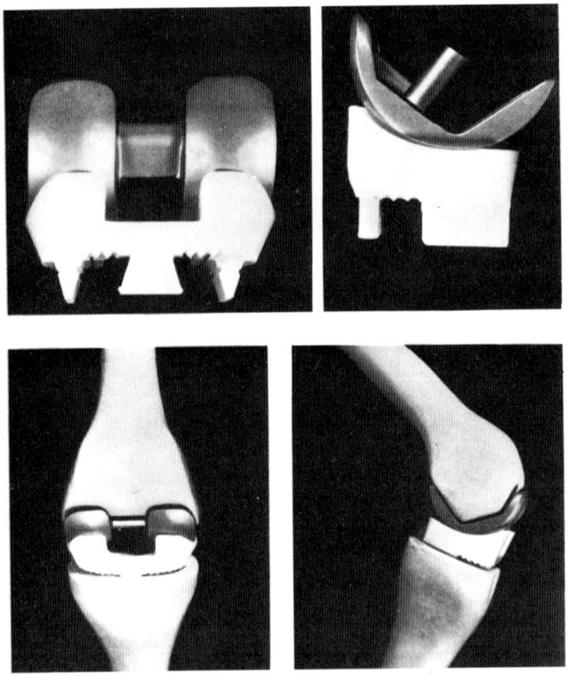

Fig. 9
Geomedic condylar prosthesis: Note anterior slope of tibial component

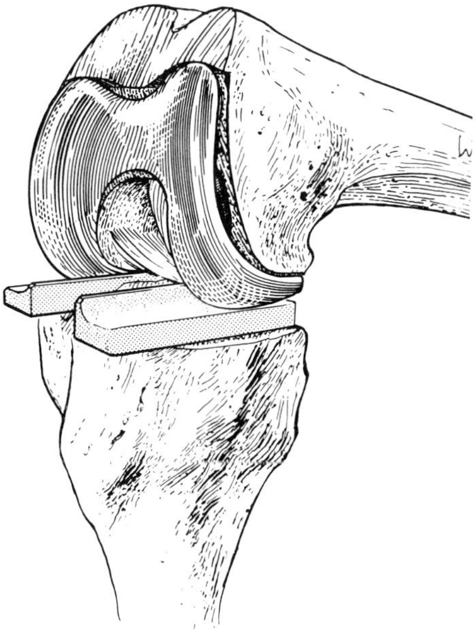

Fig. 10
UCI condylar prosthesis: Note medial slope of tibial prosthesis

Several designs try to imitate the changing radii of curvature of the femur: polycentric prosthesis designed by Gunston (10), the St. Georg sledge-type prosthesis, Marmor modular prosthesis, Special surgery design, UCI prosthesis devised by Waugh et al. (25), Townley prosthesis, etc. They are available in 2-3 different sizes for adaptation to individual anatomical variations. However they do not essentially take account the varying medial and lateral conditions. Differences between the individual types exist with respect to the radii of curvature, the changing width ventrally and dorsally (to enable rotation in flexion as in the case of the special surgery design), the existence or absence of a connection between the medial and lateral part of the prosthesis, symmetry, the width of the bearing surface, and the mode of fixation. The associated tibial components also exhibit greater variations.

Other designs reduce the sliding surface to a unicentric motion system: With this type, the radius of curvature of the dorsal part of the prosthesis is longer than in the normal knee joint, so that the ligaments, in particular the posterior cruciate ligament, are subjected to increased tension with increasing flexion of the knee: geomedic knee designed by Coventry et al. (4), unicentric joint by Kodama (14).

Both types of condylar prostheses allow, in cases that are not too severe, the existing instability of the collateral ligaments to be compensated for at least in extension, by raising the artificial tibial plateau or by lowering the femoral component to a greater or lesser degree. The cruciate ligaments are retained. These condylar prostheses can be uni- or duocondylar, the medial and lateral component being linked or unlinked.

The many variations of condylar prostheses differ, however, in the shape, size and curvature of the tibial component as well. It is either flat (St. Georg sledge-type prosthesis) or more or less concave. Slightly concave and wide is the Marmor prosthesis. On the other hand, designers of both the polycentric (Gunston, UCI, Special surgery design) and

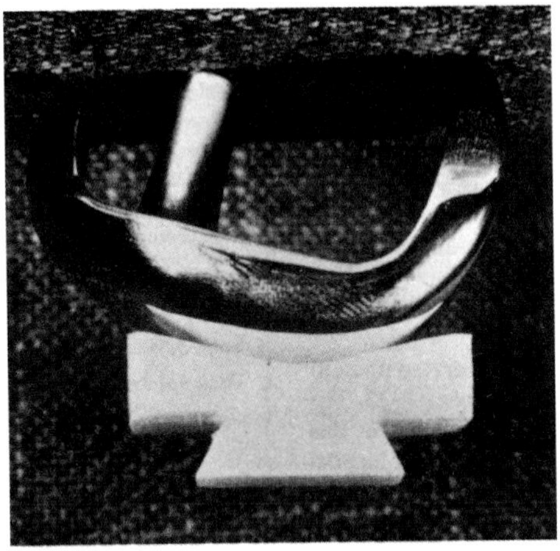

Fig. 11
Freeman-Swanson prosthesis

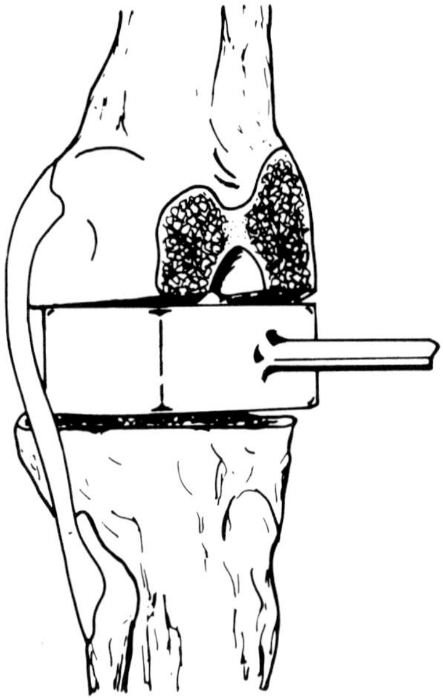

Fig. 12
Freeman-Swanson prosthesis: Resection as in arthrodesis, prosthesis serves also as a block between the bony surfaces, which restores tension in the collateral ligaments

the unicentric system (Coventry et al., Kodama) endeavour to give the artificial motion system increased inherent stability and guidance by providing a more or less marked ventral (Coventry et al.), dorsal (Gunston), medial (Special surgery) or lateral slope, or to reduce or check certain movement directions and to substitute – at least in part – the function of damaged ligaments.

Condylar prostheses such as those of Freeman-Swanson are applied irrespective of the state of the ligaments (Figs. 11,12). An attempt is made to provide stability by eliminating the space that becomes "free" as a result of resection, and by passive stretching of all the lateral structures of the knee joint. A wide contact surface of the prosthetic components, only slightly curved in extended position, serves the same purpose. All condylar prostheses reckon in addition with the stabilizing effect of the muscles moving the leg.

HINGE JOINTS

On the other hand, hinge joints were developed largely on the assumption that it is not possible to imitate the normal knee joint, or that the articular surface and ligaments are irreparably destroyed. These joints deliberately make no attempt to simulate a normal knee joint; they have only one degree of freedom as regards movement, and try to meet the increased requirements for stability by extending the anchorage in the medullary canal. The individual types differ essentially only in the position and the size of the axis, and the extent of bone resection. Thus, to name just some of the most frequently used hinge prostheses, the axis of the Walldius prosthesis (Fig. 13) lies in the continuation of the femoral and tibial axis, which results in a premature dorsal stop. This later logically induced the author to block flexion at 90 ^{o} in his earlier models. Shiers, who places the axis of his hinge prosthesis dorsally, i.e. behind the tibial axis, dispenses with a stop of the flexed artificial joint, but on the other hand deliberately accepts wide resection of the femoral condyles (Fig. 14). In order to retain as much bone as possible, and thus to

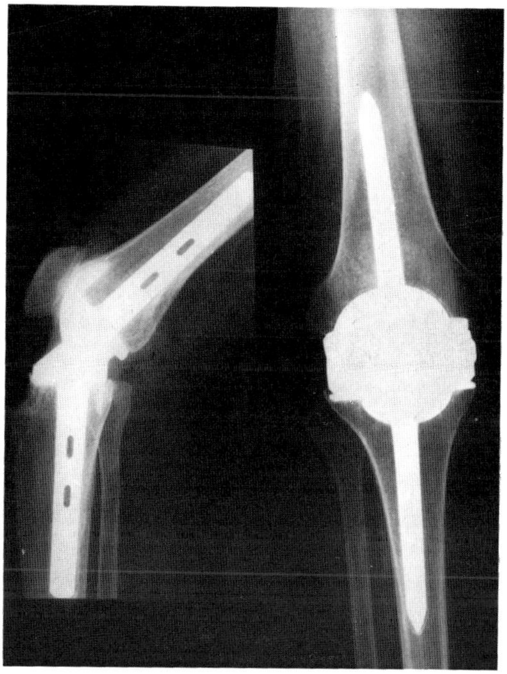

Fig. 13
Walldius prosthesis: The axis is in line with the stem of the tibial and femoral components

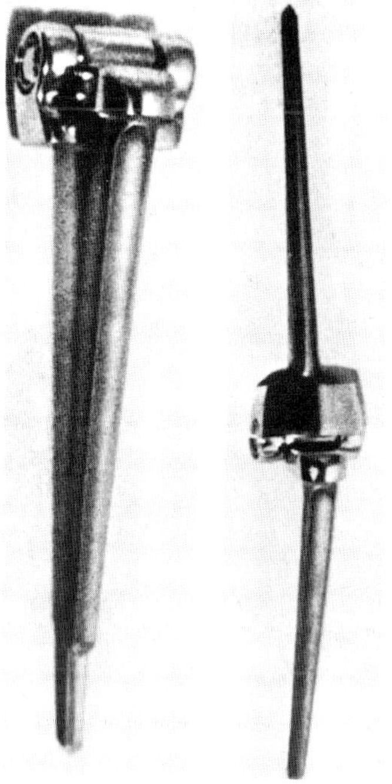

Fig. 14
Shiers prosthesis: The axis lies behind the tibial stem and in the line of the femoral stem

ensure the greatest possible chance of resorting to a salvage procedure should this become necessary, the group of orthopaedic surgeons who developed the Guepar prosthesis moved the axis even farther dorsally (i.e. not merely behind the tibial but also behind the femoral axis) and, in addition, displaced it proximally (Fig. 15). Consequently, with a relatively sparing bone resection (2.5 cm), a bony stop in the dorsal aspect can be largely avoided (i.e. in the usually attained flexion range). On the other hand, as in the case of a book being opened, the tension increases in the extensor apparatus with increasing flexion. Endeavouring to resect even less bone, the St. Georg group, Lagrange and Letournel and Devas recess their prosthesis in the femur (Fig. 16), whereby – depending

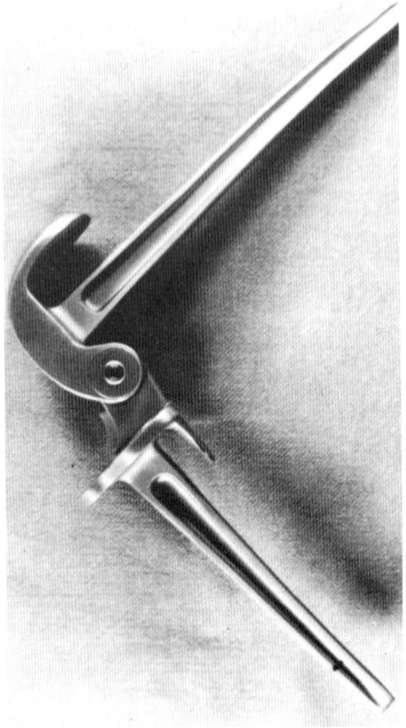

Fig. 15
Guepar prosthesis: The axis lies posteriorly to the femoral and tibial stems

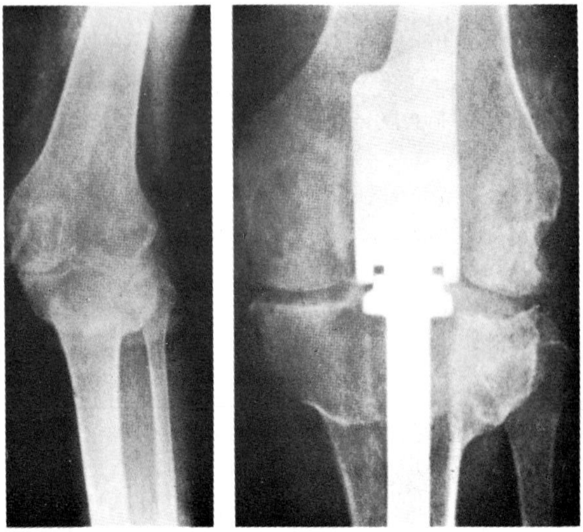

Fig. 16
Devas prosthesis: The very narrow prosthesis lies between the condyles, it does not rest on the femoral or tibial condyles

on the different types – frequently even very little condylar cortical bone is left. The smallest amount of bone is resected by Blauth (3), who uses an axis laid in polyethylene and shifted dorsocranially, but distributes the load additionally among the sliding surfaces, which imitate the shape of the femoral condyles. As is to be expected, the flexion of the prosthesis must be limited (at 120 ^{o}).

A special position is occupied by hinge prostheses where rotation is additionally incorporated in the system, e.g. in those designed by Trillat, Herbert and Blietz (Figs. 17,18). While Trillat's prosthesis attains this only by means of a wide (4 cm!) bone resection owing to a rather complicated construction, Herbert and Blietz obtain the combination movement by means of a truncated sphere, recessed between the femoral condyles.

NEW DESIGNS

Endeavouring to combine the advantages of the condylar prosthesis with those of the hinge joints offering inherent stability, several designers have developed new prostheses. Their objectives can be summarized in five points:

– The function of the artificial joint should approximate that of the normal knee joint as closely as possible.

– Any degree of destruction, and any deformity of the knee should be eliminable with the prosthesis.
– Minimum bone resection should be necessary in order that a second line of defense may be left open for possible subsequent salvage procedures in the event of infectious complications.
– The prosthesis surface coming into contact with soft tissues should be as small as possible.

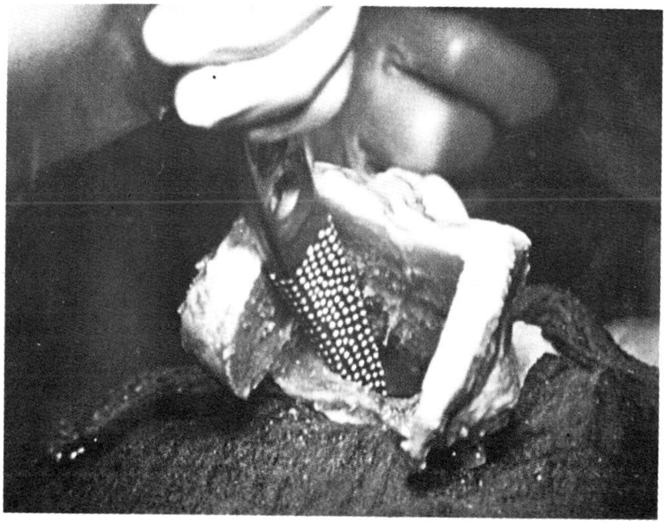

Fig. 17 St. Georg total hinge prosthesis: Note the very large amount of bone resection required for implantation of this prosthesis

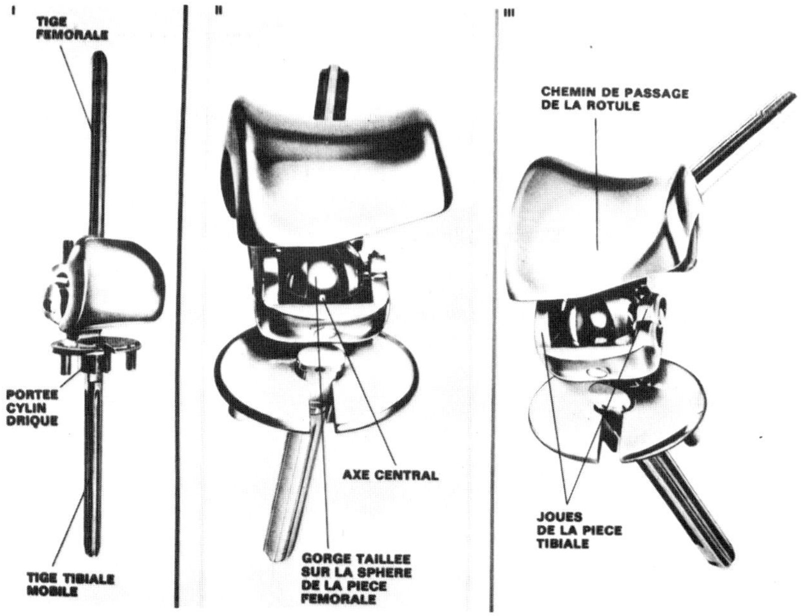

Fig. 18 Trillat prosthesis which provides the hinge prosthesis with an additional rotational motion

– The operation should be technically as easy as possible, involving very few possibilities of error, and the success rate of the operation should be high.

Sheehan has designed a prosthesis that complies with these requirements (Fig. 19). The femoral articular surface of his design exhibits changing radii of curvature and permits a flexion/extension movement of -5 ° to 130 °. A fin-shaped central eminence of the tibial component made of high-density polyethylene interlocks with a dorsally extending

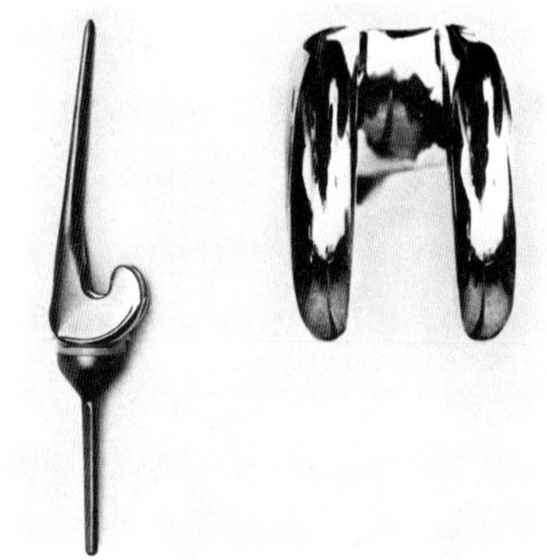

Fig. 19
Sheehan prosthesis, a "physiological" hinge joint: Note the enlargement of the gap between the condylar surfaces of the femoral component. This provides an additional rotational motion

notch of the femoral component made of a chromium-cobalt alloy. This results in stability in extension, whereas with increasing flexion it provides the possibility of rotation to 20 ° (from 60 ° flexion). The loose linkage between the femoral and the tibial component, moreover, prevents tensile forces from acting on the intramedullary anchorage, which, in the event of flexion beyond 90 °, could give rise to a loosening of the prosthesis. Lateral tilting movements are excluded but drawer-like movements are possible to a small extent (2 ° in full extension, 6-7 ° in slight flexion). The bearing surfaces of the femoral component, which are supported on the femoral condyles, are small, the cup-shaped metallic socket housing the polyethylene is relatively large. Fixation in the bone is effected by means of intramedullary pins and cement.

Using a different method, Attenborough (1) has tried to combine the physiological flexion/extension and rotation movements with the inherent stability (Figs. 20,21). The femoral sliding surfaces are also polycentric. There is a slight possibility of rotation, facilitated by the reduction of the dorsal curvature and the narrowing of the slide bar. Stability in the bone is provided by two relatively short intramedullary pins, of which the tibial pin is made of polyethylene. Between femur and tibia, a semi-rigid connection is ensured by a central metal pin. Depending on the flexion of the knee joint, the pin sinks to a varying depth into the bone along a selflubricating groove and permits not only rotation but also a limited degree of lateral and back and forth movement, since its proximal end is spherical and freely movable in the centre of the femoral component.

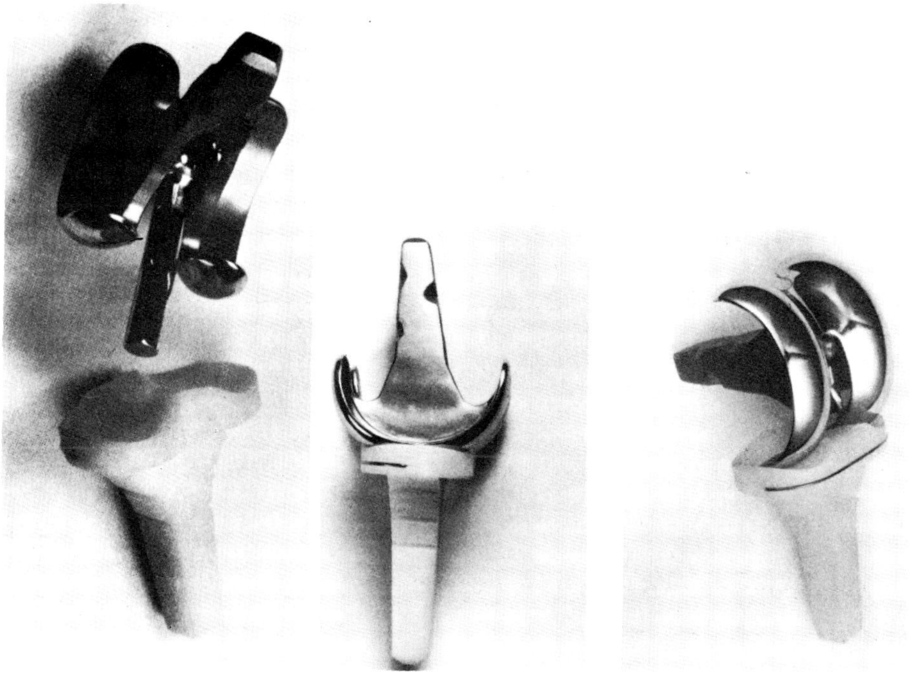

Figs. 20,21 Attenborough joint: Between the polycentric runner there is a hollow, into which is fitted a ball on the end of a rounded stem. This runs in a gap which widens at the back. The lining stem fits in a hole in the tibial component which has 2 lubrication channels

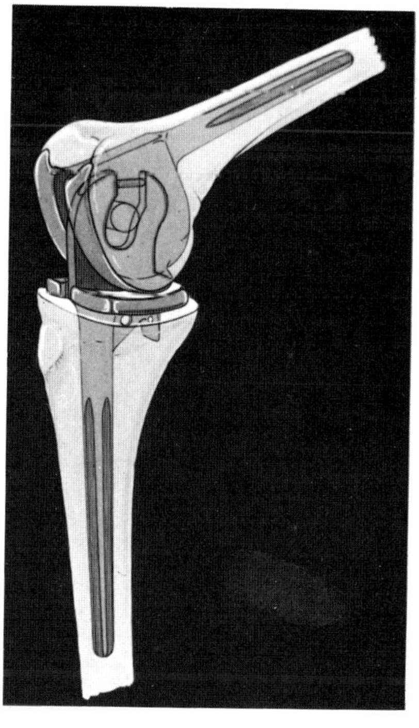

Fig. 22
GSB knee joint showing the low degree of exposure to soft tissues, the intramedullary fixation, the areas of support on the bone and the slot in the tibial bridge with the non-weight-bearing migrating axis

With the GSB prosthesis designed by us, we have also endeavoured to comply with the five objectives mentioned earlier (Figs. 22-26). It is also polycentric. The connection between the femoral and the tibial component is effected by a central bridge, in which there is a slightly curved slot running from below anterior to above posterior. The slot

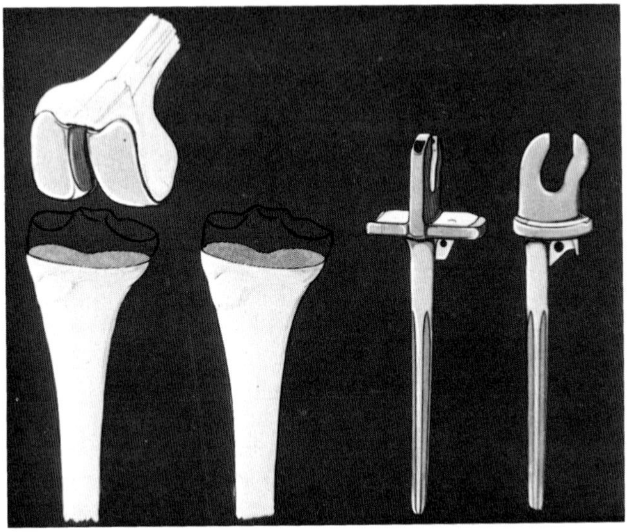

Fig. 23 GSB knee joint: Tibial components with polyethylene surface and the bridge with the slot for the migrating axis

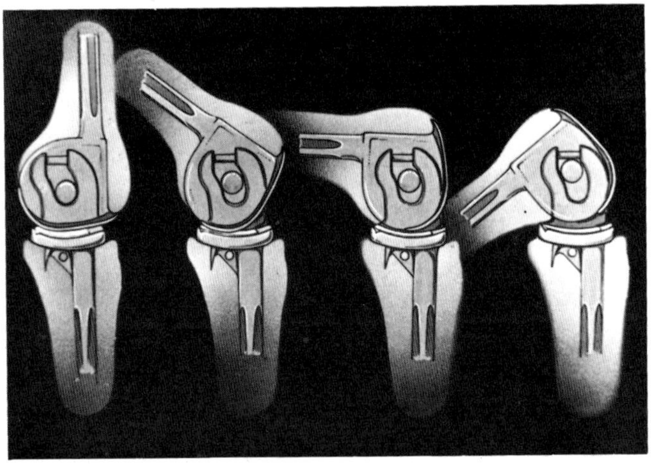

Fig. 24 GSB knee joint: Note the different positions of the axis during flexion. At the far right it can be seen how, at maximal flexion, the femoral component is lifted from the tibial component thus avoiding a posterior bone impact

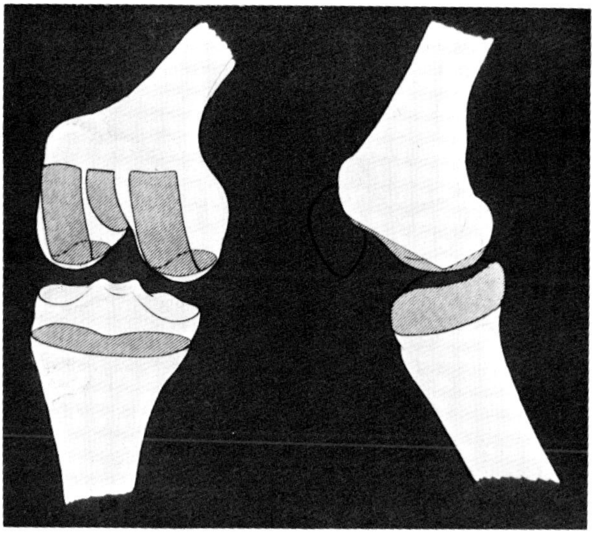

Fig. 25
GSB knee joint: Minimal resection of bone is required, on the tibial component 1 cm in average, on the femoral component few millimetres

serves as guide for the non-load-bearing axis of the femoral component. Rotation proper is absent, but there is some clearance in terms of a limited lateral and back and forth movement. In addition, the femoral component can – in analogy to a normal knee joint – be lifted off the tibial component in maximal flexion without disturbing the functional relationship between the two components. Bone resection is minimal and the bearing surface of the prosthesis on the bone very wide. Only a minimum portion of the artificial joint is in direct contact with the soft tissues.

A fundamentally different approach has been adopted by Deane (5), who has retained from the three prosthesis types just described the bridge-like central connection of the

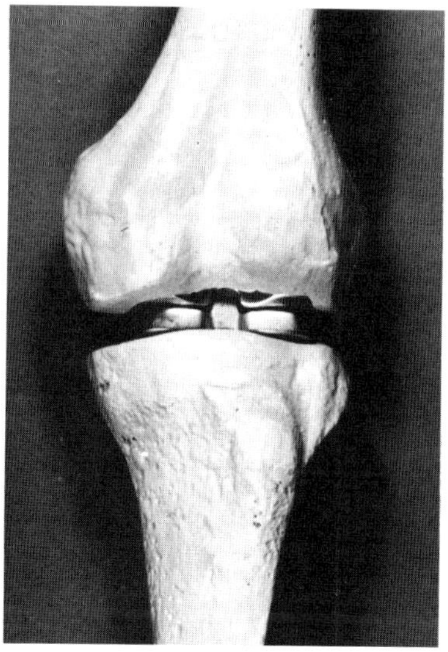

Fig. 26
Minimal exposure of the artificial joint to the soft tissues

tibial and femoral components but believes that he can dispense with their intramedullary anchorage. The sliding surface principle comes into play in the first 40 $^{\circ}$ of the movement but then, between 40-110 $^{\circ}$, passes over to a joint mechanism that works like a ball joint.

OPERATIVE TECHNIQUE

The operative technique depends – with respect to the degree of difficulty – on:

- the physiologically accurate imitation of the knee joint,
- the extent of bone resection,
- the attempt to retain or to reconstruct the ligaments,
- the actual knee deformity,
- the quality of bone,
- the replacement of the patellofemoral joint, and
- the mode of anchoring.

The degree of difficulty encountered with the implantation of an endoprosthesis is in general the lower, the less the surgeon attempts to imitate the physiology of the knee joint. It furthermore depends on the extent of destruction of the joint and the external deformation. In other words: hinge prostheses with wide bone resection can be implanted more easily (Walldius, Shiers). The greatest problems are encountered when the surgeon tries to replace a more severely deformed knee joint (flexion contracture, varus-valgus deformity) with a condylar prosthesis. The more we strive to retain the ligaments or restore its physiological function, the greater the problems. As is to be expected, the degree of deformity and the extent of damage to the ligaments set limits to most condylar prostheses. These limits are the narrower, the more sparing the bone resection performed and the more we strive to retain the cruciate ligament system. Condylar prostheses with a small bearing surface and with no connection between the medial and the lateral components encounter further difficulties when they are applied in severely osteoporotic bones. Here surgeons try to solve the problems involved either by lengthening, varying the orientation of or profiling, the anchorage pins, or by inserting the bone cement in such a way that it is supported by the cortical bone. An attempt to replace the patellofemoral joint will result in additional problems, not merely because a further articular surface has to be dealt with, but on account of the fact that the preparation of the slide bearing situated in another plane, viz. the frontal plane, may lead to new possibilities of error, which in turn may affect the correct position of the other gliding planes as well. Furthermore, the normally occurring variations in the shape of the posterior surface of the patella appear to point to the doubtful value of any prefabricated patellar slide bearing for the femoral condyle, unless the posterior surface of the patella is also properly replaced by a suitably fashioned prosthesis. The mode of anchoring the prosthetic components also has an influence on the degree of difficulty of the operation. In general, it is the smaller, the deeper the anchoring parts of the prosthesis are set in the intramedullary cavity. This allows us not only to leave the ligaments out of consideration and thus to correct malpositions of any kind, but also permits an easier correct orientation of the prosthetic components.

Consequently, the accessory instruments required for implantation of an artificial joint are in general more numerous and complicated with condylar prostheses than those that are to be anchored in the intramedullary cavity (Fig. 27). In the case of these latter, the formation of two parallel bone surfaces located one against the other at the physiological valgus angle will suffice in most cases, in other words, a procedure that is customary in arthrodesis of the knee. Of the commercially available condylar prostheses, only the design produced by Freeman and Swanson permits a similar procedure. This is possible only because the cruciate ligaments, and together with them the intercondylar eminence, are sacrificed.

INDICATIONS

Prior to attempting to analyze the specific indications associated with the individual types, it is absolutely necessary to emphasize that arthroplasty should at present still be performed with utmost care. This is demanded by a sense of responsibility towards the patient, who should be informed before every arthroplasty that

1. a still fairly new operative procedure is to be carried out,
2. it is associated with the disadvantages of all methods using plastics materials:

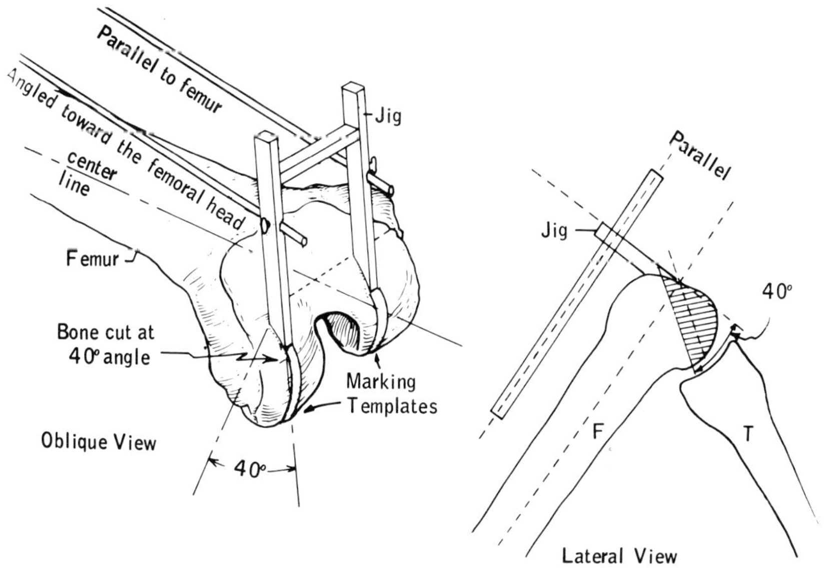

Fig. 27 Tools for correct implantation of a condylar knee joint (type Gunston)

- risk of foreign body reaction
- attrition (wear) and/or absence of any regeneration possibility (unknown late effects and complications)
- moreover, it is still in the process of development

3. it might soon be superseded by still better procedures,
4. it offers only a rather limited chance of recourse to salvage procedures in the event of complications.

Arthroplasty of the knee should therefore be performed exclusively in cases in which severe disability endangers the patient's ability to walk and arthrodesis constitutes the only possible alternative. On no account must this procedure be carried out instead of an osteotomy that still holds promise of success. The principal indication for arthroplasty of the knee is a polyarticular destruction in elderly patients (over 60 years). In the case of rheumatic arthritis, it might be more advisable to lower the age limit than in osteoarthritis. In monoarticular destruction of joints in young patients and in those who are predominantly employed in occupations involving a lot of standing and walking, preference should at this time be still given to arthrodesis, as a simple, safe, effective and ultimate salvage procedure, unless the patient insists on arthroplasty, although he is fully aware of the risks and complications involved and the uncertain late result of the operation. In such cases, however, the orthopaedic surgeon's choice should preferably fall on endoprosthesis types that provide the possibility of an easy and safe retreat to arthrodesis, the ultimate, and frequently the only possible, salvage procedure.

After this more general introduction, let us now deal with the question whether and to what extent the specific indications can be associated with the individual prosthesis types. The answer to this question – and this is pointed out in advance – can by no means be given definitively and with absolute certainty, for at this time it is still based on more or less uncertain premises. Among these is, in the first place, the authors' concept of the mechanism of functioning, which by no means corresponds to reality. In the second place, and at the same time as proof of the soundness of the design principle, comes the success rate. It might be concluded that a comparison of the results obtained with different models should enable us to establish clearer indications. This is, however, not true, because

1. with most prosthesis models, the actual long-term results of larger series are rather scarce or not yet available,
2. a fairly heterogeneous patient material in respect of primary disease, degree of severity of joint destruction, age, profession and weight of patient, the intactness of the remaining locomotor system and loading of the operated joint is involved, and – last, but not least –
3. proper evaluation of these models and consequently their comparison is rather difficult, or impossible, on account of the different criteria used.

In my opinion it is, rather, the number and mode of the failures that may allow conclusions to be drawn as to the correctness of the indication, this, however, only on condition that the implantation technique used corresponds with that of the author.

CONTRAINDICATIONS

If we try to draw conclusions from the contraindications defined by the designers of the most frequently used prostheses (Table 1, Figs. 28-36), it becomes apparent that:

Table 1 Contraindications:
– none, (+) relative, + absolute

	Instability	Flexion-Def.	Varus-Valgus	Recurvatum	Subluxation	Osteoporosis	Ankylosis
1. Hinges (Walldius, Shiers, Guepar)	–	–	–		–	(+)	–
2. Gunston	+	+	(<20°)		+	–	
"St.Georg" sledge	+	(>20°)	(>20°)		+		
Geomedic	(+)	(>40°)	(>30°)	(+)	(+)	(+)	
Special Surgery-D	–	(>25°)	(>15°)	(+)	(+)	(+)	
3. Freeman-Swanson	–	–	(<40°)		–		(+)
4. "Physiological" hinges (Sheehan, Attenborough, GSB)	–	–	–	–	–	–	–

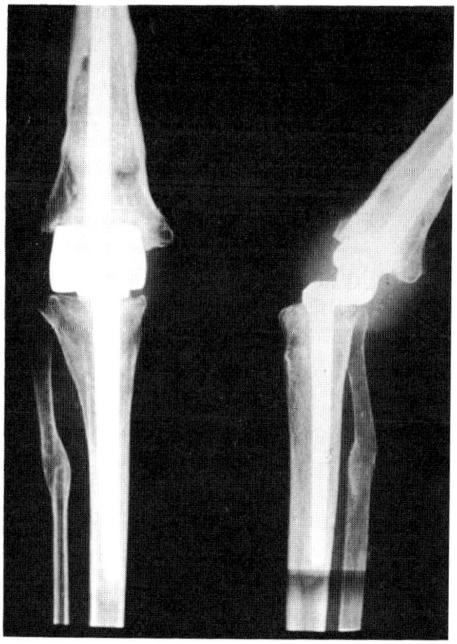

Fig. 28
Complications of constrained hinge joints: sinking-in of the prosthesis and loosening

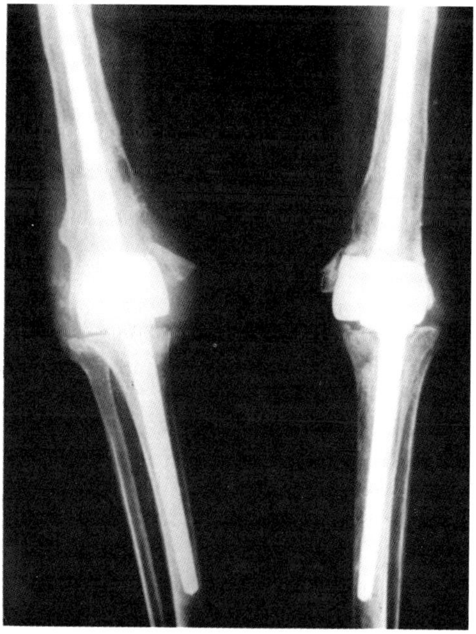

Fig. 29
Complications of constrained hinge joints: sinking-in of the prosthesis and loosening, with spontaneous fractures and rarefaction of the bone

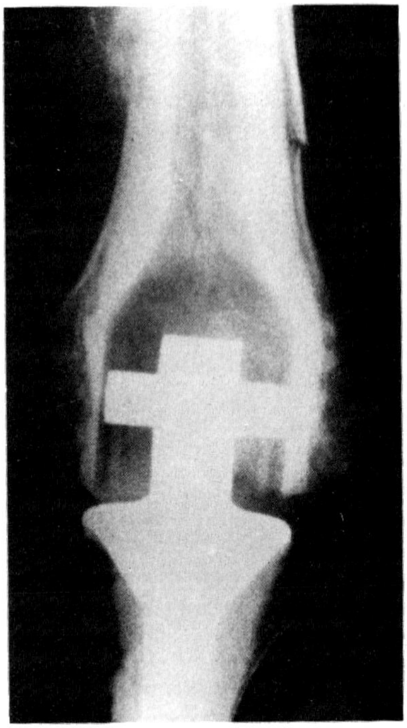

Fig. 30
Complications of constrained hinge joints with intramedullary site: Due to an abnormal stress fatigue fractures can occur

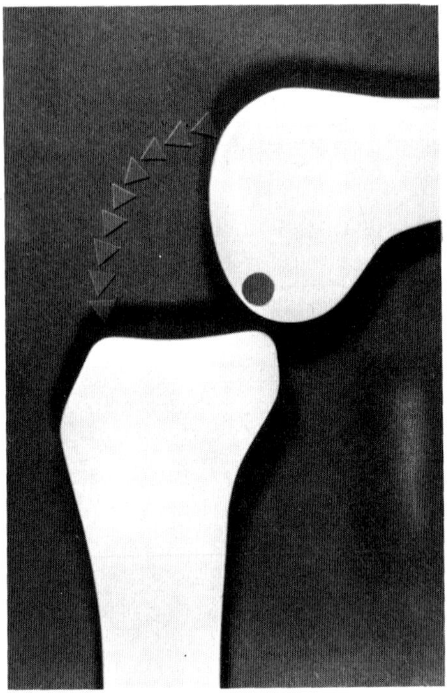

Fig. 31
Constrained hinge joints with an axis lying posteriorly and dorsally require less bone resection but increase the tension on the extensor mechanism during flexion

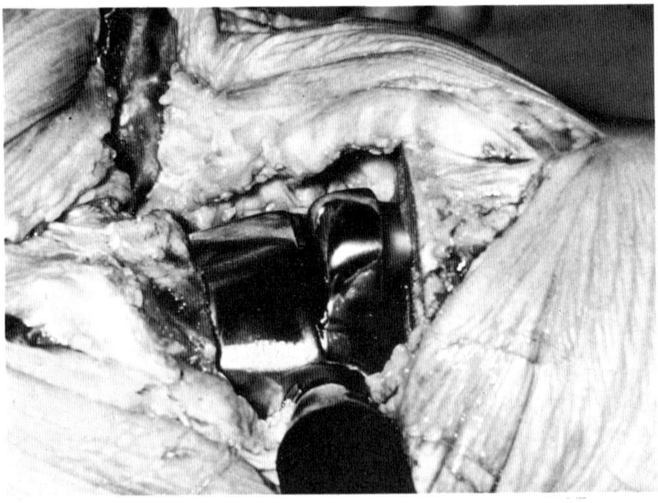

Fig. 32 Disadvantage of constrained hinge joints: greater bone resection required

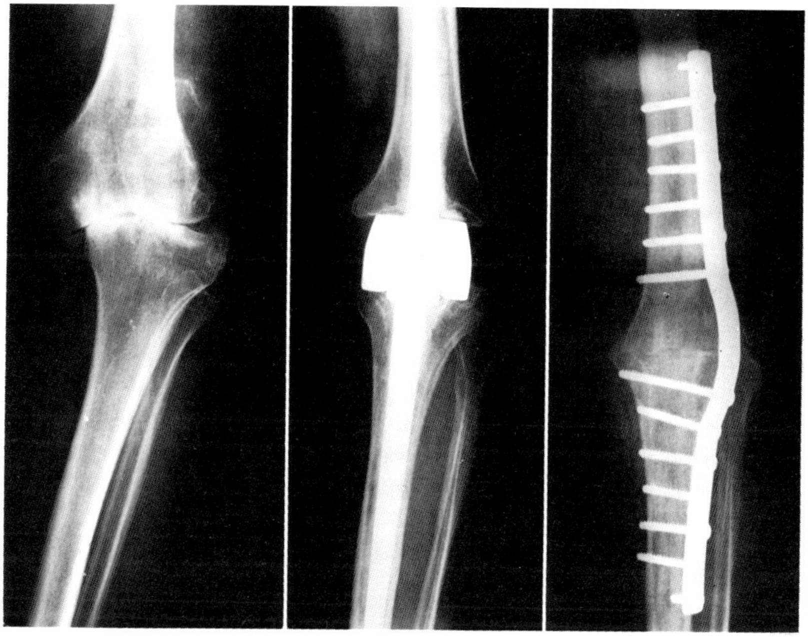

Fig. 33 Constrained hinge joints: In case of failure the best second approach is a stable arthrodesis with long plate fixation. In severe osteoporotic and non-infected cases the cement may be left in place in order to give a better grip to the screws

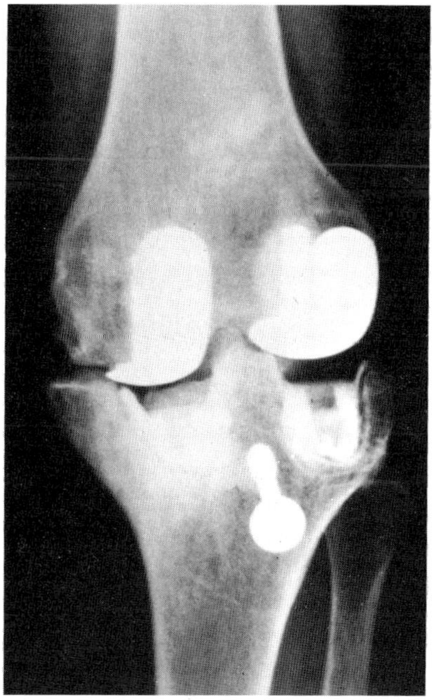

Fig. 34
Condylar prosthesis type sledge St. Georg: Tibial component on lateral side loose, varus deformity not corrected

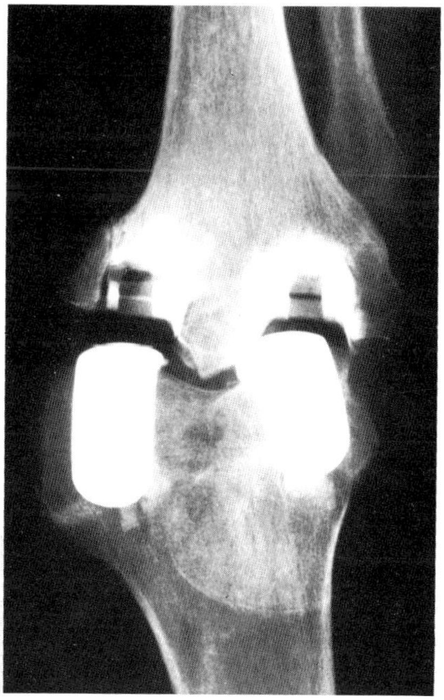

Fig. 35
Condylar prosthesis type sledge St. Georg: Note the fatigue fracture on the medial aspect of the tibial plateau

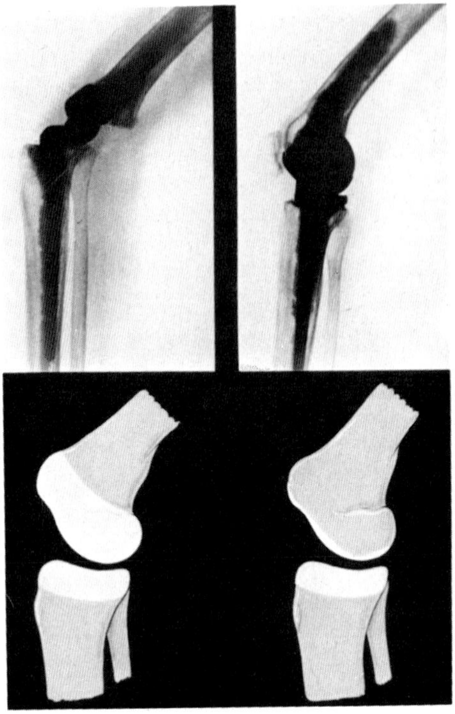

Fig. 36
Constrained hinge joint (type Shiers) versus "physiological" hinge joint (type GSB): Note the relationship between femur and tibia and the amount of bone resection

HINGE PROSTHESES

Constrained hinge prostheses and their so-called "physiological" variants allow us to correct every kind of deformity, destruction of the articular surfaces and ligament insufficiency without any major operative-technical problems (increased risk of nerve lesions and circulatory disturbances when correcting severe valgus and flexion deformities).

The problems associated with constrained hinge prostheses, however, are to be found:

1. In the increased loading of the anchoring parts and – in connection with this – the risk of loosening and fracture of the implanted prosthesis.
2. Wide bone resection (Shiers) or the intercondylar placement of the prosthesis with narrow bearing surfaces (Devas, Total-prosthesis St. Georg) enhance the risk of possible sinking in of the prosthesis.
3. Prostheses that are implanted intercondylarly in an attempt to sacrifice as little bone as possible, incur not only the risk of sinking in but also of femur shaft fracture as a result of the unphysiological flow of forces and the wedge effect produced.
4. The attempt to enable a sparing bone resection by shifting the pivot dorsocranially, and to avoid a premature bony stop (Guepar prosthesis), inevitably results in an unphysiologically severe stretching of the extensor mechanism (comparable to a book that is being opened), which sets limits to further flexion or augments the pressure on the dorsal surface of the patella. On the other hand, through the prolongation of the lever arm of the knee extensors, less force is required for the active extension of the Guepar knee than for that of the Walldius or even Shiers knee prosthesis.

5. The chance of retreat in case of complications (loosening or infection) is the more difficult, the more bone has been resected. In the event of an arthrodesis, one must consequently reckon with a greater shortening of the leg and with increased difficulties encountered in the attainment of a safe bony ankylosis. For this kind of case, a stable osteosynthesis with a laterally adjacent 16 or 18-hole AO plate, possibly with an additional smaller medial plate, has proved very successful. Due to the opening of the intramedullary cavity with its bone cement filling, increased difficulties may, moreover, arise during the second operation, especially with respect to the complete removal of the bone cement and the limitation of possible infection.

The prosthesis devised by Trillat not only has the disadvantage of necessitating a wide bone resection but also that of too much soft tissue exposure of its free parts.

CONDYLAR PROSTHESES

Almost at the other end of the prosthesis model range are the condylar prostheses with a narrow bearing surface, which can be implanted unicondylarly or bicondylarly, this depending on the condition of the medial and lateral articular surfaces. If the shape of the condyle is well preserved, or if there is no malposition and the ligaments are intact, a correct implantation technique enhances the chances of ample mobility and satisfactory stability. A restriction of mobility may be expected in the unicentric systems (Coventry et al., larger femoral component of the Gunston and Kodama prosthesis), where the radius of curvature of the dorsal aspect is greater than that of the resected dorsal femoral condyle. This inevitably results in increased stretching, in particular of the posterior cruciate ligaments, with restriction and/or pain when further flexion is attempted. The same phenomena are to be expected when, in endeavouring to correct a varus or valgus deformity, or to tighten slack ligaments, we raise the artificial tibial plateau more dorsally. As has been theoretically discussed in the introduction, owing to the impossibility of reproducing the strictly individual relations between the ligamentous system and the radius of curvature by means of prefabricated prosthetic elements, a normal knee joint can never be expected. Problems should consequently be anticipated with all types of condylar prostheses, where several pronounced deformities are to be corrected simultaneously, a sunken tibial plateau raised, or slack collateral ligament tightened. Thus we must reckon with a restriction of mobility and with abnormal tension in the ligaments, or – in the event of good mobility – with ligament insufficiency in some phase of motion. While with hinge prostheses it is the intramedullary anchorage that is subjected to severe stresses, with these condylar prostheses it is the intracondylar anchorage and simultaneously the ligaments. Extremely dangerous are the shearing forces as they occur when the prosthetic components are subjected to eccentric loads. The slopes mentioned earlier, which are located medially and laterally to counteract lateral instability, or placed ventrally and dorsally to compensate cruciate ligament insufficiency, allow the expected additional forces to act upon the prosthetic components and their anchorage respectively. In the case of the completely flat configuration of the plateau, these forces are transmitted to the ligament. This type of loading increases with the simultaneous correction of a deformity and is particularly high where the latter cannot be corrected. The risk of prosthesis loosening, the sinking in of the prosthesis, especially in the case of a small bearing surface, or fracture of the underlying bone, are well known facts. These risks increase with decreasing bone quality (osteoporosis). It is consequently easy to understand that limits are set to the applicability of prostheses of this type. In this connection most authors try to determine these limits in figures relative to the varus/valgus and flexion deformity.

A genu recurvatum, a pathological displacement between femur and tibia in the antero-posterior or lateral direction, is for most designers of condylar prostheses also a contraindication for an operation.

A special position between these two extremes is held by the Freeman-Swanson,prosthesis (in the group of condylar prostheses) and by the Attenborough, Sheehan and GSB prosthesis (among the unconstrained hinged types).

FREEMAN–SWANSON PROSTHESIS

The Freeman-Swanson prosthesis is characterized by a wide bearing surface on the tibia and the femur, conditioned by the deliberate sacrifice of the intercondylar eminence (not considering a later modification of the prosthesis). This permits us on the one hand to correct major deformities as well as subluxations (because wide parallel bone surfaces have to be created prior to implantation), and on the other hand, to effect a symmetric tightening of all structures that contribute to lateral stability. The large artificial articular surfaces provide additional stability through their shape (almost flat in extension) and by their resistance to friction. Stability is further enhanced by the systematically trained quadriceps muscle. As a result of the elimination of the cruciate ligaments (basic prosthesis version), the prosthesis and its anchorage points are subjected to specific stresses. Difficulties are also to be expected in the case of severe deformity, where a greater loss of bone substance on the inner side of the angle of curvature is accompanied by the shrinking of the ligaments. As with the other condylar prostheses the incomplete correction of a deformity and the insufficiency of the collateral ligament, which is by no means always compensated muscularly – and certainly not in every motion phase – could expose the prosthesis and/or its anchorage to critical peak loads.

PHYSIOLOGICAL HINGES

The situation is again different with the so-called physiological hinge prostheses: They possess the inherent stability of the hinge joints and – closely connected with this – the extension of the anchorage in the intramedullary cavity. The fundamental difference, however, lies in the possibility of some rotation (Attenborough, Sheehan) or clearance between the prosthetic components (GSB). As with the sliding surface prostheses, motion proper takes place between a femoral and a tibial contact surface having a similar shape and extent as the conventional types of condylar prostheses. The physiological relation between femur and tibia is thus retained and consequently also the tension conditions of the muscles bridging the knee. With the GSB knee prosthesis, a non-weight-bearing migrating axis guides the motion of the wide articular bearing surfaces. Lateral stability is ensured in all prosthesis types mentioned, by a bridge rising from the tibial component and locking with the femoral one.

Whereas with the constrained hinge joint the full load lies on the axis and the intramedullar anchorage, with the condylar prosthesis, however, on the retained ligaments and the short anchoring pins, in the so-called physiological hinge joints the load distribution additionally extends to the loosely connected, central tibio-femoral linking piece.

Thus, one could almost say that the newer generation of knee joint prostheses seeks to combine the advantages of the condylar prosthesis and the constrained hinge joints, without accepting their disadvantages (except for the anchorage extending into the intramedullary cavity). Since they furthermore require only a very sparing bone resection, they provide a similar chance of recourse to salvage procedure as the condylar prostheses (the quality of the metaphysial bone portions, which is especially important for arthrodesis, is even better, because they are not affected by the bone cement plug). So, we may ask whether it is still justified, on the one hand, to use constrained hinge joints with all their inherent disadvantages and, on the other hand, to prefer the condylar prostheses with the highly questionable retention and/or restoration of an adequate ligamentous system, to the so-called physiological hinge joints.

All the prosthesis types discussed here are subject to specific stresses, and another 5 to 10 years are required before we shall be able to establish which of the models can provide the most physiological function and the greatest possible degree of mobility with freedom from pain, without prematurely succumbing to peak loads that are inherent in every prosthesis.

REFERENCES

1. Attenborough, C.G.: Stabilized gliding total knee replacement. In: The Knee Joint. Int. Congress Rotterdam 1973. Excerpta Medica, Amsterdam 1974, 228

2. Aubriot, J.H., Deburge, A., Schramm, P.: La prothese Guepar. Acta Orthopaedica Belgica 39, 257 (1973)

3. Blauth, W.: Über eine neue Kniegelenk-Totalprothese. Medizinisch-Orthopädische Technik 94, 65 (1974)

4. Coventry, M.B., Finerman, G.A., Riley, L.H., Turner, R., Upshaw, J.E.: A new geometric knee for total knee arthroplasty. Clinical Orthopaedics and Related Research 83, 157 (1972)

5. Deane, S.: A new concept in knee joint design. In: The Knee Joint. Int. Congress Rotterdam 1973. Excerpta Medica, Amsterdam 1974, 244

6. Devas, M.: Link arthroplasty of the knee. In: The Knee Joint. Int. Congress Rotterdam 1973. Excerpta Medica, Amsterdam 1974, 248

7. Engelbrecht, E., Zippel, J.: The sledge prosthesis "model St. Georg". Acta Orthopaedica Belgica 39, 203 (1973)

8. Freeman, M.A., Swanson, S.A., Todd, R.C.: Total replacement of the knee, design considerations and early clinical results. Acta Orthopaedica Belgica 28, 181 (1973)

9. Gschwend, N., Scheier, H., Bähler, A.: The GSB knee prosthesis. In: The Knee Joint. Int. Congress Rotterdam 1973, Excerpta Medica, Amsterdam 1974, 261

10. Gunston, F.H.: Polycentric knee arthroplasty. Clinical Orthopaedics and Related Research 94, 128 (1973)

11. Herbert, J.J., Herbert, A.: Nouvelle prothese totale du genou. Revue de Chirurgie Orthopedique 59, 451 (1973)

12. Huson, A.: The functional anatomy of the knee joint: The closed kinematic chain as a model of the knee joint. In: The Knee Joint. Int. Congress Rotterdam 1973, Excerpta Medica, Amsterdam 1974, 163

13. Kapandji, I.A.: The Physiology of the Joints. Edinburgh and London, Churchill Livingstone 1970

14. Kodama, T., Yamamoto, S.: Total knee prothesis without hinge. In: Total Knee Replacement. September 1974, London, p. 88

15. Mathys, R.: Stand der Verwendung von Kunststoffen für künstliche Gelenke. Aktuelle Traumatologie 3, 253 (1973)

16. Menschik, A.: Mechanik des Kniegelenkes. Zeitschrift für Orthopädie 112, 481 (1974)

17. Mittelmeier, H.: Zementlose Verankerung von Endoprothesen nach dem Tragrippenprinzip. Zeitschrift für Orthopädie 112, 27 (1974)

18. Ranawat, C.S., Insell, J., Shine, J.: Total knee replacement duo-condylar and uni-condylar hospital for special surgery design. In: Conference on total knee replacement, September 1973, London, p. 84

19. Sheehan, J.M.: Arthroplasty of the knee. In: Conference on total knee replacement, September 1974, London, p. 80

20. Shiers, L.G.P.: Total replacement of the knee joint. Acta Orthopaedica Belgica 39, 252 (1973)

21. Sivash, K.M.: Development of alloplasty of the hip joint in the last 15 years. Orthop. Traum. Protez. 11, 28 (1969)

22. Townley, C., Hill, L.: Total knee replacement. Amer.J.Nursing 74, 1612 (1974)

23. Trillat, A., Dejour, H., Bousquet, G., Grammont, L.: La prothese rotataire du genou. Acta Orthopaedice Belgica 39, 296 (1973)

24. Walldius, B.: A comparative analysis of different methods for arthroplasty of the knee. In: Conference on total knee replacement. September 1974, London, p. 34

25. Waugh, T.R., Smith, R.C., Anzel, S.H., Orofino, C.F.: U.C.I.-Total knee surgical procedure. Memphis: Wright Manufacturing Comp. 1972

Chapter 2
Complications and Their Management

PEROPERATIVE COMPLICATIONS OF THE TOTAL ENDOPROSTHESIS

K.P. Schulitz and B. Gärtner

Under normally loading, the total endoprosthesis is able to achieve good results, but it is a wishful thinking to believe that it can also cope with maximum loading in special situations. Therefore, we do not consider the total endoprosthesis an ideal solution, but a possible alternative when treating a coxarthrosis surgically. This is explained by the fact that complications can considerably worsen the results obtained with the total endoprosthesis. Although the early and late complications are mainly responsible for the bad results, the chances of the prosthesis and thus of the patient can be determined already during the operation. The factors that may give rise to intraoperative complications comprise the patient himself, the operation, the anaesthesia, and above all the surgical personnel (Table 1). The complications can only be influenced by an appropriate indication, suitable pre-operative preparation, and impeccable surgical technique. Therefore the operation demands thorough training and experience in joint surgery, a good armamentarium of instruments and devices, and last but not least a biological intelligence, without which good results cannot be achieved even with a subtle operative technique. Although alloarthroplasty can today be considered a routine operation, technical difficulties will occur under certain conditions, which may lead to numerous complications. We may even maintain that the causes of the complications which arise during the postoperative phase can be more or less ascribed to incidents during the operation. The contamination of the wound with bacteria has to be regarded – strictly speaking – as a peroperative complication whose consequences will become evident only at later date. It must be surely be true to say that there are no serious offenses against the asepsis on the part of the operating team. But we know that turbulence within the operating

Table 1 Factors which may be responsible for intraoperative complications in alloarthroplastic surgery

Factors	Classes
patient	preoperative risk age
operation	operation itself bone cement drugs
anaesthesia	engineering
staff	state of training a. surgeon b. anaesthetist

theatre endanger the operating area. The loosening of a prosthesis can in some cases be ascribed to an insufficient reconditioning of the acetabular base, to the fact that clots of blood fibrin have been left with an increased spongy after-bleeding or to the prolonged pressure of the prosthesis during the plastic phase of hardening of the bone cement. Periarticular calcifications are the sequelae of a traumatic intra-operative lesion of the tissue. Dislocations of the prosthesis result from an unfavourable position of the cup and of the prosthesis in the medullary space of the femur or they are due to an inadequate muscular tonus. Some of these incidents can be avoided, but many of them cannot because of the site of the operation and the general reactions of the organism.

With increasing experience the complications naturally decrease. For about ten years we have been implanting total prostheses into the hip joint and have nevertheless had per-operative complications in about three per cent of the cases. Strictly speaking the complications during the operation comprise:

1. nerve lesions,
2. perforation of the acetabulum,
3. perforation of the shaft,
4. fractures of the shaft,
5. cardiovascular complications, and
6. dislocations of the prosthesis.

In the scientific literature, these complications are counted among the peroperative complications, although some of them become evident and are of importance only after the operation. The complications shall be dealt with in the sequence of their appearance.

The cause of the nerve lesions has not yet been completely clarified, but will certainly not be merely a single incident. It may arise during the preparative phase of the hip joint or during reduction of the joint.

Altogether we have 1.33 % pareses out of 902 evaluated hip joints. A breakdown shows one paresis of the sciatic nerve, seven pareses of the peroneal nerve and five pareses of the femoral nerve. Coventry (1) stated 12 pareses of the sciatic nerve and five pareses of the femoral nerve out of 2.012 hip joints. Lubinus (7) had 24 cases a paresis of the peroneal nerve among 852 patients. The nature of the lesion is certainly also determined by the operative approach.

The individual reasons for the nerve lesions can be shortly listed as follows:

1. strangulation by sterile towel,
2. pressure on the peroneal nerve,
3. injury caused during preparation (perforator, Hohmann's elevator),
4. haematoma in the iliac muscle,
5. injury caused by traction, and
6. contact with cement.

The sterile towels, when bending the knee, can lead to a fold just above the head of the fibula when stretching the knee. The pressure of the thumb of the assistant on the knee joint can possibly compress the nerve, too.

In most cases, however, the reason for the lesion of the sciatic nerve and the femoral nerve is seen in injuries caused during preparation. This is especially possible in the dorsal approach of the sciatic or the peroneal nerve and for the lateral approach to the femoral nerve (5). In the case of a lateral approach an injury of the femoral nerve may be possible during the removal of medioventral parts of the capsule, if the protecting iliopsoas is also cut through. Above all, however, the femoral nerve can be irritated by Hohmann's elevator inserted above the anterior iliac spine. The nerve is protected by the thick iliacus, and it can therefore hardly be stretched by Hohmann's elevator. But it might happen, if the leg is adducted and externally rotated for the introduction of the rasp or for the insertion of the endoprosthesis. It is known that the femoral nerve as well as the sciatic nerve react very sensitively to overstretching. This is known from injuries of the knee joint and of the ankle joint, too. After the removal of the femoral head the leg can be pulled down by several centimetres with Hohmann's elevator; as a result the nerves can also be overstretched (Fig. 1). Often the extension becomes necessary in order to be able to reduce the hip joint. This is especially necessary in cases of high dislocations, where the head of the prosthesis must be inserted opposite to the original acetabulum during the operation. The elongation of a nerve to the point, where a damage will occur, is variously assessed. Liu et al. (6) assume a 6 % elongation and Sunderland and Bradley (12) 20 to 32 %. As soon as the nerve is stretched beyond its elasticity, i.e. as soon as the resistance caused by the epineurium is broken, a neuropraxia or an axonotmesis will occur. It is important to explore the nerve at the right time. We are of opinion that the nerve must be laid bare as soon as there is no indication for a restitution.

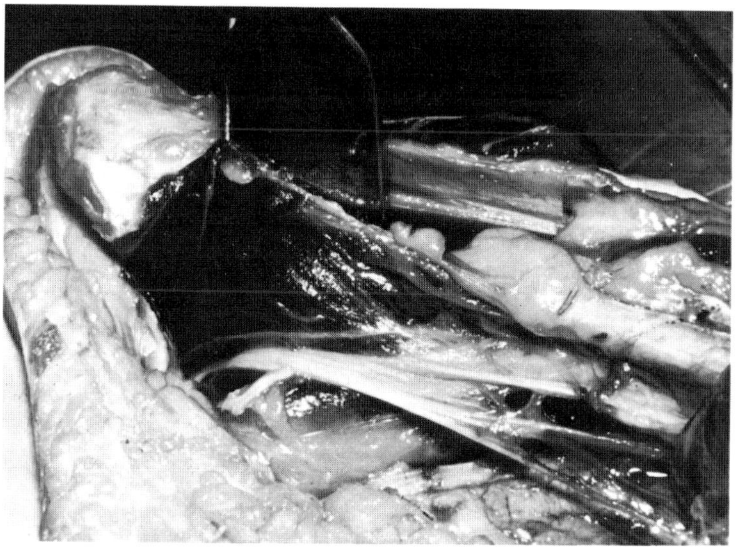

Fig. 1 Overstretching of femoral nerve by Hohmann's elevator inserted in the region of incisura lacunaris lateralis

It is worth considering how seriously manipulations of the leg may injure the iliac muscle or can lead to a haematoma after the removal of the femoral head. Such movements are, for example, necessary for the reduction of the joint or for the insertion of the shaft of the prosthesis into the medular space of the femur. The haematoma in the psoas sheath can compress the nerve underneath the fibrous ring. It may be possible that a particular tendency to bleed supports the bleeding (Fig. 2). Ruptures of the musculotendinous region after traumata of overextension with pareses of the femoral nerve have been reported in the scientific literature. In these cases the existence of a haematogenesis is supported by the fact that the paresis of the femoral nerve can only be established during the first postoperative day. In most cases of lesions the pareses is of a temporary nature. From 12 pareses out of our cases, only one paresis of the sciatic nerve and one of the femoral nerve as well as two pareses of the peroneal nerve were of lasting importance.

Hardly ever was damage caused by compression observed, which was due to a large quantity of bone cement, pressed dorsally during the insertion of the acetabulum and which could not be removed afterwards (2).

Usually the perforation of the acetabulum does not include any complication which hampers the operation in any way. Only greater damage can endanger the anchorage of the acetabulum, little holes are usually unimportant for the stability and they can be covered by a metal mesh. Some cases, however, have been reported in German and foreign scientific literature, where the borer had broken through the anteromedial aspect of the acetabulum and had injured the iliac artery and vein. Above all the osteoporotic acetabulum demands skilful handling of the motor-driven borer. This device can cause disastrous injuries in an unguarded moment. The medial protrusion in case of an advanced rheumatoid arthritis or idiopathic protrusion are especially endangered in this connexion.

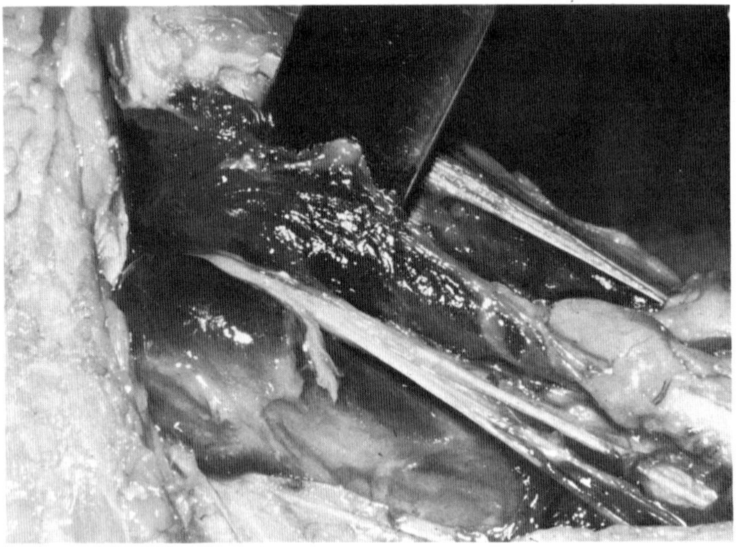

Fig. 2 Compressing and overstretching of femoral nerve by a haematoma in iliac muscle

The bone cement in the small pelvis usually does not lead to any irritation of muscles, vessels, and nerves. In scientific literature, however, one case has been reported, in which an aneurysm of the femoral artery had been produced by the sharp tip of a protruding cement block (3).

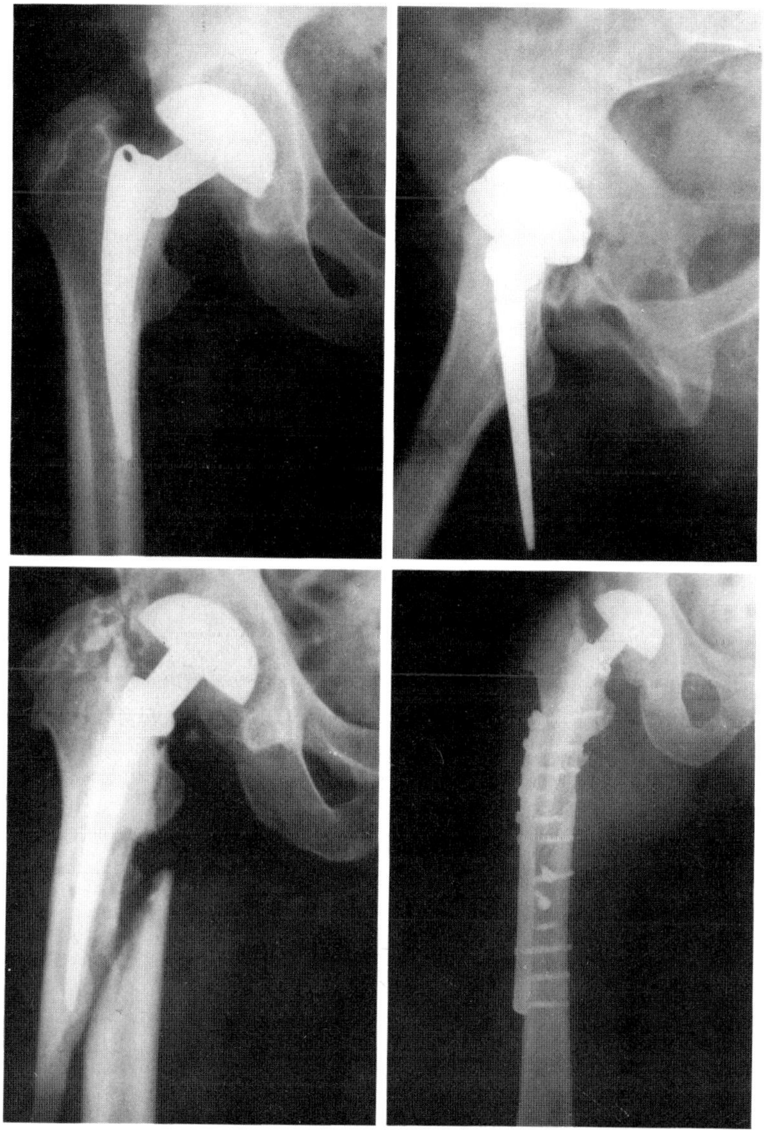

Fig. 3 Z.C., male *17.6.05. Irritation and pain when sitting. In second operation fracture of the thigh because the perforation was a locus minoris resistentiae

The perforation of the cortical substance shall not be dealt with in more detail. On the whole, this is of little importance, if it is noticed in time. It also appears in cases of osteoporotic bones and of limited view of the operation area. In difficult cases one can manage with a flexible double borer (4). The situation becomes awkward only if the hardened bone cement has to be removed together with the prosthesis. Once we had to reoperate because the protruded shaft of the prosthesis lead to an irritation of the soft parts and thus caused pain when sitting (Fig. 3). On a second occasion the perforation was the locus minoris resistentiae for a fracture of the thigh. It is important that the radiographs be taken from the front and from the side, because the protruded tip of the prosthesis can easily be overlocked.

Usually the assistant surgeons are charged with the fractures of the diaphysis and not the operator, who had arranged for the extreme position of adduction and external rotation of the leg because of an insufficient operative approach. We had five fractures of the thigh, one of them during the changing of a prosthesis; additionally a longitudinal fracture of the shaft of the thigh bone occurred during the deeper insertion (Fig. 4) of the shaft of the prosthesis. In all cases we had stabilized the fracture with an ASIF-plate during the same operation (Fig. 5).

While the complications described are, on the whole, particularly important incidents during the operation, anaesthiological and above all cardiovascular complications can give rise to dramatic incidents. 57 % of the patients had intra-operative complications, which were almost all managed. From this total, 51 % had two complications, 21 % three, 22 % four and more. It is quite understandable that with increasing age the patient's factors of risk and thus the complications will grow. Only a few complications shall be mentioned here.

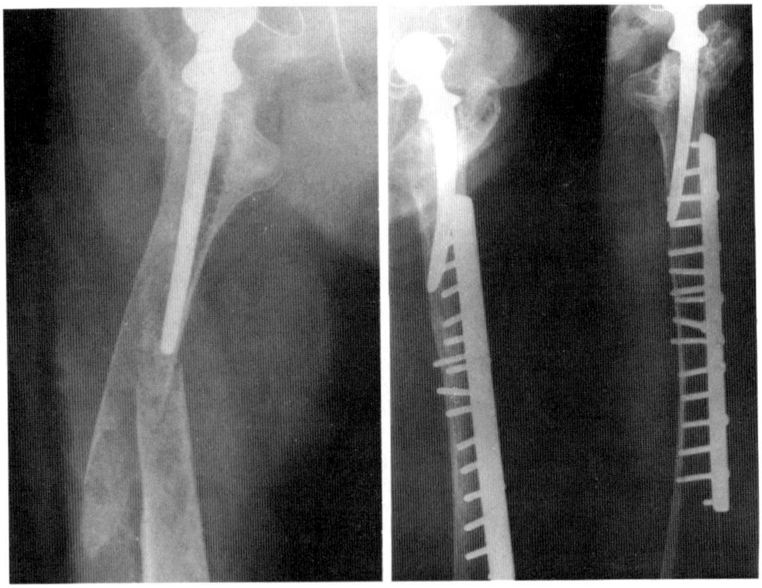

Fig. 4 M.E., female *27.9.90. Fracture of the thigh during the change of prosthesis, stabilized with an ASIF-plate

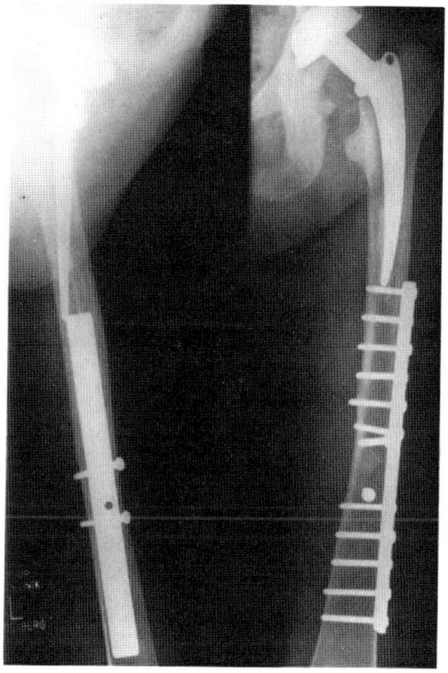

Fig. 5
G.B., female *4.12.06. Fracture of the thigh during reposition stabilized with an ASIF-plate

It is known that the blood pressure falls during the minutes after the insertion of the bone cement. The characteristic decrease in blood pressure takes place during the implantation of the acrylic cement into the acetabulum as well as during the insertion into the marrow cavity of the femur (Fig. 6). Incidents involving the anaesthesia occur more often during these operations than is generally assumed. They may represent a complication ending with the patient's death (11). From 395 patients that we evaluated in 1971 because of the frequent crises of blood pressure, we had four circulatory collapses, of which three ended with the patient's death. A check of the records of the anaesthesia

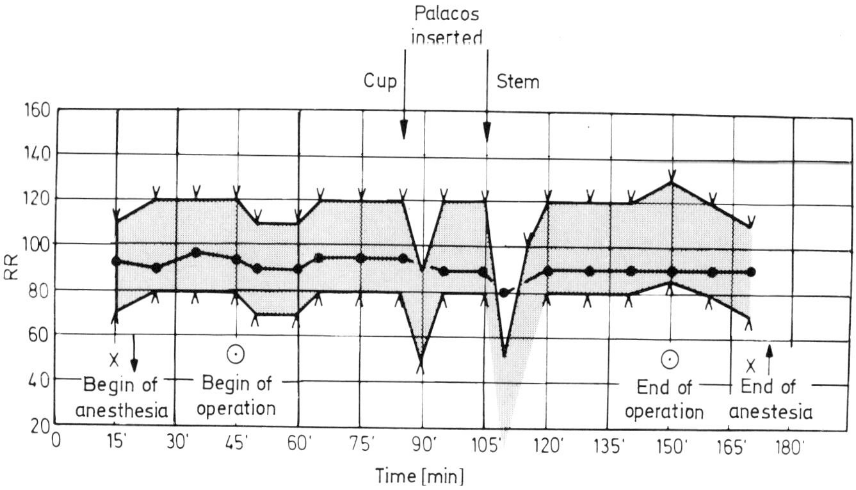

Fig. 6 Characteristic intraoperative decrease of blood pressure after insertion of the acrylic cement into the acetabulum and into the shaft of the femur

revealed that even in 50 % of the cases, in part considerable, decreases in blood pressure and disturbances of cardiac rythm had taken place during the cementation of the prosthesis (Fig. 7).

It was astonishing that these immediate cardiovascular complications had never been registrated during comparable operations of the hip. At first we thought that the fatalities were the sequel of an acutely serious cardiac infarction. In case of the patient who died at least an embolic occlusion of multiple pulmonary branches was demonstrated by angiography. The autopsy showed that the cause of death was a massive fat embolism of the lung with dilatation of the right heart. Only in the light of this finding was it possible to interpret the persistent massive cyanosis that lasted for hours, as a restriction of the alveolar gaseous interchange caused by the fat embolism of the lung. The sudden decrease in arterial blood pressure, too, and the disturbance of cardiac rythm could now be attributed to an acute insufficiency of the right heart due to a blocking of the pulmonary circulation. In the case of a successfully resuscitated female patient the subsequent disturbances of thermoregulation, the cerebral confusion, and a renal insufficiency could now be interpreted as typical sequel of a fat embolism in the general circulation, especially since the symptoms of an infarction had disappeared from the ECG after several months.

In 70 cats we have checked the cause of these phenonema in experimental examinations (4,10). According to our clinic experience and on the basis of our experiments, we believe that during the process of polymerization of the bone cement residual monomers which are liberated pass from the shaft of the femur into the blood, favoured by the heat and the increase of pressure and that they thus represent the reason for the precipitation of the fat. After the insertion of the bone cement or of fluid monomers into the shaft of the femur the animals constantly showed an increase of the central venous pressure measured in the pulmonary trunk and, simultaneously, a strong decrease in the peripheric pressure measured in the femoral artery as a sign of a pulmonarily conditioned overloading of the right heart (Fig. 8). Histologically a massive fat embolism was always be proved. We have, of course, like Pelling and Butterworth (8) also carried out a filling of the shaft of the femur only with plasticine, however, in only one case did a useful increase in pressure occur in the right heart; the fat embolism was in all cases very seldom.

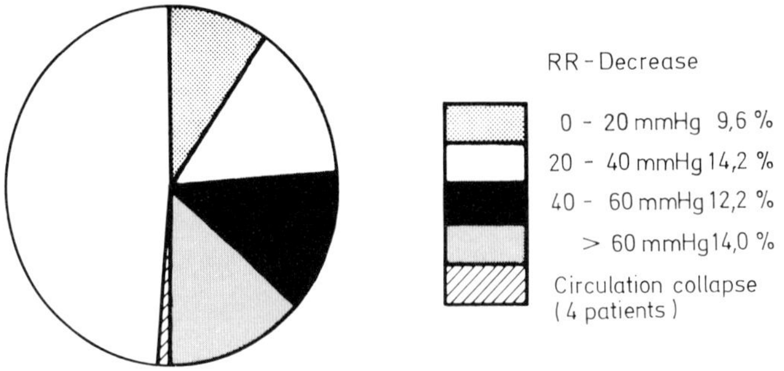

Fig. 7 Intraoperative decrease of blood pressure in 50 % of 395 patients after insertion of acrylic cement into the acetabulum and into the shaft of the femur

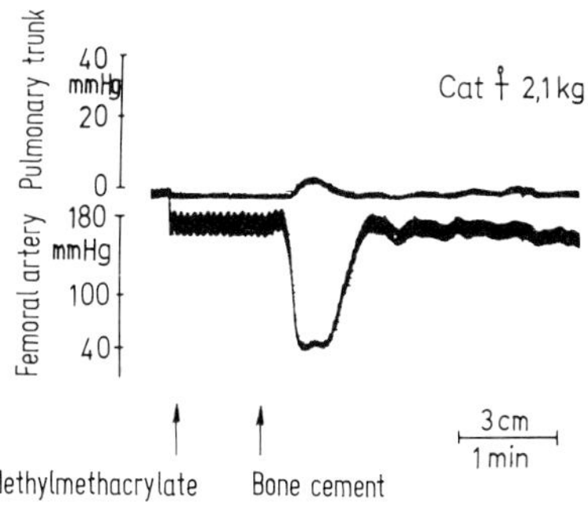

Fig. 8
Increase of the central venous pressure and strong decrease of the peripheric pressure after insertion of acrylic cement or of fluid monomers into the shaft of the femur are typical signs of a pulmonarily affected overloading of the right heart caused by fat embolism

Our observations also agree with the colloid theory of the fat embolism which says that monomers and tertiary amines liberated during the polymerization of the bone cement have effects similar to those of catecholamines.

Of course excessive blood lesses may trigger reversible incidents during the anaesthesia. Our average blood loss – i.e. in 68 % of the cases – was 1,200 $\pm$ 600 ml; in 16 % it increased to 3,000 ml. The increased blood loss does not represent a serious intra-operative complication.

The most serious complication is exitus in tabula. Up to now seven patients have died intra-operatively in total of 1,600 operations. The cause of death was in three cases the fat embolism mentioned above, twice pulmonary oedema and once cardiac infarction. In scientific literature the intra-operative mortality is given as between 0.1 % (9) and 1 %.

Although many peroperative complications do not influence the final result of the operation, we contribute to the decrease of the total rate of complications by a strict selection of the patients before the operation and by observing strict discipline during the operation. Thus we are able to influence the patient's destiny, which in most cases is determined by the durability of the prosthesis.

REFERENCES

1. Coventry, M.B., Beckenbaugh, R.D., Nolan, D.R., Ilstrup, D.M.: 2.012 Total hip arthroplasties: A study of postoperative course and early complications. Journal of Bone and Joint Surgery 56-A, 273 (1974)

2. Casagrande, P.A., Danahy, P.R.: Delayed sciatic-nerve entrapment following the use of self-curing acrylic. Journal of Bone and Joint Surgery 53-A, 167 (1972)

3. Dorr, L.P., Conaty, J.P., Kohl, R., Harvey, J.P.: False aneurysm of the femoral artery following total hip surgery. Journal of Bone and Joint Surgery 56-A, 1059 (1974)

4. Dustmann, H.O., Schulitz, K.P., Koch, H.: Fettembolie nach Anwendung von Knochenzement bei Hüftgelenkersatz. Tierexperimentelle Untersuchungen. Archiv der orthoädischen und Unfall-Chirurgie, 72, 114 (1972)

5. Green, J.P.: Proximal avulsion of the iliacus with paralysis of the femoral nerve. Journal of Bone and Joint Surgery 54-B, 154 (1972)

6. Liu, C.T., Benda, C.E., Lewey, F.H.: Tensile strength of human nerves. Archives of Neurology and Psychiatry 59, 322 (1948)

7. Lubinus, H.H., Jacobsen, U.: Erfahrungen mit dem totalen Gelenkersatz unter Verwendung des Systems Brunswik und eines dorsolateralen Zuganges. In: H. Cotta und K.P. Schulitz, edit., Der totale Hüftgelenkersatz, Stuttgart: Thieme Verlag 1973

8. Pelling, G., Butterworth, K.R.: Cardiovascular effects of acrylic bone cement in rabbits and cats. British Medical Journal 2, 628 (1973)

9. Saint-Maurice, C.: Les complications mortelles des arthroplasties. Revue de chirurgie orthopedique, Supplement 11, 61, 47 (1975)

10. Schulitz, K.P., Dustmann, H.O., Koch, H.: Fettembolie beim Einsetzen von Totalendoprothesen mit Acrylzement. In: H. Cotta und K.P. Schulitz, edit., Der totale Hüftgelenkersatz, Stuttgart: Thieme Verlag 1973

11. Schulitz, K.P., Koch, H., Dustmann, H.O.: Lebensbedrohliche Sofortkomplikationen durch Fettembolie nach Einsetzen von Totalendoprothesen mit Polymethylmethacrylat. Archiv für orthopädische und Unfall-Chirurgie 71, 307 (1971)

12. Sunderland, S., Bradley, K.C.: Stress-strain phenomena in human peripheral nerve trunks. Brain 84, 102 (1961)

SOME DISADVANTAGES OF CEMENTED INTRAMEDULLARY STEM FIXATION AND THEIR REMEDIES

M.A.R. Freeman

Many prostheses now in use are fixed to the skeleton by means of cemented intramedullary stems. It is the purpose of this paper to trace the origin of this method of fixation, to consider its advantages and disadvantages, and insofar as the latter may be thought to predominate, to consider alternatives.

Intramedullary stem fixation had its origin at the hip. The first implant for the replacement of the femoral head (the Judet prosthesis) was attached to the skeleton by means of a straight spike passing down the neck of the femur and through the lateral femoral cortex. This design reflected the use at that time of pins such as the Smith-Peterson for the fixation of fractures of the neck of the femur. It became apparent however that the loads applied to the femoral head in life were such as to depress the proximal end of such an implant, bending it as a cantilever relative to the femur. For this reason, the method of fixation used in the Judet prosthesis was modified by surgeons such as Thompson and Moore, to the now familiar alternative of an uncemented long metallic stem passing down the intramedullary canal of the femur. Clinical experience over the years demonstrated that although this method of fixation was adequate in the sense that the prosthesis did not migrate grossly so as to cause total failure of the arthroplasty, some motion frequently occurred between the intramedullary stem and the femur and that such motion was associated with pain. For this reason, Charnley introduced the use of a bonding agent, polymethylmethacrylate, for use between the intramedullary stem and the inner aspect of the cortex of the femur. With the use of this material, gross motion was eliminated between the implant and the skeleton and absolute freedom from pain resulted. Since the long bone shafts adjacent to most joints are tubular (exceptions being those joints in which one component, such as the acetabulum, is not part of a long bone) and since the contents of the tube can be dispensed with, this method of prosthetic fixation has found widespread acceptance in orthopaedic surgery. It is particularly attractive in view of its simplicity and the apparently obvious fact that an implant bonded in this way will be very securely fixed to the skeleton.

Unfortunately, although the strength of fixation is unquestionably considerable, there are now grounds for supposing that the cyclical application of the loads encountered in everyday life may nevertheless be great enough to produce fatigue failure of the elements making up the bond, and hence eventual loosening of the prosthesis, or fracture of one of the prosthetic components. Thus experience in the future may show that the fixation of prostheses with cemented intramedullary stems is convenient and satisfactory in the short-term, but that in the long-term this is an unsatisfactory method of attaching a prosthesis to the skeleton. Should this be the case, the disadvantages of cemented intramedullary stem fixation will raise serious problems in orthopaedics.

THE DISADVANTAGES OF CEMENTED INTRAMEDULLARY STEMS

The first disadvantage of the cemented intramedullary stem is that should loosening occur at the cement/bone interface, the cement is abraded to form particulate debris. This debris appears to induce tissue necrosis so that a mass of semi-fluid foreign and necrotic material is formed around the prosthesis. Repetitive pressurization of this material via the prosthesis results in its being "pumped" through the tissues to form an extensive cavity and eventually a sinus. Thus loosening of a cemented implant may eventually lead to far more tissue damage than does loosening at a bone/metal interface.

Secondly, if the prosthesis has been misplaced or has become infected, the removal of the cement may pose great difficulty and in doing it, irremedial damage may be done to the skeleton. Thus a second disadvantage of the cemented intramedullary stem is that conversion procedures may be difficult to accomplish.

Unfortunately, the disadvantages of intramedullary stem fixation do not end there. Of necessity, stems passed into the intramedullary canal are long and therefore the area of the interface between the polymethylmethacrylate and the skeleton is large. It is this area that is most at risk from the stand-point of infection since natural host defence mechanisms and antibiotics can only reach bacterial contaminants at the interface from one of its aspects. It seems reasonable to think that

1. the larger the area of the host/implant interface, the greater the chance of contaminants introduced during surgery reaching the bond and
2. the greater the bond area, and hence the larger the number of vessels supplying it, the higher the chances of blood-borne bacteria alighting at the interface.

Thus the large bone/cement interface associated with cemented intramedullary stems seems likely to increase the risk of bacterial contamination of an area of tissue where host resistance to infection might be thought to be at a minimum.

Should the tissue at the interface become infected following contamination, it would seem desirable that the tissue in question should be one in which infection is relatively easily eradicated in normal circumstances. Cancellous bone is such a tissue, but unfortunately cortical bone is not: osteomyelitis in cortical bone is well-known for its therapeutic intractability, even in the absence of an implant. A further disadvantage of the cemented intramedullary stem, therefore, is that, of necessity, it is bonded to cortical bone.

Thus there are two disadvantages attaching to the use of cemented intramedullary stems in the context of infection:

1. It seems reasonable to think that the chances of contamination occurring at the bone/cement interface may be greater than with some possible alternatives and
2. the tissue reached by such contaminants, and hence potentially infected, is cortical bone, in which infection is difficult to eradicate even under ideal circumstances.

Finally, it is now appreciated that the introduction of a prosthetic stem into an intramedullary canal full of fluid fat and medullary contents, and sealed by unpolymerized acrylic, may pressurize the contents of the intramedullary canal sufficiently to express them into the neighbouring veins. The result may be pulmonary embolism and, occasionally, death. Although this hazard can be overcome, once its existence is recognized, by decompressing the canal as the stem is introduced, it must nevertheless be recognized that the hazard exists.

Thus, there would appear to be significant disadvantages in the use of intramedullary stems which would be important even if this method of fixation was invariably satisfactory in the long-term. It will, however, now be argued that fixation may frequently be unsatisfactory in the long-term. Thus two questions should be considered by the designers of prostheses:

1. does the argument that intramedullary stems may be expected to loosen with an unacceptable frequency in the long-term have any validity? and
2. is there any alternative and preferable method of bonding a prosthesis to the skeleton?

CAN INTRAMEDULLARY STEMS BE EXPECTED TO LOOSEN WITH UNACCEPTABLE FREQUENCY IN THE LONG–TERM?

It is important to emphasize in what follows that it is not now suggested that intramedullary stems will invariably loosen: on the contrary, clinical experience demonstrates that this is not so. On the other hand it will be suggested that the incidence of late loosening may turn out to be appreciable, especially if the functional demands placed by patients upon their prosthesis and upon the bonds between the prosthesis and the skeleton, increase with improved prosthetic design. It should be remembered in this context that some years ago two alternative material combinations were widely used for the total replacement of the hip, cobalt chrome versus cobalt chrome and metal versus high-density polyethylene. The latter has now almost supplanted the former principally because experience has demonstrated a slightly increased rate of loosening with the metal on metal prostheses (attributable perhaps to the higher friction at such bearings and hence to the greater loads placed on the bond between the prosthesis and the skeleton, and perhaps occasionally to metal sensitivity). The point to be emphasized here is not related to the cause of the loosening, but is that a difference in the incidence of loosening of two or three per cent is sufficient to make one prosthetic arrangement preferable to another in clinical practice. It is now suggested that the factors to be considered below may well result in an increased incidence of late loosening of cemented intramedullary stems (as compared with certain alternatives) of this order of magnitude.

The problem of intramedullary stem fixation can be considered at its most extreme in the context of hinge replacement of the knee where the hinge is of a simple design with a fixed axis. The bone/prosthesis bond in such an implant is stressed by loads applied in a number of different ways. Firstly, since such a prosthesis effectively "by-passes" the soft tissues, whatever torsional and bending moments are applied to the joint will be transmitted entirely through the prosthesis to stress the bone/prosthesis bond. Secondly, since the position of the axis of rotation at the knee varies during movement, normal movements tend to displace the axis of rotation of the prosthesis relative to the skeleton in such a way as to distract the prosthesis from the bone. Thirdly, compressive forces applied to the limb as a whole in weight-bearing, load the intramedullary stems in such a way that they tend to move upwards relative to the femur and downwards relative to the tibia. Thus the major loads applied to the prosthesis tend to produce translational movement of an intramedullary stem relative to the skeleton either by rotating the stem in the intramedullary canal, by moving it from side to side across the canal, or by moving it up and down the canal.

Rotational movement of the stem within the canal will result in the development of primary shear stresses in the material of the bond. Such stresses may not be great when the knee is extended, but may well be very much greater in the flexed limb: considerable turning moments can be applied to a femoral intramedullary stem by flexing the knee and loading the foot from the side. The bending moments generated by the abduction and adduction forces applied to the knee during walking will tend to produce bending moments in the prosthesis if they are applied at an angle deviating only slightly from the axis of flexion and extension (and even a force applied precisely at right-angles to the axis of rotation of the prosthesis may produce a bending moment when full extension is reached). When a bending moment is applied to the prosthesis, the bond between the intramedullary stem and the skeleton will be loaded in shear in the plane of the moment whilst in the plane at right-angles it will be in tension on one side, and in compression on the other. Finally, forces tending to move the stem up or down the canal must produce primary shear stresses in the bond.

The magnitude of the resultant stresses on the bond cannot be calculated with useful accuracy since for many joints the applied loads are unknown and since the actual size of the bond (and hence of the area carrying the loads) may vary from prosthesis to prosthesis and from one patient to another with the same prosthesis. Nevertheless the essential point remains that the bond between an intramedullary stem and the skeleton must frequently be stressed primarily in shear and in tension rather than primarily in compression. In general it is shear and tension which result in the failure of mechanical bonds of any kind, whilst compression, if anything, will support a bond (Fig. 1). Thus the bond between a cemented intramedullary stem and the skeleton might be expected to fail mechanically not because of the magnitude of the stresses applied to it but because of their nature.

It is self-evident, but may be demonstrated experimentally, that in spite of the fact that the bond is likely to be stressed in shear and tension, the strength of the bond produced by intramedullary stem fixation is sufficient to withstand a single application of the loads likely to be encountered in life. Thus, statically, the bond is sufficiently strong. The question, however, that is of clinical relevance, especially in the long-term, is not: "is the bond sufficiently strong statically? " but "is the endurance limit of the bond (i.e. its fatigue strength) adequate? ".

The bone/prosthesis bond at a cemented intramedullary stem is composed of three load-carrying materials: bone, polymethylmethacrylate and metal. Bone is certainly fatigue-prone and its fatigue life has been measured experimentally (1,2). Little is known of the

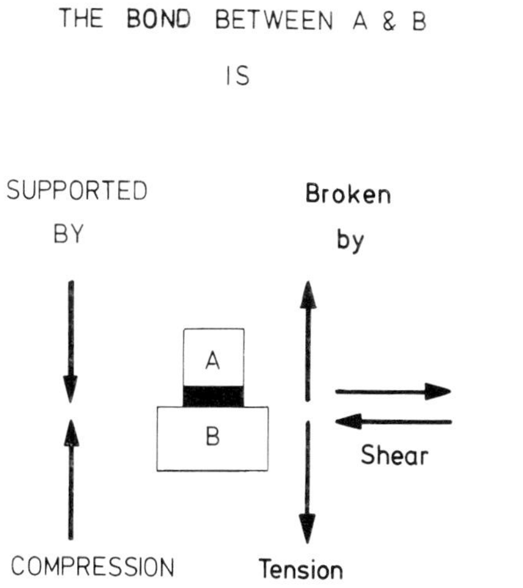

Fig. 1a This figure illustrates diagramatically the effect of compression, tension and shear upon the bond between two solids A and B. The symbols representing compression, tension and shear are used again in Figures 1b and 2

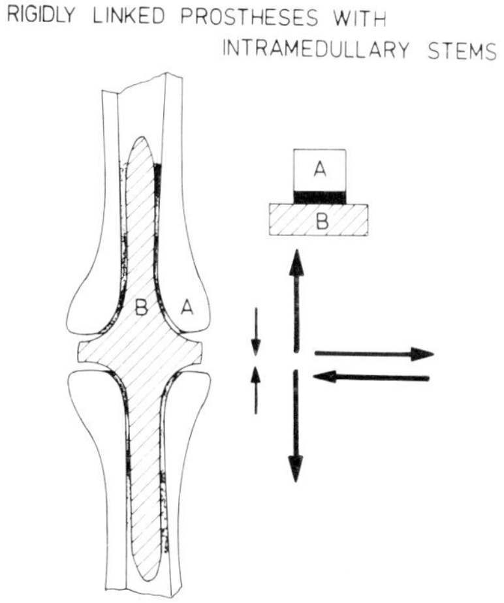

Fig. 1b This figure illustrates diagramatically the nature of the forces acting on the bond between a cemented intramedullary stem of a constrained hinge and the cortex of the shaft of a long bone. Compression is minimized, tension and shear are maximized

fatigue properties of polymethylmethacrylate but the bone-cement interface is certainly fatigue-prone (3) and cement is relatively weak in tension (4,5). Finally it is certain that all the metals used for implants are fatigue-prone. Thus the possibility clearly exists that the bond as a whole might undergo fatigue failure. In practice, the nature of the failures which occur with cemented intramedullary stems (stem fracture and more commonly loosening at the bone/cement interface) suggest that fatigue failure may occur in all three elements.

Up to this point, the argument has been illustrated in the mechanical situation which might be thought to be the worst for intramedullary stem fixation, namely that in which the knee is replaced by a uniaxial hinge. Clearly the forces acting on the bone/prosthesis bond can be reduced if the hinge is so designed, that for example, the axis of rotation can migrate in such a way as to prevent traction being applied to the intramedullary stem when the joint is flexed. Such an implant would be expected to loosen (if at all) with less frequency than a simple hinge. Further modification of the bearing can be made so as to permit rotation and even ab- or adduction. If the result of design modifications of this kind is to permit a little movement in the bearing, but when movement has been accomplished, the bearing itself is loaded, the forces referred to above will eventually be applied to the bond as they are in a simple uniaxial hinge. If, in contrast, the soft tissues check rotational motion and abduction/adduction before the bearing itself is loaded, these movements will not stress the bone/prosthesis bond. Similarly, if the prosthesis is so designed (as is the Walldius hinge) that axial compressive loads are borne by the cancellous bone ends and not by the cortex via intramedullary stems, the bond will not be stressed by weight-bearing. Thus a prosthesis could be designed through which little or no load could be passed on to intramedullary stems. Such stems should not loosen: but to cement them in place, indeed to have them at all, seems unnecessary since they would be mechanically redundant.

The conditions at a ball-and-socket articulation such as the hip approach the optimal situation described above. Hence they are favourable for the intramedullary stem geometry since movements about every axis are permitted to an essentially unlimited extent at the bearing. Thus the bending and turning moments which may be generated in a constrained hinge at the knee cannot readily be generated at the hip. Unfortunately, however, the cantilevered shape of the upper end of the femur imposes a bending moment upon the femoral prosthesis when load is transmitted through the limb. This produces tensile forces on the lateral side of the intramedullary stem and it is these forces which are almost certainly responsible for the small but increasing number of fatigue fractures that have been reported in femoral intramedullary stems at the hip. Clearly the magnitude of such stresses can be reduced by implanting larger stemmed prostheses, but the diameter of an intramedullary stem is ultimately limited by the size of the intramedullary canal and it may well be that the largest practical size will still have a finite endurance limit.

Thus the possibility must be faced that cemented intramedullary stem fixation may be associated with a gradually incrasing incidence of loosening, perhaps after 10 to 15 years of use, as a consequence of fatigue failure in the face of shear and tensile stresses at the bond. Alternatively, the metal of the stem itself may occasionally fail in fatigue. It therefore seems worthwhile to consider the question: "is there a preferable alternative to cemented intramedullary stems?"

THE ALTERNATIVE TO CEMENTED INTRAMEDULLARY STEM FIXATION

If it be accepted that the principal disadvantages of cemented intramedullary stem fixation are that the bond is loaded in tension and shear, is of large area and composed on the host side of cortical bone, and that a failed prosthesis may be hard to remove, it follows that a preferable alternative should have a bond which is loaded solely in compression, which is small in area and which is composed on the host side of cancellous bone, and the prosthesis should be easy to remove.

The normal joint surface is loaded for practical purposes only in compression. Tension is obviously never applied to the articular surface itself, tensile forces being carried by the ligaments in the joint. Minimal shear forces are generated on the normal articular surface as a consequence of friction and these may be only slightly greater between surfaces composed of prosthetic materials. Thus in principle it would seem that an attractive alternative to intramedullary stem fixation would be to resect only the surfaces of the involved joint and then to replace this limited amount of the skeleton. Provided the resection was entirely intra-articular so that the prosthesis itself did not extend beyond the bony attachments of the joint's ligaments, the bond between the prosthesis and the skeleton would, like the original articular surface, be loaded for practical purposes only in compression, scarcely at all in shear and not at all in tension (Fig. 2).

The surface area of the bonds in such a resurfacing prosthesis must be relatively limited since it cannot extend beyond the articular surfaces themselves. Thus the chances of contaminating bacteria reaching the bond at the time of surgery, or subsequently via the bloodstream, may be somewhat reduced. Furthermore, it is well-recognized that infection can be eradicated more reliably from cancellous bone than it can from cortical, so that it seems possible that even if infection developed in the bone at such an interface, conventional treatment with antibiotics might eradicate it.

Finally such a prosthesis should obviously be easy to remove in the event of failure and, having done so, most of the original skeleton would still be available for a salvage procedure. Indeed since, generally speaking, arthritis affects the articular cartilage and only the first few millimetres of subchondral bone, it seems illogical to resect large areas of the skeleton for the treatment of this disease as is done for example with conventional hip prosthesis.

Thus this type of replacement would appear to have significant advantages over intramedullary stem fixation and indeed it is becoming widely used at a number of joints. Examples at the hip, knee and ankle, with which the author has been associated are shown in Figs. 3, 4 and 5. It must, however, be appreciated that this general approach to joint replacement has problems of its own.

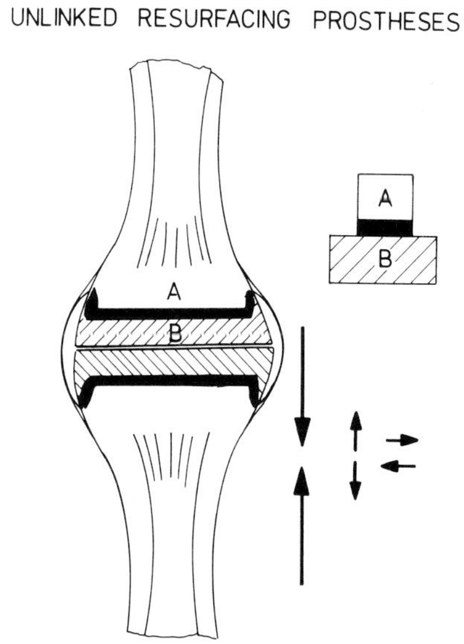

Fig. 2
This figure illustrates diagramatically the nature of the forces acting between an unlinked resurfacing prosthesis and the bone ends. Compression is maximized, tension and shear are minimized

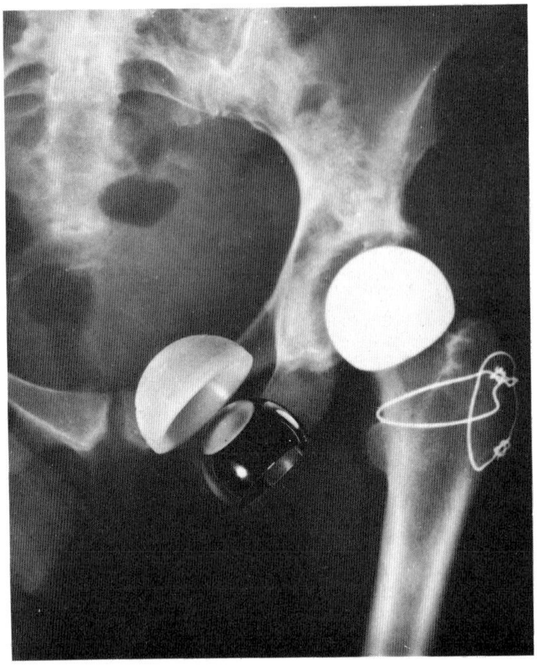

Fig. 3

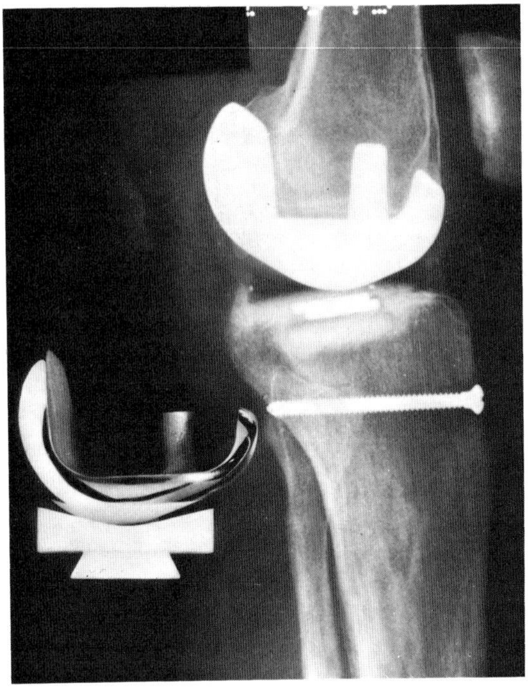

Fig. 4

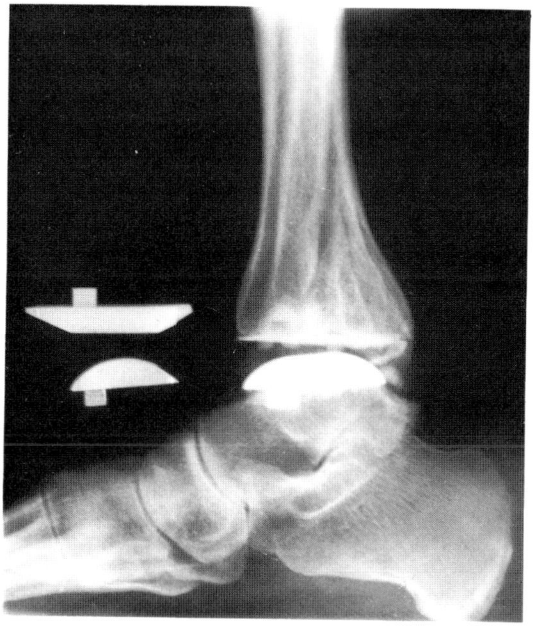

Fig. 5
The figures 3,4,5 illustrate examples of prostheses (the ICLH prostheses) designed in the author's laboratory, which avoid the use of intramedullary stems. The prostheses replace the hip (Fig. 3), the knee (Fig. 4) and the ankle (Fig. 5)

THE DISADVANTAGES OF SURFACE REPLACEMENT

Foremost amongst the disadvantages of surface replacement is the requirement for surgical precision in the forming of appropriate bone surfaces. As little bone as possible must be removed in order not to weaken the bone ends unacceptably nor to prejudice the blood supply of the residual tissue. On the other hand, bone which has been destroyed or damaged by the disease process must be replaced, and a sufficient gap must be created between the bone ends to permit the access required for implantation of the prosthesis. Thus the amount of bone removed must be precisely regulated: a situation which contrasts for example with the unrestricted removal of the femoral head, the neck and the contents of the intramedullary canal in conventional hip replacement.

Not only, however, must the amount of bone resection be appropriate in this sense; it must also be appropriately related to the thickness of the prosthesis. If for example at the knee, 3 cm of bone are resected and a prosthesis 2 cm thick is inserted, all the ligaments will have 1 cm of slack and the knee will be totally unstable. If on the other hand, only 1 cm of bone is resected, a 2 cm thick prosthesis could not be inserted at all.

Finally, the bones must be so shaped that the prosthesis can be anchored to them. Although the objective of an arthroplasty of this type is to reduce to a minimum the tensile and shear forces on the bond, it is nevertheless obviously essential to produce a bone/prosthesis bond which will resist such shear and tensile stresses as remain. The normal anatomy lends itself to this in certain situations, for example at the distal end of the femur where a prosthesis can embrace the bone, or at the acetabulum where the bone embraces the prosthesis. In other situations, however, for example at the proximal tibia, the prosthesis and the bone would be represented by two flat surfaces unless special precautions were to be taken to shape them so that they interlock.

Finally both a priori considerations and clinical experience suggest that it is unsafe to rely on only part of the juxta-articular cancellous bone for the transmission of compressive loads: to do this at the proximal tibia for example raises the risk of gradual sinkage of the prosthesis. Thus the prosthesis and the resected bone need to be so shaped that the full cross-section of the bone, including the cortex, is used to carry load.

To achieve these objectives the surgeon must resect bone accurately and may have to vary the size of the prosthesis in order to obtain a component which fits accurately. Bone cannot be resected with the required precision by eye with an osteotome: special jigs are required to determine the positions of bone section and special tools are desirable to cut the bone. Thus for surface replacement to be successful it is not sufficient simply to design a prosthesis: special tools and an appropriate surgical procedure must be developed as well.

Finally, careful attention must be given to the shaping of the articular surfaces of the prosthesis and to the correct placement of the axis of rotation of the prosthesis in relation to the axis conferred on it by the retained soft tissues. The significance of this requirement can be illustrated by reference to the hip and the ankle. If a complete capsulotomy is carried out at the hip, no soft tissues remain which will impose an axis of rotation upon a ball-and-socket prosthesis. Thus movement will not tend, for example, to force the femur (in attempting to conform to the soft tissues'axis of rotation) to move anteriorly, nor posteriorly relative to the acetabular prosthesis and in so doing to shear (on the gross scale) the bond between the acetabulum and the pelvis. In contrast, if the horizontal articular surface of the tibia at the ankle and the dome of the talus are replaced with a prosthesis shaped as a roller in a trough, and if the ligaments are sufficiently retained to impose their axis on the prosthesis, a quite different situation arises. If the prosthesis is placed with its axis posterior to that of the soft tissues, plantarflexion will tend to open the prosthesis anteriorly and drive the posterior lip of the tibial prosthesis against the back of the talar prosthesis. Dorsiflexion will be prevented by impaction between the anterior aspects of the two components. This in turn produces greater compressive forces anteriorly than posteriorly and hence tends to "squeeze" the prosthesis backwards in the ankle, thus shearing the bone/prosthesis bond. Thus a failure to ensure that the axes of the soft tissues and of the prosthesis coincide may result in the development of shear or tensile forces on the bone/prosthesis bond and may thus defeat the objective of surface replacement.

The precise location of the soft tissue axis is often difficult or impossible to determine by eye, so that to avoid this difficulty, either the soft tissues controlling the axis must be removed (as by capsulotomy at the hip, or by dividing the cruciate ligaments at the knee), or a prosthesis must be used that does not have a fixed axis (as for example a femoral roller working on a flat tibial surface at the knee), or special instruments must be developed to match the axes of the soft tissues and the prosthesis to each other (as has been done for ICLH arthroplasty at the ankle).

CONCLUSION

In this paper it has been argued that the fixation of joint replacement prostheses to the skeleton with cemented intramedullary stems may be misleadingly satisfactory in the short-term since loosening or stem fracture caused by fatigue may be not infrequent in the long-term. The alternative to the use of cemented intramedullary stems is to replace only the joint surfaces, a technique now receiving increases clinical acceptance. This technique however also has disadvantages, the nature of which have been discussed above.

REFERENCES

1. Evans, F.G., Lebow, M.: Strength of human compact bone under repetitive loading. Journal of Applied Physiology 10, 127 (1957)
2. Swanson, S.A.V., Freeman, M.A.R., Day, W.H.: The fatigue properties of human cortical bone. Medical and Biological Engineering 9, 23 (1971)
3. Kölbel, R.: Mechanische Eigenschaften einer Verbindung von spongiösem Knochen und Polymethylmetacrylat bei periodischer Belastung. Archiv für orthopädische und Unfall-Chirurgie 80, 31 (1974)
4. Charnley, J.: Acrylic cement in orthopaedic surgery, Edinburgh-London: E. & S. Livingstone 1970, p. 93 et seq.
5. Haas, S.S., Brauer, G.M., Dickson, G.: A characterization of polymethylmethacrylate bone cement. Journal of Bone and Joint Surgery 57-A, 380 (1975)

THE STRESS IN TOTAL HIP PROSTHESIS FEMORAL STEMS: A COMPARATIVE EXPERIMENTAL STUDY

B. Weightman

The incidence of stem fractures in total hip prostheses has apparently increased in recent years, to the extent that stem fracture is now a significant cause of late failure.

Charnley's figures for his own total hip prosthesis illustrate this point. There was only one stem fracture up to 1971 (1), there were six by 1973 (2), and seventeen by 1975 (4). In this latter paper Charnley reported that in his experience of some 7,000 patients the fracture rate is practically zero for patients under 64 Kg (140 lbf) in weight but can reach 6 per cent in patients over 90 Kg (200 lbf). He suggested that the primary cause of stem fracture is a defective technique in the use of cement, which can leave the proximal half of the stem unsupported while the distal half remains permanently fixed.

Müller (7) discussed the danger of fatigue fracture of femoral stems, between 50 and 70 mm from the tip, whenever a weakness is present at the level of the femoral calcar. Müller recommended the use of a special straight stemmed prosthesis in these cases.

Galante, Rostoker and Doyle (5) examined six fractured femoral stems; four cast cobalt-chromium alloy Müller prostheses, and two forged 316 L stainless steel Charnley prostheses. A third Charnley failure was mentioned but this had not been removed and so could not be examined. Six of the prostheses had fractured within two years, the seventh had lasted just over three years. All of the examined fracture surfaces exhibited fatigue striations, indicating metal fatigue as the cause of failure, and five of the six prostheses had metallurgical defects which could have initiated fatigue. Other factors which could have contributed to failure were identified as varus positioning of the stem and loosening of the stem in its cement bed, both of which would produce increased stress levels.

Markolf and Amstutz (6) studied three femoral stem failures. Metallurgical examination of a cast cobalt-chromium-molybdenum Müller prosthesis which had fractured sixteen months after insertion showed fracture surface markings typical of fatigue, but no obvious material defects. A Bechtol stem showed gross plastic deformation in the proximal region but had not fractured. A second Bechtol stem had yielded and fractured, the fracture being attributed to fatigue. Markolf and Amstutz mentioned two other fractured stems but did not give details. They also indicated the occurrence of a significant number of unreported stem fractures.

In the same paper Markolf and Amstutz present the results of a series of tests with instrumented femoral components. Strain gauged components were loaded in three types of test:

1. with the stems securely fixed into blocks of acrylic cement,
2. with the stems loose in blocks of cement, and
3. with the stems fixed in blocks of cement by the distal third only.

The results showed that the stress levels in the stems were much higher when they were loose or supported only distally, than when rigidly fixed over their full length. While these results support the conclusion of Charnley that fatigue failure occurs because of a lack of proximal support, they do not answer the question of whether or not the stresses developed in properly cemented prostheses are dangerous. This is because the stress levels measured in the stems rigidly fixed in acrylic cement were influenced by the thickness of the cement mass, and therefore may not be relevant to the in vivo situation. Markolf and Amstutz concluded that inadequate stem design, varus placement, low strength metal, and lack of adequate proximal medial support due to poor quality bone or cement fracture could all contribute to dangerously high stress levels in femoral stems.

Galante, Rostoker and Doyle (5) discussed the question of stress levels in properly orientated and cemented stems. Although these workers found that the location of fractures corresponded to the sites of maximum surface tensile stress predicted by the stress analysis of stems in a varus position or loose in cement, they concluded that, due to lack of information about the fatigue properties of implant materials, current designs of femoral stems should be regarded as marginal in relation to prolonged periods of service.

Although it is at present impossible to estimate the fatigue life of a femoral stem from a consideration of the maximum stress developed in it and the fatigue properties of the material, it is clearly the case that, as far as the stem is concerned, the lower the maximum tensile stress on the convex lateral surface the better. In any given situation of good or bad cement fixation, high or low strength bone, or valgus or varus positioning of the stem, the value of the maximum tensile stress produced in a stem is a function of the design of the stem. In recent months two major new designs of stem, both aimed at reducing the incidence of fatigue fracture, have been announced. Howmedica have introduced a computer-aided design stem (Vitallium CAD) and Thackrays are marketing the Charnley Heavy and Extra-Heavy "cobra" design.

The Howmedica design has been produced with the aid of a finite-element computer program while the Charnley design attempts to reduce the stress in the stem by transferring an increased proportion of the applied load directly to the cement.

As far as the present author is aware, not direct laboratory measurements of the stresses produced in these stems under physiological conditions have been reported to date. The remainder of this paper will therefore present the results of such a study, aimed specifically at assessing the reduction in maximum tensile stress achieved by the latest designs of stem under clinically relevant conditions.

MATERIALS AND METHODS

Five types of femoral stem were tested:

1. a Charnley (original), manufactured by Thackray Ltd.,
2. a Charnley Extra-Heavy ("cobra"), manufactured by Thackray Ltd.,
3. a CAD Standard Curved (Vitallium CAD) manufactured by Howmedica Ltd.,
4. a CAD Standard Straight (Vitallium CAD) manufactured by Howmedica Ltd., and
5. a stem designed and manufactured in the author's laboratory and designated the Imperial College stem.

Stem profiles are shown in Fig. 1, together with details of the cross-sectional shapes. As the figure shows, the Imperial College stem had the same profile as the original Charnley stem, the same neck angle as the CAD stems, and a trapezoidal cross-section. This section widened from 10 mm on the medial side to 15 mm on the lateral side.

Seven resistance strain gauges (gauge factor 1.91) were attached to the lateral face of each stem in the positions shown in Fig. 1. Each strain gauge was connected to a temperature compensating dummy gauge so as to form a bridge circuit. A carrier wave input

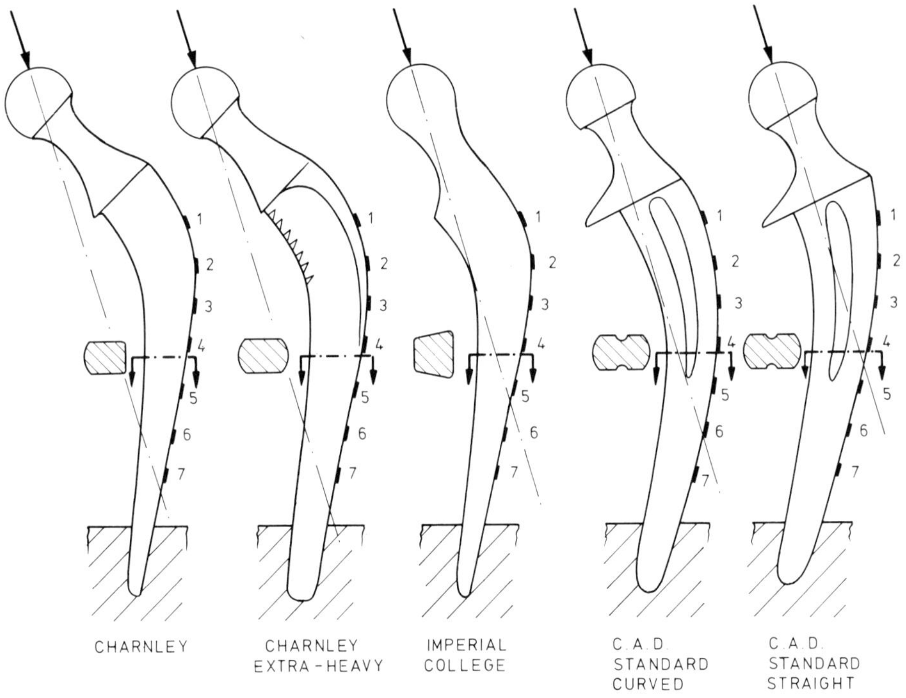

Fig. 1 Details of the five tested stems. The figure shows, (a) the stem profiles, (b) cross-section at mid-stem, (c) the position of the strain gauges, (d) the line of load action, and (e) the position of the clamp in the distal fixation tests

was provided by an oscillator, and the output signals were fed, via an amplifier/demodulator, to an ultra-violet recorder. Readings were converted to stress values using the known moduli of elasticity of the stem materials (E = 200 GN/m^2 for both stainless steel and cast cobalt-chromium alloy. Reference B.S. 3531 Part 1).

Two series of tests were carried out, both of which were designed to simulate clinical situations. In the first series each stem was clamped at the tip (approximately 25 mm) in a specially designed fixture with the stem at an angle of 24 degrees to the vertical, and loaded to 2 KN in a materials testing machine (Tensometer, Type E). The angle of 24 degrees was chosen so that a vertically applied load simulated the average angle at which the resultant force acts in vivo during normal walking. That is, the stem/femur at an angle of 10 degrees to the vertical, plus the resultant force applied at an angle of 14 degrees to the vertical. Load was applied to each femoral head through a high density polyethylene block with a flat surface so as to minimize lateral loading. This test was designed to simulate the clinical situation of complete breakdown of cement fixation over a large part of the stem.

The second series of tests was designed to simulate the ideal clinical situation of cement fixation to bone over the entire length of the stem. The five femoral components were cemented into the proximal halves of post-mortem human femurs by an orthopaedic surgeon. Radiopaque Simplex Bone Cement was used so that radiographs would show whether or not proper fixation had been achieved. Each femur plus prosthetic component was then loaded in the materials testing machine to 2 KN as before.

All tests were repeated three times with the specimens being removed from the clamping fixture between tests. After calculating the mean stresses produced by a 2 KN load, the values were doubled. The stresses shown in the following results therefore correspond to an applied load of 4 KN.

RESULTS AND DISCUSSION

The results of the first series of tests, in which the five femoral stems were clamped at their tips and loaded are shown in Fig. 2. The test simulates the clinical situation of correct orientation with complete breakdown of proximal cement fixation. Although it is unlikely that femoral stems would remain secure if the breakdown of cement extended down to the tip of the stem, the results are relevant to any level of proximal cement breakdown. That is, if the breakdown of proximal cement fixation extended to, say, the level of strain gauge 5, the tensile stresses produced in the lateral surface of the proximal stem would be as shown by strain gauges 1 to 4. Only the stresses produced in the distal stem (gauges 5 to 7) would be reduced by the reinforcement of cement and bone.

The actual stress values shown in Fig. 2 correspond to an applied load of 4 KN (approximately 400 Kgf or 900 lbf), which is perhaps four to five times the body weight of a heavy patient. At applied loads other than 4 KN the tensile stresses will be in direct pro-

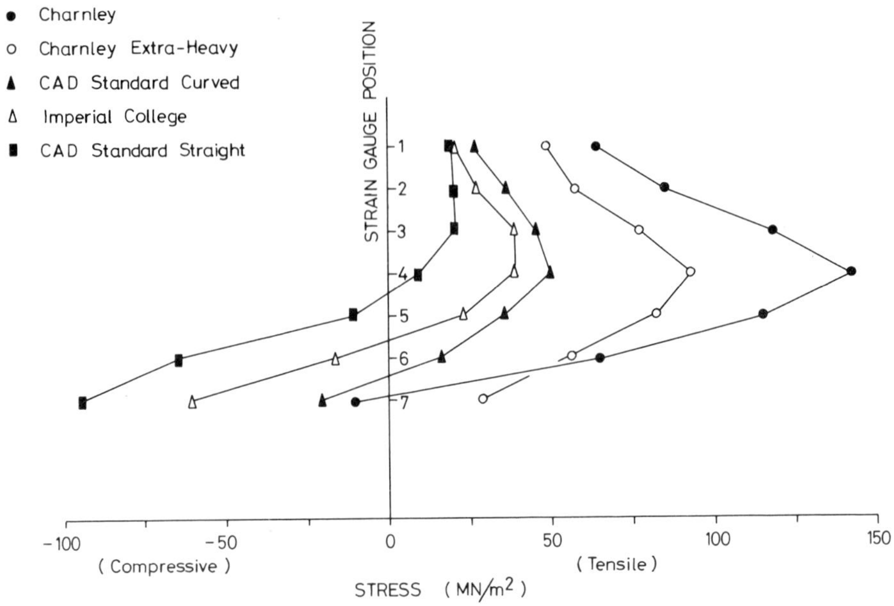

Fig. 2 Stress profiles with stems distally clamped.
Graph of stress magnitude against strain gauge position. Applied load of 4 KN

portion to the values shown in Fig. 2. For this reason the relative magnitudes of the stresses in the five stems provide a valid basis for comparison.

From the fatigue failure point of view the maximum tensile stress produced in each stem is the critical factor. The decreasing order of merit, with maximum tensile stresses in brackets, is therefore:

CAD Standard Straight (20 MN/m^2)
Imperial College (40 MN/m^2)
CAD Standard Curved (50 MN/m^2)
Charnley Extra-Heavy (95 MN/m^2)
Charnley (145 MN/m^2)

At any given load the maximum tensile stress produced in the CAD Standard Straight stem, under conditions of zero proximal support, will be a factor of 7.25 less than that produced in the Charnley stem; in the Imperial College stem a factor of 3.6 less; in the CAD Standard Curved stem a factor of 2.9 less; and in the Charnley Extra-Heavy a factor of 1.5 less.

Tensile stresses are produced on the lateral surface of the stems by the bending action of the applied load. For a given load the magnitude of the tensile stresses depends on the moment arm of the load about the stem and the resistance to bending offered by the shape of the stem cross-section. Three separate factors can therefore be identified to explain why the maximum tensile stress produced in the CAD Standard Straight stem is so much lower (by a factor of 7.25) than those produced in the Charnley stem. Firstly, the moment arm of the applied load about the proximal stem is reduced by the increased neck angle of the CAD Standard Straight stem. Secondly, the moment arm is further reduced by the decreased curvature, or "throw" of the stem itself. Thirdly, the cross-sectional area (more accurately the second moment of area) of the CAD Standard Straight stem is greater, and this gives an increased resistance to bending.

Each of the other three stems tested have some, but not all, of these stress-reducing design features. The CAD Standard Curved stem for example has a similar curvature/throw to the Charnley stem, but a greater neck angle and a larger cross-section combine to reduce the maximum tensile stress by a factor of 2.9. The Charnley Extra-Heavy stem has the same neck angle and curvature as the Charnley, so that the reduction in maximum tensile stress by a factor of 1.5 must be the result of a change in cross-sectional shape. It is relevant to note that the cobra-like flange on the Charnley Extra-Heavy stem does not extend down to the position of the maximum tensile stress. The flange does not, therefore, reduce the maximum tensile stress when the stem lacks proximal cement fixation.

Since the Imperial College stem has a similar curvature to the CAD Standard Curved stem and the same neck angle, the lower maximum tensile stress appears to result from the higher resistance to bending offered by the trapezoidal cross-section.

The high compressive stresses produced at the distal end of the CAD Standard Straight and the Imperial College stems are the direct result of reducing the moment arm of the applied load about the proximal stem. As Fig. 1 shows, design features which reduce the moment arm about the proximal stem increase the moment arm about the distal stem. Since the sense of the bending moment is reversed for the distal stem, bending produces compressive stresses on the lateral surface and tensile stresses on the medial surface. High tensile stresses at the medial surface of the distal stem are potentially dangerous from the fatigue point of view. However, the high stresses measured on the distal stems in this laboratory test are unlikely to occur in practice, since a situation where the stems are fixed only at the very tip seems unlikely to occur clinically.

It is more difficult to analyse the results of the second series of tests in which the five femoral components were cemented into post-mortem human femurs. The difficulty arises because there were undoubtedly differences, other than differences of stem design, in the five cases. For example, the femurs varied in size, and probably strength, there were differences in the positioning of the stems in the femurs, and there might also have been differences in the extent and integrity of the cement fixation.

Fig. 3 is a composite radiograph of the stems after insertion. It shows that the positioning of the stems was generally good, apart from the Imperial College stem and the CAD Standard Straight stem, both of which were in varus. Unfortunately, the radiopaque Simplex cement did not show up well in the radiographs, and for this reason each femur was split open after testing. In all cases the fixation appeared to be excellent. There was full cement packing between stems and bone, including those areas which appear to be lacking cement on the radiographs.

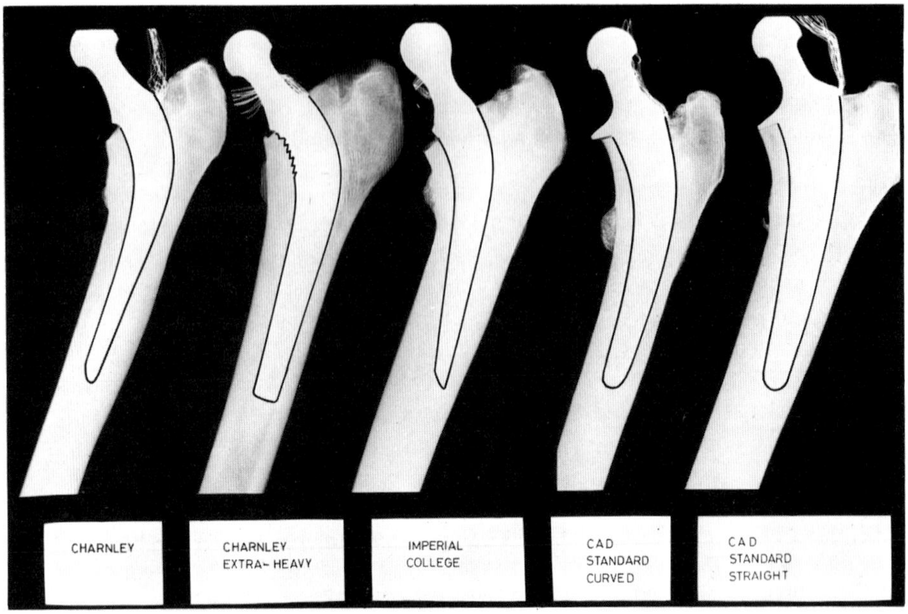

Fig. 3 Composite radiograph of the five stems cemented in bone (for clarity the stem profiles are outlined in ink)

Fig. 4 shows the results of this second series of tests with the stems cemented in bone and loaded to 4 KN. Table 1 compares the maximum tensile stress on each stem when distally clamped and when cemented in bone. Although the results of the second series of tests can only be considered as typical values, a number of interesting conclusions can be reached.

The first point to be made is that while the maximum tensile stress in the Charnley and Charnley Extra-Heavy stems were significantly lower when fully cemented in bone than when distally clamped, there was very little difference in the maximum tensile stress between the two tests for the other three stems. This general trend is predictable. In the case of a weak stem the reinforcing provided by cement and bone will be significant, and in the combined structure the cement and bone will carry a relatively high proportion of the applied load. In the case of a strong stem the addition of cement and bone will have less effect. The results shown in Table 1 illustrate this point. The maximum tensile stress in the distally clamped Charnley stem was over 100 per cent greater than when cemented. In the Charnley Extra-Heavy the maximum tensile stress was some 30 per cent greater without cement and bone support, and in the CAD Standard Curved approximately 10 per cent greater. With the Imperial College stem and the CAD Standard Straight stem the maximum tensile stress actually increased when cemented in bone, but this was almost certainly the result of the varus positioning of these stems. The increased moment arm produced by the varus positioning will produce an increased bending stress which could easily outweigh the relatively small increase in strength produced by the bone and cement. The varus positioning of the CAD Standard Straight and Imperial

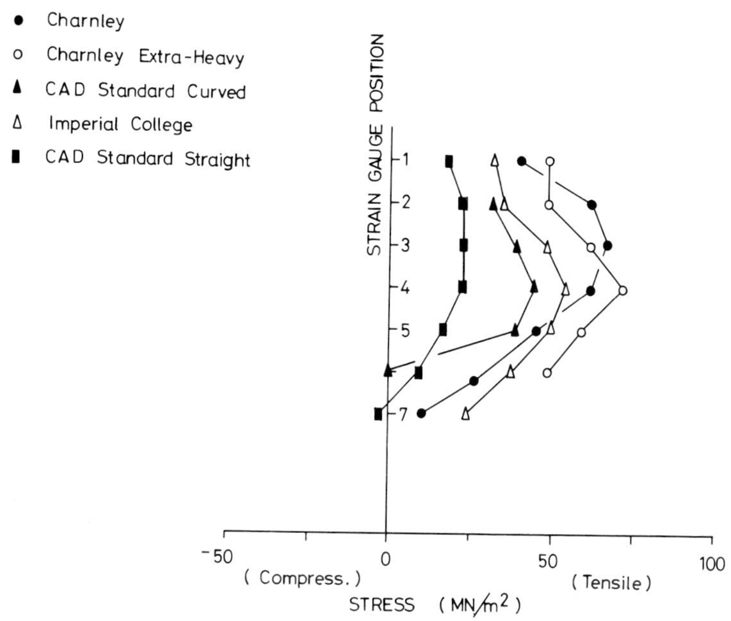

Fig. 4 Stress profiles with stems cemented in bone.
Graph of stress magnitude against strain gauge position. Applied load of 4 KN

Table 1 Comparison of peak tensile stresses with the stems distally clamped and cemented in bone

Stem	Test 1 Distally clamped	Test 2 Cemented in femur	
	Max. tensile stress (MN/m^2)	Max. tensile stress (MN/m^2)	Position
Charnley	145	68	good
Charnley Extra-Heavy	95	72	good
Imperial College	40	55	varus
CAD Standard Curved	50	45	good
CAD Standard Straight	20	22	varus

College stems also explains why high compressive stresses were not produced at the distal end of these stems as they were when the stems were distally clamped. That is, the moment arm about the proximal stem is increased by varus positioning while the moment arm about the distal stem is decreased.

The results of these tests suggest that the large neck collars on the CAD stems and the cobra-like flange on the Charnley Extra-Heavy stem have little or no effect on the stresses produced in the stems. The collars are designed to reduce the load and therefore the stress, on the stem by transferring part of the applied load directly to the cortical bone. The cobra-like flange aims to transfer part of the applied load directly to the cement, so by-passing the stem. If these design features had been effective, the tensile stresses in the stems would have been significantly lower when cemented in bone than when distally clamped. This is certainly not the case with the CAD stems, and although the stresses on the Charnley Extra-Heavy were reduced when the stem was implanted, the reduction can probably be explained by the reinforcing effect of the bone and cement.

The above results indicate that, of the commercially available femoral stems tested, the Howmedica CAD stems are the least likely to experience fatigue failure in vivo. Even with complete breakdown of proximal cement fixation the peak tensile stresses produced on the lateral surface of these stems by a load of 4 KN are remarkably low. Unfortunately, however, the observation that the peak stresses in these stems (and the Imperial College stem) were not significantly reduced when they were cemented in bone suggests a possible cause for concern. It appears that these stems are so stiff that most of the applied load is carried by the stem and very little by the cortical bone of the proximal femur. To the extent to which the normal turnover and remodelling of bone depends on mechanical stress (Wolff's Law), this could be a severe criticism. Wilson and Scales (8) have drawn attention to this problem. They state that disuse-atrophy of the calcar femoral and cervical stump can occur with a firmly cemented femoral component if the applied load is distributed to regions of bone distal to the transected neck of the femur. In the analysis of his nine and ten year results Charnley (3) found some bone resorption in 44 of the 93 cases available for follow-up. Although Charnley considered 3 to 4 mm of resorption to be the "normal" result of the interrupted blood supply, 20 cases out of the 93 showed more than 4 mm of bone resorption, and 3 showed more than 10 mm. It seems probable that in at least some of these cases resorption was the result of a decrease in the mechanical loading of the proximal femur. The problem of disuse-osteoporosis would be expected to increase with the use of stiffer stems such as the Howmedica designs, since the load, and therefore the stresses, in the proximal bone will be further reduced. Clearly more work to study the changes in stress levels produced in bone by the insertion of metallic stems is necessary. The results of such work might lead to an optimum design of stem which would minimize both fatigue failure of the stem and resorption of the bone.

REFERENCES

1. Charnley, J.: Stainless steel for femoral hip prostheses in combination with a high density polythene socket. Journal of Bone and Joint Surgery 53 B, 343 (1971)
2. Charnley, J.: Biomechanical considerations in total hip prosthetic design. In: The hip, Pub. St Louis: C.V. Mosby 1973
3. Charnley, J., Cupic, Z.: The nine and ten year results of the low-friction arthroplasty of the hip. Clinical Orthopaedics and Related Research 95, 9 (1973)
4. Charnley, J.: The histology of loosening between acrylic cement and bone. British Orthopaedic Research Society meeting held at The Nuffield Orthopaedic Centre, Oxford 1975
5. Galante, J.O., Rostoker, W., Doyle, J.M.: Failed femoral stems in total hip prostheses. Journal of Bone and Joint Surgery 57 A, 230 (1975)
6. Markolf, K.L., Amstutz, H.C.: A comparative experimental sudy of stresses in femoral total hip replacement components: The effects of prosthesis orientation and acrylic fixation. In Press, Journal of Biomechanics
7. Müller, M.E.: Total hip prostheses. Clinical Orthopaedics and Related Research 72, 46 (1970)
8. Wilson, J.N., Scales, J.T.: Loosening of total hip replacements with cement fixation. Clinical findings and laboratory studies. Clinical Orthopaedics and Related Research 72, 145 (1970)

MORPHOLOGICAL AND ANALYTICAL STUDIES OF THE TISSUES ADJACENT TO JOINT PROSTHESES: INVESTIGATIONS INTO THE CAUSES OF LOOSENING OF PROSTHESES

B. Vernon-Roberts and M.A.R. Freeman

Loosening of the prosthesis, an important cause of clinical failure following total joint replacement, may be due to faulty implantation of the prosthesis, to trauma, or to infection in the tissues adjacent to the implant. Many cases of loosening exist, however, in which the technique of implantation appears to have been satisfactory, in which there is no history of injury, and in which there is no evidence by conventional criteria of the presence of infection. Moreover, the very good results which are generally obtained immediately following total joint replacement are, regrettably, no guarantee of permanent success in the long term. Thus even if a prosthesis is firmly fixed for a short or long period after implantation, various factors can eventually lead to loosening at a later date. Clearly, at the forefront of any discussion of the causes of late prosthetic failure must be the consideration of the possible sequelae of the interaction between the body tissues and the implant materials used. It is for this reason that the biological reactions to implant materials have been actively studied in a number of centres in recent years. This chapter will attempt to review the findings in the light of current knowledge with particular regard to:

1. loosening of the bond between cement and bone,
2. reactions of the tissues to the products of wear and corrosion,
3. hypersensitivity to implant materials as a cause of prosthetic failure, and
4. the implications regarding the future design of prostheses, techniques of implantation, patient selection, and the early detection and treatment of late prosthetic failure.

LOOSENING OF THE BOND BETWEEN CEMENT AND BONE

CONSTITUENTS OF ACRYLIC CEMENTS

With the majority of total joint endoprostheses in use at the present time, one or both of the prosthetic components are fixed into bone using one of the self-curing acrylic cements. These cementing materials are essentially methylmethacrylates, and in situ polymerization is achieved by mixing powdered pre-polymerized methylmethacrylate with liquid monomer. An "initiator", usually a tertiary amine such as dimethylparatoluidine, is added to the monomer. The initiator reacts with a substance such as benzoyl peroxide which is added to the pre-polymerized methylmethacrylate as an "activator", and an activated form of the initiator then proceeds to induce the polymerization of the monomer. The reaction is exothermic and autocatalytic, takes several minutes to reach completion, and may attain temperatures in the region of 100 °C. During the polymerization process, the monomer dissolves the faces of the spheres up to 80 µm diameter which constitute the pre-polymerized methylmethacrylate and binds them into a single block by polymerization of the monomer (24). Between 2 and 5 % of the monomer is not polymerized (4, 18). Benzoyl peroxide also remains in the mixture after polymerization (28).

THE NORMAL REACTION OF BONE TO ACRYLIC CEMENT IMPLANTS IN MAN

The early and late histopathological changes in the bone adjoining acrylic cement bonding endoprostheses in place in man have been carefully studied and described by Willert and his colleagues (23, 24, 25). The findings of the present author are in general agreement with those of Willert and his co-workers who consider that the tissue reaction passes through the following three phases:

1. an initial phase lasting from the time of implantation to three weeks after operation,
2. a reparative phase commencing during the third week after operation and lasting for up to two years, and
3. a phase of stabilization beginning one to two years after operation.

While this division of the tissue reaction to implants into these phases aids the understanding of the underlying pathological processes, there are very wide variations in the duration of these phases in individual cases.

In the initial phase, there is no mobility between the cement and bone irrespective of whether the surface of the cement is relatively smooth or has multiple nodules projecting into the implant bed when examined macroscopically. However, in the author's personal experience cement surfaces having multiple protruding plugs of cement are more difficult to remove from the bone bed, and this suggests that they are more firmly bonded into the bone than is the case when the cement surface is relatively smooth. Where plugs of cement are present, they fit into spaces having a similar shape in the adjoining body tissues. When the implant bed is examined histologically, the most striking finding is the presence of a zone of dead bone and marrow tissue extending up to 5 mm from the cement surface (Fig. 1). A less constant finding is the presence of larger areas of necrosis of the cancellous bone, and necrosis of the compact cortical bone. The distribution of the dead bone indicates that the constantly-occurring zone of necrosis immediately surrounding the implant results from reaming, from heat produced during polymerization, from toxic effects of non-polymerized monomer, or from a combination of these factors; the death of other areas of the cancellous bone and of cortical bone away from the implant cannot be ascribed to the properties of the cement and clearly must be the result of interruption of the vascular supply to those areas by the operative procedure (Figs. 2a, 2b). At the junction between dead and living bone, there is reactive hyperaemia, exudation of inflammatory cells, proliferation of capillaries, and the appearance of fibroblasts, osteoclasts and osteoblasts; these are, of course, the characteristic initial

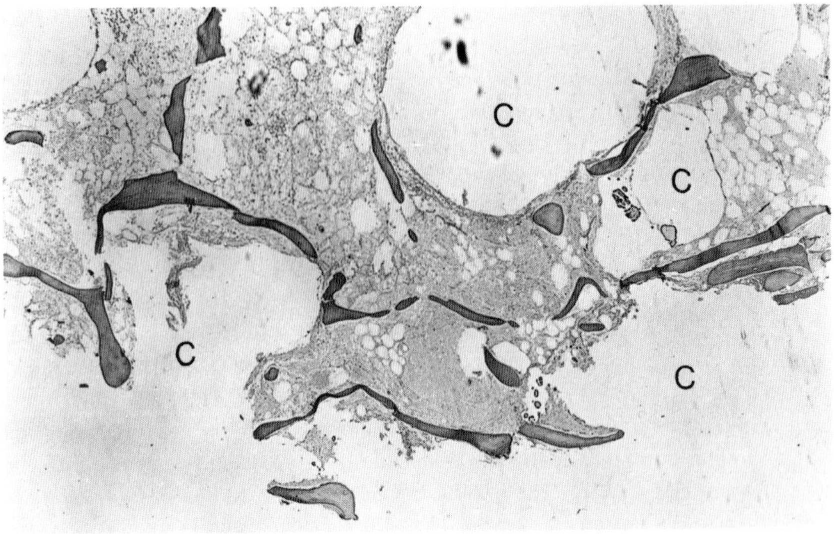

Fig. 1 Implant bed 10 days after implantation. The trabecular bone and bone marrow adjoining the cement (C) is all dead. Spaces in the tissues are occupied by cement masses separate from the cement bonding the prosthesis in place. Haematoxylin-eosin (x 15)

reactions of the living vascularized body tissues to any zone of necrosis, and, as such, are identical with the initial reaction to a bone infarct from any cause. These histological changes, therefore, herald the onset of the reparative phase of the normal reaction to the implant. During the initial phase and the early part of the reparative phase, the cement

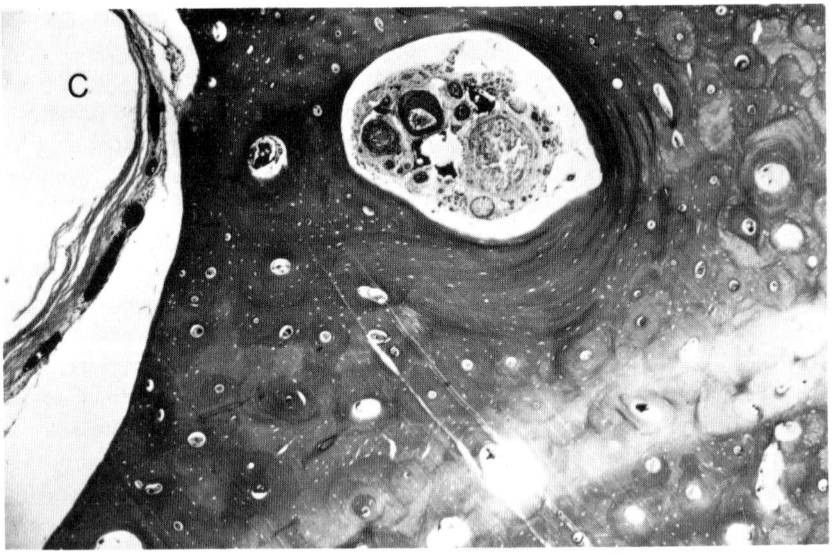

Fig. 2a Cortical bone separated from cement (C) by layer of fibrous tissue 1 year after implantation. The cortical bone exhibits death of bone around a vascular channel. Haematoxylin-eosin (x 50)

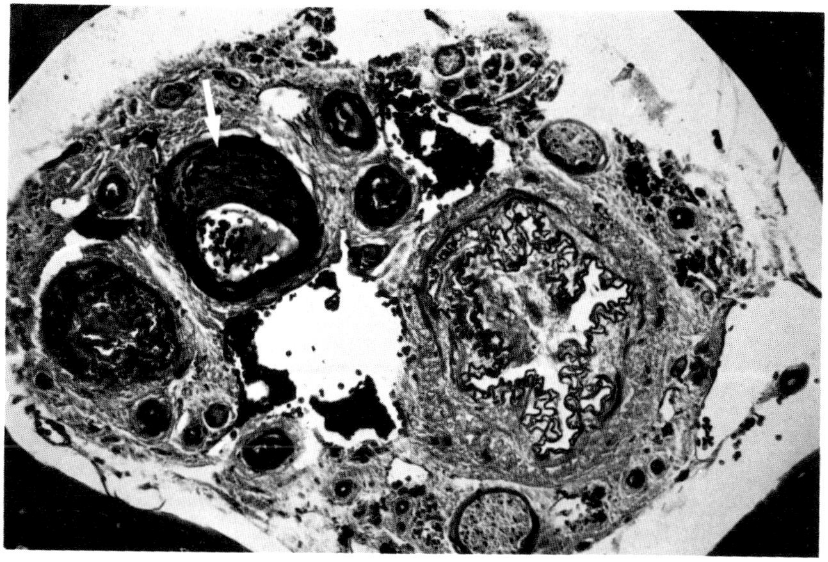

Fig. 2b Higher magnification of vascular channel shown in Fig. 2a. Shows dead original blood vessels and ingrowth of new artery (arrow) (x 120)

is obviously in contact only with dead tissue. Whether the cement surface is smooth or nodular at the macroscopic level, at the microscopic level the cement surface has the outline of large and small smooth-surfaced nodules indenting the necrotic tissues and with separate discrete "acrylic pearls" (spheres of cement up to 80 μm in diameter) lying singly or aggregated together in the necrotic tissues adjacent to the main cement mass (Fig. 1).

During the reparative phase there is progressive invasion of the dead bone by vascular granulation tissue bringing with it scavenger cells to remove the dead bone and marrow, and connective tissue cells to lay down new bone and fibrous tissue. Dead bone is removed by the activity of osteoclasts, although some dead trabeculae may gain a covering of new living bone and persist for a long period as "composite" trabeculae having cores composed of dead bone (Fig. 3); these composite trabeculae may persist for several years in the tissue immediately adjacent to the cement surface. In some cases, there is marked buttressing of dead trabeculae with nodular coverings of new bone which occurs soon after implantation at the junction of dead and living bone (Fig. 4), although it would appear that these are eventually remodelled to form normal trabeculae. At the border between the cement and implant bed, the cement is separated from the living tissue by a membranous acellular layer which may be exceedingly thin and delicate (Fig. 5) and has the appearance of fibrin; more commonly, there is an additional layer of collagenized fibrous tissue up to 1 mm thick separating the cement from the other tissues (Fig. 6). On occasions, parts of the surface abutting on to the cement are lined by numerous foreign-body giant cells (Fig. 7a) which may sometimes be seen to contain intracellular small spherules having the appearances of pre-polymerized methylmethacrylate (Fig. 7b). In this author's experience, living bone and haemopoietic tissues do not have contact

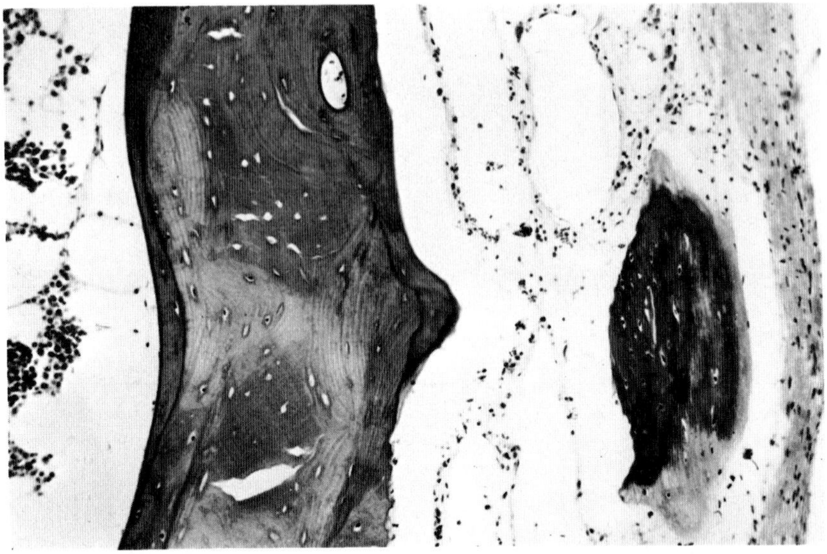

Fig. 3 Implant bed 2 years after implantation. Fibrous tissue separating cement from bone is at right of micrograph. Shows "composite" trabecula having central core of dead bone (note empty osteocyte lacunae) surrounded by living bone. Haematoxylin-eosin (x 120)

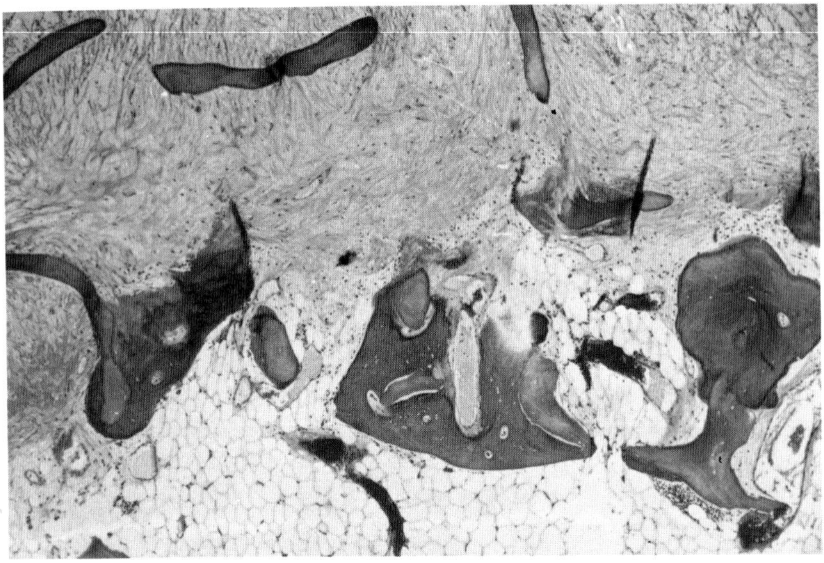

Fig. 4 Implant bed 1 year after implantation. The bone and bone marrow in the upper half of the micrograph is dead. Shows buttressing of dead trabeculae by surface apposition of new bone at the junction of living and dead tissue. Haematoxylin-eosin (x 50)

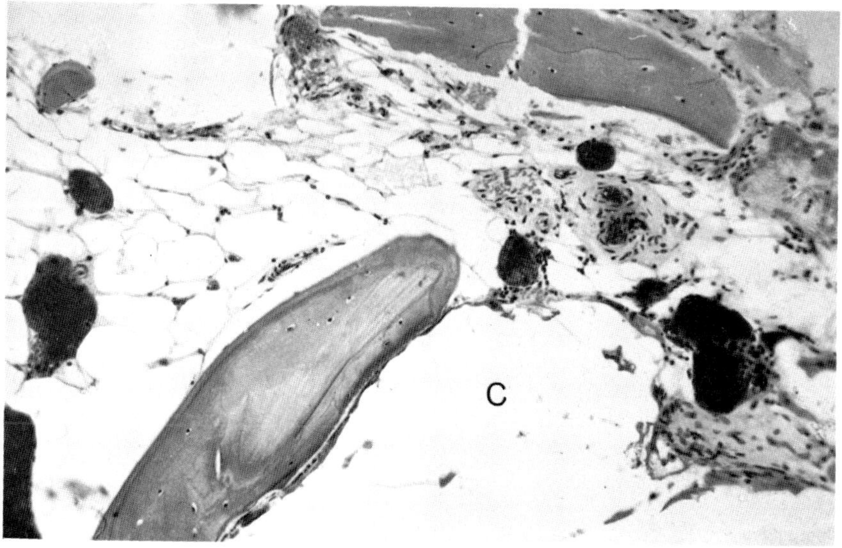

Fig. 5 Implant bed 1 year after implantation. Cement (C) is separated from the bone by a thin acellular layer. Haematoxylin-eosin (x 120)

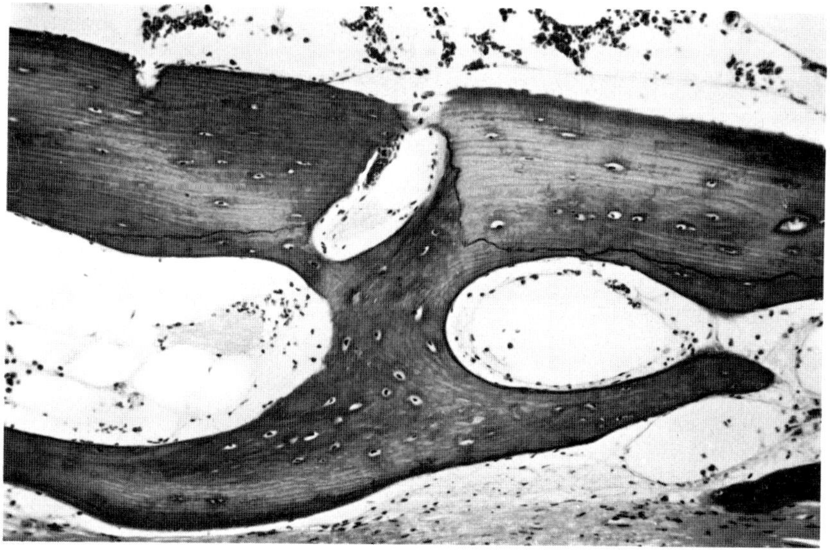

Fig. 6 Implant bed 1 year after implantation. Bone is separated from cement by the layer of heavily-collagenized fibrous tissue seen at the bottom of the micrograph. Haematoxylin-eosin (x 120)

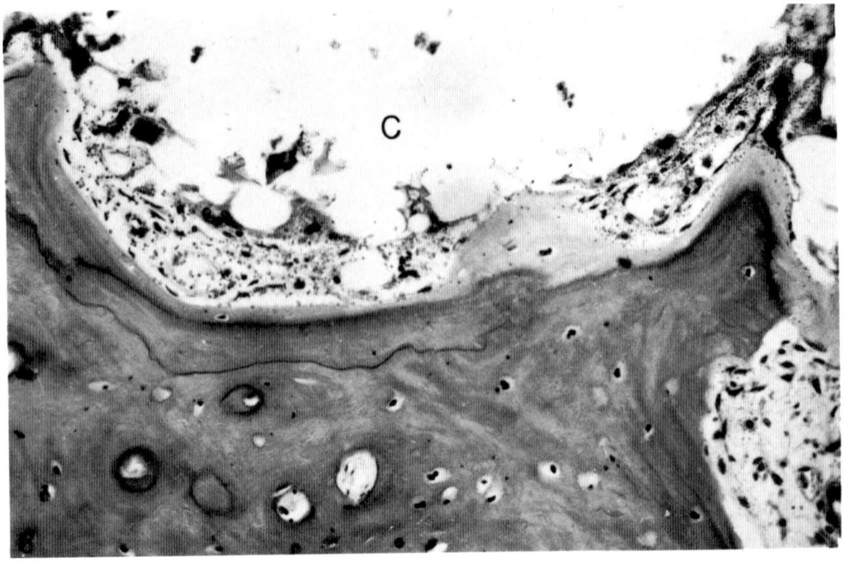

Fig. 7a Numerous giant cells in contact with cement (C) at cement-bone interface 1 year after implantation. Haematoxylin-eosin (x 50)

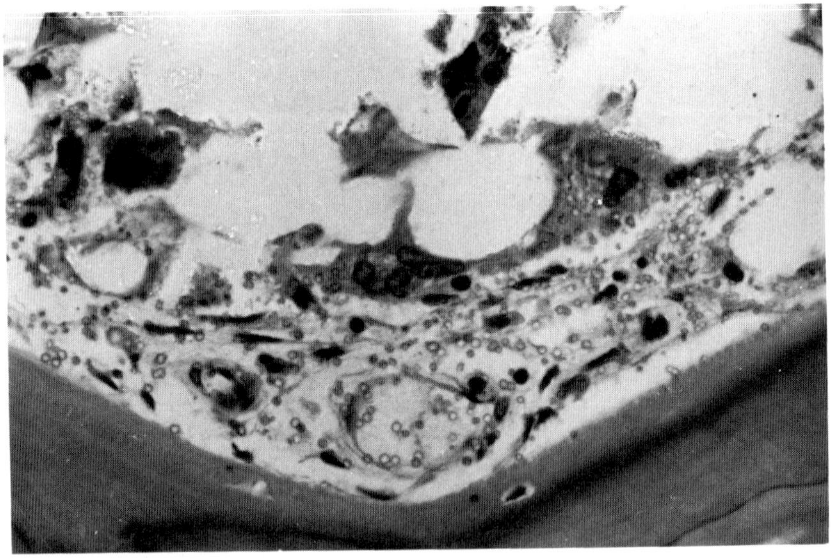

Fig. 7b Higher magnification of part of field shown in Fig. 7a. Shows numerous spherules in giant cells and tissues in interface region (x 400)

with the cement surface and remain separated from it by at least a very thin fibrinous layer a few microns in thickness. In the tissues adjacent to the cement, the discrete acrylic pearls (Fig. 8) become surrounded by multinucleate giant cells which frequently form a syncytium having few visible cell boundaries. In this area, there is also very active bone formation and remodelling, fibrous tissue formation, occasional hyaline cartilage formation, perivascular lymphocytic infiltrates (Fig. 9), and foamy macrophages and multinucleate giant cells containing acrylic cement and removing necrotic fatty marrow (Fig. 10). Haemopoietic marrow may appear early during the repair process, and may come to lie very close to the cement surface (Fig. 11). Small foci of necrotic bone and marrow tissue not infrequently persist without evidence of further efforts at repair, but these do not appear significantly to affect the stability of the implant, providing the implant has been firmly anchored into place.

The repair process proceeds until all (or almost all) the necrotic tissues have been replaced by living bone and soft tissues. Eventually, a stable state is established between the implant and its bed, and the implant may therefore be considered to be healed into place during a phase of stabilization which begins one to two years after operation (23). The "permanent" implant bed is composed of a thin "membrane" of fibrin in immediate contact with the cement with or without a surrounding layer of collagenized fibrous tissue up to 1.5 mm thick (Fig. 12). The discrete acrylic pearls persist and are surrounded by a thin syncytium of multinucleate giant cells and are often embedded in fibrous tissue. Other multinucleate giant cells may contain particles of cement. Scattered foci of perivascular lymphocytes may be present in the tissues close to the cement, but inflammatory cells are generally sparse and vascularity is minimal. The granulation tissue occupying the marrow spaces during the reparative phase becomes replaced by normal haemopoietic

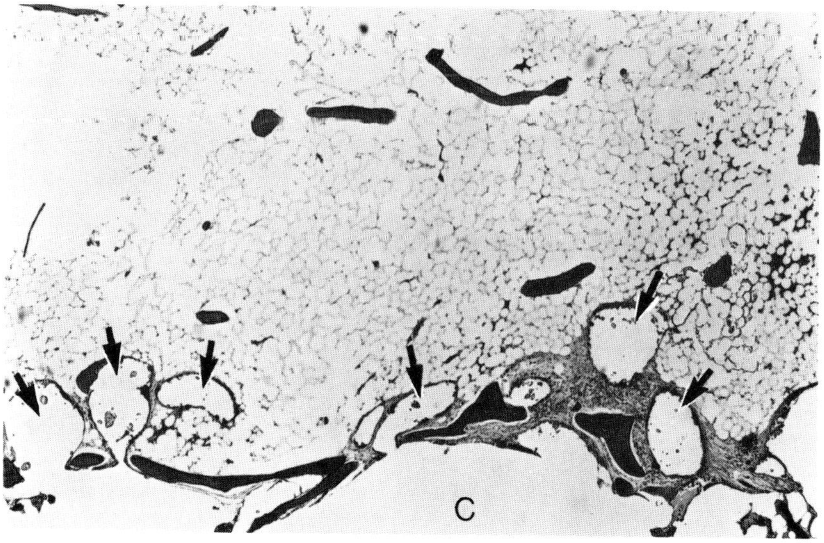

Fig. 8 Implant bed 10 months after implantation. Shows spaces (arrows) occupied by spheres of cement, some of which are extensions of the main cement mass (C). Haematoxylin-eosin (x 15)

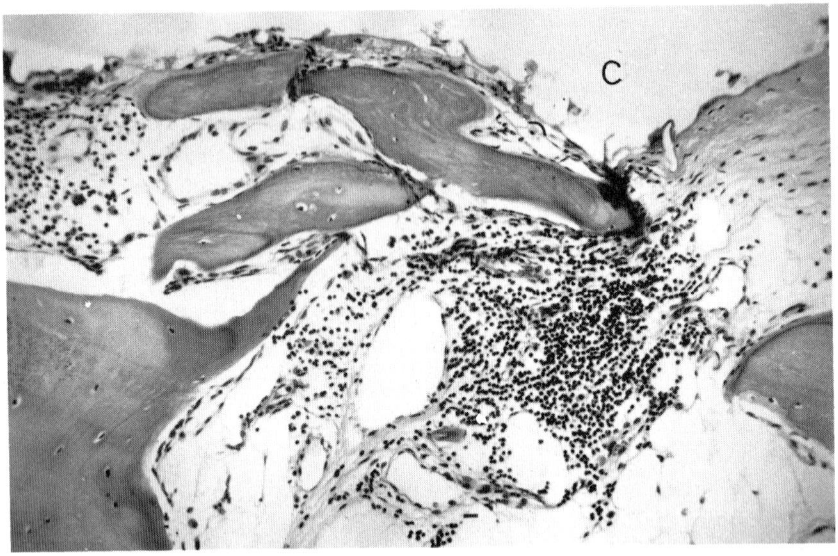

Fig. 9 Perivascular lymphocytic infiltration in soft tissue adjacent to cement (C) 1 year after implantation. Haematoxylin-eosin (x 120)

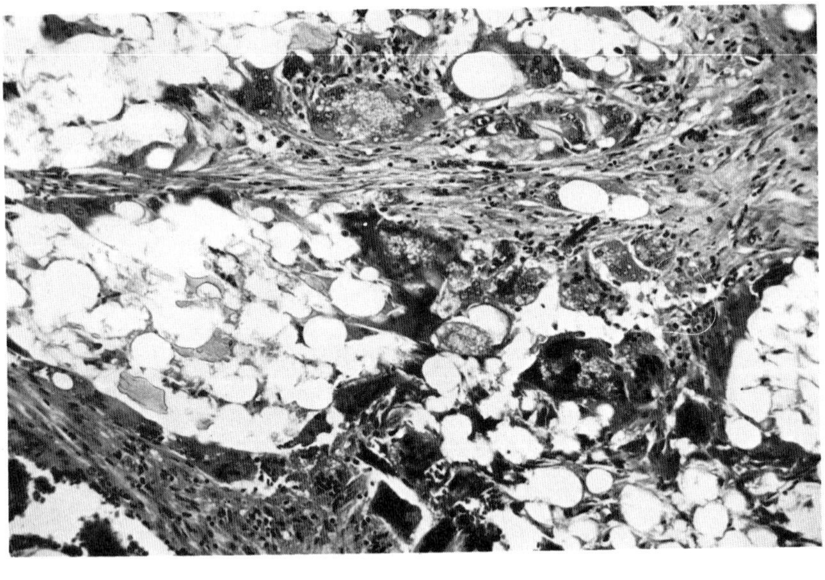

Fig. 10 Large numbers of multinucleate giant cells containing acrylic cement fragments and removing necrotic fatty marrow in implant bed surrounding a painful prosthesis 1 year after implantation. Haematoxylin-eosin (x 120)

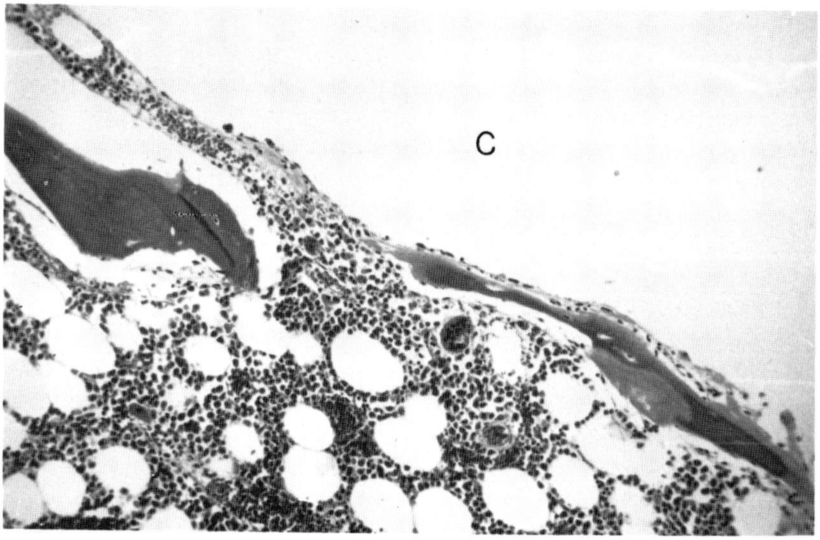

Fig. 11 Haemopoietic marrow lying close to cement (C) surface 2 years after implantation. Haematoxylin-eosin (x 120)

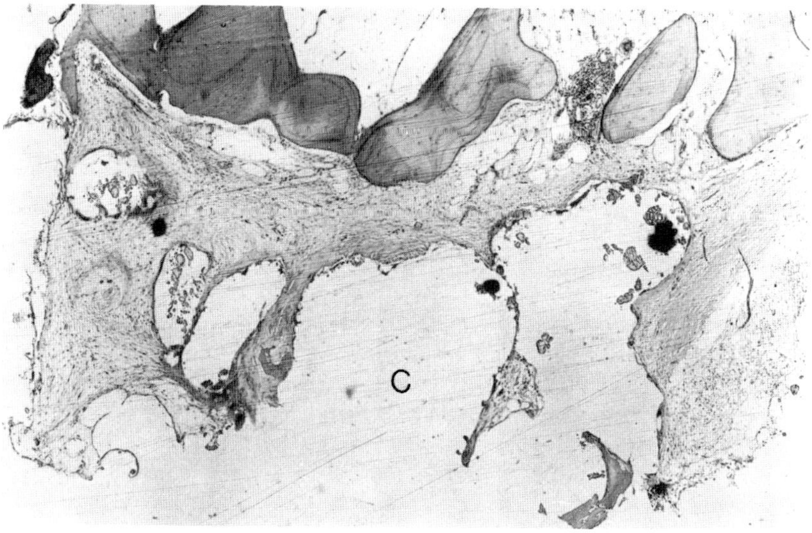

Fig. 12 Implant bed 2 years after implantation. Shows cement (C) separated from bone by a thick layer of fibrous tissue containing some isolated spheres of cement. Haematoxylin-eosin (x 30)

and fatty marrow. The dead bone and woven repair bone of the reparative phase is also replaced by healthy lamellar trabecular bone; initially, many of the trabeculae are orientated perpendicularly to the cement surface, but eventually those nearest the cement frequently become orientated parallel to the cement surface (Fig. 13). In some cases, there is a marked loss of trabecular bone from the area between the trabeculae encircling the cement and the inner region of the cortex, the inner and outer bone being apparently linked by occasional radially-orientated trabeculae (Fig. 13).

THE NORMAL BOND BETWEEN CEMENT AND BONE

As Willert (23) has pointed out, certain features of the tissue reaction around bone cement are important with respect to a lasting fixation of the endoprosthesis. There is little doubt that a firm bond between the cement and the implant bed is based upon close congruity between the cement surface and the bone, that is, between the bone trabeculae of the cancellous bone and with the inner surface of the cortex. However, it is clear that the cement does not remain in close contact with the surface reamed out during the implantation procedure, since, as stated previously, a zone of necrotic bone is always present around the cement immediately after implantation. This dead bone is removed and then replaced by new living bone during the reparative phase which follows, and the new bone tends to

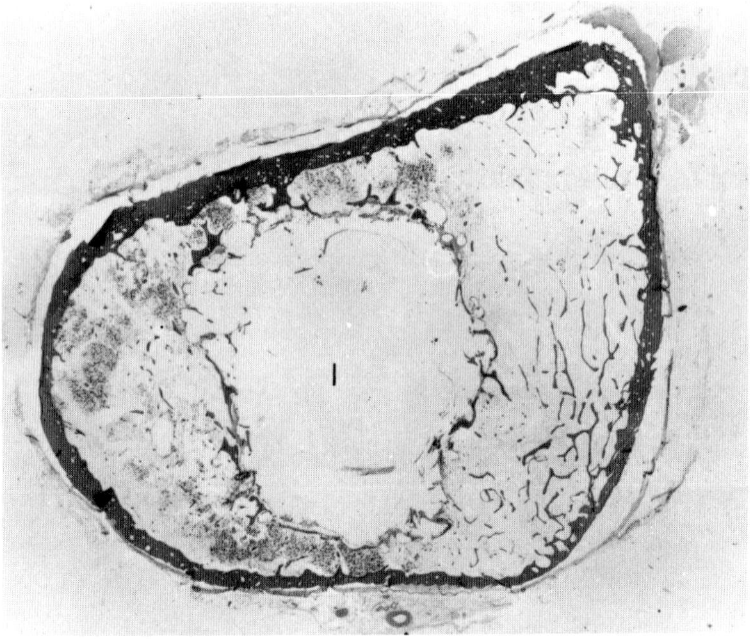

Fig. 13 Section through shaft of femur of patient who died 2 years after implantation. The implant (I) was stable. The trabeculae nearest the cement are orientated parallel to the cement surface. The remainder of the cancellous bone is porotic. The cortex is united to the trabeculae around the implant by a few radially orientated trabeculae. Haematoxylin-eosin (x 4)

form a shell around the cement with new trabeculae radiating towards the inner cortex. Although the new living bone which surrounds the cement is in close contact with it, the contact is not likely to exert the degree of pressure exerted immediately following implantation when the fresh cement has been pressed firmly against the bone anchoring the implant in place. Moreover, the cement is normally eventually separated from the adjacent bone by a layer of fibrous tissue (Fig. 12) which would appear to be capable of allowing some degree of movement between the prosthesis and its bed and thereby acts as a type of shock-absorber protecting the surrounding trabeculae from sudden stresses. The changes in the direction of the trabeculae from the initial disposition at implantation to their orientation when a state of stability has been reached, supports the view that there is a change in the direction of stresses transmitted through the bone; the frequent appearance of osteoporotic areas (Fig. 13) also favours this concept of changes in forces within the bone. These changes in the implant bed which accompany repair and stabilization are unlikely to improve the firmness of implantation; on the contrary, it would seem that the implant is most firmly anchored immediately after fixation and declines thereafter.

From the above considerations, according to Willert (23) it would seem that the greatest care must be directed towards the optimal fixation of the prosthetic components at the time of implantation, so that a part of the bond between cement and bone guarantees stability even if other parts of the bone are subjected to resorption and remodelling. The fact that the majority of endoprostheses function satisfactorily for many years without loosening, indicates that the changes described do not necessarily lead to the fixation being insufficient to meet the routine mechanical stresses of everyday life. It would therefore appear likely that additional factors must be brought to bear to bring about loosening of the bond between the cement and the surrounding tissues.

LOOSENING OF THE BOND BETWEEN CEMENT AND BONE

The factors which overload the bond could be insufficient contact between cement and bone or incomplete filling of the prepared implant bed by the use of insufficient cement, faulty positioning of the implant, high friction between the prosthetic components, excessive mechanical stresses occasioned during physical activity, and an increase in bodyweight. It is clear that, in practice, all reasonable attempts are made to exclude these factors since once the process of loosening has commenced it cannot be arrested.

Pathological studies of implants which became loose have shown that differences exist between early and late loosening. Willert et al. (25) examined the implant beds from five cases in which loosening had occurred within two years of operation, and found that there was increased removal and remodelling of bone. The question which clearly arises is, what is the cause and effect of the initial bone death in early loosening? The constant finding of a zone of dead bone immediately surrounding the cement following implantation has been previously described, together with the occasional finding of larger areas of necrotic cancellous or compact bone. While the latter changes are almost certainly the result of operative interference with the vascular supply to those areas, the cause of bone necrosis immediately surrounding the implant is less clear. It has been reported that the polymerization of self-curing acrylic resins in the marrow cavity of the rabbit femur is followed by the necrosis of bone surrounding the cement and extending to include up to one-third of the thickness of the inner cortex (16, 29); however, the bone necrosis observed in these studies was unlikely to be due to toxic reactions to free monomer or to heat produced during polymerization, since studies in the sheep have shown that, although up to one-third of the inner cortex of the femur dies during polymerization of self-curing acrylic resin in a reamed cavity, bone death occurs to the same extent after reaming alone or after reaming and packing the cavity with bone wax warmed to a temperature of 70 °C (3). The findings therefore indicate that all bone death occurring in the initial phase is due to interference with blood supply.

While, in the early stages after implantation, the cement is firmly anchored to surrounding dead bone, the dead bone is removed and then replaced by new living bone during the ensuing repair reaction. The extent of initial bone death largely determines the length of time which it takes to replace dead bone with new living bone. In the situation where extensive bone death has occurred following the implantation procedure, it is therefore likely that the cement remains anchored to dead bone for a prolonged period. Recent animal studies suggest that the bone of the experimentally infarcted femoral head exhibits marked changes in mechanical behaviour under applied stresses (20, 21), and indicates that dead bone may be more prone to fatigue failure than living bone. Thus, the situation can be envisaged in which prosthetic implants become loose in the early stages (within one to two years) because of the fatigue failure of dead trabeculae transmitting the stresses between cement and living bone. Bone death occurring at a later stage, after removal of dead bone and its replacement with living bone, could, for similar fatigue failure reasons, give rise to late loosening. The possible role of reactions to products of abrasion and corrosion in bone death and loosening are discussed in a later section but it is relevant now to examine the possible role of reactions to the cement when considering the causes of late loosening.

In cases of late loosening occurring more than two years after implantation, there are tears in the permanent implant bed with haemorrhages and fibrinous exudates in the connective tissues surrounding the cement and there is bone resorption (25). Once firm fixation is lost, loosening is usually progressive. Once loosening is marked, the cement is frequently fragmented. Bone resorption tends to occur earlier and to be more marked near to the articulating surfaces of the prosthesis; breakage of the shaft of the prosthesis may therefore occur because the distal part of the shaft is firmly anchored while the proximal part is unsupported due to loss of bone and cement.

The role in early and late loosening of the acrylic pearls constantly seen in the implant bed is speculative. Their morphological appearances by scanning electron microscopy have been described by Willert et al. (25) who found that they may become dispersed more than 0.5 cm from the cement surface. They may solely indicate improper curing of the bone cement; and Willert et al. (25) postulated that acrylic pearls found in the tissues around implants undergoing early loosening might be the result of a relative lack of monomer during the curing process due to, for example, an excess of monomer becoming dissolved in the surrounding adipose tissue during polymerization (24). Another possible factor in loosening is sensitivity to the cement, since it has been shown that it is possible to induce skin sensitization using acrylic monomer although there is a marked lack of agreement in the results obtained (4). Moreover, although Evans et al. (6) were unable to detect skin sensitivity to cement components in patients having loose prostheses, the possibility of sensitivity to methacrylate playing a part in loosening clearly merits further study. Another possible cause of loosening might be that the mechanical properties of acrylic change with time. While acrylic plastics are strong but brittle, they have good fatigue properties. There is some evidence that abrasion of the cement surface takes place at the interface between the cement and the prosthesis (28).

The majority of evidence at the present time indicates that early loosening of the bond between cement and bone occurs because the reamed cavity around the prosthesis is not properly filled with cement at operation. Early or intermediate stage loosening may also occur because widespread bone death takes place at the time of operation, and the dead bone then undergoes fatigue failure before its replacement by new living bone can be accomplished. Loosening in the absence of unusual overloads at any stage, and particularly after stabilization has apparently been achieved, may well in the majority of cases be the end-result of tissue reactions including hypersensitivity to products of wear and corrosion of the articulating surfaces of the prosthesis. It is clearly important that the tissue reactions to the products of wear and corrosion should therefore be considered in some detail.

TISSUE REACTIONS TO THE PRODUCTS OF WEAR AND CORROSION

WEAR AND CORROSION

Some degree of wear of the bearing surfaces of total joint replacements is inevitable. Particulate products of wear are thus formed from the bearing surfaces of both metal and plastic components, but the degree and rate of wear differs markedly between different types of prosthesis and in different patients.

Corrosion of metal components and of metallic wear particles leads to the formation of soluble and insoluble compounds. Studies of the metal levels in tissues surrounding implanted cylinders have shown that the constituent metals of cobalt-chrome and stainless steel are detectable in the tissues four to six months after implantation (7), and this indicates that wear is not essential for metal release. Moreover, Coleman et al. (5) found that in nine patients with prostheses composed of cobalt-chrome articulating with cobalt-chrome, both blood and urinary cobalt and chromium levels were persistently raised: by contrast, they were unable to detect a significant elevation of blood and urinary cobalt and chromium in three patients with cobalt-chrome articulating against high density polyethylene. This clinical observation was in agreement with the findings of Swanson et al. (19) who showed that in laboratory simulators prostheses in which both components were composed of cobalt-chrome, the alloy released both cobalt and chromium into the solution bathing them during the test; metal release could not be detected when cobalt-chrome or stainless steel was articulated against high density polyethylene.

In all patients who have joint endoprostheses the situation therefore exists in which components of the endoprostheses are being liberated into the body tissues by wear and corrosion. It is thus important to examine the nature of the tissue reactions to metallic and plastic materials, with particular attention to the possible role of these materials in pain and loosening.

MORPHOLOGY OF TISSUE REACTIONS TO PARTICLES CONTAINING METAL AND TO PARTICLES OF POLYETHYLENE

There have been a number of recent studies describing the cellular reactions to the products of wear and corrosion in the connective tissues of the joint cavity (6, 17, 23, 25, 30). The morphological findings described are in general agreement and are summarized below.

Following the implantation of a prosthesis, if the original articular capsule has been excised, a new fibrous connective tissue capsule is formed around the articulating parts of the prosthesis. Whether the joint is surrounded by the original capsule or a new capsule, the general structure of the lining soon resembles synovial membrane and may continue to do so for a long period. However, it is now evident that the morphology of the connective tissues internal to the joint capsule and lying in close proximity to the endoprosthesis may undergo marked changes associated with the presence of foreign material in those tissues. When these changes are present to the most marked degree, the most striking feature is the presence of large sheets of macrophages and multinucleate giant cells (Fig. 14) which may be arranged in nodules separated by thick or thin bands of fibrous

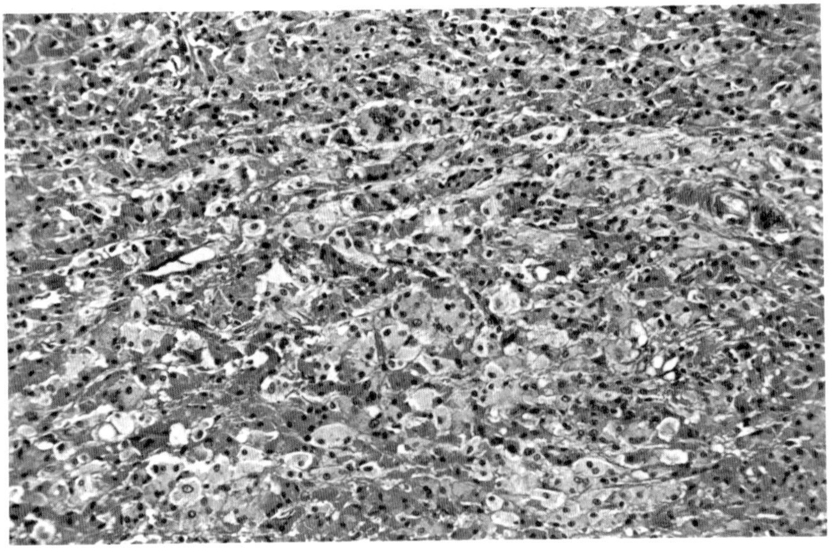

Fig. 14 Sheet of macrophages and giant cells in articular tissues 15 months after implantation of a cobalt-chrome against high-density polyethylene knee prosthesis which became painful. Haematoxylin-eosin (x 120)

tissue. Not infrequently, there are also some lymphocytes and plasma cells among the macrophages, particularly around blood vessels; occasional neutrophil and eosinophil polymorphs may also be observed but they are not a marked or constant feature. Using a combination of ordinary light and polarized light microscopy it is easy to see that the macrophages and giant cells constituting this tissue reaction contain variable quantities of foreign material. The foreign material which may be visualized is of three types (Table 1):

1. Metal-containing particles appear as discrete and distinct brown-black or black granules, rods and needles up to 3 μm maximum dimension (Fig. 15a) which are strongly birefringent when viewed between crossed polars (Fig. 15b).
2. Polyethylene particles are not visible in ordinary transmitted light, but are strongly birefringent when viewed between crossed polars. The presence of smaller particles may be revealed by a diffuse intracytoplasmic birefringence (Figs. 16a, 16b), but larger fragments are in the form of granules, spears, splinters, ovoids and rectangles up to 50 μm in maximum dimension (Figs. 17a, 17b).
3. Acrylic cement fragments are commonly seen, sometimes in large quantity, the size of the particles varying up to several millimetres in maximum dimension. They are usually seen in the form of "acrylic pearls" which may be clustered together and frequently embedded in fibrous tissue (Fig. 18) with each pearl having a diameter of up to 80 μm. They appear to provoke a predominantly giant cell reaction, with the giant cells forming a syncytium having ill-defined cell boundaries. The particles may also be present as granules, splinters and irregular fragments. Polymethylmethacrylate is distinguished from metal and polyethylene by the fact that it is readily soluble in the solvents used in normal tissue processing procedures, and its location is therefore indicated by empty spaces in the tissues and cells. When present, it is only weakly birefringent when viewed between crossed polars.

The macrophages and giant cells comprising the tissue reaction around prostheses frequently contain large amounts of iron which becomes visible when sections are examined after staining by the Perls technique. Winter (30) visually assessed the iron content in the tissues from around 44 cobalt-chrome implants and 44 stainless steel implants, and formed the opinion that about 50 % of the cobalt-chrome cases contained iron to a minor degree only, while 75 % of stainless steel cases contained iron, which was frequently present in large amounts: he concluded that haemosiderinlike granules are a specific feature of the tissue reaction to stainless steel implants. The present author is unable to agree with the conclusions of Winter (30), and has found very large amounts of iron in the macrophages reacting to both cobalt-chrome and stainless steel implants in a high proportion of cases, and has found haemosiderin-type granules in the tissues reacting to cobalt-chrome. Moreover, there are frequently large amounts of iron in the cells reacting to polyethylene particles despite the fact that metal analysis reveals very low levels of cobalt, chrome and nickel in the tissues. The significance of the frequent presence of large amounts of iron in the tissue reactions to prosthetic implants is at present obscure since the iron deposition could be the result of haemoglobin breakdown following bleeding due to operative trauma or, more likely, repeated trauma to the articular tissues following implantation. In this connection, large amounts of iron, sometimes amounting to haemosiderosis of the tissues, are a frequent finding in rheumatoid synovial tissues (14,15) and this is thought to result from the constant oozing of blood into the joint cavity.

Table 1 Light microscopic appearances of intracellular foreign material in tissues adjacent to joint prostheses

Prosthesis material	Type of tissue reaction				Morphology of intracellular material	Maximum dimensions of particles	Birefringence
	Macrophages	Giant cells	Necrosis	Fibrosis			
Metal (cobalt-chrome or stainless steel)	++++	++	++++	++	black granules, rods and needles	0.1 – 3.0 /um	strong-granules, rods and needles
Polyethylene	+++	++++	–	++++	colourless	0.5 – 50 /um	strong-diffuse intracellular mottling, spears, splinters, sheets
Polymethyl-methacrylate	++	++++	–	+	empty spaces * in form of spheres, ovoids and splinters	0.5 – 80 /um	very weak

* readily soluble in solvents used in routine processing

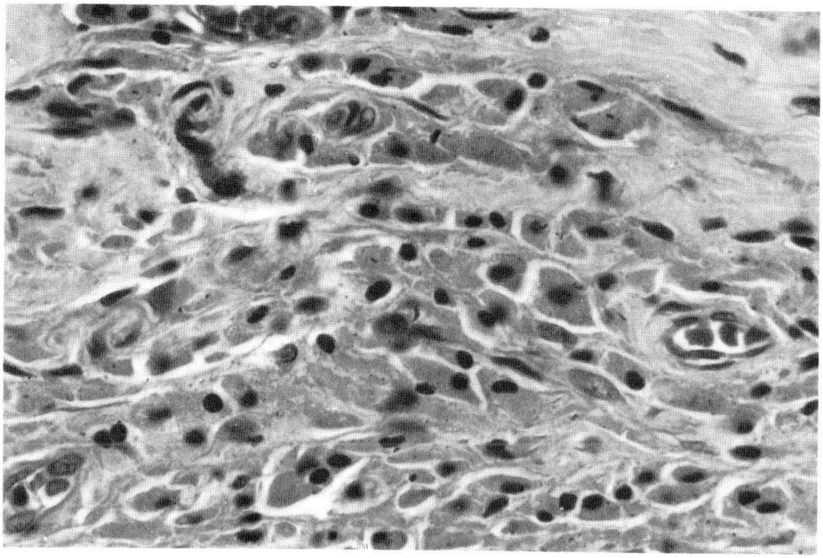

Fig. 15a Numerous small black metallic particles in macrophages and giant cells in articular tissues 1 year after implantation of an all-cobalt-chrome knee prosthesis which became persistently painful. Haematoxylin-eosin (x 400)

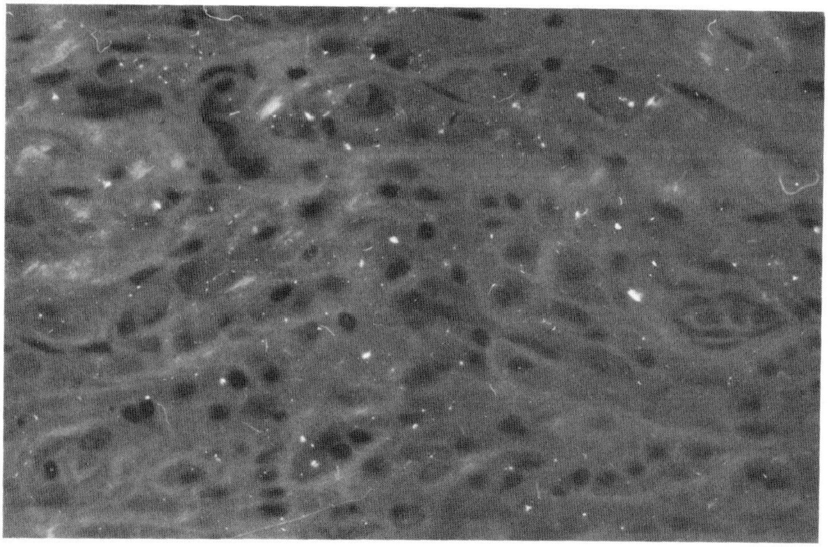

Fig. 15b Same field as Fig. 15a viewed between crossed polars. Shows strong birefringence of the intracellular crystalline particles

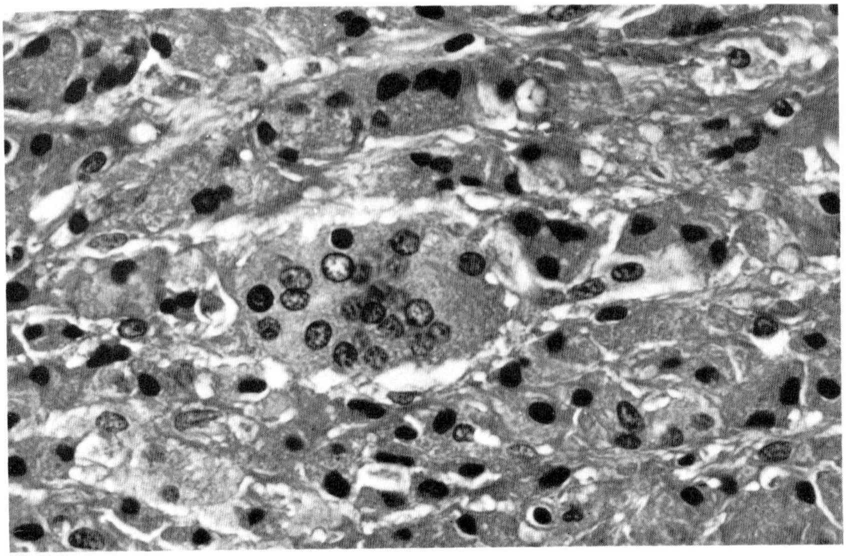

Fig. 16a Macrophage and giant cell reaction in articular tissues 15 months after implantation of a cobalt-chrome against high density polyethylene knee prosthesis which became painful. No intracellular material is visible. Haematoxylin-eosin (x 400)

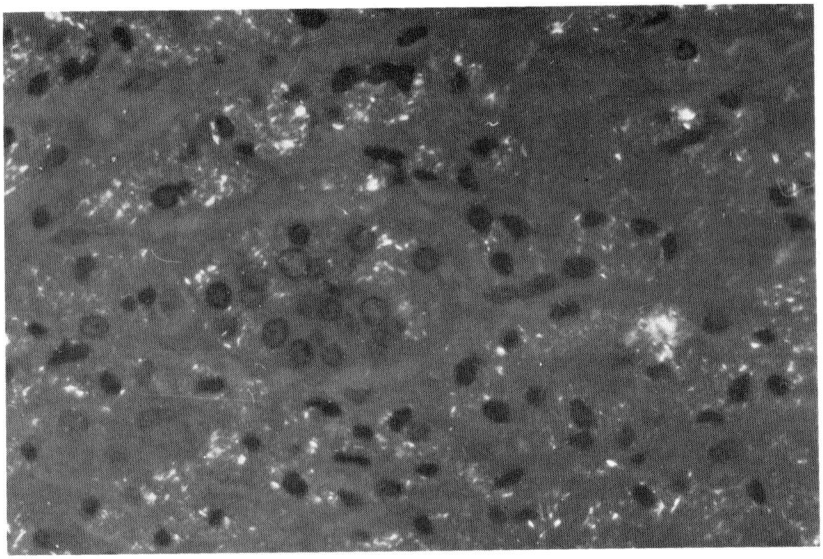

Fig. 16b Same field as Fig. 16a viewed between crossed polars. Shows diffuse mottled birefringence of small intracellular particles of polyethylene

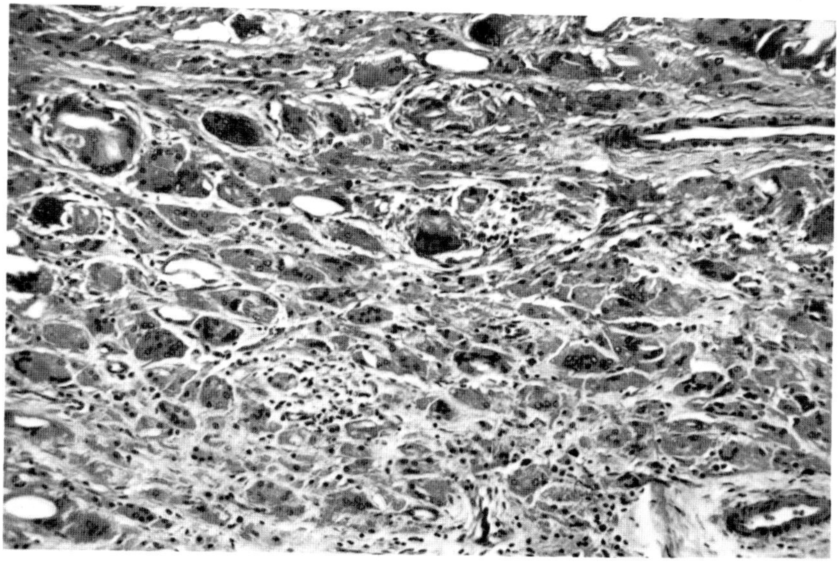

Fig. 17a Many multinucleate giant cells and bands of fibrous tissue in articular tissues 2 years after implantation of a cobalt-chrome against a high-density polyethylene knee prosthesis which became painful and unstable. Haematoxylin-eosin (x 120)

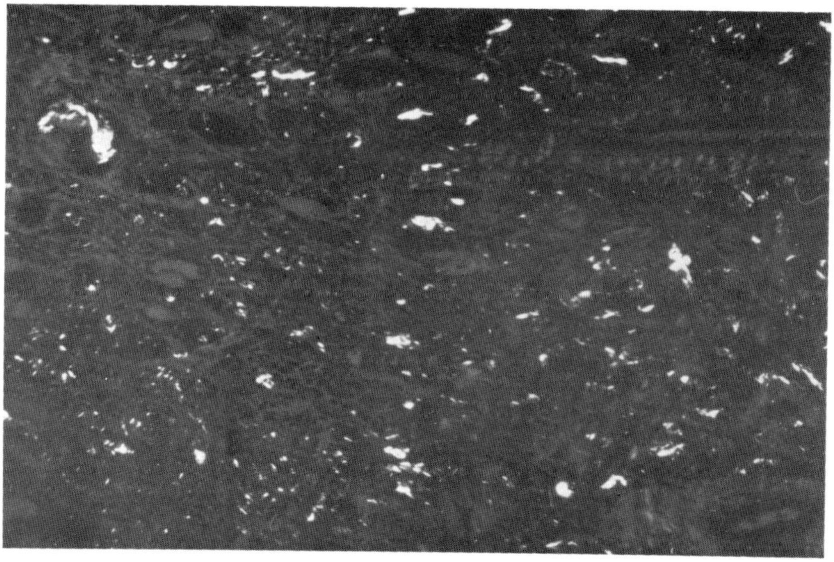

Fig. 17b Same field as Fig. 17a viewed between crossed polars. Shows numerous birefringent fragments of polyethylene within giant cells and embedded in fibrous tissue

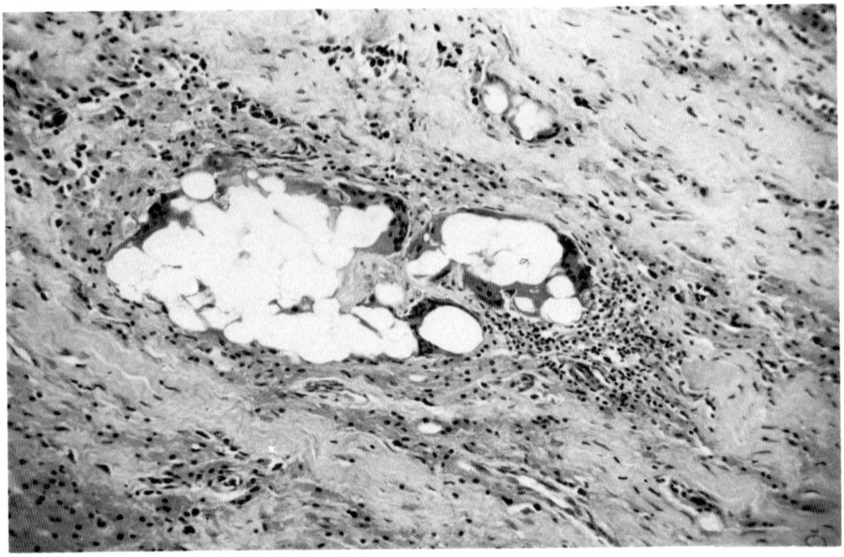

Fig. 18 Spaces representing site of cluster of "acrylic pearls" of polymethylmethacrylate which is surrounded by syncytial giant cells and embedded in fibrous tissue in articular tissue around knee prosthesis. Haematoxylin-eosin (x 120)

The degree of macrophage and giant cell proliferation in response to the presence of foreign material depends on the amount of that material formed by wear and corrosion. The fact that foreign material having the characteristics of metal-containing particles and of polyethylene may be found within lymph nodes draining the region of the prosthesis (Figs. 19a, 19b) indicates that some of this material is normally mobilized away from the articular tissues. Thus, one can postulate that, in the majority of patients with successful prostheses not undergoing pain or loosening, a "stabilized" situation of equilibrium is reached where the amount of foreign material being released into the articular tissues from the implant is balanced by the macrophages and giant cells being replaced by fibrous tissue and by mobilization of foreign material to lymph nodes. This state of equilibrium is much more likely to exist in the case of prostheses in which metal articulates against polyethylene. When larger amounts of foreign material are generated, as in the case of prostheses in which metal articulates against metal, the tissue appears not to be capable of eliminating or sequestering all of the foreign material in many instances. The macrophage and giant cell reaction is therefore intensified so that all, or almost all, of the articular tissues are involved in the reaction. In such cases, it is common to find areas of cell death in the granulation tissue. These areas of necrosis may be small and scattered or extensive and diffuse (Figs. 20, 21) and may also involve areas of collagenized fibrous connective tissues. The breakdown of the granulation tissue and fibrous tissue may result in pultaceous white or grey necrotic tissue, similar to caseous tuberculous debris, filling the joint cavity.

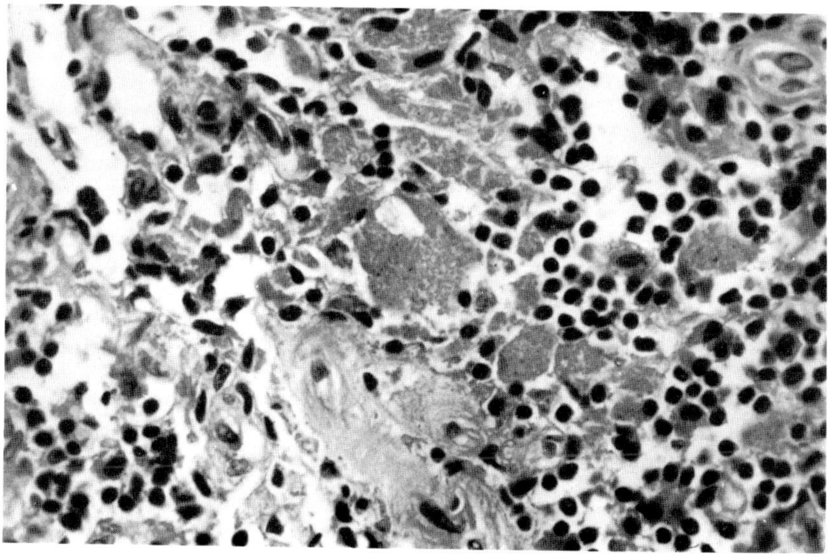

Fig. 19a Macrophages of cortico-medullary sinus of iliac lymph node from patient who died 18 months after implantation of a cobalt-chrome against high-density polyethylene knee prosthesis which was stable and painless. The macrophages contain black metallic-type particles. Haematoxylin-eosin (x 400)

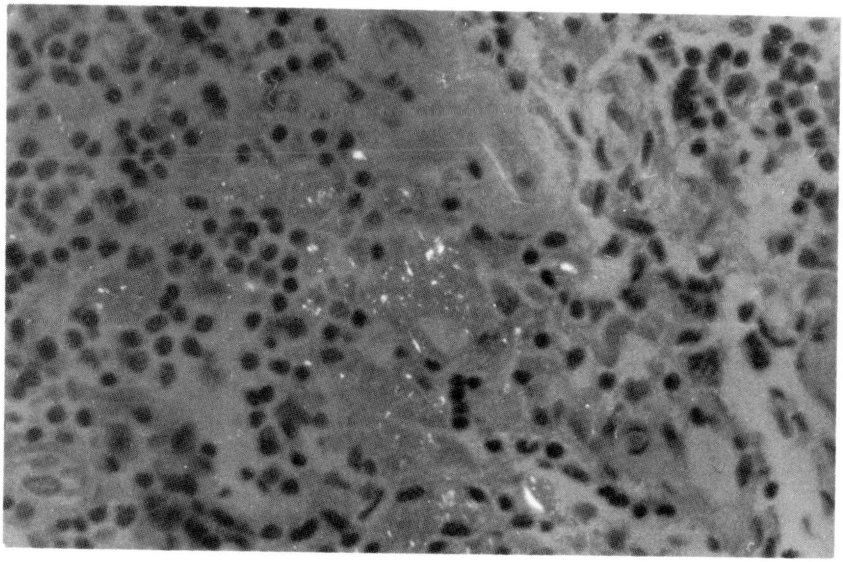

Fig. 19b Same field as Fig. 19a viewed between crossed polars. Shows that both metallic and polyethylene particles are present in the cells

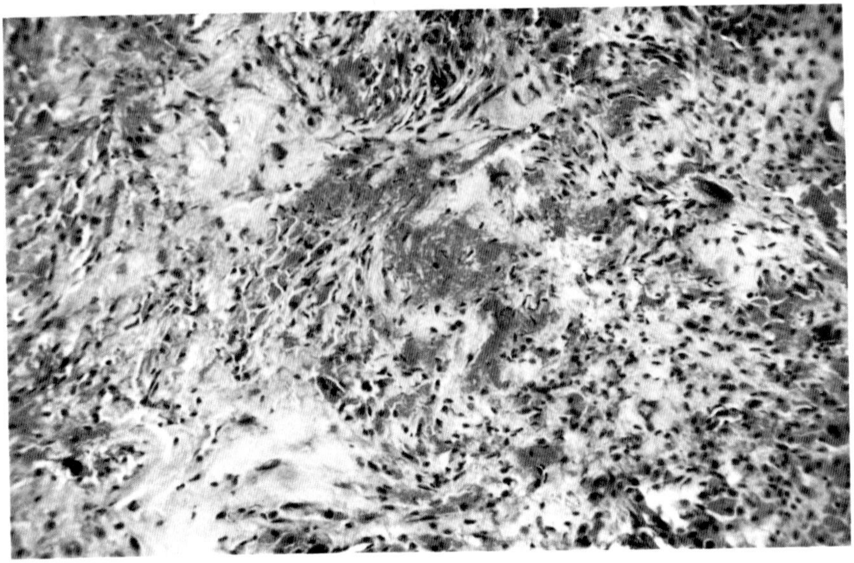

Fig. 20 Scattered areas of necrosis in articular granulation tissue 4 years after implantation of an all-cobalt-chrome hinged knee prosthesis which became loose. Haematoxylin-eosin (x 120)

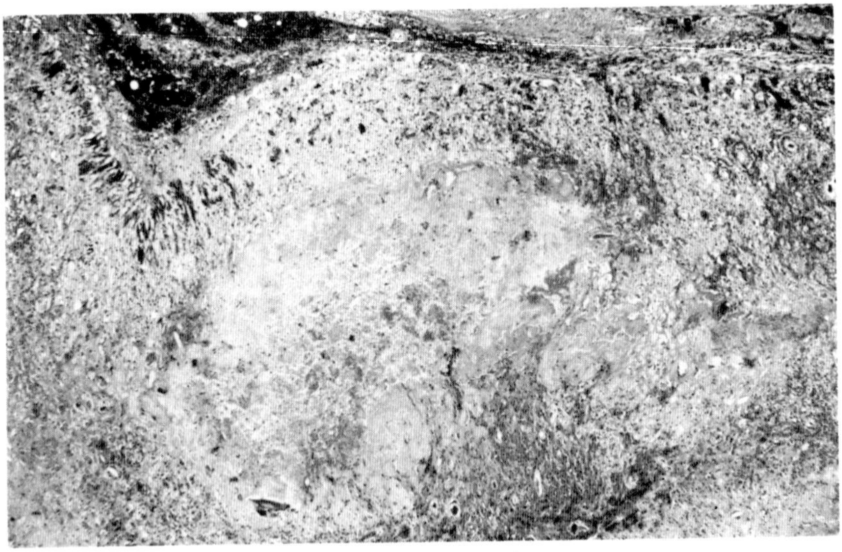

Fig. 21 Extensive necrosis of articular granulation tissue 9 years after implantation of an all-cobalt-chrome hip prosthesis which had been increasingly painful for 2 years. Haematoxylin-eosin (x 50)

In many cases where the prostheses have been removed because of pain or loosening, the proliferation of granulation tissue containing foreign material is restricted to the articular tissues and does not extend to involve bone. However, in the majority of cases in which loosening has taken place, the granulation tissue composed of macrophages and giant cells containing foreign material extends into the bone surrounding the prosthesis and its cement (Figs. 22, 23). At first, the granulation tissue appears to infiltrate the marrow spaces without the loss of bone (Fig. 22), but later there is active removal of living and dead trabecular bone by the infiltrating tissues (Fig. 24). The result of bone removal and its replacement by granulation tissue is the destruction of the osseous anchors necessary for the fixation of the implanted bone cement (Fig. 25) which is most marked in the region around the joint articulation. It would seem to be inevitable that this process should lead to loosening of the prosthesis. Since, not infrequently, the prosthesis initially becomes unsupported near its articulation while the remaining part of the shaft is still firmly cemented in place, the shaft of the implant may fracture.

From light microscopic studies it is evident that a direct correlation exists between the amount of foreign particulate matter in the articular tissue surrounding an implant and the degree of macrophage and giant cell proliferation; and the greater the degree of macrophage and giant cell proliferation, the greater is the tendency towards the invasion and replacement of bone by granulation tissue.

Since the stability of an implant depends ultimately upon the integrity of the bone into which it is cemented, it is clearly of the greatest importance to clarify the exact identity of the foreign particulate matter which appears to be playing a major role in bone resorption; moreover, since the amount of particulate foreign material in the tissues also appears

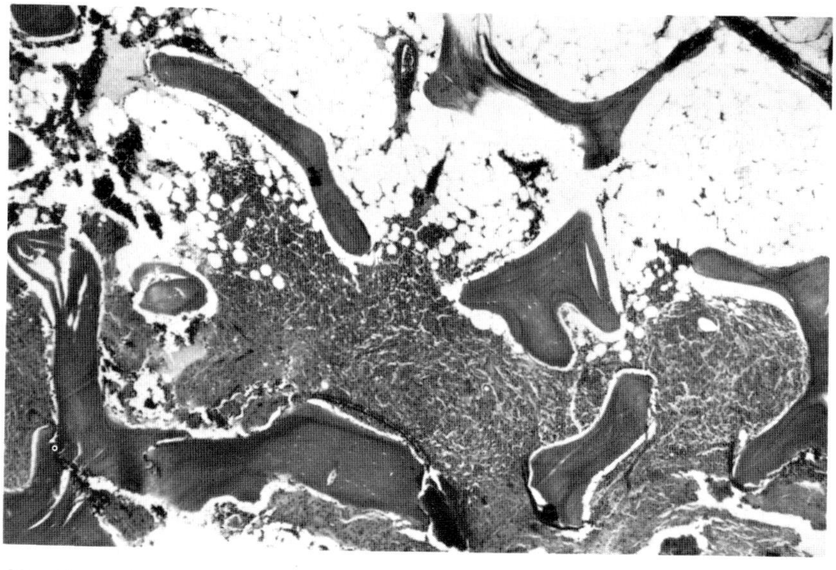

Fig. 22 Granulation tissue extending from articular tissue into peri-articular bone 4 years after implantation of an all-cobalt-chrome hinged knee prosthesis which became loose. Haematoxylin-eosin (x 50)

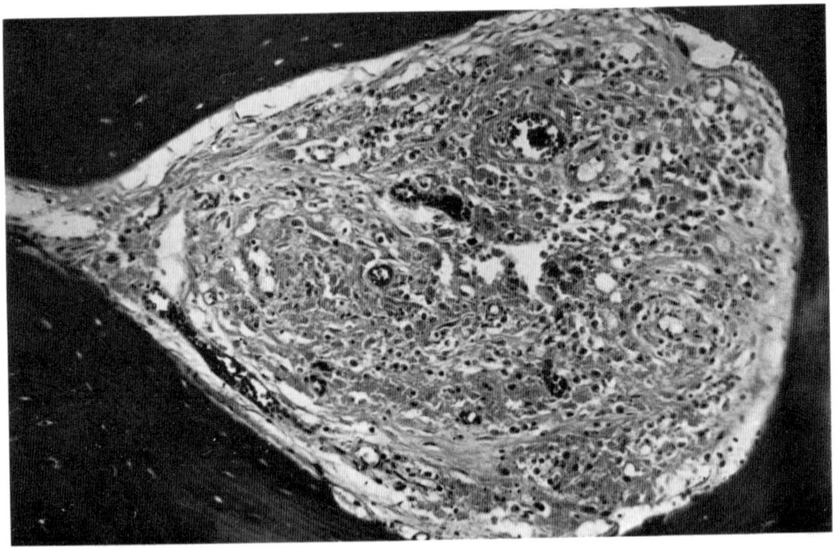

Fig. 23 Granulation tissue with numerous macrophages containing metallic particles occupying a vascular channel in the cortical bone of the femur adjacent to a loose cobalt-chrome against bone hip prosthesis 14 years after implantation. The bone is dead. Haematoxylin-eosin (x 120)

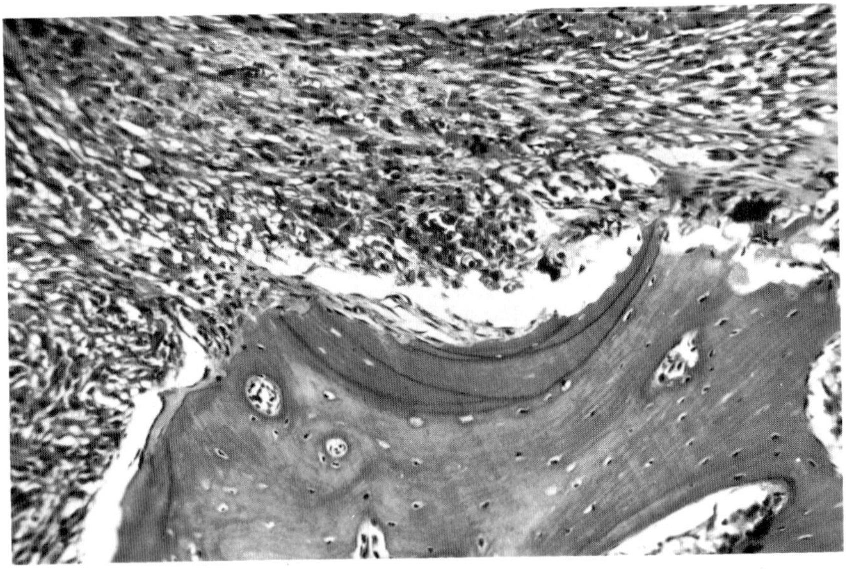

Fig. 24 Living and dead peri-articular bone being removed by infiltrating granulation tissue 4 years after implantation of an all-cobalt-chrome hinged knee prosthesis which became loose. Haematoxylin-eosin (x 120)

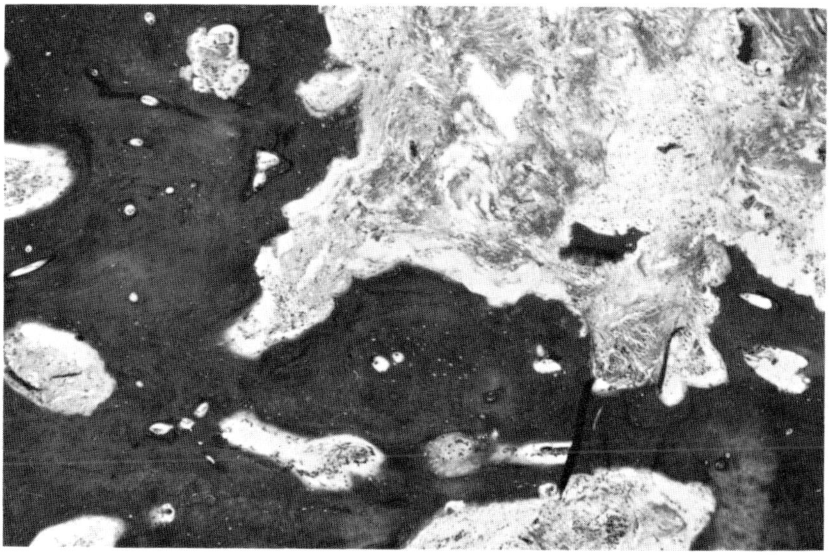

Fig. 25 Death and disappearance of cortical and cancellous bone and their replacement by partly-necrotic granulation tissue in femur 14 years after implantation of cobalt-chrome against bone hip prosthesis which became loose. Haematoxylin-eosin (x 50)

to be a significant factor in loosening, it also appears to be important to ascertain which types of prostheses predispose to the formation of large amounts of foreign material.

ANALYTICAL STUDIES OF METALLIC CONSTITUENTS OF INTRACELLULAR CRYSTALLINE STRUCTURES

Hitherto, there has been little published information regarding the electron microscopy of the tissues surrounding joint prostheses. Winter (30) found very small fragments of highly crystalline foreign material in phagosomes within macrophages in the tissue surrounding an all-cobalt-chrome total hip prosthesis, and the Debye-Scherrer diffraction pattern indicated that these were unchanged cobalt-chromium alloy particles. In two other tissue samples from around cobalt chrome knee and elbow prostheses, Winter found very small intracytoplasmic agglomerates having electron diffraction patterns, indicating that they were carbides of chromium and cobalt. We have observed similar very small electron-dense particles in the tissues around all-cobalt-chrome prostheses, but their size is such that they could not be responsible for the crystalline particulate material seen in the light microscope. However, we have observed intracytoplasmic electron-lucent crystalline structures having approximately the same dimensions as the particles seen in the light microscope (Fig. 26). Electron microscopy of tissues containing abundant particles of polyethylene reveal the presence of irregular plates of crystalline material (Fig. 27).

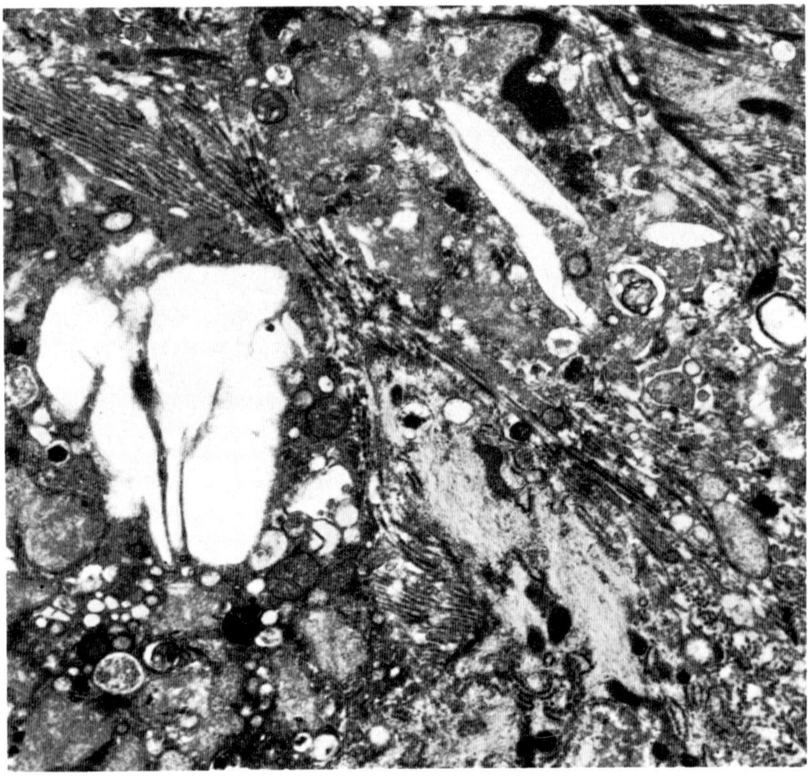

Fig. 26 Electron-lucent foreign material within macrophages in articular granulation tissue around an all-cobalt-chrome knee prosthesis which had become loose with extensive bone loss 9 years after implantation. Light microscopy had revealed the presence of numerous black intracellular crystalline particles of "metallic" type in the granulation tissue. Electron micrograph (x 15,000)

We have also carried out preliminary studies of the intracytoplasmic foreign particles using electron microscope micro-analysis (EMMA), and the initial findings are summarized in Table 2. It will be seen from the table that the patients E.B., E.L., C.B., and F.S. had all revealed very high concentrations of cobalt, chromium or nickel in the articular tissues analysed by neutron activation analysis (NAA), and light microscopy had revealed numerous black intracellular foreign particles; in these four patients, EMMA of the particles confirmed the presence of nickel, titanium and iron in all four, other elements including chromium were variably present, but cobalt was not detected in any. By contrast, in the patients E.E. and N.T. having much lower concentrations of metal in the articular tissues, and in whom the light microscopy indicated large quantities of polyethylene, EMMA revealed that nickel and iron were absent from the inclusions. It is of interest that cobalt could not be detected in the crystals examined in any of the six cases; and in this connection, it is of interest that Semlitsch et al. (17) also found virtually no cobalt or chrome in the connective tissues around all-metal hip prostheses using electron probe micro-analysis (EPMA), but this was not the case for hip joints in which a metallic ball articulated with a mica-reinforced Teflon socket.

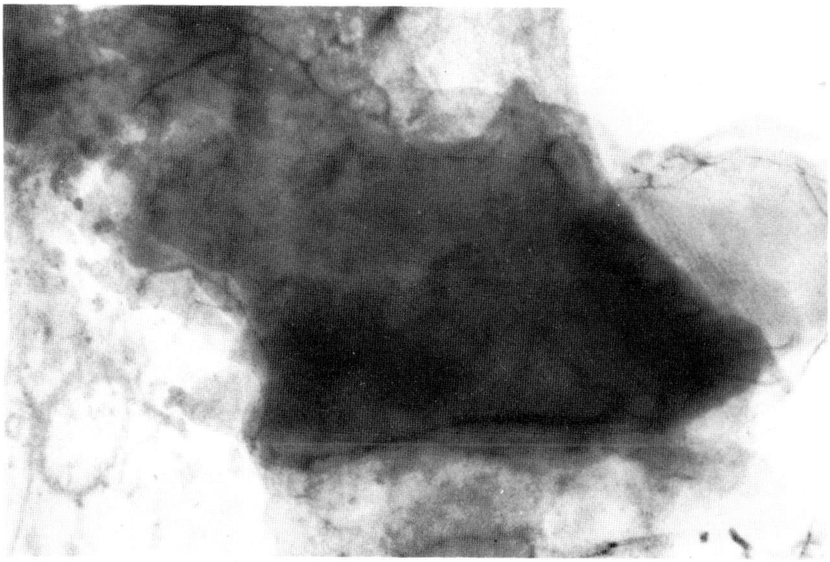

Fig. 27 Moderately electron-dense crystalline material within macrophage in articular granulation tissue around a cobalt-chrome against high-density polyethylene knee prosthesis implanted for 15 months and which had become painful. Polarized light microscopy had revealed the presence of abundant intracellular particles of "polyethylene" type. Electron micrograph (x 60,000)

The variable presence of chromium, and the complete absence of detectable cobalt in these EMMA studies of intracellular particles, despite the NAA findings of high levels of one or both elements in the tissues generally in some cases, could be accounted for by the solubility of cobalt and chrome compounds resulting in their removal from intracellular crystalline structures during tissue processing, although analytical studies tend to exclude this possibility, or that they normally exist as soluble salts of cobalt and chromium. Until further EMMA and EPMA studies are carried out, the situation therefore exists in which it is possible that cobalt and chrome do not contribute to the formation of intracellular crystalline structures, at least not in every case. In contrast our data suggest a more important role for nickel and titanium in forming crystalline structures. Nickel is present in a concentration of 10-15 % in stainless steel and thus its presence around stainless steel implants is not surprising. On the other hand no more than 2.5 % of nickel is permitted in the specification of cast cobalt-chrome alloy. Thus the presence of nickel in significant quantities in the tissue and its invariable presence in particles around cobalt-chrome as well as stainless steel prostheses supports the view, presented here, that the metal in such tissues and particles is not simply wear debris but rather is the end result of wear, corrosion, chemical inter-action with other substances (for example protein) and phagocytosis. The presence of titanium is harder to explain and is indeed at present inexplicable: its origin and significance remain a topic for further study.

Table 2 Electron microscope micro-analysis (EMMA) of elements in intracellular particles in tissues adjacent to joint prostheses

Case	Articulating surfaces of prosthesis	Parts per million in tissue (NAA)			Elements detected (EMMA)
		cobalt	chromium	nickel	
E.B.	cobalt-chrome on cobalt-chrome	12.0	30.0	1.4	Ni, Ti, Fe, Zn,
E.L.	cobalt-chrome on cobalt-chrome	0.3	0.72	40.0	Ni, Ti, Fe, Cr
E.E.	cobalt-chrome on polyethylene	2.2	2.0	0.4	AlSi
C.B.	stainless steel on polyethylene	0.49	86.0	313.0	Ni, Ti, Fe, Mn
F.S.	stainless steel on polyethylene	0.14	13.3	14.0	Ni, Ti, Fe, Zn, Cr, AlSi, Mg
N.T.	stainless steel on polyethylene	0.025	0.26	0.76	Ti

RELATIONSHIP BETWEEN LOOSENING, METAL SENSITIVITY AND TISSUE METAL CONCENTRATION

It is well known that the skin may become sensitive to certain metals and that such sensitivity can be demonstrated by epicutaneous patch tests in which a positive response is denoted by an eczematous reaction in the skin occurring when a solution of the relevant metal is placed on it. Epicutaneous tests may in fact give falsely negative results, and intracutaneous tests are possibly more reliable, particularly in the case of trivalent chromium (9). Cobalt, chromium and nickel are capable of exciting skin sensitivity. For all three elements the readiness with which sensitivity can be induced and demonstrated depends upon the solubility of the element in the form presented to the tissue, and thus upon the nature of the anion when the element is presented as a salt or upon the nature of the alloy when it is presented as the metal (9, 10). The incidence of skin sensitivity to cobalt, chromium and nickel in the general population is unknown, but Fregert and Rorsman (10), studying a group of 5,416 patients suspected of having contact dermatitis, found an incidence of epicutaneous sensitivity in women to nickel of 2.5 %, to cobalt of 1.7 % and to chromium of 0.8 %. By contrast, men displayed an incidence of sensitivity to chromium of 3.8 %, to cobalt of 1.6 % and to nickel of 0.9 %.

The development of skin sensitivity following the implantation of metal in the tissues has been observed. Thus, Laugier and Foussereau (12) described four cases in which dermatitis had developed in patients who had stainless steel pins or plates inserted. Brendlinger and Tarsitano (2) reported a case of dermatitis due to sensitivity to a cobalt-chrome denture, and McKenzie et al. (13) a case of urticaria following the insertion of a cobalt-chrome nail for a femoral fracture.

An association between epicutaneous skin sensitivity to metal and late loosening of prostheses was first demonstrated by Evans et al. (6). They found (Table 3) that of a total of fourteen patients having loose prostheses, nine had positive skin sensitivity tests to metal (seven to cobalt, one to chromium, and one to both nickel and cobalt); by contrast, twenty-four patients with normally functioning securely fixed prostheses were not sensitive to metal. The findings suggested that there was a strong association between metal sensitivity and loosening of prostheses composed entirely of cobalt-chrome alloy. These findings have received recent support from the studies of Jones et al. (11) who found positive skin sensitivity to cobalt in six patients having late failure of all-cobalt-chrome McKee hip arthroplasties, and negative skin tests in thirty patients in whom McKee hip arthroplasties were functioning satisfactorily.

The above clinical findings clearly show that after the implantation of a prosthesis in which cobalt-chrome articulates with cobalt-chrome, certain patients are sensitive to cobalt, and less frequently to chromium or nickel. Sensitivity may also be present in patients having prostheses in which cobalt-chrome articulates against bone (6), but the position regarding sensitivity to cobalt, chromium and nickel after the implantation of a prosthesis in which cobalt-chrome or stainless steel articulates with polyethylene is not yet known.

Table 3 Results of skin sensitivity tests to cobalt, chromium and nickel in thirty-nine patients with uninfected cobalt-chrome prostheses (6)

State of prosthesis	Skin	
	sensitive	insensitive
loose	9 (11 prostheses)	5
not loose	0	24

The findings of these studies (6, 11) do not allow a distinction to be made between the possibilities

- that the patients were metalsensitive before implantation of the prosthesis, or
- that they became sensitive after implantation, or
- that one or other sequence of events was common to all cases.

Nevertheless, it would appear to be of great significance, even in these selected cases, that every metal-sensitive patient had a loose prosthesis and this suggests a causal relationship between metal sensitivity and loosening. A number of controlled prospective studies using epicutaneous skin testing for metal sensitivity are currently in progress both in patients having satisfactorily functioning prostheses and in patients before arthroplasty has been performed. Since it is conceivable that the patch testing procedure itself could lead to sensitization, it would seem unwise to perform this investigation as a routine pre-implantation or post-implantation procedure. It is to be hoped that current attempts to perfect in vitro tests for detecting metal sensitivity using lymphocytes from patients will result in a safe method of detecting pre- and post-implant metal sensitivity.

Histopathological studies of articular tissues in patients having loosening and metal sensitivity (6, 11) have revealed widespread necrosis of tissues in addition to the proliferation of macrophages and giant cells containing abundant particulate matter of metallic type. This group of patients tend to have marked vascular changes in the form of lymphocytic vasculitis, fibrinoid necrosis and fibrous intimal proliferation (Figs. 28a, 28b, 28c). While some of these vascular changes could be secondary to tissue death from other causes, their presence in tissues still alive or undergoing early degenerative changes indicate that tissue death may be due largely or partly to deprivation of blood supply. This group of

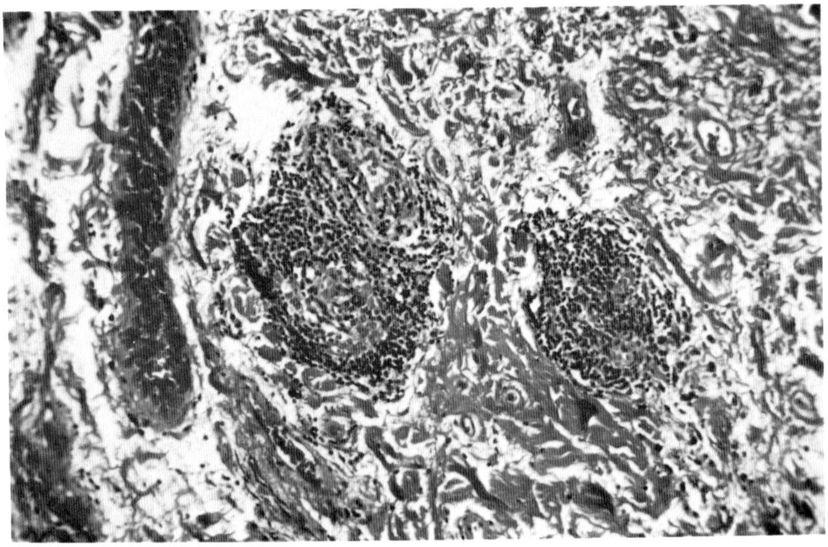

Fig. 28a Lymphocytic vasculitis and degenerate connective tissue in articular tissue of patient sensitive to cobalt. Haematoxylin-eosin (x 120)

patients also tend to have marked invasion of the bone marrow by granulation tissue containing much particulate foreign material, with extensive death of the granulation tissue and replacement and death of bone.

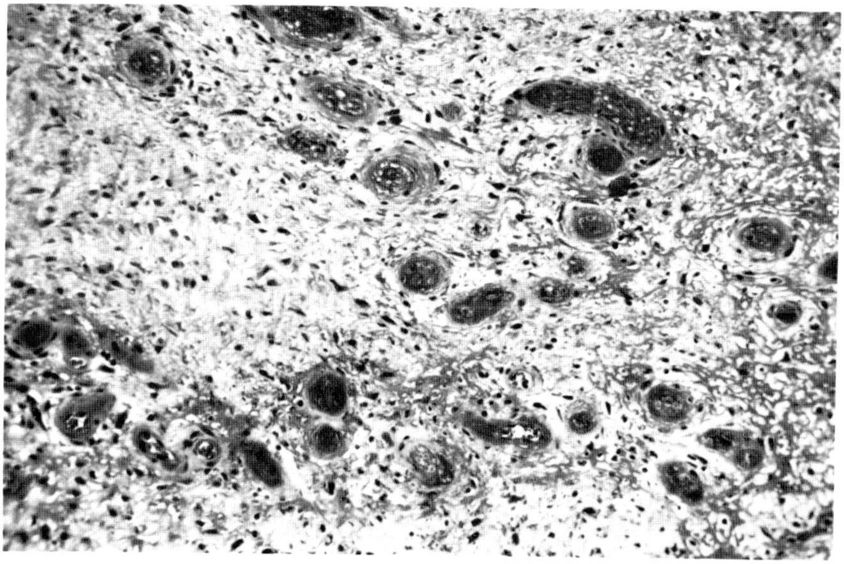

Fig. 28b Fibrinoid necrosis of arterioles in articular connective tissues of patient sensitive to cobalt. Haematoxylin-eosin (x 120)

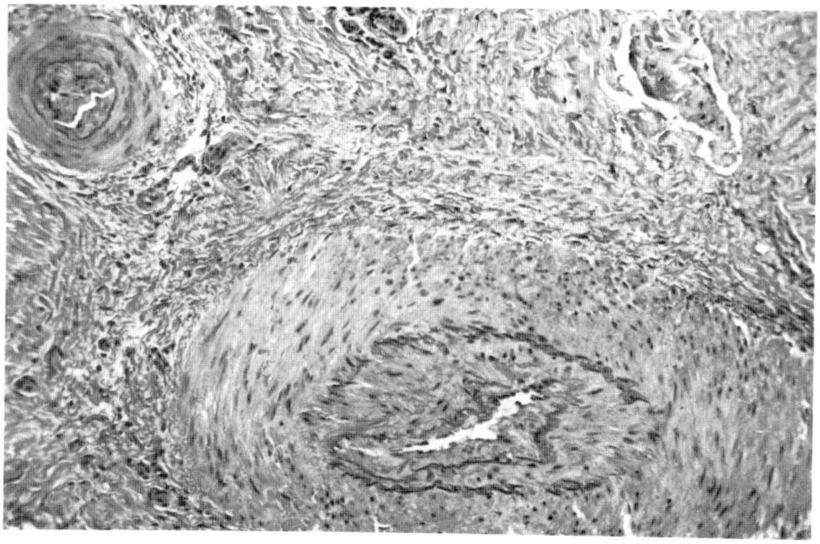

Fig. 28c Articular connective tissue showing obliteration of lumen of large and small arteries by fibrous intimal proliferation in patient sensitive to cobalt. Haematoxylin-eosin (x 120)

There is evidence, therefore, that in metal-sensitive patients the tissue reaction to the products of wear and corrosion is exaggerated, tissue death is associated with large amounts of foreign intracellular material and obliterative vascular changes, and bone death and replacement by living and dead granulation tissue is rapid and widespread. These changes are progressive and removal of the prosthesis is indicated (6).

While there is evidence of an association between metal sensitivity and loosening in the studies of selected cases so far carried out, the following questions need to be answered:

1. what is the relationship between tissue metal concentration and the development of metal sensitivity and
2. is there a relationship between metal concentration and loosening due to a direct toxic effect of metal on the soft tissues and bone?

Studies of metal concentration in the tissues adjacent to loose prostheses showed (6) that in five specimens (four patients) with all-cobalt-chrome prostheses, both cobalt and chromium levels were considerably elevated as compared with control tissue taken from patients in whom no prosthesis had been inserted. In specimens taken from three patients who had cobalt-chrome articulating against bone, cobalt and chromium levels were also elevated although not to the levels seen with all-cobalt-chrome prostheses. Much lower levels of cobalt and chromium, approaching the levels seen in controls, were found in specimens taken from around three prostheses in which cobalt-chrome articulated against polyethylene. Our latest results (22) confirm and extend the above observations. They show (Table 4) that cobalt, chromium and nickel levels are markedly elevated in the tissues around prostheses in which cobalt-chrome articulates against cobalt-chrome; chromium and nickel, and to a lesser degree cobalt, levels are elevated in the tissues around prostheses in which cobalt-chrome articulates against bone, but to much lower levels than with all-cobalt-chrome prostheses; while generally low levels of all three metals are found in the tissues around prostheses in which cobalt-chrome or stainless steel articulates against polyethylene. These and our previous findings tend to show that the higher levels of cobalt and chrome are seen in those cases which also exhibit skin sensitivity to one of these metals, but we do not yet know if sensitivity leads to higher metal release or vice versa. The fact that loosening is not restricted to cases in which metal concentrations in the tissue are high indicates that a direct toxic effect of high concentrations of metals on the tissues is unlikely to be the only mechanism involved, although our results indicate that pain without definite evidence of loosening may be the commonest complaint in those patients having medium to low metal concentrations in the tissues. In fact, the analytical and histopathological studies tend to show that pain or loosening in patients having low metal levels around prostheses in which metal articulates against polyethylene is usually associated with the presence of large amounts of polyethylene particles in the tissues.

At the present state of knowledge, the situation may be summarized as follows:

1. the rate of release of cobalt, chromium and nickel is much higher from prostheses in which cobalt-chrome alloy articulates with itself than when cobalt-chrome articulates with HDP,
2. the rate of release of metal may also be moderately high from prostheses in which cobalt-chrome articulates against bone,

Table 4 Concentration of cobalt, chromium and nickel in tissues adjacent to painful or loose prostheses

Articulating surfaces of prosthesis	Number of patients	Parts per million in tissues		
		cobalt	chromium	nickel
Cobalt-chrome on cobalt-chrome	8	43.1 (11 – 230)	57.2 (25 – 103)	2.3 (0.1 – 6.0)
Cobalt-chrome on bone	9	0.7 (0.02 – 2.5)	3.4 (0.12 – 9.3)	4.0 (0.4 – 20)
Cobalt-chrome on polyethylene	9	0.56 (0.02 – 2.2)	0.86 (0.15 – 2.0)	0.31 (0.2 – 0.6)
Stainless steel on polyethylene	12	0.06 (0.05 – 0.5)	0.56 (1.0 – 3.3)	0.76 (0.10 – 2.0)

3. the rate of release of metal from prostheses in which cobalt-chrome or stainless steel articulates against polyethylene is usually low,
4. skin sensitivity to cobalt, chromium or nickel is frequently associated with high concentrations of these metals in the tissues around the prosthesis,
5. patients with skin sensitivity to cobalt, chromium or nickel and high concentrations of these metals in the tissues around the prostheses are liable to develop progressive loosening of the prosthesis.

PRACTICAL IMPLICATIONS

Certain practical implications follow from the present information regarding metal sensitivity and metal concentrations in tissues.

First, since the rate of release of metal is much higher from prostheses in which cobalt-chrome alloy articulates with itself, it would be better to use a metal-to-polyethylene combination wherever possible. In this respect, on the basis of metal levels in the tissues, there are no grounds for preferring a combination of stainless steel and polyethylene to a combination of cobalt-chrome and polyethylene.

Second, it is highly desirable that a safe method of sensitivity to cobalt, chromium and nickel should be applied in every patient before the implantation of an alloy containing one of these metals. If a patient proves sensitive to one of these metals, the prosthesis used must be free of that metal. Sensitivity to chromium would currently pose a difficult problem since both cobalt-chrome and stainless steel contain this element.

Third, all patients in whom the prosthesis becomes loose should be tested for sensitivity to the relevant metals. If they are found to be sensitive, the condition can be expected to be progressive and removal of the prosthesis is indicated.

Fourth, since in many publications prosthetic loosening with the production of necrotic pultaceous debris around the prosthesis is regarded as being due to infection even though no pathogenic organism is cultured, and since it is now suggested that tissue necrosis in some of these cases is due to metal sensitivity or to excessive wear-particle formation, the figures now in the literature for the incidence of infection following joint replacement may now have to be revised. Indeed, it seems possible that necrotic debris resulting from metal sensitivity or excessive wear-particle formation may become secondarily infected, so that even in some infected joints the failure may primarily be due to metal sensitivity.

THE PATHOGENESIS OF LATE LOOSENING: AN HYPOTHESIS

Based upon the information available at the present time regarding the histopathological, analytical and clinical findings in patients in whom late loosening of joint prostheses takes place, it is possible to formulate an hypothesis to explain the sequence of events which brings about pain and loosening in these cases. This hypothesis is illustrated in diagrammatic form in Figs. 29–31.

First, it is now clear that all types of prostheses having bearing surfaces release products of wear into the joint cavity surrounding the articulating components (Fig. 29). Abundant metal is released from the surfaces of prostheses in which metal articulates against metal, lesser amounts of metal are released from prostheses in which metal articulates against bone, and small amounts of metal are released from prostheses in which metal articulates against a plastic surface such as polyethylene. Plastic articulating surfaces normally release small amounts of plastic, but occasionally abundant plastic wear products are formed. Metal is also released from the surfaces of prostheses by corrosion, and there is almost certainly rapid "corrosion" of metallic wear particles. Thus, under normal circumstances, there are variable amounts of metal and/or plastic wear particles and metal salts in solution within the joint cavity surrounding a prosthesis.

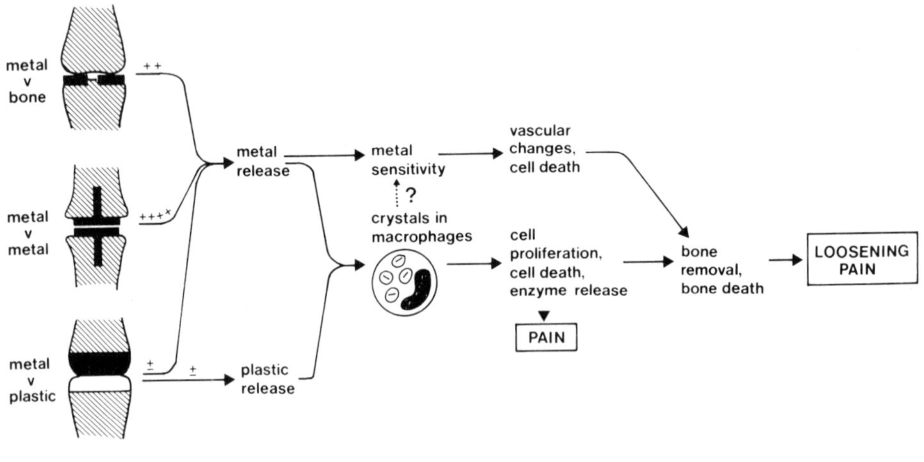

Fig. 29 Diagram to illustrate possible sequence of events leading to pain and loosening

Second, crystalline structures of metallic and/or plastic type appear within macrophages and giant cells in the articular tissues (Fig. 29). The larger the amounts of metallic or plastic crystalline material, the greater is the degree of proliferation of macrophages and giant cells. The ultrastructure and analysis of the metallic crystals suggests that they are formed within the phagocytic cells from the products of corrosion of bearing surfaces and wear particles, and indicates that they are not themselves the wear particles in unchanged form.

Third, when particles of metal or plastic are particularly abundant in the tissues, there is frequently evidence of cell and tissue death; the death of tissue is more extensive in the case of metallic particles. It is already known that there are certain exceptions to the generally harmless effects of the phagocytosis of inorganic materials by macrophages; thus it is well established that silica particles are intensely toxic for macrophages and kill them during a process in which the phagolysosomes containing the silica particles rupture and release the lysosomal enzymes into the cell cytoplasm (1). After death, the macrophages containing silica disintegrate and the material is then re-phagocytosed; the cycle is then repeated and a strong stimulus to fibrogenesis is exerted. If intracellular particles containing metal (and, to a lesser degree, plastic wear particles) have a similar effect, particularly when present in large numbers, this could account for cell and tissues around some prostheses (Fig. 30). The release of lysosomal enzymes not only leads to further tissue damage, including death of bone, but would also release pain-producing factors.

Fourth, when there are large amounts of metallic or polyethylene particles present, the granulation tissue extends into adjoining bone and induces death and resorption of bone. Bone removal results in loosening of the prosthesis due to loss of the bond between cement and bone (Fig. 31).

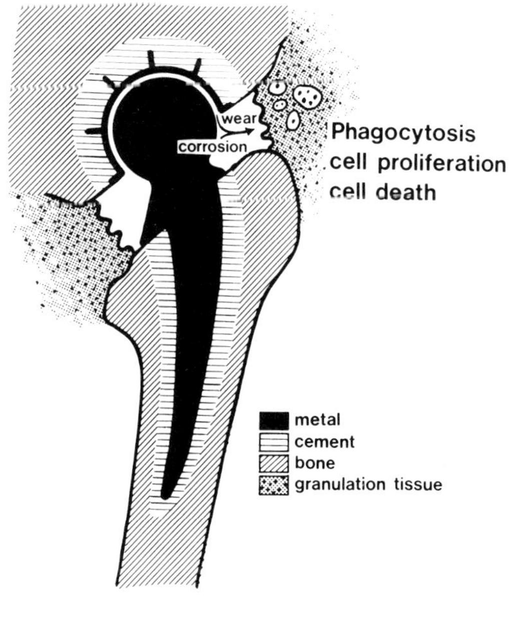

Fig. 30 Diagram illustrating proliferation of macrophages and giant cells in articular tissues in response to products of wear and corrosion

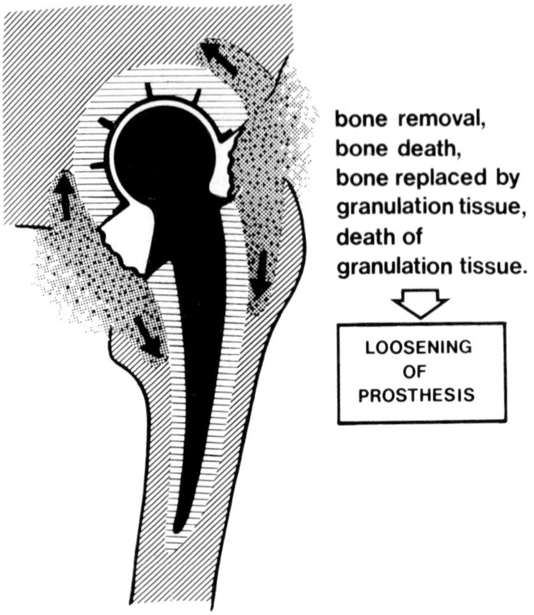

Fig. 31 Diagram illustrating how loosening of prosthesis arises from the extension of articular granulation tissue into the bone and from the removal of bone around the cement which bonds the prosthesis in position

Fifth, when large amounts of metal are released from the prosthesis, a state of hypersensitivity to one or more of the constituent metals may be induced. Patients are more prone to become hypersensitive to cobalt than to nickel or chromium. When a state of hypersensitivity to a metal is present, there is widespread tissue death due to marked obliterative vascular changes and, possibly, to cytotoxic effects on cells containing metals as crystals or soluble salts. The death of bone and other tissues is accompanied by pain due perhaps, partly to the release of lysosomal enzymes and pain-producing factors and partly to loosening due to death and resorption of bone.

REFERENCES

1. Allison, A.C., Harington, J.S., Birbeck, M.: An examination of the cytotoxic effects of silica on macrophages. Journal of Experimental Medicine 124, 141 (1966)
2. Brendlinger, D.L., Tarsitano, J.J.: Generalized dermatitis due to sensitivity to a chrome cobalt removable partial denture. Journal of the American Dental Association 81, 392 (1970)
3. Challis, J., Freeman, M.A.R., Vernon-Roberts, B.: unpublished observations (1975)
4. Charnley, J.: Acrylic cement in orthopaedic surgery. Edinburgh-London: Livingstone 1970
5. Coleman, R.F., Herrington, J., Scales, J.T.: Concentration of wear products in hair, blood, and urine after total hip replacement. British Medical Journal 1, 527 (1973)
6. Evans, E.M., Freeman, M.A.R., Miller, A.J., Vernon-Roberts, B.: Metal sensitivity as a cause of bone necrosis and loosening of the prosthesis in total joint replacement. Journal of Bone and Joint Surgery 56-B, 626 (1974)

7. Ferguson, A.B., Laing, P.G., Hodge, E.S.: The ionization of metal implants in living tissues. Journal of Bone and Joint Surgery 42-A, 77 (1960)

8. Freeman, M.A.R., Vernon-Roberts, B.: Unpublished observations (1975)

9. Fregert, S., Rorsman, H.: Allergic reactions to trivalent chromium compounds. Archives of Dermatology 93, 711 (1966)

10. Fregert, S., Rorsman, H.: Allergy to chromium, nickel and cobalt. Acta dermato-venerologica 46, 144-148 (1966)

11. Jones, D.A., Lucas, H.K., O'Driscoll, M., Price, C.H.G., Wibberly, B.: Cobalt toxicity after McKee hip arthroplasty. Journal of Bone and Joint Surgery 57-B, 289 (1975)

12. Laugier, P., Foussereau, J.: Les dermites allergiques a distance provoquees par le materiel d'osteosynthese. Gazette Medicale de France 73, 3409 (1966)

13. McKenzie, A.W., Aitken, C.V.E., Risdill-Smith, R.: Urticaria after insertion of Smith-Petersen Vitallium nail. British Medical Journal 4, 36 (1967)

14. Mowat, A.G., Hothersall, T.E.: Nature of anaemia in rheumatoid arthritis — VIII. Iron content of synovial tissue in patients with rheumatoid arthritis and in normal individuals. Annals of the Rheumatic Diseases 27, 345 (1968)

15. Muirden, K.D., Senator, G.B.: Iron in the synovial membrane in rheumatoid arthritis and other joint diseases. Annals of the Rheumatic Diseases 27, 38 (1968)

16. Scales, J.T., Duff-Barclay, I., Jackson Burrows, H.: Proceedings of Biomechanics and Related Bioengineering Topics (Glasgow Symposium) p. 205, Oxford-New York: Pergamon 1965

17. Semlitsch, M., Vogel, A., Willert, H.-G.: Investigation of joint endoprostheses abrasion products in the connective tissue of the joint cavity. Sulzer Technical Review 2, 137 (1972)

18. Smith, D.C., Bains, M.E.D.: The detection and estimation of residual monomer in polymethyl methacrylate. Journal of Dental Research 35, 16 (1956)

19. Swanson, S.A.V., Freeman, M.A.R., Heath, J.C.: Laboratory tests in total joint replacement prostheses. Journal of Bone and Joint Surgery 55-B, 759 (1973)

20. Szepesi, K., Kapitany, S.: Druckprobe zur Beurteilung der Tragfähigkeit des Femurkopfes in Tierversuchen. Archiv für Orthopädische und Unfallchirurgie 79, 21 (1974)

21. Szepesi, K., Kapitany, S., Czorba, E.: Tragfähigkeit des Femurkopfes nach experimenteller ischämischer Nekrose der Epiphyse. Archiv für Orthopädische und Unfallchirurgie 80, 283 (1974)

22. Vernon-Roberts, B., Freeman, M.A.R., Sculco, J.: In preparation 1975

23. Willert, H.-G.: Tissue reactions around joint implants and bone cement. In: Arthroplasty of the Hip (ed. G. Chapchal) pp. 11-21, Stuttgart: Thieme Verlag 1973

24. Willert, H. G., Frech, H.-A., Bechtel, A.: Measurements of the quantity of monomer leaching out of acrylic cement into the surrounding tissues during the process of polymerization. Read at the 166th National Meeting of the American Chemical Society, Chicago, Illinois, 1973

25. Willert, H.-G., Ludwig, J., Semlitsch, M.: Reaction of bone to methacrylate after hip arthroplasty. Journal of Bone and Joint Surgery 56-A, 1368 (1974)

26. Willert, H.-G., Puls, P.: Die Reaktion des Knochens auf Knochenzement bei der Alloarthroplastik der Hüfte. Archiv für Orthopädische und Unfallchirurgie 72, 33 (1972)

27. Willert, H.-G., Semlitsch, M.: Articular capsule reactions associated with joint endoprostheses. Paper read at the Congress of Dutch-Swiss Orthopaedic Societies, Lausanne 1974 (abstract published by Sulzer Brothers Limited)

28. Williams, D.F.: The selection of implant materials. In: D.F. Williams, R. Roaf, edit., Implants in Surgery pp. 299, London-Philadelphia-Toronto: Saunders 1973

29. Wiltse, L.L., Hall, R.H., Stenehjem, J.C.: Experimental studies regarding the possible use of self-curing acrylic in orthopaedic surgery. Journal of Bone and Joint Surgery 39-A, 961 (1957)

30. Winter, G.D.: Tissue reactions to metallic wear and corrosion products in human patients. Journal of Biomedical Materials Research 8, 11 (1974)

COMPLICATIONS AFTER JOINT REPLACEMENT – LONGTERM FOLLOW–UP, CLINICAL FINDINGS, AND BIOMECHANICAL RESEARCH

A. Schreiber, A.H. Huggler, C. Dietschi, and H. Jacob

Authors of world-wide orthopaedic literature are unanimous on the nature of the main complications that arise from hip joint replacement, viz. infection, loosening of the implant (including material failure) and wear, together with the thereby induced reaction of the surrounding tissue, which in turn may lead to loosening of the implant or stiffening of the joint. The presented figures, however, giving the number of cases associated with each of the above-mentioned causes vary considerably, depending on the number of endoprostheses inserted, the types employed (materials) and the length of the follow-up period.

At the Department of Orthopaedic Surgery of the University of Zurich, Balgrist, 1552 prostheses of the hip have been inserted between 1962 and 1974.

Of all these cases, a follow-up was possible in 1136. The 1136 replacements were grouped into 577 from 1962 to 1971 and the remaining 559 from 1972 to 1974. The first group of 577 belonged to a period prior to the introduction of the greenhouse and must be regarded as examples of long-term results. The second group, however, has furnished only short-term results.

Table 1 shows the percentage of clinical results classified according to type of prosthesis and period of follow-up and showing the corresponding rate of infection, loosening and number of re-operation. Table 2 shows the clinical assessment.

Some important facts in connection with long-term results are as follows:

1. The number of clinically "unsatisfactory" to "bad" results is matched by the proportion of infections, loosenings and re-operations.
2. The first prosthesis of the Charnley fluorosint and teflon type shows a significantly higher rate of infection (20 %) and loosening (57 %) than all other types employed. The loosening was caused mainly by material failure of the fluorosint socket.
3. Another significant rise in loosenings was registered with the metal-to-metal types (19.6 %), chiefly because of failures of the shaft.
4. The infection and loosening rate of the Charnley polyethylene type should perhaps be considered as being no higher than that with the Müller-Charnley type since the postoperative follow-up period of the former was 8 to 10 years compared with 3 to 7 years in the case of the latter.
5. Today, of course, we may ask why it was decided to abandon the relatively successful Charnley polyethylene type and go over to metal-to-metal prostheses. The answer is that the tendency to follow a new trend was particularly appealing at that time.

Table 1 Follow-up of 1136 prostheses of the hip (577 from 1962 to 1972, 559 from 1972 to 1974)

Type, year of operation	Postop. follow-up period (in years)	Total number	Clinical results in % good	satis-factory	unsatis-factory	bad	Long-term results (prior to "greenhouse") 62-71: Complications in % infections	loosenings (+ material failure)	reoperations
Charnley fluorosint + teflon 62-65	10-14	21	19	19	9.5	52	20	57	77
			38		62				
Charnley polyethylene 65-67 (68)	8-10	35	37	40	14	9	3.4	5.1	8.5
			77		23				
metal/metal 67-69	6-9	137	35.8	29.9	16	18.7	3.8	19.6	23.4
			65.7		34.7				
Müller-Charnley Protasul 2 69-71	3-7	384	51	23.4	12	11.5	2.3	1.7	4
			74.5		23.5				
							Short-term results (with "greenhouse") 72-74		
Müller-Charnley Protasul 2 modified shaft 72-74 (75)	1-3	559	56.3	26.5	11.1	6.1	1.2	0.9	2.1
			82.8		17.2				

Table 2 Clinical assessment

Criteria	Points
No pain	1
Flexion of 90 ^{o}	1
Manner of walking and ability	1
good	3 Points
satisfactory	2 "
unsatisfactory	1 "
bad	0 "

6. Finally, it should be mentioned that of a total of 1552 prostheses 416 (including death not directly related to the hip operation), or a little over one quarter, could not be followed-up. It must be assumed that the results might well fall into the "unsatisfactory" or even "bad" class, so that the figures in Table 1 should be considered as being a bit on the optimistic side.

The present results of re-operations (prosthesis replacement) performed by us are not encouraging; there appears to be no significant advantage over Girdlestone or Milch-Batcheler resection.

Some brief observations regarding radiological changes in long-term follow-up are as follows:

1. Over 80 % of "good" and satisfactory clinical results, show, in the course of time, an increase in alteration of bone and cement in the region of the trochanters (minor and major) as well as in the area surrounding the socket (Fig. 1). One certainly wonders whether this should be defined as potential loosening which, however, would manifest itself clinically only at a later date. At this point we must define and differentiate the terms "clinical loosening" and "radiological loosening". By the former we mean all signs of loosening exclusively accompanied by pain, whereas in the latter case pain is not necessarily felt by the patient.
2. Two examples of a long-term follow-up (one of over 20 years and one of over 10 years) are radiologically demonstrated. These have been classified as clinically "bad" (Figs. 2,3).

In the immediate past the infection rate and complications due to implant materials have dropped off steeply, but the loosening of implants has remained constant. Therefore, we decided to investigate the mechanical behaviour of the surrounding bone by means of experimental stress-analysis as well as in a hip-joint simulator (dynamic testing).

The idea that the acetabulum might deform under physiological load is not a new one. When standing on one leg, three principal forces influence the pelvis: body weight, abductor muscles and resultant force, which acts via the femoral head on the acetabulum.

These three forces cause an elastic deformation of the acetabulum which can freely take place, due to the flexible articular cartilage in the loaded acetabulum. The elliptical shape tends to adopt a spherical form (Fig. 4).

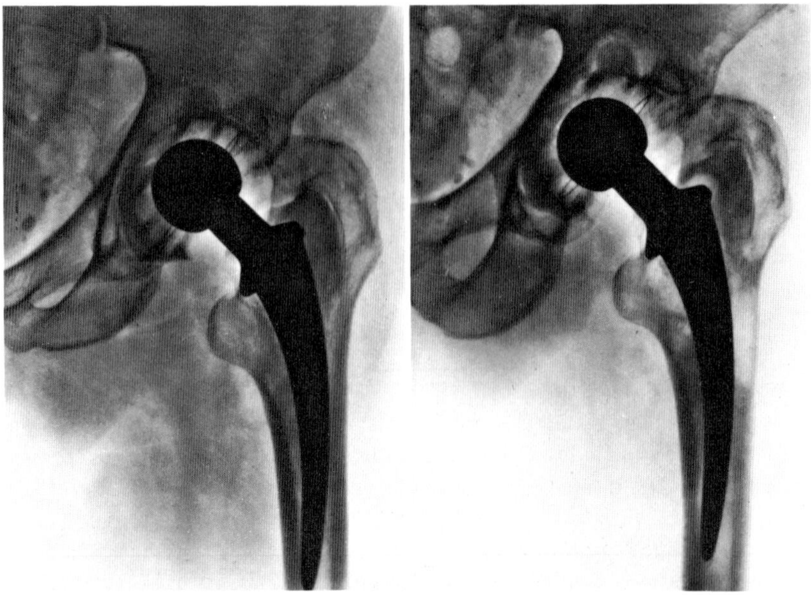

1971 1975

Fig. 1 Time dependent increase of bone and cement in the region of the trochanters and in the area surrounding the socket

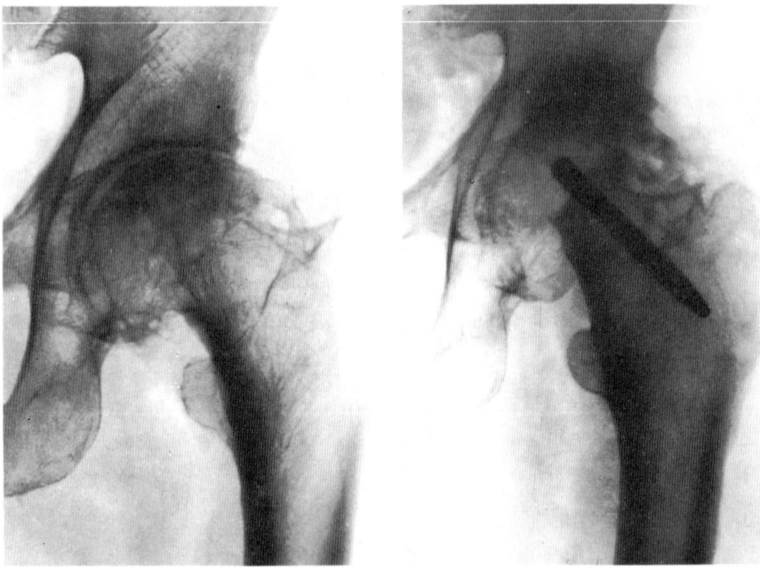

a b

Fig. 2 23 year follow-up period, within which the prosthesis had been changed 6 times

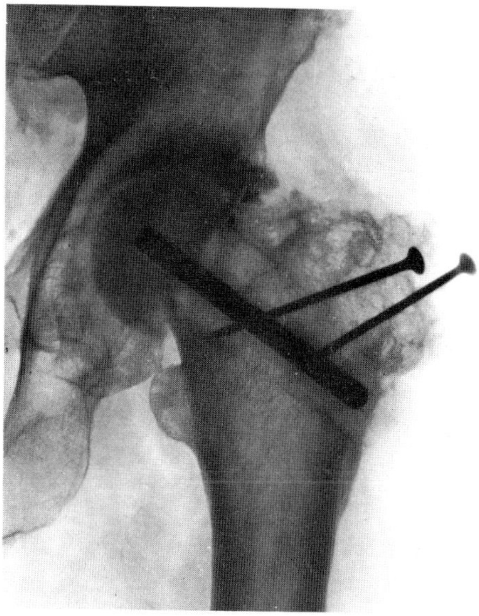

Fig. 2c

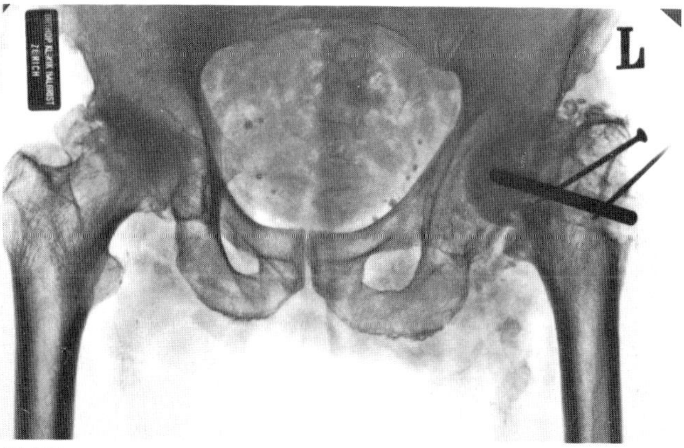

Fig. 2d
1965

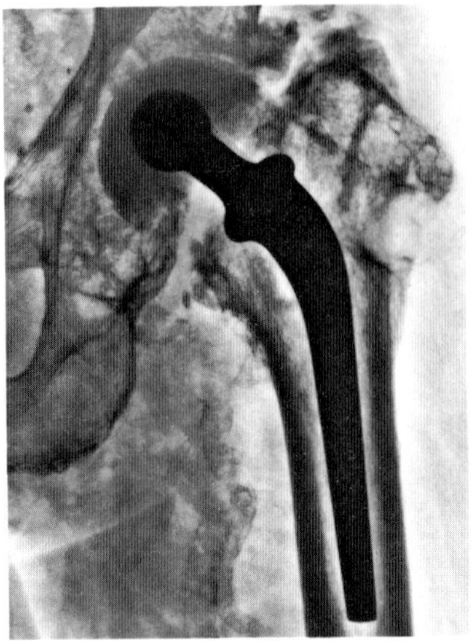

Fig. 2e

1965

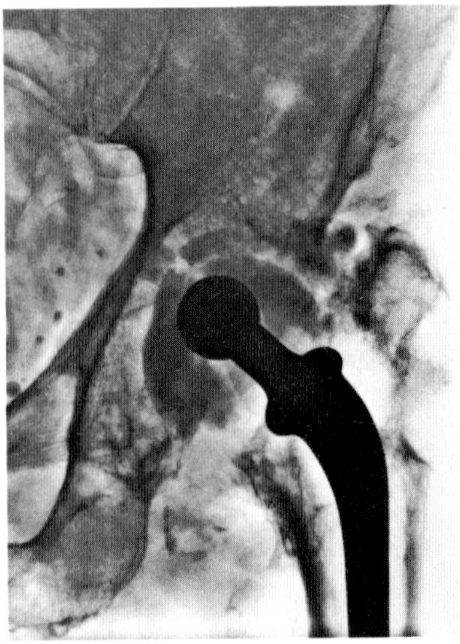

1967

Fig. 2g

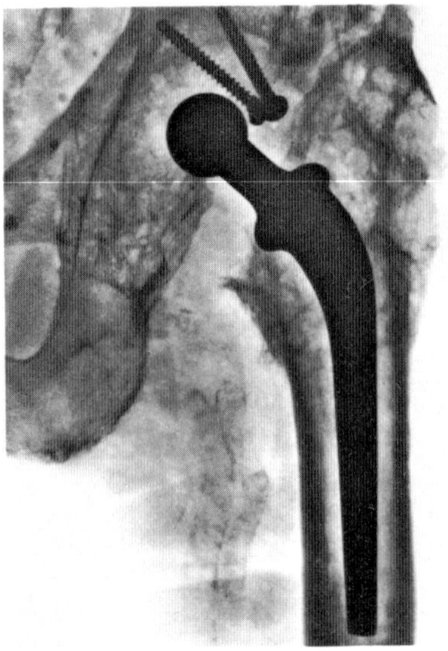

Fig. 2f

1969

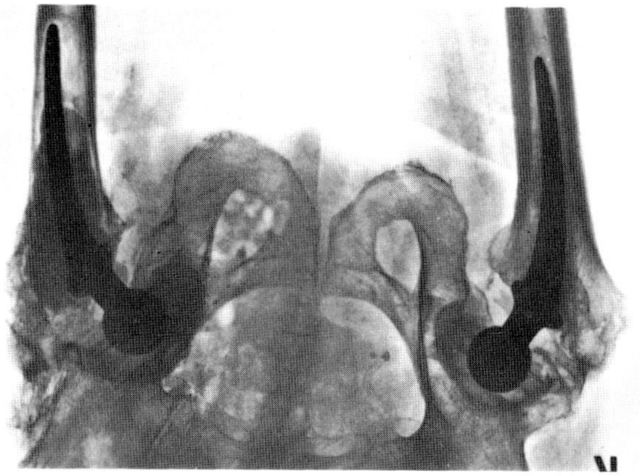

Fig. 2h

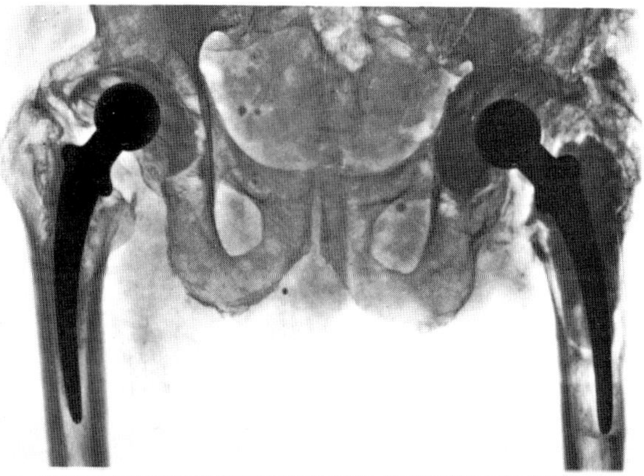

Fig. 2i

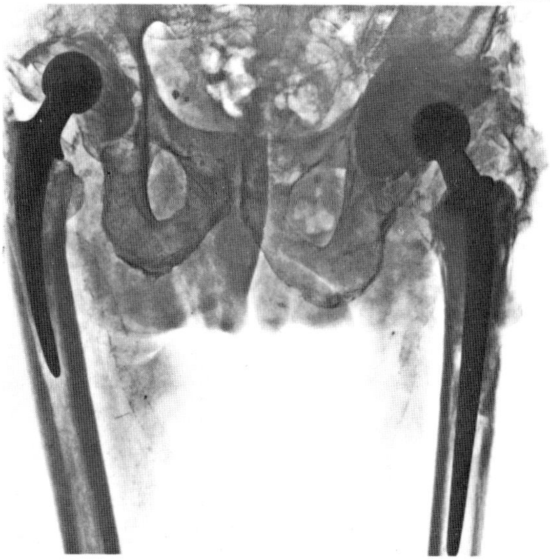

Fig. 2k

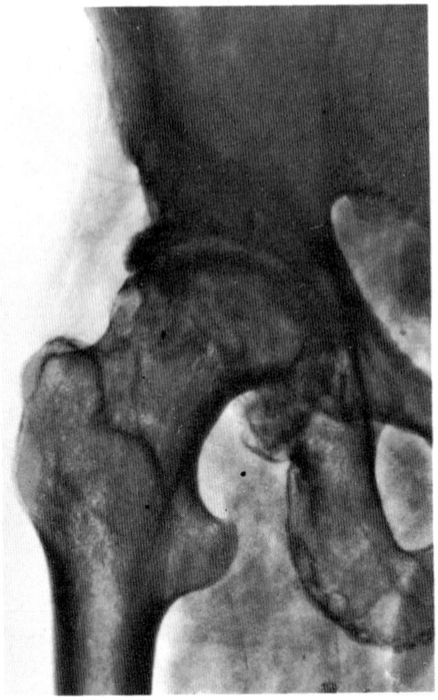

Fig. 3a

4 / 62

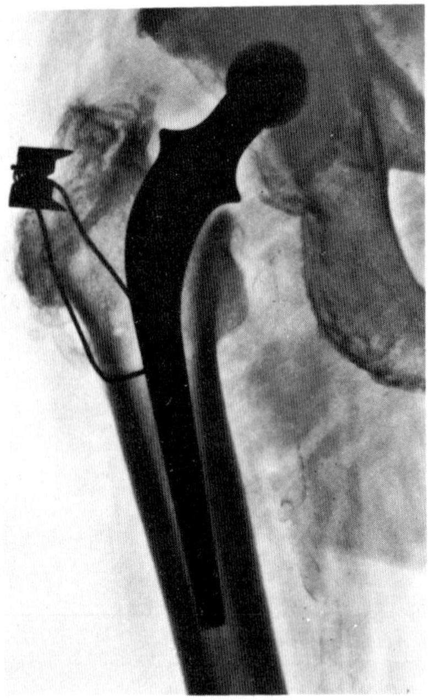

Fig. 3b

9 / 62

Fig. 3 14 year follow-up period, during which time extensive tissue reactions occurred because of wear despite the removal of the implants. The last two X-rays seem to indicate a malignant process which, however, could not be confirmed histologically

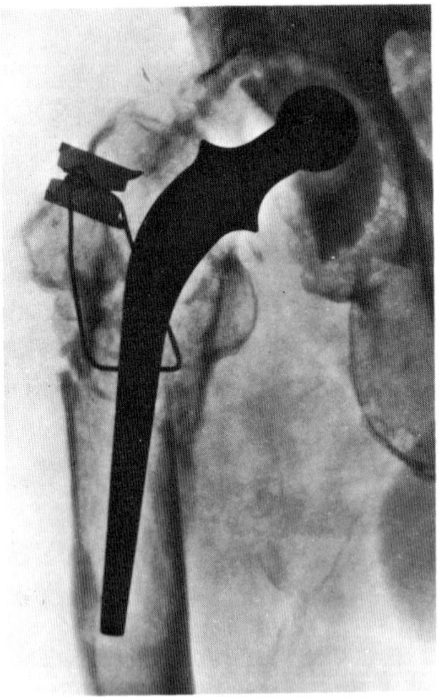

Fig. 3c

11 / 65

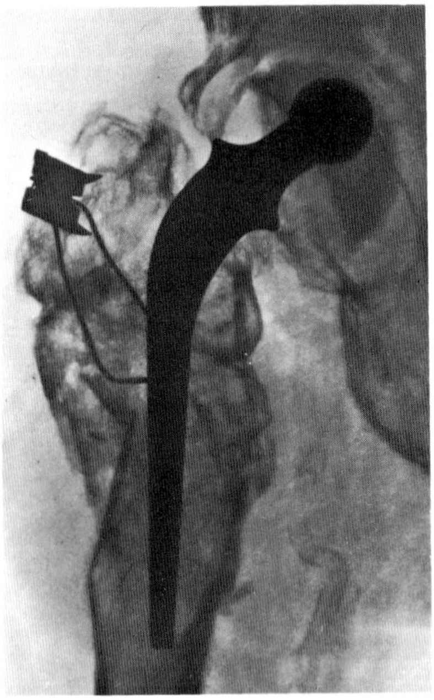

Fig. 3d

4 / 69

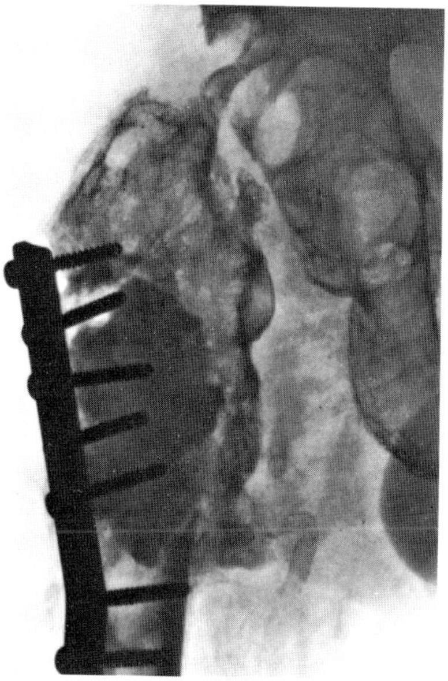

Fig. 3e

1969

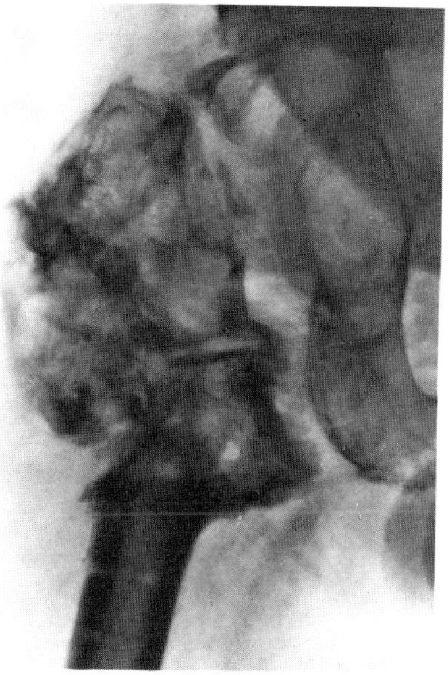

Fig. 3f

1972

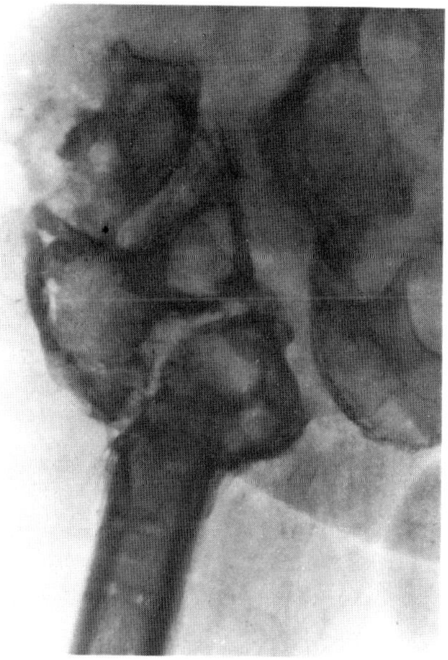

Fig. 3g

1975

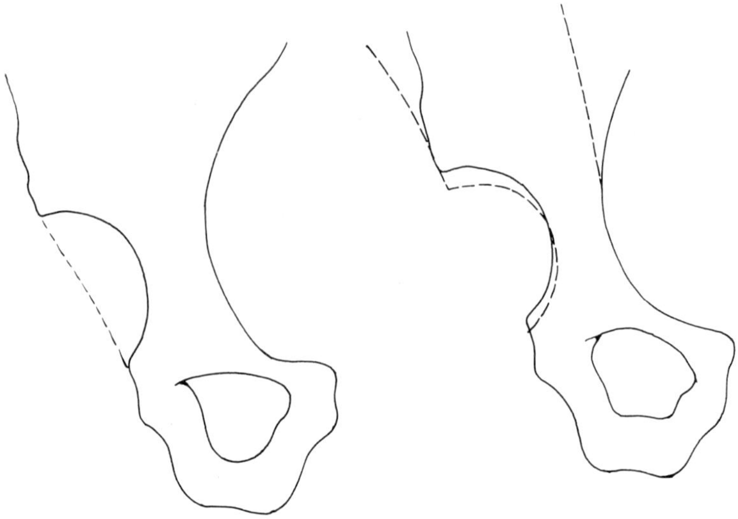

Fig. 4 Elastic deformation of the pelvis
left: unloaded
right: loaded

After the implantation of a rigid socket, the original degree of deformation is hindered, and therefore secondary compressive stresses occur. These stresses tend to push the socket out (Fig. 5).

Since it is difficult to measure strains and deformation directly in a physiological pelvis, we first examined the direction and magnitude of the principal stresses and strains on a loaded epoxy model. The body weight, the abductor muscles, and the layer of cartilage between acetabulum and femoral head have all been simulated in this model (Fig. 6).

Eighty rosette-shaped strain gauges were placed in previously determined points. If the principal strains and stresses of an isotropic pelvis coincide with the trabecular structure of an anisotropic one, like the bony pelvis, a comparable analysis is justified.

In this epoxy model several measurements with various loads have been made; resulting tensile and compressive stresses were reproducible at the corresponding measuring points.

On the outside of the pelvis (Fig. 7), mainly compressive stresses can be found in the region above the acetabulum. On the inner side of the pelvis as well as on the inside of the acetabulum, tensile stresses prevail. Table 3 shows some values of measured compressive stresses in the principal directions.

In, for example A 3, with 60 Kp weight bearing, a value of 0.82 Kp/mm^2 or 82 Kp/cm^2 compressive stress would occur. This value, for example, is about three times above the ultimate static strength of cancellous bone.

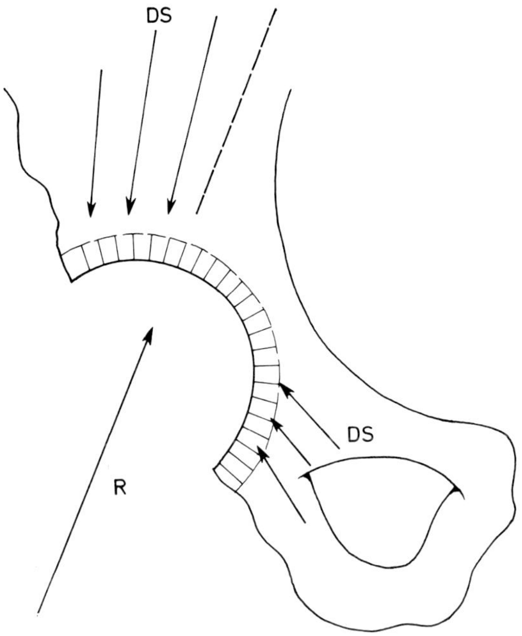

Fig. 5
Resultant force due to gravity, muscles, and compressive forces after implantation of a rigid socket

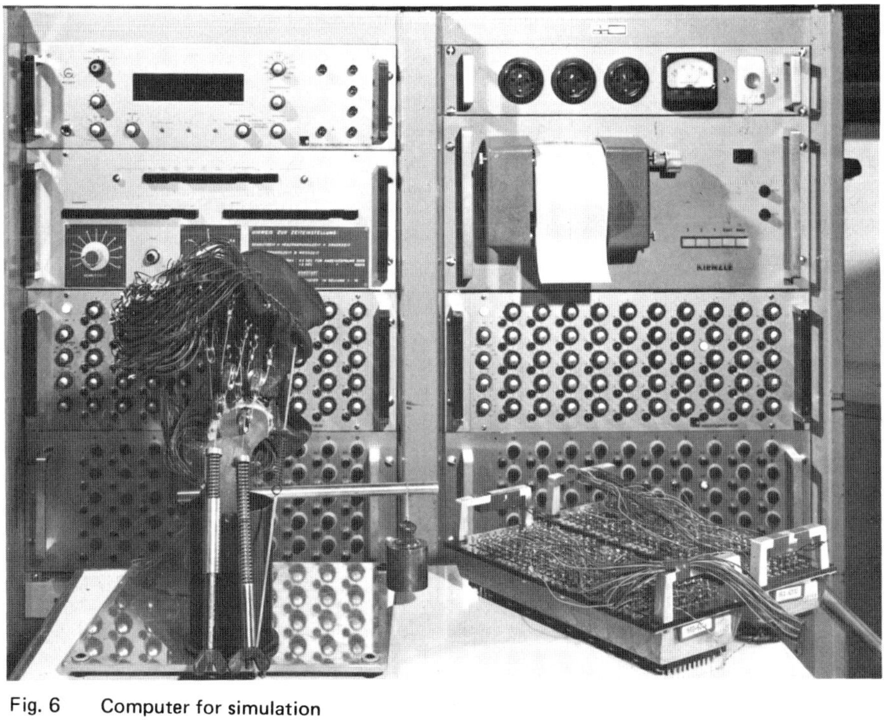

Fig. 6 Computer for simulation

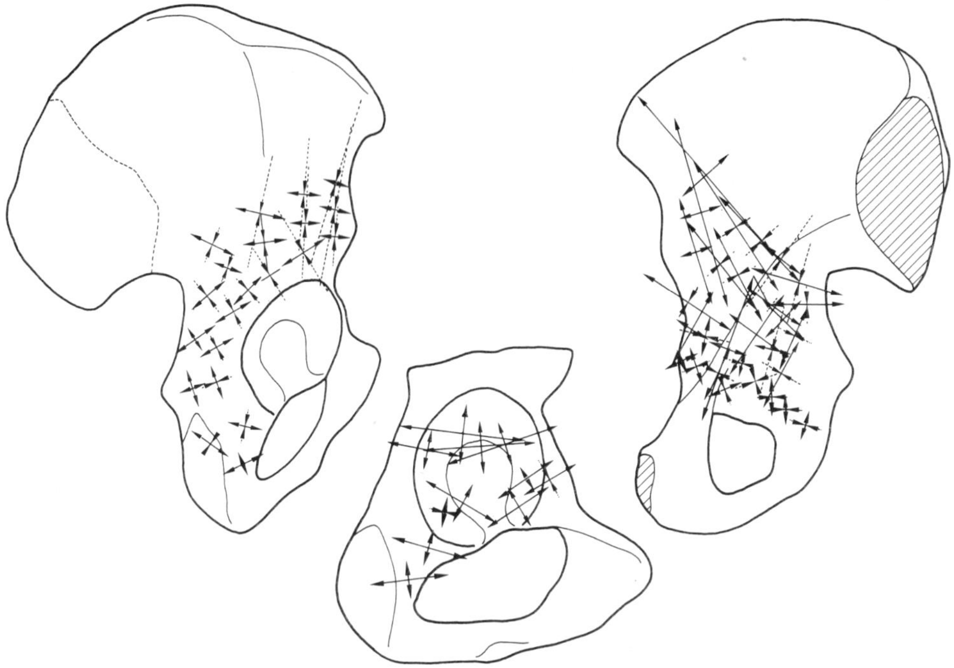

Fig. 7 Compressive and tensile stresses acting at the pelvis, weight bearing on one leg

Table 3 Values of some compressive stresses in a loaded epoxy pelvis (pelvis loaded with 6 Kp)

A_2:	– 0.079 Kp/mm^2	=	– 7.9 Kp/cm^2
A_3:	– 0.082 Kp/mm^2	=	– 8.2 Kp/cm^2
A_4:	– 0.070 Kp/mm^2	=	– 7.0 Kp/cm^2
B_2:	– 0.072 Kp/mm^2	=	– 7.2 Kp/cm^2
B_3:	– 0.066 Kp/mm^2	=	– 6.6 Kp/cm^2
B_4:	– 0.051 Kp/mm^2	=	– 5.1 Kp/cm^2
C_2:	– 0.062 Kp/mm^2	=	– 6.2 Kp/cm^2

We expect that when a rigid socket is implanted the maximum compressive stress-values must be even higher. It is probable that, due to such high compressive stress values, micro-fractures occur in the soft cancellous bone.

Such micro-fractures have indeed been recently observed on several occasions as follows:

1. Histological investigations of the boundary zone in the proximity of the socket-cement complex in patients who had to be re-operated because of loosening of the socket, often showed fracturing of the cancellous bone with subsequent healing as indicated by callus formation in the trabecular structure.

2. Dynamic loading of prosthesis implanted in pelvis and femoral bone, as tested in a hip joint simulator (Fig. 8a), induced micro-fractures in the cancellous bone, even extending to macro-fractures and implant-loosening in some cases. The maximum value of the alternating load in all the tests was about three times the body weight. The frequency was 2 Hz and the test specimens (implant, cement and bone) were immersed in Ringer's solution (Fig. 8b).

Altogether we have carried out three different tests on the hip simulator.

1. In the first test the socket was placed deep within the cancellous region of the pelvic bone (Fig. 9a). After three million cycles macro-fracturing of the cancellous bone in the immediate vicinity of the cement surface was observed, accompanied by a severe loosening of the implanted socket.

2. The second test was carried out with a natural hip joint that exhibited an absolutely intact cartilage (Fig. 9b). On completion of seven million cycles, testing was stopped because of damage that occurred to cartilage within the acetabulum as well as to the femoral head.

3. In the third test we removed only the cartilage, so that the socket came to bear directly on the cortical bone of the acetabulum (Fig. 9c). After seven million cycles, testing was discontinued because of destruction of the bearing surface. No loosening of the socket whatsoever occurred.

A comparison of the state of the cancellous bone after completion of the third test (Fig. 9c) with that of the first test (Fig. 9a) showed that fewer defects occurred within the cancellous region in the former case. This clearly indicates that a rigid implant certainly induces fracturing of the cancellous bone in the boundary area when the compact cortical layer is removed.

Fig. 10 shows a clear indication of this happening, protrusion of the socket and loosening was the result.

Of course, we are quite aware that the behaviour of bone "in vitro" is very different from that "in vivo" since no tissue reactions etc., can occur but, under given similar conditions, we have shown that the deeply inserted socket (Fig. 9a) is inferior to the one which is made to bear against the cortical bone (Fig. 9c). Therefore we suggest using – whenever possible – a small-sized socket in order not to have to remove a lot of the subchondrial bone from the acetabulum. We are of the opinion that the best choice available today is a special ball of alumina (Al_2O_3 = ceramic) paired with a small-sized socket of polyethylene. The excellent tribological properties of alumina moving against polyethylene has been demonstrated recently in several simulator tests.

Preliminary experiments have shown that cancellous bones exhibit a Young's modulus of approximately 70 Kp/mm^2, whereas the layer of cortical bone has a value of about 800 Kp/mm^2.

This has been taken into consideration in some very recent experimental investigations, we have carried out, in which the sandwich structure of the pelvic bone has been taken into account. We believe that:

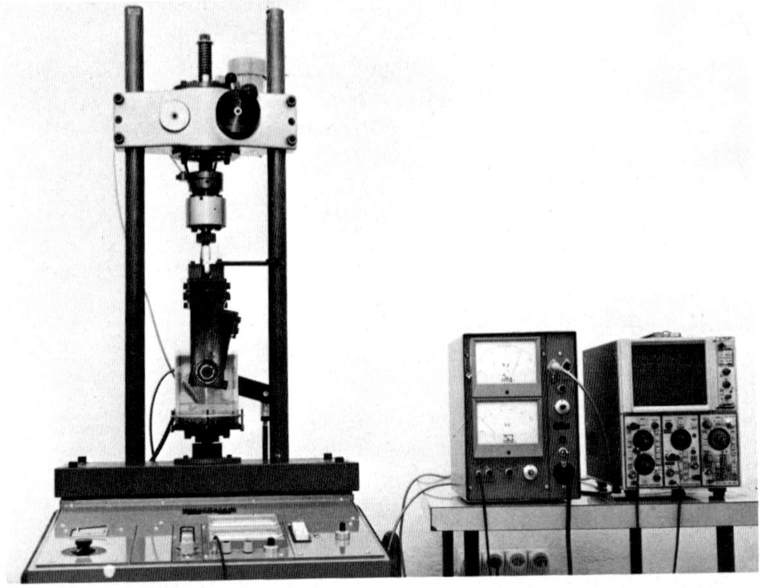

a

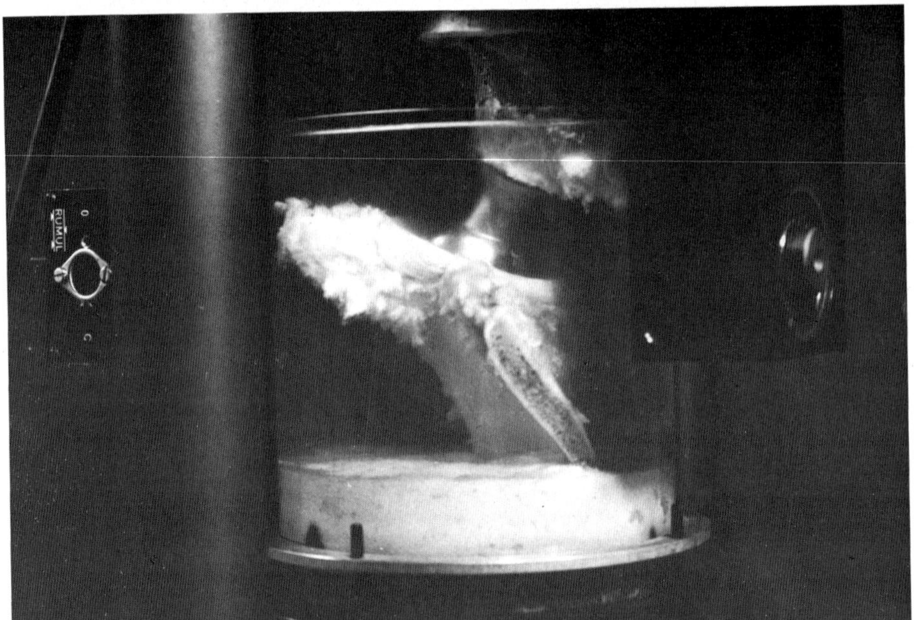

b

Fig. 8a,b Hip simulator

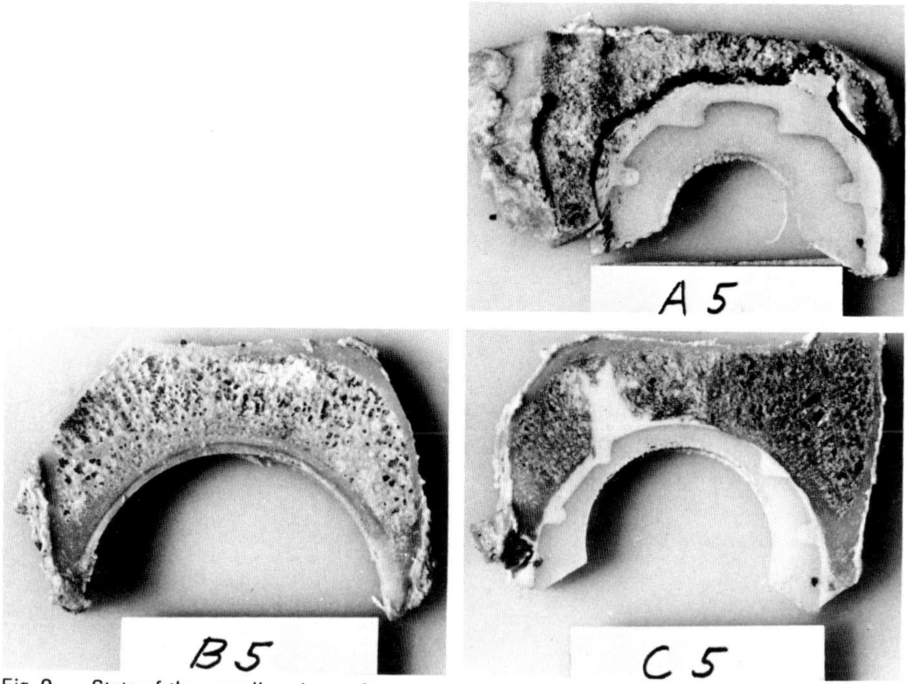

Fig. 9 State of the cancellous bone after test

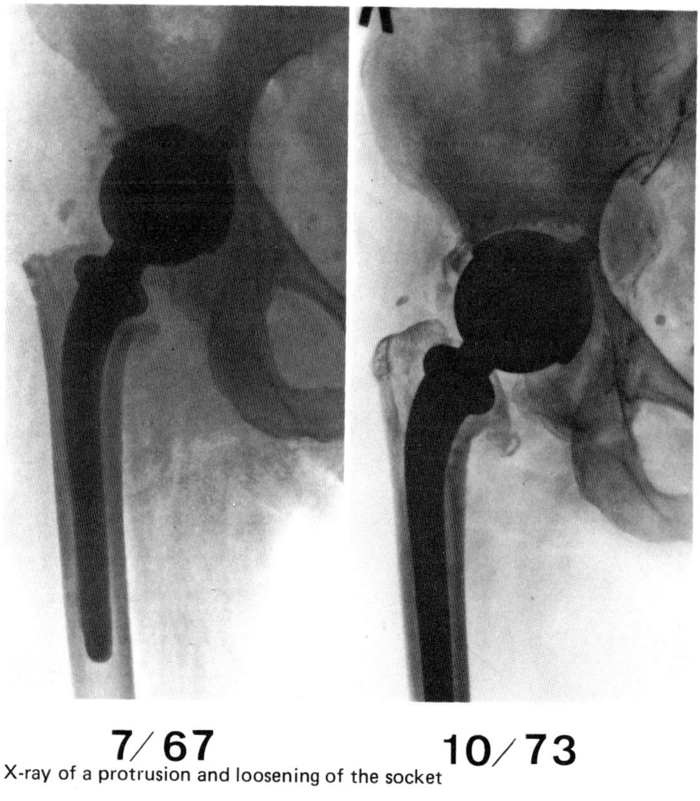

Fig. 10 X-ray of a protrusion and loosening of the socket

1. A rigid implant that is brought to bear directly on the relatively flexible bone must inevitably lead to failure through loosening.

2. Removal of the cortical layer enforces direct load bearing of the trabecular structure and this would also lead to failure.

3. In order to attain measure of success, the socket must be compatible with its immediate environment, that is, close attention must be paid to the material selected, its shape and rigidity, not forgetting the tribological and mechanical requirements necessary for a proper ball and socket joint.

4. The implantation technique must be chosen so as to ensure that the natural stress pattern in the pelvis is not adversely effected in any way.

5. It has recently been discovered that certain ceramics exhibit excellent tribological properties when moving against polyethylene and therefore, on the basis of all that has been said above, we believe that a relatively small sized socket (which would not require any of the subchondrial bone to be removed) of polyethylene paired with a special ball of alumina (Al_2O_3) is about the best choice available today.

THE TRUNNION BEARING TOTAL HIP PROSTHESIS

B.G. Weber and G. Stühmer

The trunnion bearing total hip prosthesis was designed in 1961. Challenging the inevitable phenomenon of wear, a femoral head made of plastic material mated with a femoral component on a trunnion, with a pelvic component in a ball and socket joint, the two peripheral components being made of chromium cobalt alloy (1-8). Wear would be restricted to the interpositum, thus allowing easy replacement, leaving the cemented main components untouched (Fig. 1).

Technologists had suggested polyester for the femoral head, a resin of phthalic acid, a material which had given most satisfactory wear resistance in certain machines. Polyester was tested in tissue cultures and implanted in animals. Both tests showed good tissue tolerance as for high density polyethylene.

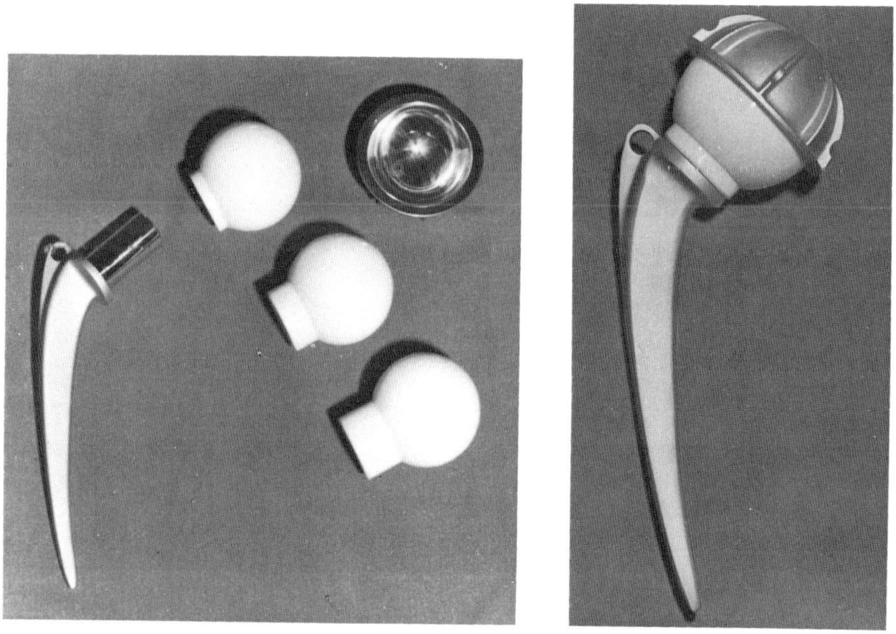

Fig. 1 The trunnion bearing total hip joint with polyester head.
a. The 3 components: Femoral component and cup made of chromium cobalt alloy, the heads with different neck lengths made of polyester (Sulester)
b. The assembled prosthesis, the head rotating on the trunnion

The prosthesis tested in the simulator behaved most satisfactorily. Based on such preclinical results, the trunnion bearing prosthesis was implanted 1049 times at our hospital between 1968 and 1972.

PROBLEMS OF THE POLYESTER TRUNNION BEARING TOTAL HIP JOINT

During the first 3-4 years after the operation, patients with a polyester prosthesis are happy with the result. In 30 % of the cases, however, the result is then compromised by an unexpected deterioration, appearing either spontaneously or after a minor accident involving a shock to the hip joint. Such patients complain of pain when starting to walk and weakness in the hip joint during ambulation. At rest they feel no pain.

At the beginning of deterioration, the X-ray picture of the hip joint already shows definite signs of loosening of the socket, while the femoral component is still firm. However there is a certain degree of resorption of the calcar femoris to be registered.

Loosening is a progressive process, as the bone of the pelvis and the calcar are progressively resorbed (Fig. 2).

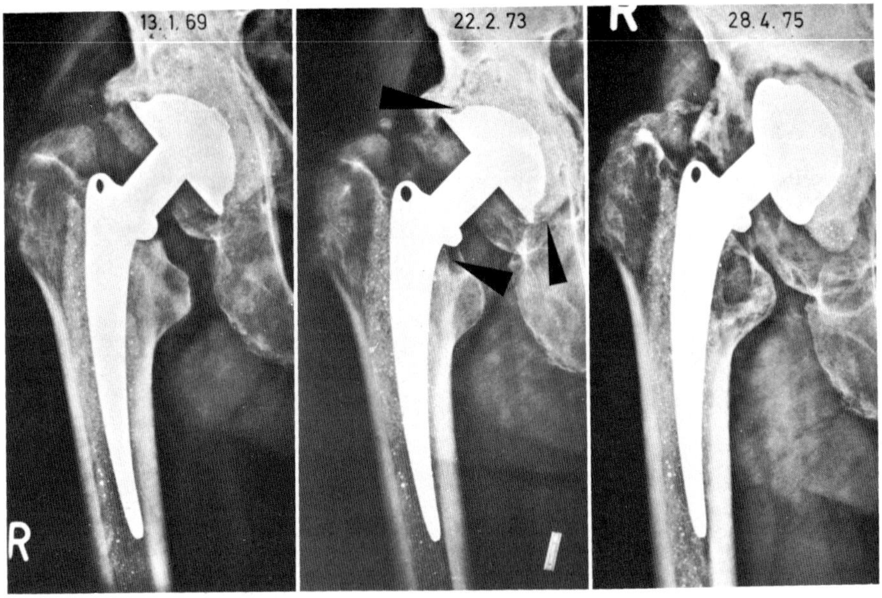

Fig. 2 Implant loosening, a progressive process (F.H., 1907, male, Nr. 121 966)

a. X-ray after hip replacement: The prosthesis is firmly bonded.
b. 4 years after surgery: To date, patient has had no complaints, however, loosening has started with bone resorption (►).
c. 6 years after surgery: For a year the patient has been complaining of pain when starting to walk, weakness, need of a stick

Such observations suggested the necessity for an alternative prosthesis. Revision operations offered material for investigation. The results were as follows:

1. The metal components showed no measurable wear at the time of revision, i.e. 3-4 years after operation.
2. The polyester showed little wear along the hole and the head surface. The wear pattern is uniform, proving that the head was able to rotate all the time.
3. Willert and Semlitsch (9) found in specimens that bone resorption and loosening are the effect of a foreign body reaction against very fine polyester powder, smaller than 20 microns in diameter. The tissue reaction is the same, as had been observed in other loose prostheses made of different materials, i.e. is unspecific.
4. It is evident that in our prosthesis the socket becomes loose first and the femoral component much later.
5. The femoral component was broken in only 1 case of the whole series. This positive finding is to be attributed to the sound geometry of the shaft, providing optimal hold in the cement and in the cavity of the femur.

HOW TO REVISE A LOOSE POLYESTER TRUNNION BEARING TOTAL HIP JOINT?

The loosening of the prosthesis is a progressive pathological process. Therefore it is most important to change the loose components as soon as symptoms arise. The sooner the revision is carried out, the less resorption of bone occurs, the easier the reoperation can be done, the more successful the result will be (Fig. 3).

In most cases, the socket is loose and the femoral part still firm. After osteotomy of the greater trochanter, the hypertrophic capsule is removed, the hip joint dislocated, the polyester head discarded from the trunnion. The trunnion is protected from scratching with a small plastic cap. The loose socket is extracted and the cement removed.

Between cement and bone, there is a membrane of connective tissue which has to be removed. The remaining sclerotic and very well vascularized bony socket is left intact. With a 6 mm drill, numerous holes are made to offer stability for the new socket. A polyethylene socket of adequate size and depth is then inserted using bone cement. In the case of a bony defect, this must first be closed with a bone graft, employing a cement shell and a metal mesh, depending on the size, shape and localization of the defect.

The trunnion protector is now removed. A chromiumcobalt head with the optimal neck length is fitted to the trunnion and the hip is reduced.

The greater trochanter is refixed to the shaft with tensionband-wiring. The postoperative treatment is the same as for primary operation.

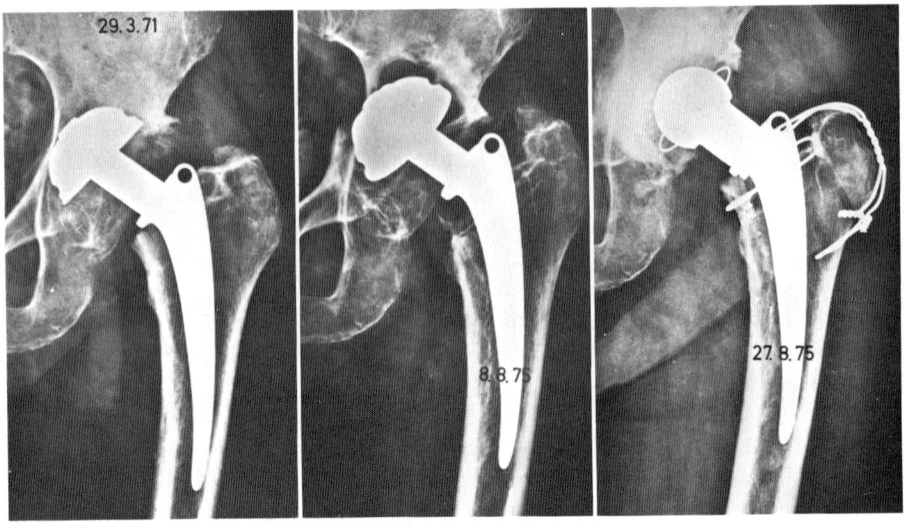

Fig. 3 Changing of a loose cup in a polyester-head total hip (B.L., 1906, female, Nr. 147 673)

a. X-ray after hip replacement. The prosthesis is firmly bonded.
b. 4 1/2 years after surgery: For 6 months the patient has had symptoms of loosening. Bone resorption around the cup with infraction of the floor of the socket and resorption of the femoral spur.
c. X-ray after revision operation: The firm femoral component has been left in place, the femoral spur has been reconstructed with a piece of the greater trochanter. The bony defect of the pelvic floor has been filled up with cancellous bone, the loose metallic socket has been replaced by a polyethylene cup and fixed with bone cement. The polyester head has been replaced by a 32 mm metal head. The osteotomized greater trochanter has been fixed with wire

THE PRIMARY HIP JOINT REPLACEMENT

The prosthesis described is not only suitable for the exchange operation, but also for primary procedure (Fig. 4). Now there are 4 stems available, 3 heads with different neck lengths and 3 pairs of polyethylene sockets, plus one very large socket.

With such a "building block" system, all individual variations of the patient's anatomical situation can be dealt with (Fig. 5).

Appropriate instruments make the operation easier in the case of primary or revision operation.

From 1972-1974, 700 32 mm trunnion bearing total hip joints were implanted, 260 to convert loose polyester prostheses, 440 as primary procedures. The continuous follow-up of as many patients as possible is on the way. Table 1 shows the early results of those cases which have had the new prosthesis for more than 2 years.

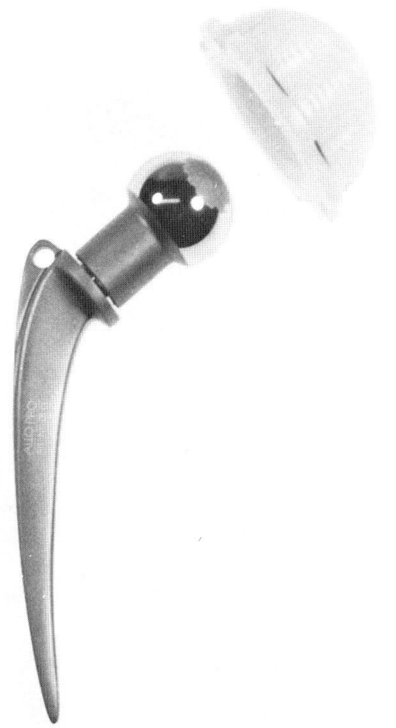

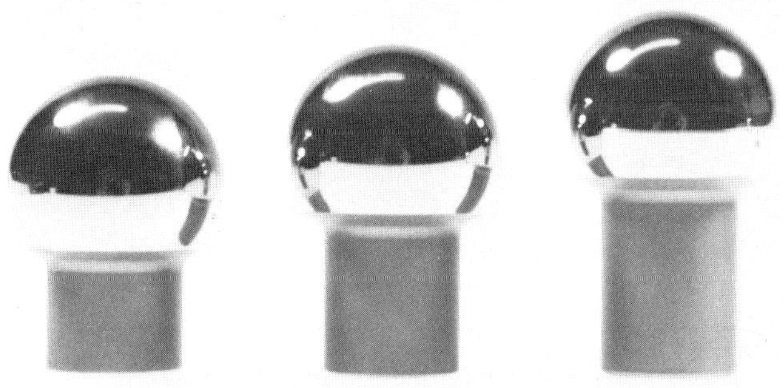

Fig. 4 The trunnion bearing total hip joint with 32 mm metallic head and polyethylene cup
a. The 3 components permitting relative motion against one an other.
b. The 32 mm heads with selectable different neck lengths

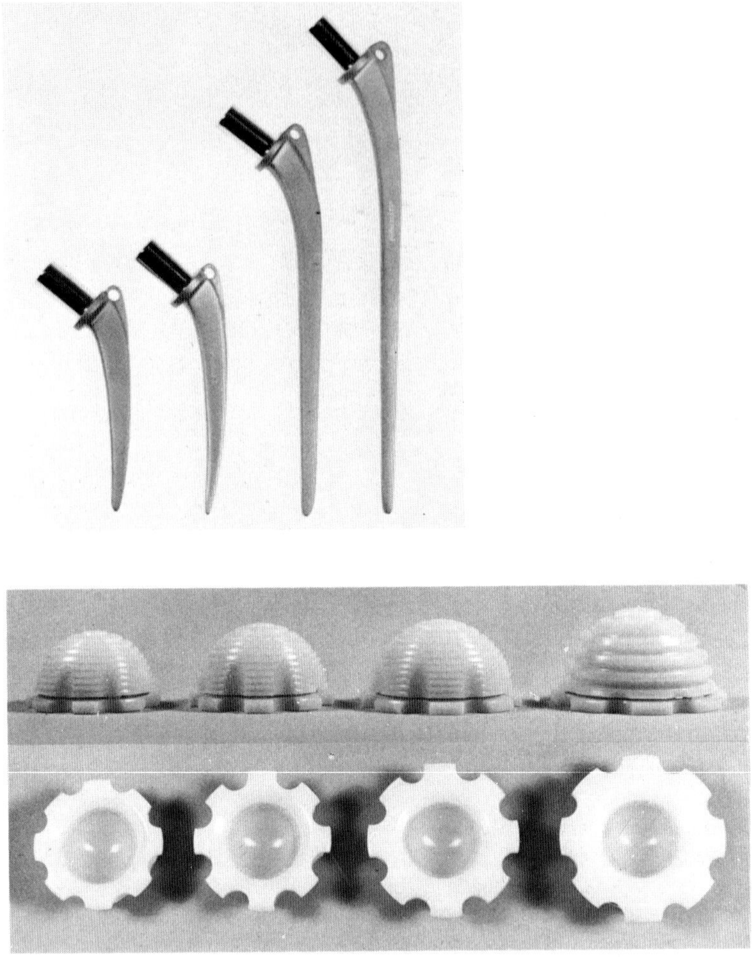

Fig. 5 Building block system of the total hip joint
a. Various dimensions and configurations of the shaft and
b. various sizes and configurations of cups are available to meet the requirements

Table 1 Early results of the 32 mm trunnion bearing total hip joint

	66 cases converting polyester- into 32 mm-type	100 cases of primary procedure with 32 mm-type
good	80.0 %	90.5 %
fair	17.5 %	9.5 %
bad	2.5 %	–

It is not surprising that the primary prostheses are superior to the repair-procedures. The anatomical situation is more favourable in the one group than in the other. In the primary procedure group, loosening symptoms are present in less than 5 % in contrast to 18 % in the repair-group.

DISCUSSION

Loosening of the implant in total hip replacement has several causes. One is a foreign body reaction of the host tissue to abraded material, a reaction of the joint capsule tissue and of the bone to which the implant is anchored.

Willert and Semlitsch (9) come to the conclusion, that different materials abraded from total hip joints, teflon, polyethylene, polyester, bone-cement, produce the same pattern of tissue reaction. The reaction to polyester is therefore unspecific, but more violent. It seems that not the material itself, but its quantity determines whether loosening appears earlier or later. Loosening is to be characterized as follows: The loosening of a polyester prosthesis starts after 3-4 years, initially the pelvic component, leaving the femoral component intact. Bone resorption is progressive, giving rise to a very well-vascularized enlarged bony socket. This is in contrast to infection, where bone resorption is accompanied by a rather poorly vascular or avascular bone bed.

The loose socket with a firm femoral part lends itself to a repair procedure leaving the femoral stem in place. Because loosening is a progressive process, repair should be done as soon as possible. At a later stage, bone resorption may be of such an extent, that a refixation is impossible, leaving the patient crippled, without any hip joint at all.

The 3-piece prosthesis may have an advantage: Rotation of the head on the trunnion protects the head socket joint from wear to an unknown degree. This would result in a longer "life" of the polyethylene cup than in the case of the ordinary 2-piece implants.

REFERENCES

1. Weber, B.G.: Die Rotations-Totalendoprothese des Hüftgelenkes. Zeitschrift für Orthopädie 107, 304 (1970)
2. Weber, B.G.: Total hip replacement with rotation-endoprosthesis (Trunnion-bearing prosthesis). Clinical Orthopaedics and Related Research 72, 79 (1970)
3. Weber, B.G.: Hip arthroplasty. Complications after total hip replacement by rotation endoprosthesis. Acta Orthopaedica Scandinavica 42, 429 (1971)
4. Weber, B.G.: Total hip replacement with rotation endoprosthesis. Int. Congress Series 291, Proceedings of the 12th Congress of the International Society of Orthopaedic Surgery and Traumatology, Tel Aviv 1972

5. Weber, B.G.: Total hip replacement: Problem of implant-loosening. In: Chapchal, G., edit., Arthroplasty of the hip, Stuttgart: Thieme 1973, p. 203

6. Weber, B.G., Stühmer, G.: Gute und schlechte Erfahrungen mit der Totalprothese des Hüftgelenkes. In: Cotta, H., Schulitz, K.P., edit., Der totale Hüftgelenksersatz, Stuttgart: Thieme 1973, p. 118

7. Weber, B.G., Stühmer, G.: Erfahrungen und Ergebnisse mit der Rotations-Totalprothese für das Hüftgelenk. Acta Traumatologica 3, 225 (1973)

8. Weber, B.G., Stühmer, G., Semlitsch, M.: Erfahrungen mit dem Kunststoff Polyester als Komponente der Rotationstotalprothese des Hüftgelenkes. Zeitschrift für Orthopädie 112, 1106 (1974)

9. Willert, H.G., Semlitsch, M.: Kapselreaktionen auf Kunststoff- und Metallabrieb bei Gelenkendoprothesen. Technische Rundschau Sulzer 2 (1975)

CLINICAL REQUIREMENTS OF ARTIFICIAL JOINTS

D. Hohmann

Long-term follow-ups of the last few years have shown that the number of late disorders of artificial joints is disturbingly high despite many improvements.

Reasons for the failure of joint endoprostheses are only partly known. Improved materials and designs have not fulfilled the requirements for long-term use under load bearing conditions. New principles of design and new biomaterials are now being tested.

This chapter is an attempt to define the clinical requirements to be met by artificial joints, and to find out what conditions for satisfactory long-term results have already been realized and where there are still important gaps in our knowledge.

In the main, there is a considerable lack of information on the behaviour of some biomaterials in situ, the bone reactions associated with them and the changed biomechanical conditions (12,22,33).

The primary requirement to be met by an artificial joint is unlimited easy moving. In most hip and knee endoprostheses these important functional requirements are fulfilled.

The way of moving of total hip prostheses imitates the physiological way of moving at a virtually unchanged centre of rotation. EMG-examinations, however, show a clear deviation of the physiological muscle actions of the type of "standing gait" in nearly two thirds of the cases. This most probably means a change in the resultant forces during the dynamic process of function. The shock absorption of the kinetic chain is thereby also changed.

In knee prostheses a relatively physiological moving sequence is only to be expected in prostheses of the condylar type (15) or the sledge-type (13) and e.g. in the Sheehan or Deane prostheses (9,31). A compromise would be the migrating axis of the GSB prosthesis (17). Hinge-type prostheses have an axis more dorsaly situated in order to obtain a greater range of flexion. This is always achieved at the expense of an increased tension of the extensor tendon. Limited rotational movement in flexion is permitted by only few designs (2,9,31). Rotation means an advantage, not so much for walking comfort, but for the stress of the anchorage.

The design of condylar or hinge type prostheses must always take account of the soft tissue, mainly the ligaments of the joint, in the case of a changed center of moving.

Charnley has coined the term "low friction arthroplasty" (8). Without any doubt, we are far from being able to imitate the ideal lubricational properties of a natural joint (12). Increased friction means increased torque and shear stress at the implant-bone interface and may lead to an increased rate of loosening. According to Anderson, Freeman, Swanson, Wilson and Scales, however, it is doubtful whether low friction, apart low wear, has any real importance for the anchorage of prostheses as is assumed by Ruckelshausen (27) and others. For the loosening of a cemented socket, twisting forces of 140-180 Nm are needed, whereas frictional moments between socket and head are about 9.5-16 Nm (1,4,19,22).

A low moment of friction however may be of vital importance if it is assumed that the functional differentiation of the interface tissue is improved if shearing forces are avoided during the phase of stabilization of implant healing. Bone ingrowth in structured surface, or repair of fractured or necrotic bone spicules require "mechanical rest", which will be disturbed by any kind of micro-movement. Avoiding this would be one of the preconditions for a real continuity of implant and bone by ingrowth in order to cope with acting forces through tension in the material (22).

A vital condition for good long-term results is stability, security and wear-resistance of the implant. Fractures of the implant have become rare with the types of prostheses in current use, given a valgus position of the hip prosthesis. Improvements of the material properties and stem geometry have reduced fatigue fractures and tissue damage due to metal wear and corrosive products (30). From this point of view the requirements of materials and design seem to have been fulfilled better then others.

Inadequately clarified is the mechanical behaviour of new biomaterials e.g. ceramics, to which, right from the beginning, new principles of design based on their known properties have to be applied. It seems possible that, for example, the brittleness of ceramics requires certain principles of design which also meet biomechanical requirements.

There is no danger of dislocation in any of the hip and knee prostheses in current use, provided a proper implantation technique is used. Loss of muscular balance may mean an increased danger of dislocation even in cases with correct fit of the joint. This is more a question of indication or operative technique than of joint design.

In contrast, in particular snap-sockets may leed to additional stress on the anchorage. There will never be completely ideal implants. Precise informations about the biomechanical background of the prosthesis, simple designs, big head diameters to prevent dislocation, and optimally adapted, easy-to-handle tools for insertion will minimize the failure of operative technique. The main problem which affects the future of an endoprosthesis is the inherent danger of loosening. All artificial joints known to date have no absolutely stable anchorage. There is always a layer of connective tissue on the interface between bone and cement, which develops in the process of repair of the damaged bone (5,6,7,24,32).

Given biologically inert material, it will become fibrocartilage under certain mechanical stress, and bone under "mechanical rest". Such connective tissue can take upon load. It is doubtful whether it can work as a shockabsorber as Charnley assumes. In current designs it is possibly necessary for the coexistance of bone and implant.

Shear forces are unavoidable at the interface between bone and implant, as a separation of continuity will always exist. It is not easy to forsee the conditions, under which this apparently necessary layer of connective tissue creates a sufficiently long-term connection, or when an increasing loss of fixation is to be expected. Certain stress forces make probable early insufficiency of this connection, in part also with destruction of cement (16, 20,21,26).

The quality of the compound depends on the congruence between bone and implant. Good congruence will be maintained by cementing, despite shrinkage of self curing polymers (11). Penetration of the cement into the cancellous bone effects an extraordinary large surface, yet without straightened structures (5,32).

The stress distribution on a large surface suffices in some cases to maintain a long-term balance. Thermal and toxic damage to the tissue, on the other hand, can be so great that adequate repair at the load-bearing interface does not occur — the prosthesis remains instable and can loosen further. It is not yet clear whether special structures at the surface of the implant effect an equally good or even better long-term fixation if a congruent cementless implantation is performed (23,24,25). Here the slight fretting between materials of identical or different elasticity which do not permit "mechanical rest" has to be considered.

These problems are relevant for both stem and socket anchorage, especially under dynamic, less so under static, conditions. A basic requirement for an improvement of this situation is a more precise knowledge of the direction and size of the forces acting in the environment of the implant, and the adequate differentiation of tissue related to them.

The examination of tissue reactions due to wear products of joint surfaces and PMMA has become of special importance. Loosening is not always due to thermal, toxic or mechanical damage. According to Duff-Barclay, Willert and others polymers can behave as biologically inert materials. But the amount and the grain size of abrasive particles can cause serious tissue damage. Chemical influences can be of equal importance if the surface of the abraded material is immensely enlarged. Metal sensivity, toxic reactions due to metal wear, foreign body reactions to HDPE and tissue necrosis due to PETP and PMMA are known (12,14,32,33) As these wear products can be part of a reason for implant loosening it is absolutely necessary to reduce wear. It is possible to imagine that there may be a balance between the amount and type of the wear particles and the tissue reactions related to it. Cementless implantation will help avoid debris due to abraided PMMA. This may be of some importance, because bone resorption at the femur shaft has never been observed in non-infected, loose Moore prostheses — rare cases with metal sensivity excluded.

Ceramic joint surfaces are said to have high wear resistence after a certain initial period of "running in". Chemical stability seems to be beyond any doubt. In addition to electrochemical stability, a porous structure of the implant means a scaffolding for bone ingrowth, which provides a very firm anchorage at an enlarged surface. Pore diameters greater than 0.1 - 0.2 mm show ingrowth of mineralized bone (28,29). Whether the amount of ingrowing bone in special structures of the surface of ceramic implants differs from the ingrowth rate in, for example, porous metal or polymers is not yet properly known. The ingrowth rate in inert material seems to depend more on size and profile of these structures (10).

The chemical bond between bone and the so-called "bioglasses" make these to a most promising material on the way to a cementless implantation. Such a very tight compound of bone and implant, on the other hand, will not develop merely with the aid of a chemical reaction, but only if "mechanical rest" obtains at the same time. Local "mechanical rest" at the bone-implant interface will be achieved only by avoiding all forces that lead to shearing stress. This means an absolutely stable implantation and a minimum of elastic bone deformation. This may afford a postoperative immobilization of the patient for about 3 months and it leads to the necessity of an extremely precise congruence between bone and prosthesis. This provides special instruments, high accuracy in operative technique and a wide range of dimensions of implants.

It can bee argued, however, that such a bone-to-implant bond may also loosen in time, if bending or shearing forces under weight-bearing lead to resorption of overloaded bone "anchors". It must be emphasized that the design of an implant for long-term use should provide a transmission possibly of tensile and shearing forces into compressive forces to the bone layer. In this case, the load should be distributed to a plane as large as the load-bearing surface of the joint to be replaced (15).

The size and direction of such only-compression-stressed zones are known in the growing skeleton. The structure and direction of the epiphyseal plate, for example, are adjusted perpendicular to the resultant forces. The epiphyseal scar in adult bone may indicate such a zone of compression equilibrium. Some endoprostheses, for example, the Freeman-Swanson knee-joint are designed to meet these basic requirements. A femoral head replacement of this type is under construction. The deformation of bone under load-bearing and muscle force stress in the layer of the implant has to be investigated, since shearing forces at the interface will prevent the ingrowth of mature bone (18).

Preconditions for a widespread utilization of special types of prostheses are simple design for easy and speedy implantability in order to avoid infections, adaptation to all varieties of the skeleton and all degrees of pathological disorders. Under certain circumstances this must be based on a great variety of dimensions of the implants. For the time being an overall good replacement for extreme sizes and forms of joints is not possible with any of the prosthesis systems in current use. Hospitals therefore have to keep in store a variety of different prosthesis systems together with the instruments needed for implantation. This makes joint replacement more expensive and means additional work for the surgical staff. A standardized design for example, would be one solution to this problem.

These difficulties may be tolerated as long as cement fixation is in general use.

Apart from subtle operative techniques, cementless anchorage will also require an even wide range of prosthesis dimensions in order to make possible an absolutely stable implantation. The replacement of a prosthesis in the case of fracture or loosening, must not be made additionally difficult by the design of the implant.

Among other things, the preservation of bony substance is the reason for the further follow-up of an exchanged prosthesis. Each loosening and each removal of cement, especially in the environment of the stem, is connected with loss of bony substance.

Either a bone-saving method of removal of cement has to be found or else we must get away from the intramedullary cemented fixation. This means at the same time an implant has to be developed, which can be fixed on the head or neck of the femur, with a desirable reduction of the amount of resection. This will give a more favourable second line of defense. In knee joints arthrodesis for the salvation of failed prostheses is no problem.

CONCLUSION

We find that we get closer to the goal of a satisfying long-term result only by better consideration of size and direction of biomechanically acting forces, and the behaviour of deformation of bone, and by more clearly interpreting the reaction of the living tissue to these forces and to incorporated materials. Otherwise we will not have self locking but self loosening prostheses. It is to be expected that one day, we shall find materials and designs that represent a more favourable compromise between living tissue and implant.

REFERENCES

1. Andersson, G.B.J., Freeman, M.A.R., Swanson, S.A.V.: Loosening of the cemented acetabular cup in total hip replacement. Journal of Bone and Joint Surgery 54-B, 590 (1972)
2. Attenborough, C.G.: Stabilized gliding total knee replacement. In: The knee joint, Amsterdam: Excerpta Medica 228, 1974
3. Boutin, P.: Arthroplastie totale de la hanche par prosthese en alumine fritee. Revue de Chirurgie Orthopedique 58, 229 (1972)
4. Chen, S.C., Lowe, S.A., Scales, J.T., Ansell, R.H.: An in vitro experiment to determine the efficiency of fixation of the McKee-Farrar acetabular component in relation to torsional force. Acta Orthopaedica Scandinavica 45, 429 (1974)
5. Charnley, J.: Anchorage of the femoral head prosthesis to the shaft of femur. Journal of Bone and Joint Surgery 42-B, 28 (1960)
6. Charnley, J.: A biomechanical analysis of the use of cement to anchor the femoral head prostheses. Journal of Bone and Joint Surgery 47-B, 354 (1965)
7. Charnley, J.: Acrylic cement in orthopaedic surgery. Edinbourgh-London: Churchill-Livingstone 1970
8. Charnley, J.: Low friction arthroplasty of the hip joint. Journal of Bone and Joint Surgery 53-B, 149 (1971)
9. Deane, S.: A new concept in knee joint design. In: The knee joint, Amsterdam: Excerpta Medica 244, 1974
10. Debrunner, H.U., Eulenberger, J.: Der Einbau von Fremdkörpern aus Kunststoff in Spongiosa. Aktuelle Traumatologie 4, 277 (1974)
11. Debrunner, H.U.: Die Volumenänderung von Knochenzementen während der Härtung. Archiv für orthopädische und Unfall-Chirurgie 81, 37 (1975)

12. Duff-Barclay, I.: Total human hip prostheses – a laboratory study of friction and wear, London: The Institution of Mechanical Engineers, 181/III, 90 (1967)

13. Engelbrecht, E., Zippel, J.: The sledge prostheses "model St. Georg". Acta Orthopaedica Belgica 39, 203 (1973)

14. Evans, E.M., Freeman, M.A.R., Miller, A.J., Vernon-Roberts, B.: Metal sensivity as a cause of bone necrosis and loosening of the prostheses in total joint replacement. Journal of Bone and Joint Surgery 56-B, 626 (1974)

15. Freeman, M.A.R., Swanson, S.A., Todd, R.C.: Total replacement of the knee, design considerations and early clinical results. Acta Orthopaedica Belgica 28, 181 (1973)

16. Grünert, A., Ritter, G.: Experimentelle Untersuchungen zum Problem der Verankerung von Hüftendoprothesen. Archiv für orthopädische und Unfallchirurgie 77, 149 (1973)

17. Gschwend, N., Schreier, H., Bähler, A.: The GSB knee prostheses. In: The Knee joint, Amsterdam: Excerpta Medica 261, 1974

18. Huggler, A.H., Schreiber, A., Dietschi, C., Jacob, H.: Experimentelle Untersuchungen über das Deformationsverhalten des Hüftazetabulums unter Belastung. Zeitschrift für Orthopädie 112, 34 (1974)

19. Jäger, M.W., Küßwetter, W., Rütt, J., Ungethüm, M., Burkhardt, R.: Torsionslockerung technisch verschieden implantierter Hüftendoprothesenpfannen. Zeitschrift für Orthopädie 112, 34 (1974)

20. Kölbel, R., Boenick, U.: Mechanische Eigenschaften der Verbindung von spongiösem Knochen mit Polymethylmethacrylat. 1. Zugfestigkeit. Archiv für orthopädische und Unfallchirurgie 73, 89 (1972)

21. Kölbel, R., Boenick, U.: Mechanische Eigenschaften der Verbindung von spongiösem Knochen und Polymethylmethacrylat. II. Scherfestigkeit. Archiv für orthopädische und Unfallchirurgie 77, 339 (1973)

22. Kölbel, R., Boenick, U.: Biomechanische Probleme der Implantatchirurgie. Der Orthopäde 3, 152 (1974)

23. McBride, E.D.: A metallic femoral head prosthesis of the hip joint. Int. Coll. Surg. 4, 15 (1952)

24. Mittelmeier, H.: Zementlose Verankerung von Endoprothesen nach dem Tragrippenprinzip. Zeitschrift für Orthopädie 112, 27 (1974)

25. Morscher, E.: Erste Erfahrungen mit einer zementlosen, isoelastischen Totalprothese der Hüfte. Kongress der Niederländisch-Schweizerischen Gesellschaften für Orthopädie, Lausanne 1974

26. Ritter, G., Grünert, A., Schweikert, C.H.: Biomechanische Ursachen von Lockerung und Bruch der Hüftendoprothesen. Archiv für othopädische und Unfallchirurgie 77, 154 (1973)

27. Ruckelshausen, M.C.: Haltbarkeitserwartung von Hüfttotalprothesen in Abhängigkeit von Verschleiß, Reibungskoeffizient und Kopfdurchmesser. In: Cotta-Schulitz, Der totale Hüftgelenksersatz, Stuttgart: Thieme 28, 1973

28. Sauer, B.W., Weinst, A.M., Klawitter, J.J., Hulbert, S.F., Leonard, R.B., Bagwell, J.G.: The role of porous polymeric materials prosthesis attachment. Journal of Biomedical Materials Research Symposium 5, 145 (1974)

29. Sauer, B.W., Spector, M., Fleming, W.R.: Ingrowth kinetics of bone in porous high-density polyethylene. Proceedings of the 28th Annual Conference of Engineering in Medicine and Biology, New Orleans 38 (1975)

30. Semlitsch, M.: Implantatmetalle für Platten, Schrauben und künstliche Gelenke in der Knochenchirurgie. Technische Rundschau Sulzer 54, 245 (1972)

31. Sheehan, J.M.: Arthroplasty of the knee. In: The knee joint, Amsterdam: Excerpta Medica 296, 1974

32. Willert, H.G., Puls, P.: Die Reaktion des Knochens auf Knochenzement bei der Alloarthroplastik der Hüfte. Archiv für orthopädische und Unfallchirurgie 72, 33 (1972)

33. Willert, H.G., Semlitsch, M.: Die Reaktion der periartikulären Weichteile auf Verschleißprodukte von Endoprothesenwerkstoffen. In: Cotta-Schulitz: Der totale Hüftgelenkersatz, Stuttgart: Thieme 1973

ISSUES OF LAW IN CONNECTION WITH ARTIFICIAL JOINT REPLACEMENT

F.-J. Knappen

This is an attempt to give you a short general view of the legal situation concerning medical liability, particularly with respect to operations involving artificial joints.

The law in foreign countries, especially in the English-speaking world, in many cases deviates from German practice. However, on the basis of the English and American law book to which I have had access, I believe that the general situation is roughly the same in the United States and in Germany, particularly with respect to the rules requiring the attending physician to properly inform the patient of the risks of the treatment, and to obtain from the patient what is called his "informed consent" to the operation.

Under the present German law on medical malpractice it not only is a very high standard of care required of a doctor, but he must also fully disclose to the patient the risks and possible consequences of the treatment to be carried out.

This is the reason why questions of liability are becoming more important, the more so since the risks of liability are constantly increasing, especially in our field, because of the introduction of new types of surgical techniques and complicated new therapeutic methods. The number of liability claims against physicians is, therefore, increasing from year to year, and sensational journalism on medical questions is, unfortunately, contributing to this development by interfering in pending proceedings prior to the final judgment of the court.

In principle, according to the case law handed down by the German appeal courts, a surgical operation, if carried out without the patient's prior consent, is considered unlawful bodily injury as defined in section 823, subsection 1, of the German Civil Code. This applies even where the operation has been carried out successfully. Thus, if a doctor removes a uterus without having obtained the patient's prior consent, he will be liable, even though the operation has been carried out in accordance with the standard of care required from a doctor under the circumstances. I shall discuss the prerequisites of what is called "valid informed consent" more fully later on.

Supposing that the necessary prior consent has been obtained a doctor will be liable in damages only where it can be shown that he has violated the standard of care required by law, and that this violation was the cause of the injuries the patient has suffered. It is true that a doctor does not guarantee the outcome of his treatment. On the other hand, by undertaking to render medical services, the doctor will be held to act according to the skill and learning commonly possessed by members of his profession in good standing, and he will be liable if harm results because he does not have these skills and learning. It is not sufficient if the doctor can show that he has acted like any "average" member of his profession, since only those in good professional standing are to be considered. If the doctor represents himself as having greater skill, as for example where he claims to be a specialist, the standard of care will be modified accordingly. In general, it can be said that the standards of care established by the courts in the field of medical liability are extremely strict.

In principle, it is the patient who has to show that the doctor has violated the standard of care required of him. The burden of proof of the doctor's negligence rests, therefore, with the plaintiff. However, the patient's burden of proof is alleviated by the rule, under which it is sufficient, in many situations, to adduce what is called "prima facie evidence". In other words, if the patient can show that, in accordance with general medical experience, an injury of the type which has occurred is caused by negligence on the part of the doctor, it will then be the doctor who has to show either that no such general medical experience exists or that despite such experience, under the circumstances of the case at hand, the injury may have occurred without his negligence. If this proof cannot be furnished by the defending doctor the court will hold him liable.

The courts have held that there is no basis for prima facie evidence if small objects, such as plugs, have been left in the operation wound. However, if the injury has resulted from the fact that a larger object has been left in the operation wound it will be up to the doctor to show why he has not been negligent.

Normally, it is also the patient who has to prove that the defendant's negligence has caused the injury for which compensation is claimed. In many cases, therefore, the doctor's first line of defense is the contention that he acted in accordance with the required standard of care; the second line of defense is the allegation that, irrespective of whether or not he complied with the standard of care, the plaintiff would in any case have died, or would have suffered the injuries in question. If the causal relationship between the breach of care and the harm suffered remains in doubt, the plaintiff's action will be dismissed. However, the courts have held that the burden of proof as to the causal relationship will be shifted to the doctor if there has been gross negligence on his part. Accordingly, in these cases, it is the doctor who must prove that the patient's death or injury was not a consequence of his conduct.

The district court of Rottweil recently decided a case in which a child after anaesthesia died on the operation table for reasons unknown. The court shifted the burden of proof to the doctor even though no gross negligence had been shown, simply because a complicated medical instrument had been used. The doctor could not furnish the necessary proof and was found liable. If this judgement becomes final, then in many cases of injury caused by fate, there will be a shift from pure negligence liability to absolute liability (Gefährdungshaftung). We are not at all sure, whether this development will, in the last resort, be to the advantage of the patient.

Unfortunately, there is a clear tendency in case law to shift the burden of proof as to the causal relationship to the doctor by calling gross negligence what had hitherto been considered as simple negligence. It is clear that these decisions tend to increase the risks of medical activity, particularly in cases where the exact course of events that led to the injury remains in doubt.

Let me now say a few words on the physician's duty to obtain the patient's prior "informed consent".

The increasing mobility of the population has led to a situation in which the individual patient more frequently changes his physician and where medical advice is more frequently taken from a specialist. It is no longer the rule that there is a confidential relationship of many years standing between doctor and patient. Accordingly, patients no longer place reliance in receiving the right treatment from the physician whom they have been consulting for a number of years. Instead, patients now ask for detailed information and an explanation of the methods of treatment, and of the various risks connected with such treatment. If complications arise, the patient is nowadays more frequently inclined to complain that he was not properly informed about the risks of the treatment, and to base his claims on an alleged lack of proper information.

The advances of medical science have also contributed to the change in the relationship between doctor and patient. The hopes and expectations of the patient have risen enormously, and they have risen more than is justified by the results of the new techniques. The well-known gynaecologist Römer of the University of Tübingen aptly described the situation when he said that the risk of disease is decreasing but that the risks of treatment are increasing. He pointed out that, while formerly, 95 deaths out of 100 cancer patients were considered inexorable fate and the 5 living were looked on as the achievement of the physician, nowadays, 50 percent will be cured almost as a matter of course and the 5 percent cured but with complications will begin to be looked on as victims of the doctor's malpractice. Increased confidence in the achievements of modern medicine seems to have led to a loss of confidence in the attending physician.

Also, there is little doubt that the increase of diagnostic and therapeutic methods and of available drugs has also increased the danger of mistakes. Medical specialization requires more and more collaboration between various doctors and technical helpers, and this, in turn, increases the danger of blunders caused by imperfect communication between the individuals involved in the treatment.

The physician's duty to fully disclose to the patient the risks of the treatment proposed, creates particular problems in the area in which he is working. It is in this area that there is sometimes a number of different procedures that may be adopted in order to achieve the same result. At the same time, it is not clear which of these procedures will be the safest for the patient and will carry the least risk of complications. The District Court of Aachen recently had to answer the question whether a physician had violated the standard of care required of him by using in 1969 a prosthesis of the coxa designed by McKee-Farrar rather than a prosthesis of another type.

Even now the development of the endoprosthesis of the coxa is not at an end. Even today metal/metal prostheses like the McKee-Farrar prosthesis are used. Here the acetabulum and the os coxae both consist of metal. On the other hand prostheses are used in which either the one or the other are of either metal or plastics.

There are now exact investigations as to the rate of loosenings of the various types of endoprostheses. These complications are therefore known. In the cases decided by the German courts, it is absolutely necessary to expressly explain the risk of loosening to the patient.

On the other hand, it is, of course, true that the various types of prostheses can be evaluated with respect to their performance only after many years. In the case I have just referred to, the court found that various types of prostheses were in use in various hospitals, and that sometimes those various types were used even in the same hospital. The court, therefore, held that using a McKee-Farrar prosthesis did not constitute a failure to provide the standard of care in 1969. I would add that even today there is no unanimous opinion in school medicine on this problem. Sometimes a surgeon believes, on the basis of his experience with his own patients, that one type of prosthesis is better than another. However, even in that case, there is no statistical evidence to support this conclusion and, accordingly, a doctor who has used another type of prosthesis cannot be held negligent on the basis of his colleague's diverging experience.

Let me now make the following general observations on the physician's duty to inform the patient of the possible risks of the treatment envisaged.

In many legal proceedings the plaintiff originally bases his claim on malpractice on the part of the physician, but subsequently changes his tactics to allege a violation of the physician's duty to furnish proper information about the risks of the planned operation. Every lawyer, therefore, will advise his client to found his claim not only on the allegation of malpractice but also on the contention that no or inadequate information on the risks involved has been given. As stated above, there will be no basis for a tort claim on this ground if the patient has consented to the treatment. Valid consent will be held by the courts to exist only where the patient has been given all the information necessary to assess the possible consequences and risks of the treatment. This regularly requires that the patient be advised by his physician as to the procedure, risks and consequences of the treatment in question. According to the decisions of some higher courts, it is not possible to say that the probability of complications must exceed a certain defined percentage in order to make it obligatory for the physician to inform the patient accordingly.

Even in cases where the probability of complications is very low, it is not for the doctor but for the patient to decide whether or not he wishes to run the risk. Informing the patient is not necessary only in cases, in which the possibility of injury would be of no importance in the decision by a reasonable patient to consent to the operation.

A decision made by the court of appeal at Stuttgart in 1973 states that "it is impermissible for a doctor to use, even with the best of intentions, the authority of his knowledge and ability to relieve the patient of his own decision and thus to treat him like a mere physical object".

In orthopaedics, for instance, the question arises as to what age limit the patient should have reached before knee endoprostheses may be implanted. Before the patient has reached the age of 60 such implantation is justifiable only where this is the only way to prevent the patient from losing his ability to walk. It is, of course, in such a case imperative that the patient be told prior to the operation about the danger of loosening and other complications, such as a serious intraoperative drop of blood pressure as a reaction to filling bone cement into the shafts of tibia or femur. The patient must be told about this risk as well as about dangers resulting from the brittleness of his bones and from material fatigue.

You know best what difficulties may arise from chemo-therapeutic problems and how serious associated complications may be. If endoprostheses are being implanted, the patient must always be informed in detail that no guarantee can be given for the complete fixation of the metal or plastic parts and that, according to present experience, implants will be accepted by the body only for a period of 5 to 10 years. In addition, the patient must be informed of the possibility of fractures to the long bones and the pelvis. This information must be given even though the probability of the complications mentioned is, statistically speaking, very low. The courts have always held that serious risks must be disclosed to the patient even though their probability may be very low.

Therefore, if an operation involving artificial joint replacement is to be carried out, the following information should be given to the patient:

1. Explanation of the kind of disease presenting (diagnosis) and of the consequences of not carrying out the operation (prognosis).
2. Description of the surgical measures involved in a generally understandable form, and a description of the result sought to be achieved thereby.
3. Information as to possible detrimental consequences of the intended operation with respect to
   a. the general risks of the treatment;
   b. the typical risks of the operation planned;
   c. the individual risk of the patient with particular regard to his personal physical condition.
4. Information as to other possible methods of treatment, their advantages and disadvantages, their chances of success and their risks.

If an action for malpractice is brought against the doctor, it is up to the defendant to provide facts to show that the patient had been given all the information required and that the patient had consented to the operation on the basis of that information. In other words, as far as the patient's informed consent is concerned, the burden of proof is on the physician. If the physician can show that he adhered to the above scheme, there will be no liability on the grounds of a failure to properly inform the patient.

There is still one more question to be discussed: To what extent is the physician responsible for injuries arising from defects of the material used in the treatment, particularly of the material implanted in the patient's body? In principle, a physician must carefully select the material he uses. If the material used breaks because of fissures or other defects not apparent to a reasonably careful physician there will be no liability.

As far as the producer of the material is concerned, there is, in principle, no liability under present German law unless it is established that the producer failed to use ordinary care in the production of the material. However, the burden of proof is on the producer. In other words, it is the producer who, in such a case, must show that he acted in accordance with the extremely high standard of care required from a producer of medical appliances to be implanted in a patient's body. At the present time a bill is being prepared by the Federal Ministry of Justice that would change the law so as to make the producer strictly liable for all damage caused by defects of his products. Thus, German law would take the position already reached in the United States under the doctrine of "strict products liability".

Let me conclude by saying that, despite the recent developments tending to impose on the physician a very strict liability, it cannot be said that the courts are generally hostile to the medical profession. The liability for malpractice is still a liability based on the court's finding that the doctor has failed to provide the standard of care required from members of his profession in good standing, and there are many cases where harm has occurred following the treatment but where the doctor has not been held liable. On the other hand, as far as the physician's duty to inform the patient is concerned, it has been recognized that the duty to disclose all material facts is restricted if it can be shown that complete information of the patient might provoke a heavy emotional shock or might severely weaken the patient's physical or psychological ability to withstand the risks involved in the operation.

You all know that not all patients are able to bear the full truth they ought to know in order to understand the necessity of the operation and to accept its risks. The dilemma in which the physician finds himself was well known to Goethe who introduced his collection of poems called "West-Eastern Divan" with the following words:

"If there is anything I thank Allah for, it is that he divided pain from knowledge:
all sick people would despair if they had to know the evil as their doctors do."

Chapter 3
Criteria and Selection of Materials for Implants in Orthopaedic Surgery

THE SUITABILITY OF METALS FOR SURGICAL IMPLANTS

H. Zitter

Before taking a look at a particular group of materials, for example the metals, consideration should be given to the requirements that have to be met by implants in general. With respect to the manufacture of implants, the first requirement to be met is the workability of the material so as to provide a multitude of parts with, in some cases, complicated shapes.

The demands on the functionability of an implant can be compared with those required in mechanical engineering, where a basic differentiation is made between static and dynamic stress. In both cases, the optimal properties of a constructional element are determined not only by the properties of the material, but also by appropriate shape and dimension. It is the task of the construction designer to combine these two aspects. In the development of implants, the designer is highly restricted by the situation within the organism and the requirements of the surgeon. This fact should, however, never give rise to the idea that the constructor might be dispensed with. That such cases frequently occur may be illustrated by the case of a plate, the screw holes in which reduce its cross-section by more than a half, thus giving rise to a point of weakness (Fig. 1). The resistance of the material to mechanical stress is, in the main, characterized by its resistance to tensile, compressive and impact forces. In particular the latter presupposes a certain elastic and plastic deformability of the material. This means, with regard to an optimal choice of materials, that tensile strength and toughness should match the given stress situation. Especially in these points opinions as to what are the absolutely necessary requirements vary considerably, even with the very same implant. In consequence of the movements of the body, implants are predominantly subject to alternating stress, for which static tensile properties cannot be taken into account. With increasing frequency of stress alternation, the material is submitted to fatigue which manifests itself as a loss of tensile properties. This loss of tensile properties is furthermore increased with increasing corrosivity of agents (Fig. 2). On the other hand, the development of a fracture due to corrosion fatigue is promoted by any abrupt change in cross-section as well as notch effects and rough surfaces.

As important as mechanical stability is the chemical resistance of the implant against body fluids and tissues. This requirement is on the one hand important for the implant which, as a result of corrosion, can suffer a loss of tensile properties, and on the other hand for the organism, which can suffer damage from corrosion products.

Last but not least, it must be taken into account that even implants should not become too expensive, a point which concerns not only the selection of alloys, but also the manufacturing process. As is shown in practice, this question concerns less the use of noble metals, than the irresponsible economizing on relatively inexpensive alloying elements. This tendency, unfortunately, is even expressed in standards proposals.

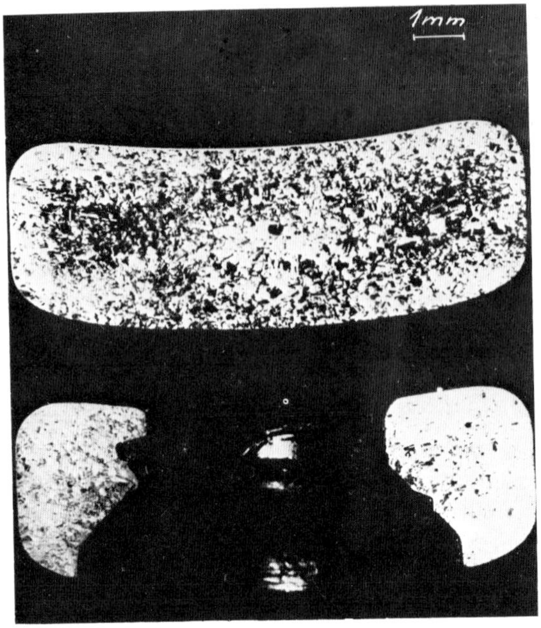

Fig. 1
Constructionally impermissible reduction of the bearing section of a plate by a hole

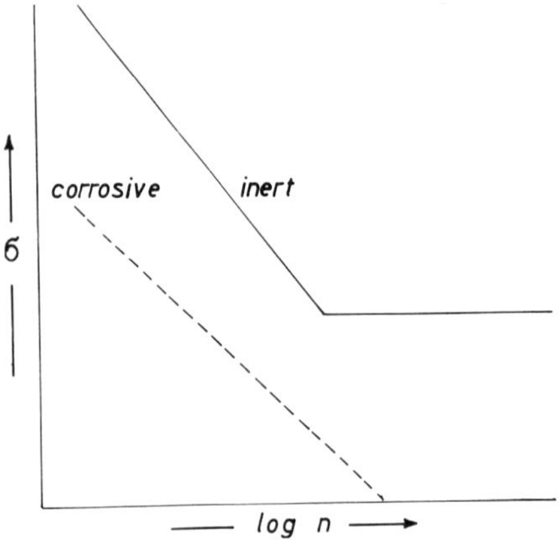

Fig. 2
Change in stress-life diagrams due to corrosion

COMPARISON BETWEEN REQUIREMENTS AND PROPERTIES OF TECHNICAL MATERIALS

It would be obvious to develop materials specifically for implants which, very probably, would best comply with the demands made on them. In practice, however, implants have always been made of materials that were developed and used for completely different purposes. The reason for this is that, on the one hand, the development of a material for the exclusive manufacture of implants would probably be too expensive, while on the other such a development does not seem necessary – at least until the particular suitability of a multitude of existing technical materials has been adequately investigated. Of the various materials that might be considered for implants, we can differentiate three important groups: ceramics and glass, plastics and metals.

Ceramic materials and glasses are manufactured by sintering, casting or drawing. They are characterized by a high resistance to compression, but low resistance to tensile stress and impact as well as low ductility. Compared with metals and plastics, these oxidic materials show higher resistance to corrosion. The thermodynamic stability arises from their chemical composition, which can be compared with that of corrosion products. Consequently with ceramics and glasses an improved tissue compatibility may be expected.

Plastics are, in general, manufactured by extrusion and casting. Their tensile properties are inferior to those of ceramic materials and metals, especially with regard to alternating stress. Their chemical stability varies, depending upon composition, within a wide range. The most stable kinds of plastics promise a favourable behaviour in body fluids.

Metals and their alloys can be manufactured by casting, forging or sintering. Compared with ceramic materials, metals are characterized by better workability with respect to drawing, turning, grinding and polishing. By means of appropriate alloying, tensile properties of metals can be varied within wide limits. Within these limits, the alloys are characterized by an opposing tendency of strength and ductility. Their chemical stability ranges between that of noble to that of base metals. A considerable difference to other materials and also to biological tissue can be seen in the high electrical and thermal conductivity of metals. These properties have, in particular in dentistry, given rise to many discussions. As long as no electrical current flows between metal and tissue, this property is probably without influence on tissue. The thermal conductivity of these materials, at least in the case of implants located at some distance from the surface of the body, is unlikely to have any negative effects since the entire implant is, so to speak, within a thermostat.

Due to the large variety of metals and the possibility of combining their technologically interesting properties by alloying, the variety of implant requirements is most likely to be met by this group of materials.

CORROSION PROPERTIES OF METALS

Considerable changes in the mechanical properties of a large number of metals can be achieved by relatively small additions of other alloying elements. Thus we can differentiate soft iron and hard steel, soft copper and hard bronze or ductile and hardenable titanium alloys. Heat treatment and/or cold working can furthermore considerably change mechanical properties of one and the same alloy.

In contrast to this, corrosion resistance is generally not attainable by small additions of alloying elements. Stainless steels acquire their corrosion resistance with about 18 % chromium. Similar percentages are required for corrosion resistant nickel and cobalt alloys. Corrosion properties of one and the same alloy are influenced by heat treatment and cold working in a varying manner, as a consequence of changes in structure and texture. Cold working the materials causes a deformation of the structure, which results in a lowering of the corrosion resistance.

In contrast to all other materials, the corrosion of metals in electrolytes, i.e. in ion-conducting liquids, usually involves an electrochemical process. The actual corrosion process, that is the dissolution of the metal, corresponds to an oxidation and takes place at the anode, where electrons are transferred to the metal (Fig. 3). For reasons of electroneutrality, a reduction process must proceed at the same time, which runs with the equivalent number of electrons as the oxidation. In body fluids, the reduction of dissolved oxygen takes place at an uncorroded part of the metal (Fig. 3).

Due to liberated OH—ions, an alkalization takes place at the cathode which influences the behaviour of the corrosion products. As a result of the electron conductivity of metals, anodic and cathodic processes can occur at different sites. As a result, the anodic area can be locally "fixed". This fact is the cause of specific forms of localized corrosion.

Since high demands of corrosion resistance must be fulfilled by implants, only two groups of alloys should be considered:

The noble metals with their complete stability with respect to body fluids, and passivable metals, which owe their stability to protective films.

The resistance of individual metals and their chemical compounds can best be compared with the corrosive conditions in body fluids on the basis of potential—pH diagrams (1). The aggressivity of body fluids is marked by pH values of approximately 7.3 and rH values of 8 to 16, corresponding to a redox potential of -150 to +100 mV (2-5).

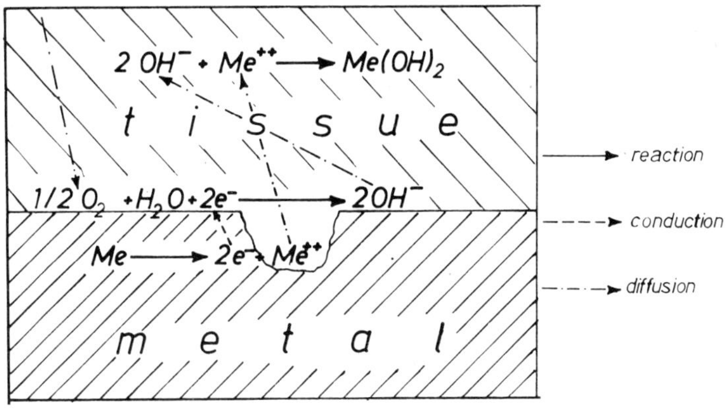

Fig. 3 Local corrosion of metals: separate oxidation and reduction

Comparing these conditions with the stability range of a noble metal, it can be seen that the most stable phase is the metal. For base metals such as iron, chromium or titanium, the corrosive conditions lie within the stability range of an oxide; the metal would thus be oxidized in body fluids (Fig. 4). If this reaction between metal and dissolved oxygen is fast enough, the oxide formed can develop as a film directly on the metal surface and thus prevent further oxidation. This ability of a metal to protect itself from oxidation is called passivability. It is interesting to note that this qualification is characteristic for base metals and is less marked the nobler the metal.

The danger involved in the use of passivable metals is the extremely thin passivating layer, which can be damaged. Such damage can be effected mechanically or chemically. Localized corrosion is dangerous since, as mentioned above, the electrochemical corrosion mechanism permits a separation of anodic oxidation and cathodic reduction areas. A considerable acceleration of the localized corrosion process usually occurs on account of the fact that a relatively large cathodic surface is available. In addition, a localized accumulation of dissolved metal ions is more unfavourable for the surrounding tissue than a uniform distribution of corrosion products.

Normally, passivable alloys are used in manufacturing implants. The only exception – virtually without practical importance – are a few noble metals. The most important alloys owe their good passivation properties to the alloying element chromium, which is able to confer its own passivation properties on other heavy metals.

According to the basis metal, iron alloys, well known as stainless steels, are distinguished from nickel and cobalt alloys. The latter are characterized by higher resistance under conditions which do not permit the development of a passivating layer. Alloys of the much less noble titanium have, on account of their excellent passivation properties, also come into widespread use. Table 1 shows specifications for a number of alloys, which are presently recommended for implants with their guide analysis and tensile properties.

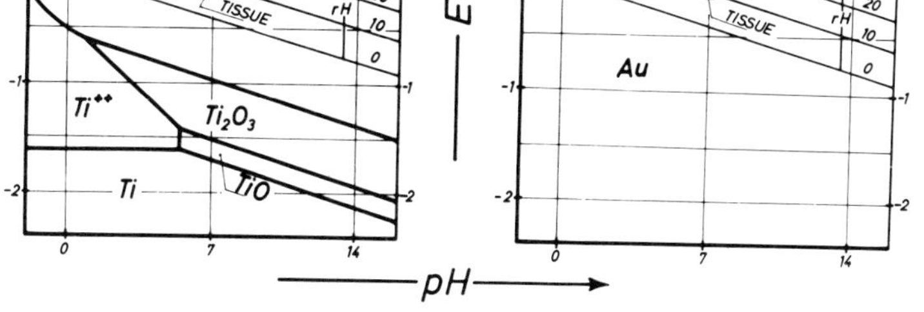

Fig. 4 Comparison of stability of titanium and gold with the electrochemical properties of body fluids

Table 1 Alloys for surgical implants

Kind of alloy	Basis	Alloying elements (%)				UTS (Kp/mm^2)		Standard	Ref.
		Cr	Mo	Ni	others	min.	high tensile		
wrought	Fe	16.5-18.5	2-3	10.5-14.5		—	—	DIN	6
austenitic	Fe	16.5-19.5	2.25-4	10-15		—	—	BS	7
stainless steels	Fe	17-20	2-4	10-14		~50	~90	ASTM	8
	Fe	17-19	2.5-3.5	12-16		45	110	SNV	9
	Fe	17.5-19.5	2.5-3	13-15		65	—	AUVA	10
cast CoCrMo-alloy	Co	27-30	5-7	2.5 max.		~67	—	ASTM,BS,SNV	11,7,18
wrought CoCr-alloy	Co	19-21	—	9-11	W: 14-16	~90	—	ASTM,BS	12,7
wrought CoNi-alloy	Co	19-21	9-10.5	33-37	Ti: 1	80	160	SNV	15
wrought CoNiCr-alloy	Co	18-22	+W: 6-8	15-25	Fe: 5-15, Ti: 0.5-2.5	60	130	SNV	16
wrought Ti	Ti	min.: 99 %				~45	56	ASTM,BS,SNV	13,7,17
wrought Ti-alloy	Ti				Al: 5.5-6.5, V: 3.5-4.5	88	—	ASTM	14

The large majority of implants are, probably on account of the low price, made of low-carbon, chemically resistant chromium-nickel-molybdenum steels. The use of this type of steel started after massive failures had been observed in implants made of molybdenum-free chromium-nickel steels and corresponding alloys with higher carbon content.

It is in this very point of the molybdenum content that steels standardized for implants still differ today. Undoubtedly, the best protection against local corrosion is guaranteed by steels with the higher percentages of molybdenum and chromium. However, a content of 2.5 % molybdenum should be considered as absolute minimum (10).

The cobalt-chromium alloys have been incorporated into the field of dentistry as cast alloys, and are also successfully used for implants. Their disadvantage as compared to wrought alloys is a higher degree of brittleness due to the structure of the cast state, which is not adequately controlled by all manufacturers. For this reason, ductility values of these alloys found in literature vary (19-20). Better ductility is provided by wrought alloys, a nickel-containing type of which is characterized by high tensile values.

DAMAGE TO METALLIC IMPLANTS

Mechanical damage of implants resulting from a single act of force seems, for the duration of its application, to play an insignificant role. An analysis of a wide variety of complaints (21) indicates that such damage occurs, in particular, during implantation or explantation, the majority of cases involving screws (Fig. 5). This very example would seem to be evidence for the fact that the manufacturer and the user are not clear as to the optimum of tensile properties, and that many surgeons overestimate the mechanical properties of an implant. Nor are there any recommandations on this, so that it is not surprising that these products are manufactured with widely differing tensile properties (Fig. 6). Cases of corrosion failures of implants are still to be observed to a virtually

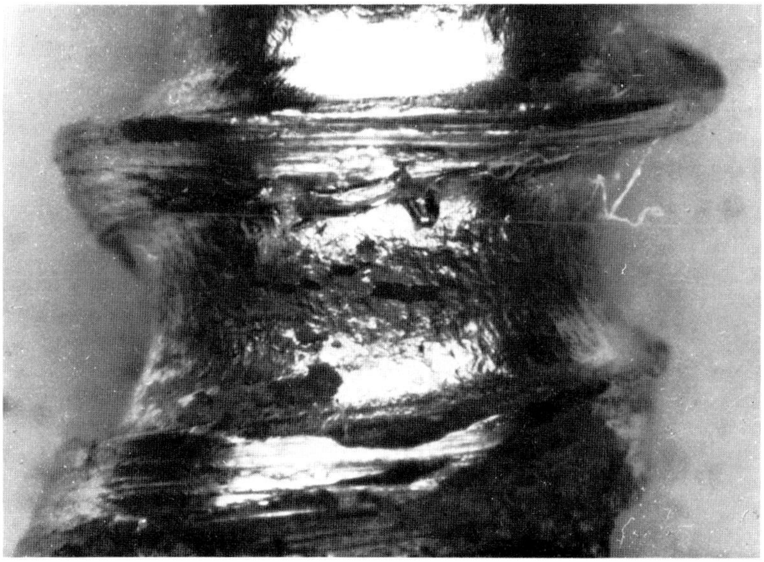

Fig. 5 Mechanical damage to a screw during surgery

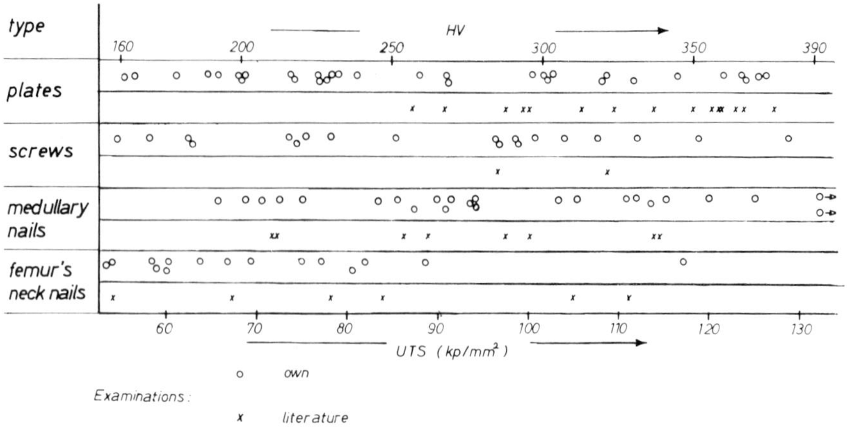

Fig. 6 Mechanical properties of commercial implants

unchanged extent. They involve, almost exclusively, local corrosion. Today, after the negative experiences of early decades (22), galvanic corrosion between metals with different electrochemical potentials is less frequently observed. Passivable metals, that are now used almost exclusively, seem less endangered, since they manifest no characteristic stable potentials and can thus be more easily matched to one another. In the last few years, however, the percentage of pitting corrosion has increased. This kind of attack is limited to austenitic chromium-nickel-molybdenum steels containing too little chromium or molybdenum, which, unfortunately, are still listed in many standards. As a striking example, Fig. 7 shows typical pitting corrosion of an inadequate implant.

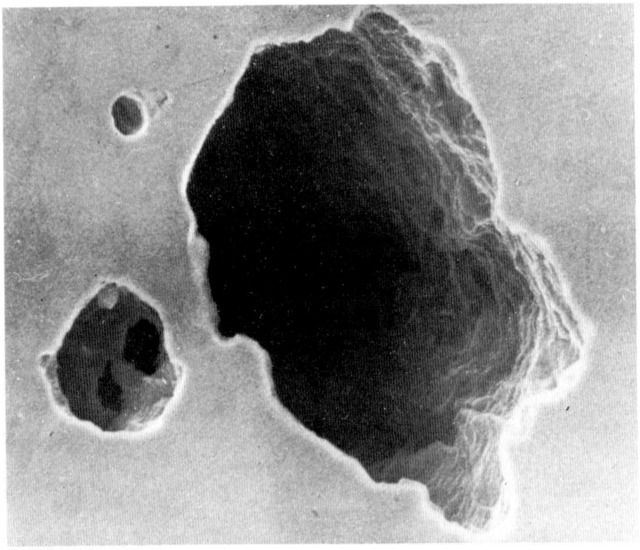

Fig. 7 Pitting corrosion in an inadequate implant

More dangerous than pure corrosion processes is the combined effect of corrosion and mechanical stress. This applies in particular to fretting corrosion which, even with noble metals, cannot be avoided completely and involves especially heads of screws, countersunk holes (Fig. 8) or serrations (Fig. 9). This type of corrosion can largerly be avoided by ensuring a good fit. Thus, it is a matter of designing and implantation technique.

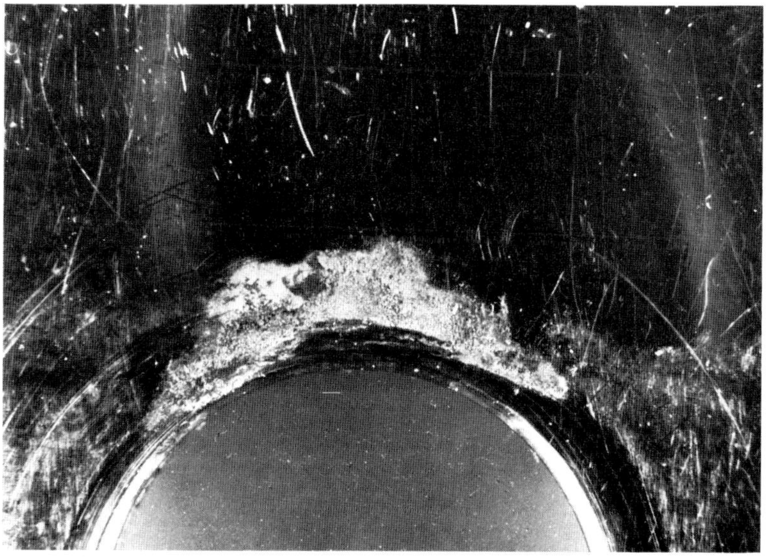

Fig. 8 Fretting corrosion between plate and screw

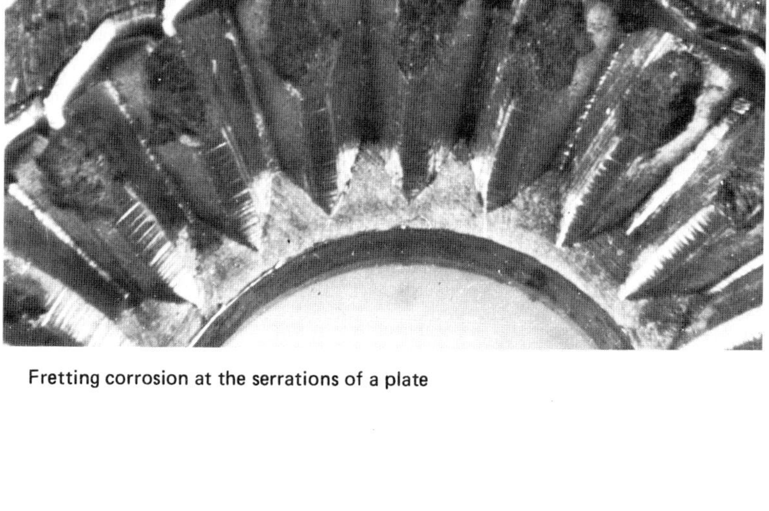

Fig. 9 Fretting corrosion at the serrations of a plate

Stress corrosion cracking is also said to occur in implants (23). This is unlikely, since temperature and chloride concentration in tissue are relatively low (21). The greatest danger for a breakdown of an implant is corrosion fatigue which, in general, originates in notches in the surface. Predominantly, the following initiating factors of corrosion fatigue have been observed: sharp edges, surface faults and local corrosion. Fig. 10 illustrates a typical example of the effects of a sharp edge. The clearly recognizable striation of the fracture's surface indicates the initiation of the fracture. This striation is not always so clearly marked, but can usually be identified with the aid of a scanning electron microscope (Fig. 11). Fig. 12 shows an example of a surface fault in a plate, from which a corrosion fatigue fracture has started. Particularly noteworthy is the third case, in which the fracture originates from a site of a local corrosion – usually pitting corrosion – and progresses from hole to hole (Fig. 13). In the last few years, such cases have frequently been observed and should provide food for thought, especially since they could easily be avoided by selecting more resistant alloys.

DAMAGE TO TISSUE BY CORROSION PRODUCTS

Damage to tissue by the corrosion products of metallic implants is generally described as metalosis, although this term also includes any other kind of influence on tissue by metals (24). As preceeding remarks show, the greater part of corrosion damage in metallic implants is caused by local corrosion. As a result, high local concentrations of corrosion products build up in the tissue. The primary products are soluble (Fig. 3), but can react

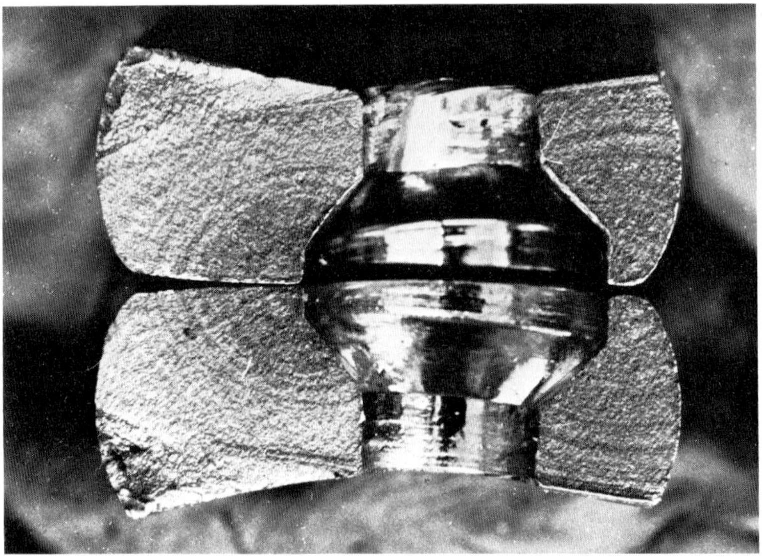

Fig. 10 Fracture of a plate due to corrosion fatigue initiated at a sharp inner edge of a hole

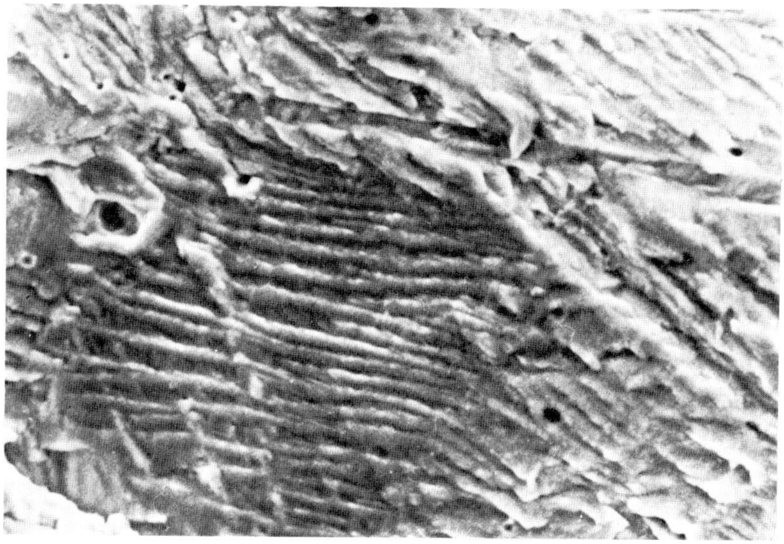

Fig. 11 Typical striation of a fracture surface as a consequence of corrosion fatigue

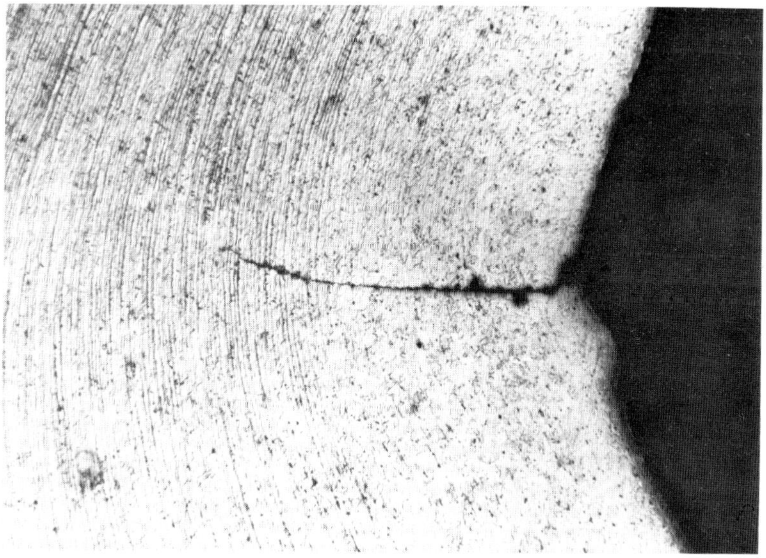

Fig. 12 Initiation of a corrosion fracture in a surface fault in a plate

with tissue to produce various deposits. These can be observed at various distances from the implant and exhibit differing densities (Figs. 14 and 15). The quantity and composition of the deposits depend upon the specific reactions of the alloying elements and on the solubilities of the respective secondary corrosion products. A chemical analysis of tissue around an alloyed implant is therefore likely to show a relative enrichment of

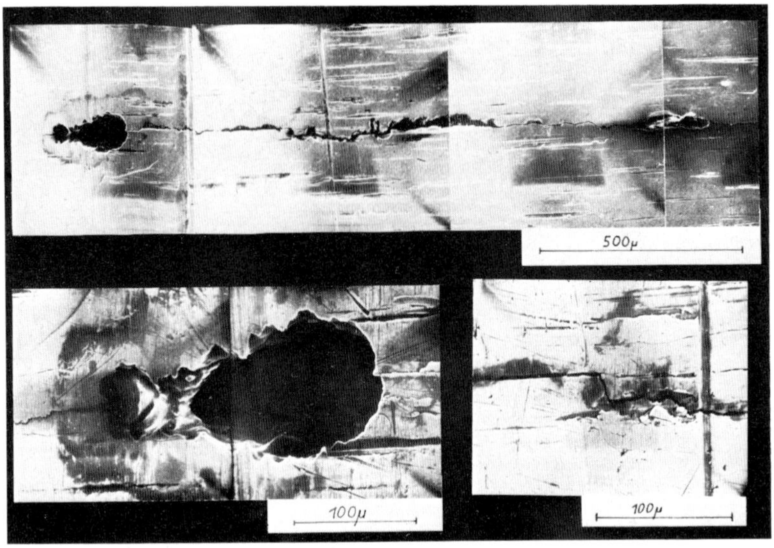

Fig. 13 Initiation and progress of a corrosion fracture at pitted corrosion sites of a nail (Ender, Simon, Waidner)

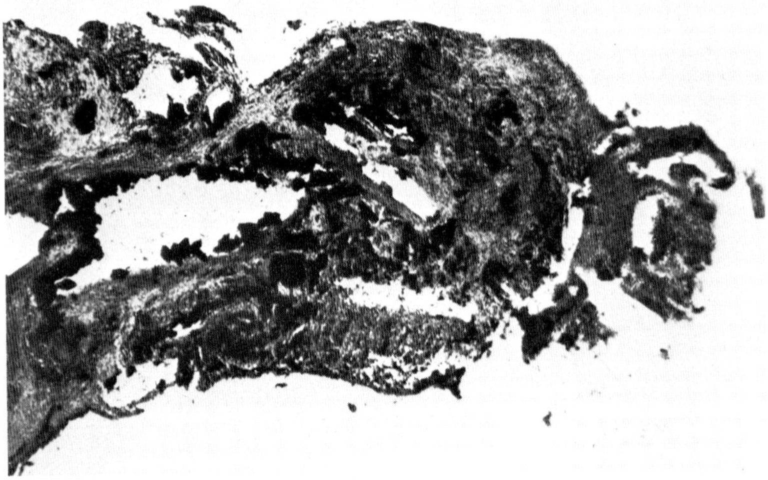

Fig. 14 Massive rust granuloma in connective tissue

the elements forming insoluble compounds and an impoverishment of the elements of more soluble compounds. For that reason the ionic composition of the corrosion products vary from the composition of the alloy the more the distance to the corroding surface increases (Fig. 16). The question as to whether the metals deposited in the area of the implant or those which remain in solution for a longer period represent the greater danger to the organism has not been sufficiently investigated.

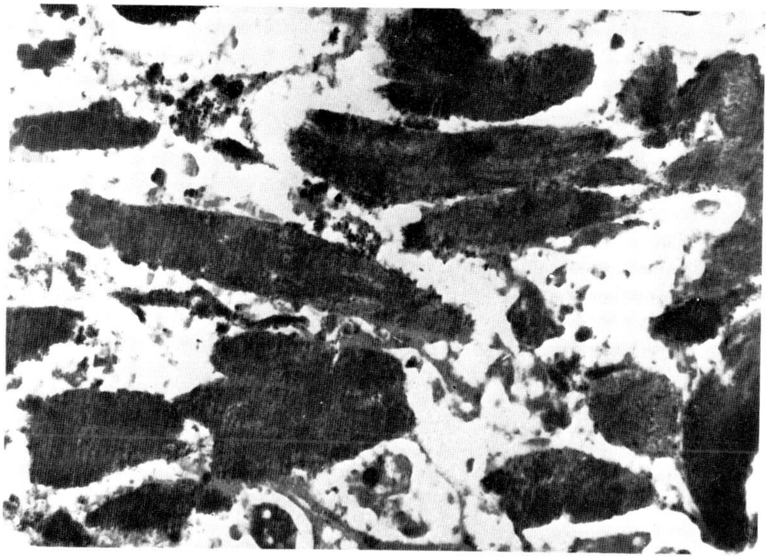

Fig. 15 Agglomerates of "precipitated" corrosion products with striated structure

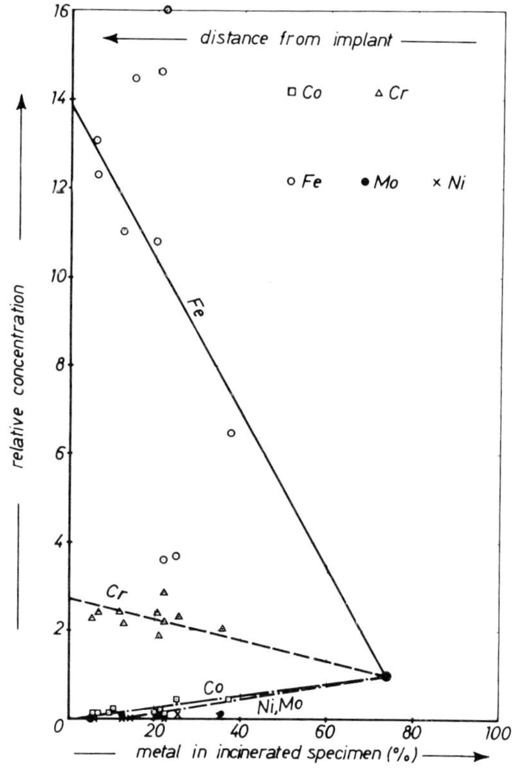

Fig. 16
Relative concentration of deposits of a Co-Cr-Mo-Ni-Fe-alloy in tissue according to analysis of (25)

MEASURES TO REDUCE FAILURES OF METALLIC IMPLANTS

Considering the possibilities of failures described, three main ways of reducing damages to metallic implants should be implemented:

First of all, the selection of proper materials. This should be carried out by a materials expert exclusively on the basis of the specific mechanical requirements and the aggressivity of tissue. In a considerable number of inadequate implants these prerequisites were obviously not met.

The next important measure should be the implant design, which still leaves much to be desired. A proper design requires the cooperation of designer and surgeon, in order to match the technical and biological situations and to secure the functionability of the system implant-organism.

The third measure involves correct selection and proper fixation of the implant.

The simplest preventive measure is evidently the selection of suitable materials, with which a considerable portion of the damage observed could have been avoided.

A reduction of the fractures quota presupposes the resolute contribution of a designer. At the same time a designer could reduce the unnecessarily large number of different designs to a degree that would favourably affect the production economy of implants.

REFERENCES

1. Pourbaix, M.: Atlas d'Equilibres electrochimiques, Paris: Gauthier-Villars 1963
2. Rauen, H.M.: Biochemisches Taschenbuch, Wien-New York: Springer 1964
3. Geigg, J.R.: Wissenschaftliche Tabellen, Basel: Verlag der Pharma AG. 1968
4. Damm, H.C., King, J.W.: Handbook of chemical laboratory data, Cleveland Ohio: The Chemical Rubber Co. 1965
5. Netter, H.: Theoretische Biochemie, New York-Wien: Springer Verlag 1959, p. 455
6. DIN 58 800: Implantate aus nichtrostendem Stahl, 11 (1971)
7. British Standard 3531: Specification for metal implants and tools used in bone surgery, Part 1 (1968)
8. ASTM Designation F 55-71: Standard specification for stainless steel bars and wire for surgical implants
9. SNV, Reg.Nr. 056/506, Dez. 1974, 3. Entwurf: Chirurgische Implantate, Werkstoff: Nichtrostender Stahl
10. Frank, E., Zitter, H.: Metallische Implantate in der Knochenchirurgie, Wien-New York: Springer Verlag 1971, pp. 126-128
11. ASTM Designation F 75-67: Standard Specification for Cast Cobalt-Chromium-Molybdenum Alloys for Surgical Implants

12. ASTM Designation F 90-68: Standard Specification for Wrought Cobalt-Chromium Alloy for Surgical Implants

13. ASTM Designation F 67-66: Standard Specification for Titanium for Surgical Implants

14. ASTM Designation F 136-70: Standard Specification for Titanium 6 Al 4 V ELI Alloy for Use in Clinical Evaluations as a Surgical Implant Material

15. SNV, Reg.Nr. 056/509, Dez. 1974, 3. Entwurf Chirurgische Implantate, Werkstoff: Kobalt/Nickel/Chrom/Molybdän/Titan-Schmiedelegierungen

16. SNV, Reg. Nr. 056/510, Dez. 1974, 3. Entwurf Chirurgische Implantate, Werkstoff: Duktile Kobalt/Nickel/Chrom/Molybdän/Wolfram/Eisen-Legierungen

17. SNV, Reg. Nr. 056/507, Dez. 1974, 3. Entwurf Chirurgische Implantate, Werkstoff: Unlegiertes Titan

18. SNV, Reg.Nr. 056/508, Dez. 1974, 3. Entwurf Chirurgische Implantate, Kobalt/Chrom/ Molybdän-Gußlegierungen

19. Asgar, K., Peyton, F.A.: Effect of microstructure on the physical properties of cobalt-base alloys and effect of casting conditions on some mechanical properties of cobalt-base alloys. Journal of Dental Research 40, 63 (1961)

20. Morral, F.R.: Cobalt alloys as implants in humans. Journal of Materials 1, 384 (1966)

21. Zitter, H.: Schadensfälle bei osteosynthetischen Implantaten und ihre Ursachen. Werkstoffe und Korrosion 22, 598 (1971)

22. Ludwigson, D.C.: Today's prosthetic metals. Journal of Metals 16, 226 (1964)

23. Lux, F., Zeisler, R.: Instrumentelle Multi-Element-Aktivierungsanalyse von biologischem Gewebe und ihre Anwendung zur Metallose-Untersuchung. Zeitschrift für analytische Chemie 261, 314 (1972)

24. Nicole, R.: Metallschädigung bei der Osteosynthese. Basel: Schwabe Verlag 1947

25. Semlitsch, M., Willert, M.G.: Gewebsveränderungen im Bereiche metallischer Hüftgelenke; mikroanalytische Untersuchungen mittels Spektralphotometrie, Elektronenmikroskopie und der Elektronenstrahl-Mikrosonde. Microchimica Acta 1, 21 (1971)

CORROSION OF HIGHLY STRESSED ORTHOPEDIC JOINT REPLACEMENTS

R. Thull and M. Schaldach

The success of an artificial joint in the locomotor system depends, aside from clinical factors, on a series of mechanical and physico-chemical parameters of the metallic material involved, and also on the particular design properties of the implant. Not all the influencing factors act simultaneously on the implant. Loosening of the prosthesis, which often occurs within the first three years, is still the most important problem that limits the functional life of the prosthesis, including implant fracture or rejection. This will, however, change decisively when work presently being undertaken at many different institutions, with the objective of improving implant anchorage, finally meets with success. Then, prosthesis fractures resulting from corrosion fatigue and damage to tissue attributable to corrosion and abrasion products may well prove to be the primary complications associated with this form of therapy.

Corrosion products and corrosion fractures result from the interaction of metallic materials and the highly aggressive body electrolytes in the presence of high mechanical stressing from body weight, muscular forces and acceleration forces acting on the artificial joint. These forces act primarily through the anchorage of the joint implant, on the long bones of the extremities where they lead in connection with the agressive body fluid to corrosion fracture of the stem of artificial joints (1-3). In addition, as a result of mechanical friction in the joint, abrasion particles are found to accumulate largely in the zone proximal to the joint (4-7); further, corrosion products in the form of ions develop and, if they are not removed quickly enough by metabolic processes, can lead to abacterial infections by interacting with the tissue (8,9) and to loosening of the implant (10). These foreseeable consequences emphasize the importance of investigating the electrochemical aspects of corrosive changes by carrying laboratory examinations of the materials used and of manufactured finished implants, and also tissue examinations in cases in which explantation of the joint has become necessary.

FORMS OF CORROSION

In the case of mechanically induced forms of corrosion, the effects of forces (which are either present in the material as a result of the manufacturing process or which act on the implant from outside) on the oxide layer protecting the surface of metallic materials are investigated, consideration being given to the electrochemical reactions involving the body electrolytes.

Shearing forces acting on articulating surfaces lead to more or less extensive destruction of the oxide layer, so that at this point, the metallic material is in an active state and releases ions to the electrolyte. This process, known as fretting corrosion, must be considered the most important cause of the concentration of corrosive products in the region proximal to the joint. Other local forms of corrosion, resulting from cold-forming of the structure or from particular properties of the material and forming, an additional source of metallic ions, are of less importance.

Tensile forces periodically occurring in the body of the joint and acting in particular in the anchoring stems, cause local disruption of the passivating layer and lead to electrochemical destruction of the metal structure, known as corrosion fatigue – a state that in numerous cases has already been responsible, aided by an unfavourable pattern of forces in the implant and errors in the design of the prosthesis, for the fracture of the prosthetic stem.

CORROSION FATIGUE

As already mentioned, corrosion fatigue is the combined attack on metallic materials, in which, at the same time as the mechanical interactive stressing, an electrochemical reaction occurs. For the quantitative theory of the electrolytic influences, there are at present only tentative beginnings, which are largely modelled on the mechanisms of stress corrosion. The primary differences with respect to corrosion fatigue lie in the fact that the mechanical stressing is not periodic but results from a constant force or a force "locked" into the material of the joint during the manufacturing process. Although the two forms of corrosion are thus based on different mechanisms, the fracture that occurs as a consequence of corrosion fatigue may, nevertheless, in some materials be hastened by weaknesses in the surface structure which, in turn, are caused by stress corrosion. Other metal alloys, for example, austenitic steel alloys, may reveal corrosion fatigue in physiological saline solutions, but stress corrosion cannot be demonstrated (11).

The susceptibility of various implant materials to corrosion fatigue is determined in revolving fatigue testing machines, in which the material to be tested, in the form of a rod, is stressed one-side, while being rapidly rotated in the test electrolyte. In the procedure utilized by Wöhler, a number of identical samples of material were loaded to fracture by using an alternating stress, increasing in intensity in predetermined increments. The load values are entered in a coordinate system against the number of alternating loads leading to fracture to give a Wöhler curve; the abscissa scale is logarithmic, the ordinate scale is arithmetic.

The mechanisms for fracture formation depend primarily on the composition of the metallic material. Of interest is the fact that elementary metal is generally not susceptible to stress corrosion. Even minute concentrations, or changes in concentration of contaminations or alloy components, considerably change the susceptibility of the material towards corrosion fatigue. Fig. 1 shows as an example, the influence of small quantities

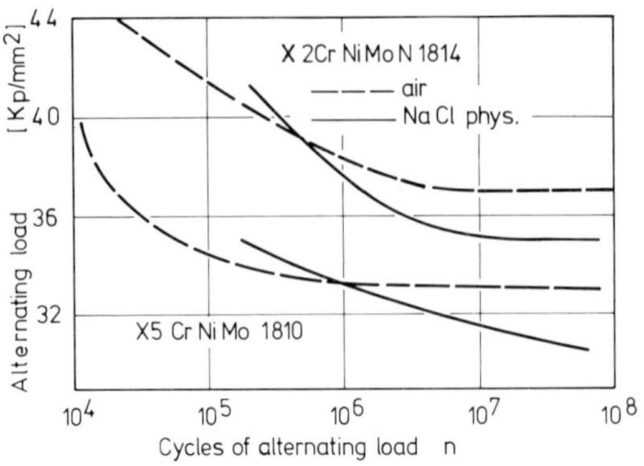

Fig. 1 Results of fatigue tests (steel alloys) (12)

of nitrogen in a steel alloy, and the susceptibility of the material to corrosion fatigue in a physiological saline solution (12); for comparative purposes, the alternating load resistance in air is also indicated. The nitrogen-free alloy is an austenitic steel containing 17 % chromium, 12 % nickel, 2.1 % molybdenum, and 0.056 % carbon. In comparison, the nitrogen-containing alloy has 18.5 % chromium, 13.8 % nickel, 2.8 % molybdenum and 0.021 % carbon. The higher fatigue strength in air and the increased resistance towards corrosion fatigue of the nitrogen-containing material as compared with the nitrogen-free steel, can clearly be recognized.

It would seem obvious to make the state of the surface responsible for corrosion fatigue and, in particular, for the formation of the first crack. Thus, it can be shown that corrosion fatigue can be effectively delayed (13,14) if the active centers of the surface, from which the fractures can originate, can successfully be eliminated. Thus, for example, polished metallic surfaces are less susceptible towards fracture formation depending on the finesse of the polishing agent used, and, therefore, the smoother and finer the surface finish (15).

There seems to be much to say for the simplistic solution to the problem, namely that the primary formation of cracks originates in the mechanically produced microdestruction or in electrochemically induced local centers on the surface, for example, the result of pitting corrosion or intergranular disintegration. In accordance with this postulation, implant materials that are immune to pitting corrosion and intergranular disintegration in chloride-containing electrolytes, should considerably reduce corrosion fatigue.

Although this assumption does not represent any attempt at an interpretation of the mechanism of corrosion fatigue, a number of test results obtained with an austenitic steel complying with AISI type 316, and in titanium in Ringer's solution (16) point in this direction. The differing initial electrochemical conditions were "set" by potentiostatic polarization of the samples. The mechanical pretreatment took the form either of mechanical polishing (60 μm) or by electropolishing.

Fig. 2 shows that the prolonged alternating stress strength fatigue decreases sharply with positive-going polarization of the surface in the steel samples as compared with the

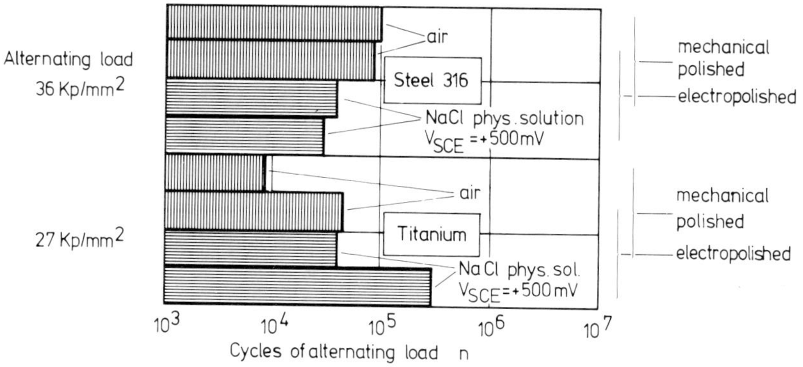

Fig. 2 Fatigue life of steel (AISI 316) and titanium in air and electrolyte (16)

titanium samples. This behavior of the two materials with respect to the mechanical surface treatment is reversed. Here, titanium shows a much higher dependency than does the steel alloy, so that it must be assumed that the ability of the titanium to repassivate is less marked in the scratches and grooves than with steel.

For cobalt-base alloys, little information is at present available, so that the resistance of this prosthetic material to corrosion fatigue can only be approximately assessed. The small degree of susceptibility to intergranular corrosion and pitting corrosion (17) suggests that the fatigue strength will be high.

Although fatigue testing is being widely used to assess the susceptibility of given materials to corrosion fatigue, it must not be forgotten that the results are only of limited value for an objective estimation of the long-term stability of orthopedic joint prostheses. An expedient interpretation of results that can be extrapolated to the joint, is possible only in those cases in which the susceptibility for corrosion fatigue depends entirely on the material and the mechanical treatment of its surface. If, however, in addition, a primary corrosive attack which has a "promoting effect" on the fatigue fracture also has to be considered, fatigue testing of the finished implant is completely without any practical usefulness. In situ, primary damage to the surface which occurs postoperatively, only after a relatively lengthy period, as a result of pitting corrosion or intergranular disintegration — in the case of anchoring stems also crevice corrosion — may represent just the very factor that sets a limit to the useful life of the artificial joint. For this reason, fatigue tests should always be conducted with simultaneous electrochemical simulation of primary forms.

In this discussion, it has already been shown that repassivation of primary passivated materials after destruction of the oxide layer is of particular significance for the useful life of implants, not merely for the mechanically promoted forms of stress corrosion, corrosion fatigue, and fretting corrosion, but also for pitting corrosion. The rate of repassivation is the decisive factor for the time-dependent degree of destruction of the material. Thus, before artificial joints are designed, accurate information on the kinetics of oxide layer formation should be available so that an assessment of potential failure of the implant by corrosion damage can be made before implantation in humans is effected.

Fundamental studies in the laboratory on the influences determining corrosion in the passive state cannot be replaced even by preclinical tests on the materials or on the finished prostheses. Such accelerated tests provide information only on the effects of corrosion but not on their genesis. For the development of reliable orthopedic implants, the trial-and-error methods, so popular today, represent no genuine possibility for the future if a responsible evaluation of the medical and economical damage resulting from a failure of the prosthesis is to be made. Thus, the development of an artificial joint should always begin with the establishment of physical and physico-chemical material criteria which must be oriented to the required function of the implant. The importance of this preliminary work is on a par with the generally recognized requirement for intensive preliminary studies on the biological tolerability of the material.

FRETTING CORROSION

Material destruction resulting from the attacks of fretting corrosion can be observed in the artificial joints whenever shearing forces disrupt the oxide layer of the primarily passivated metal surface, and the basic metal is, at least for a short period, exposed to the body electrolytes in the active state. In this condition, the articulating joint surfaces and anchoring stems of the femoral head and knee joint prostheses that move relative to the bone cement beds, are particularly at risk.

The partial activation of the metallic surface can, with respect to aspects of measuring techniques, be recognized by the change in electrical potential in the electrolyte, a change that, as a function of joint loading, can be determined with reference to the comparative potential of a standard electrode. In the nonstressed state, the resting or mixed potential of the prosthesis assumes a value that is characteristic for the passive material surface and which is always more positive than the potential of the active surface. A drop in the mixed potential under function, indicates at least partially activated surface regions of the stressed prosthesis.

As an example of change in the electrochemical state of the forcetransmitting surfaces of a Guepar knee joint, Fig. 3 shows the change in mixed potential of the prosthetic material in a simulator. Depending upon the set load, the potential changes with respect, to the state of equilibrium in the nonstressed state, changes successively with each cycle of movement towards more negative values, becoming more negative as higher forces act on the joint. Sensitive potential measurements in the subsequent more-or-less steady state, that is, on conclusion of the partial activation, reveal the interaction between activation and repassivation in the periodic pattern of the potential and synchronous with the stressing cycle. Even at this stage, important information can be deduced with accumulation of corrosion products in the region proximal to the joint:

A hip or knee prosthesis moved under load is always in the partially activated state. Complete repassivation is effected only in the resting state and with the joint unstressed.

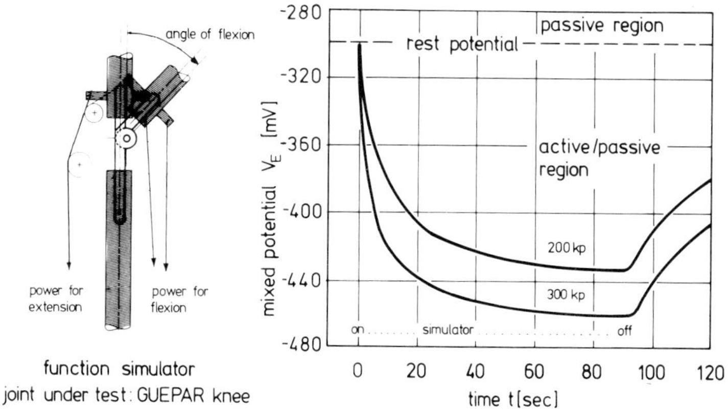

Fig. 3 Mechanical influence on the properties in the passivated state of articulating surfaces

The quantity of ions passed into the tissue, however, depends not only on the design of the implant and the degree of stressing, but is also largely determined by:

1. The physical properties of the articulating components, that is, the extent of the active surface regions depends upon whether the articulating surfaces are metal on metal, metal on ceramic, metal on bone cement, or metal on plastic, and on the degree of hardness of the oxide layers forming on the materials involved.
2. The kinetics of the formation of the oxide layer, that is, as the quantity of ions released increases, the repassivation rate leading to complete formation of the protective passivated layer on the metal decreases.

Because in all knee joint prostheses investigated to date in the simulator, a partial reactivation under stressing occurred, the influence of oxide layer hardness has been ignored in this study; rather, here, attention has been directed to investigatative methods and results which allow an assessment of the electrochemical course of re-passivation of various implant metals.

Figs. 4,5 show the condition of the metallic surface in the activated and in passivated state. In both cases, electrochemical reactions can occur on the surface only as long as, in the individual partial reactions at the metal, just as many charge carriers are released as are captured, that is, the system as a whole is in electrical equilibrium.

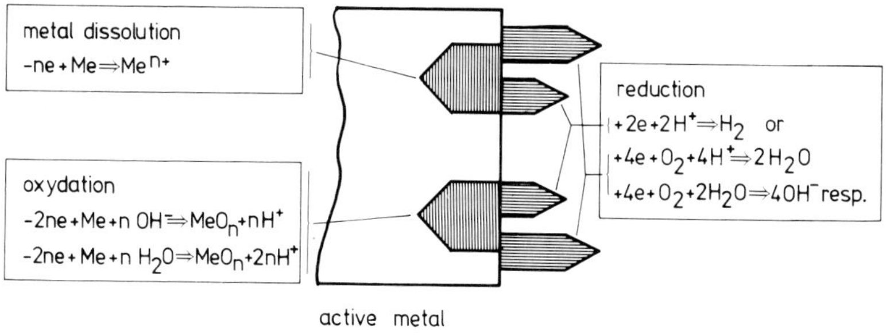

Fig. 4 Electrochemical reactions at the activated metal surface

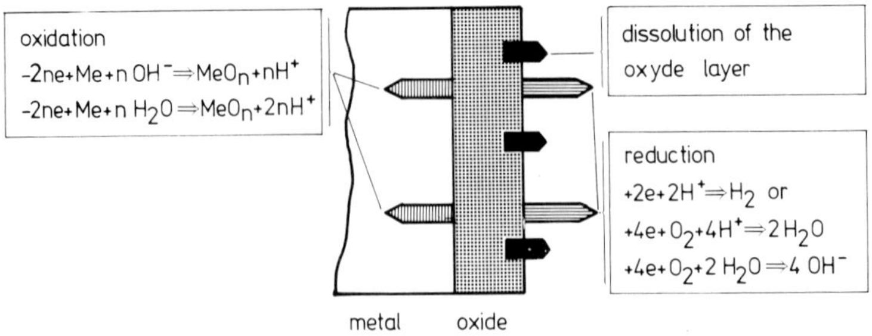

Fig. 5 Chemical and electrochemical reactions at the passivated metal surface

As electron releasing reactions, we may consider:

1. The active corrosion of the metallic material:

$$-ne + Me \rightarrow Me^{n+}$$

2. The oxidation of metal to the metal oxide with accompanying release of hydrogen ions:

$$-2ne + Me + nH_2O \rightarrow MeO_n + 2nH^+$$
$$-2ne + Me + nOH^- \rightarrow MeO_n + nH^+$$

3. The oxidation of adsorbed hydrogen at the surface of the metal:

$$-e + H_{ad} \rightarrow H^+$$

In contrast, the following are electron-absorbing reactions:

1. The reduction of hydrogen,

$$+e + H^+ \rightarrow H \quad \text{Volmer reaction}$$

to a hydrogen atom which is adsorbed on the surface as H_{ad} or which recombines with a second hydrogen atom (Tafel reaction) and is released as gaseous molecular hydrogen H_2. The hydrogen atoms adsorbed at the surface can also, by capturing or absorbing an additional electron and combination with a further H^+ ion, be further reduced to molecular hydrogen in accordance with the equation

$$+e + H^+ + H \rightarrow H_2 \quad \text{Heyrowsky reaction}$$

A diffusion of atomic hydrogen along the grain boundaries associated with a local disruption of the lattice in the vicinity of the surface is also possible. This mechanism must be considered, in addition to the already mentioned primary damage to the surface, as the triggering condition for corrosion fatigue (18).

2. The reduction of the oxygen in accordance with the overall reduction formulae

$$+4e + O_2 + 4H^+ \rightarrow 2H_2O$$
$$+4e + O_2 + 2H_2O \rightarrow 4OH^-$$

In the first of the two reactions, oxygen perioxide can be produced as an intermediate product.

In cases in which oxygen is present, dissolved in the electrolyte, the rate-determining electron-absorbing reaction will always proceed via a reduction of the oxygen.

The minus sign before the electron term means a transfer of electrons to the metal (anode); the corresponding reaction is termed an anodic reaction. The positive sign before the electron term means the absorbing of electrons from the metal (cathode); the corresponding reaction is designated a cathodic reaction.

The dissolution mechanisms in the active and passive conditions of the surface differ clearly from each other. In the active state (Fig. 4), obtained after mechanical removal of the passivating metallic-oxide layer, metal dissolution and the repassivation reaction occur at the surface as electron-releasing reactions, and the reduction of the hydrogen ions and the dissolution of oxygen as electron-absorbing reactions. Because the total electrons absorbed by the implant material must equal the total released electrons, the dissolution of metal in the active state, and also repassivation of the surface, does not depend entirely upon the electrochemical properties of the metal but, in addition, also on the kinetics of the reduction reaction occurring simultaneously. This means that the more rapidly repassivation of the implant material occurs, the more negative the potential of the associated oxide electrode becomes. The current density of the hydrogen ion reduction increases exponentially towards increasingly negative potential so that this reaction should not limit the repassivation rate, whereas the current density of the reduction of oxygen dissolved in the electrolyte depends upon the diffusion of oxygen to the surface of the electrode and can be a limiting factor, although the reduction potential is much more positive than for the hydrogen system. Implant surfaces which, after mechanical disruption of the oxide, must repassivate rapidly to inhibit the active dissolution of metal and must, therefore, meet the following requirements:

1. The potential of the associated oxide electrode should, with respect to the reduction/oxidation potential of the hydrogen, manifest a high negative value. Table 1 shows potentials for various oxide electrodes of passivatable metals. Because the thermo-

Table 1 Redox potentials of investigated oxide-electrodes

Oxide-electrode	Charge carriers per atom	Potential $_{SCE}$ of the oxide electrode pH=7
Al/Al_2O_3	3	− 1.95 V
V/V_2O_3	3	− 1.65 V
Ti/TiO_2	4	− 1.5 V
Cr/Cr_2O_3	3	− 1.24 V
Fe/Fe_3O_4	8/3	− 0.72 V
Mo/MoO_2	4	− 0.68 V
Ni/NiO	2	− 0.56 V
Co/CoO	2	− 0.54 V

dynamic magnitudes forming the basis for the calculations are, in part, available in only a very equivocal form, and moreover, for the metal alloys examined here, mixed potentials that are individually not forseeable, become established, the potentials given can only serve as a guide.

2. The active metal surface should, as far as possible, represent no inhibition for the reduction reaction.

The two requirements are mutually independent and are thus, in many cases, not both met at the same time by the implant material.

Corrosion of the passive surface (Fig. 5) depends primarily upon the solubility of the surface oxide. The electrochemical reformation of the passivating layer to the thickness obtaining at equilibrium, is effected only in accordance with this reaction. The condition, namely that the electrons released during oxidation of the material must be absorbed by the simultaneously occurring reduction reactions, applies here, too. For this reason, concentration gradients, for example of the dissolved oxygen at the surface, can lead to different equilibria and can thus be the cause for formation of local elements.

The transition from active to passive surface can be followed in the laboratory by electrochemical measuring procedures. For this purpose, the material sample to be investigated is introduced into an electrochemical cell as a measuring electrode. Electrical polarization of the material sample, required for simulation of the active or passive state, is effected by means of a counter electrode with the aid of an electronic potentiostat/galvanostat. The potential obtaining at the sample surface is indicated with respect to the reference electrode in the electrolytic vessel (Fig. 6).

Observations of the passivation of an active metal surface are carried out with the aid of intensiostatic tests. As shown in the lower part of Fig. 7, at a fixed time t = 0, the cathodic current required to maintain the active state, is switched to an anodic current. The resulting potential change at the material surface as a function of time, provides information as to the passivation properties, in particular with respect to the influence of oxygen on the rate of repassivation. Obviously, the results obtained in such a laboratory investigation under, in part, simplified measuring conditions, cannot be directly extra-

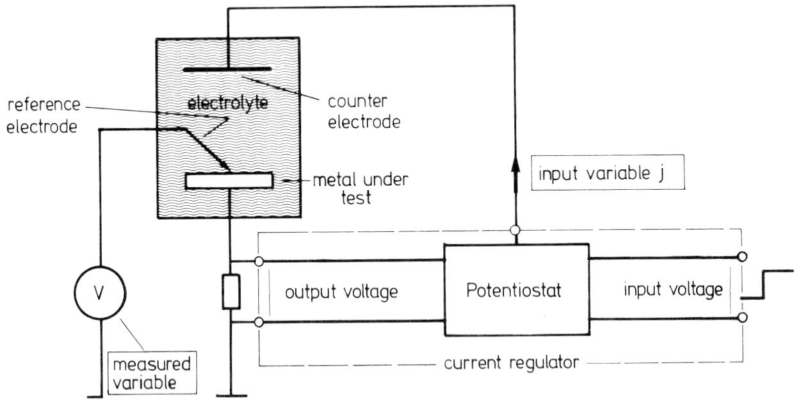

Fig. 6 Experimental set-up for intensiostatic tests

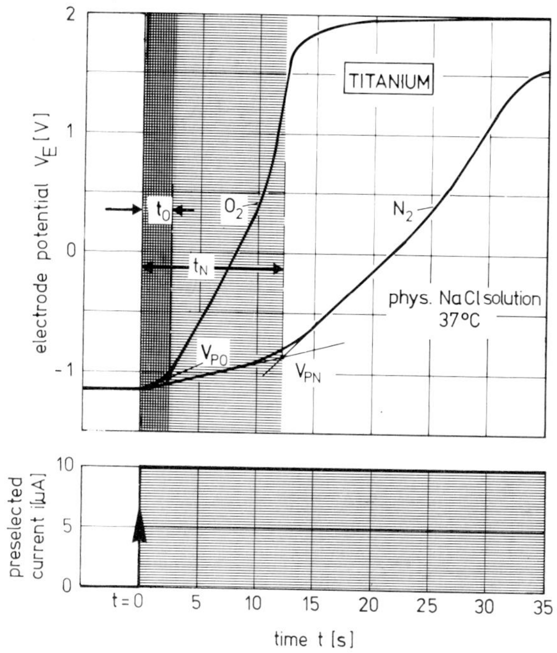

Fig. 7 Determination of oxygen dependent repassivation time

polated to the in-vivo condition; nevertheless, they do allow individual materials to be classified in a certain order with respect to their repassivation properties following mechanical disruption of the surface, and thus provide the basis for the interpretation of results from in-vitro functional tests of artificial joints in the simulator.

Fig. 7 shows the potential pattern of a titanium electrode after switching from a cathodic to an anodic current. Beginning at time t = 0, the electrode potential increases at an approximately constant rate, until the entire surface has been passivated, to the passivation potential V_{po}. Since it describes a condition of the electrode, the passivation potential is largely independent of aeration of the electrolyte. In contrast to this, the passivation times clearly depend upon whether the electrolyte is flushed with oxygen (t_O) or with nitrogen (t_N).

The passivation of titanium in a physiological saline solution free from oxygen is slight, so that, despite the strongly negative potential of the Ti/TiO_2 electrode, the surface can remain active. For this, the strongly inhibited reduction of hydrogen can be responsible. When the neutral electrolyte is aerated with oxygen, however, passivation improves considerably.

The quotient obtained from the passivation times with nitrogen and oxygen flushing for tianium and other alloys used in the manufacture of implants is shown in Table 2. High t_N/t_O values indicate a markedly variable passivation behavior while low values infer an oxygen-independent formation of the oxide layer. Among the materials investigated, the cobalt-based alloys and steel manifest an oxygen-independent behaviour as compared with the titanium-base materials. Since high oxygen gradients are encountered

Table 2 Oxygen dependency of repassivation of different metals

Metal	t_N/t_O	
Ti	6.7	strong O_2 dependent passivation
TiAlV	5.2	↓
TiAlMo	3.6	↓
316 L	2.9	↓
CoCrMo	1.6	weak O_2 dependent
CoCrNiMoTi	1.6	passivation

at the interface between the implant stem and the bone cement, local elements can be formed in the case of titanium alloys.

More strongly practice-oriented results are obtained when simulation of the passivation process is more closely matched to the actual in-situ situation by eliminating the impressed anodic current. Partial removal of the oxide layer can be effected either mechanically (19,20) or electrochemically (21,22). Since with mechanical scraping of the surface, or by breaking material samples, the layer-free state is poorly reproducible, the investigations described below were carried out on electrochemically polished partially activated surfaces.

The case seen in practice, namely, that the active part of the surface produced by friction is associated with a residual part of the implant that has remained in the passive state, is simulated by a dual-cell electrolyte system in which each cell approximates to the

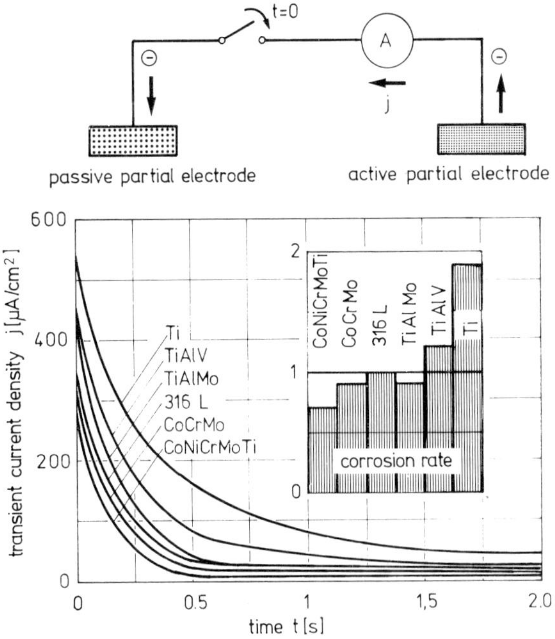

Fig. 8 Transient current density due to repassivation

experimental set-up shown in Fig. 6. The experimental set-up permits the initially galvanically separated samples of identical material to be adjusted to active and passive states by suitable polarization. At a fixed time t = 0, the two partial areas are separated from the galvanostat/potentiostat and, as shown in the upper part of Fig. 8 are galvanically coupled. At this point, the condition representing a partially activated surface such as occurs in the joint implant during each movement cycle is simulated. In the experiment, current flowing between the active and passive surfaces can be measured. The time-dependent behavior of this transient current provides important information on the repassivation process.

Fig. 8 shows the respective transient current densities for the alloys investigated. All measurements were taken in physiological saline solution saturated with oxygen, at a temperature of 37 ^{o}C. Here, too, titanium manifested a more unfavorable behavior than other alloys because restoration of the passive equilibrium required a particularly long time. The current densities, which reach values of 500 $\mu A/cm^2$, show that the destruction of material at the activated parts of the surface is greater by several orders of magnitude than that at corrosion current densities, which range between 100 nA/cm^2 and 10 $\mu A/cm^2$, measurable in the passive state of the same materials. Thus, the repassivation properties of alloys represent an important criterion for the selection of implant materials for artificial joints. The quantities of material dissolved during repassivation or "consumed" to build-up the passivating layer, can be compared for the various materials by dividing the charge required for establishing the passive state of equilibriums by the electrochemical valence of the elements contained in the oxide. The averaged values of the valences are shown in Table 3, together with respective compositions of the alloys. The corrosion rate established in this way standardized with reference to the steel alloy AISI 316 are shown in Fig. 8.

Fig. 9 shows the reactions occurring at a partially activated surface. In contrast to the electrochemical processes at an active (Fig. 4) and a passive (Fig. 5) electrode, at a mixed electrode, the reduction of surface oxide of the passivated surface must also be considered. This partial disruption of the surface oxide of the passivated part of the surface during the repassivation process of the active part of the surface, results in the fact that, in artificial joints, parts of the surface not subjected to mechanically stressing are also involved in disruption of the surface oxide.

Table 3 Composition of the investigated metals and average electrochemical valences

Metal/Elements	Fe	Co	Cr	Ni	Mo	Ti	Al	V	Z
CoCrNiMoTi	1%	33%	20%	35%	10%	1%	–	–	2.4
CoCrMo	1%	60%	28%	2%	6%	–	–	–	2.4
TiAlMo	–	–	–	–	–	90%	7%	3%	3.9
TiAlV	–	–	–	–	–	89%	6%	3%	3.9
Ti	–	–	–	–	–	100%	–	–	4.0
Steel (AISI 316)	65%	–	18%	14%	3%	–	–	–	2.7

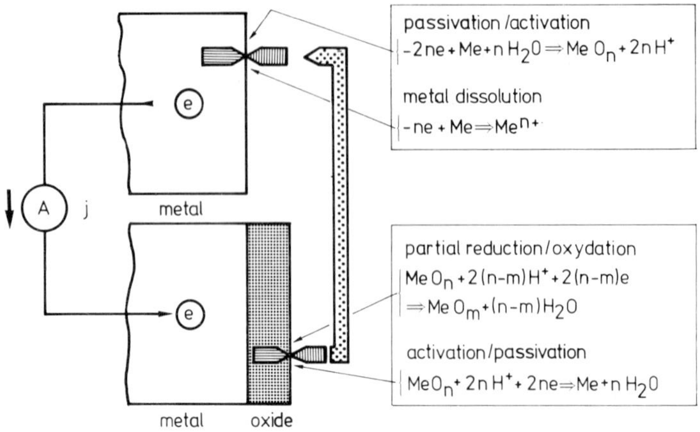

Fig. 9 Electrochemical reactions after partial activation

In the general cases of stainless steel or cobalt alloys, materials with electron conducting passive oxide layers, the repassivation rate is determined primarily by the velocity of the reduction/oxydation reaction at the surface. The rate-determining step of this reaction is the passing of electrons through the solid/electrolyte interface, which is much more faster than the diffusion of ions or atoms through the surface oxide of ionconducting passive layers. This step, however, the diffusion of oxygen in the nonelectron conducting titanium oxide, is the limiting function and the reason for the generally unexpected slow repassivation rate of pure titanium and the investigated TiAlV-alloy. The diffusion of oxygen or of metal atoms limitates the current density in the circuit consisting of the active and passive electrode and the connecting wire and electrolyte path. An improvement of the corrosion properties especially with reference to fretting corrosion should be possible with an increase of the electron conductivity in the oxide layers of titanium alloys.

The behavior of transient currents with time lead us to conclude that, in artificial joint implants in the locomotor apparatus, the establishment of passive equilibrium of mechanically activated parts of the surface is not effected within the period of a cycle of movement of approximately 1 sec. This assumption is confirmed by tests on artificial joints carried out in the simulator (Fig. 3). The change in equilibrium potential to negative values is unequivocally due to a partial activation of the joint implant. This means that, together with metallic abrasion products, corrosion products, too, are imparted to the tissue in considerable quantities.

Although we are evaluating measurements taken under laboratory conditions, we can safely assume that the corrosion rates of periodically stressed surfaces are higher those in nonstressed implants by several orders of magnitude. Thus, measurements of the uniformly affective or only locally affective corrosion are not adequate to permit a satisfactory assessment of corrosion properties of materials in use for implants.

The necessity for continuing work on the development of materials with better abrasion and repassivation properties and better fatigue strength in corrosive media is emphasized by laboratory tests on artificial hip and knee joints carried out by Swanson, Freeman and Heath (23). Although the test conditions were certainly more severe than the requirements normally expected to be met by joints, the results clearly show that the current technology in corrosion-resistant alloys for stressed implants is not yet satisfactory.

REFERENCES

1. Hughes, A.N., Jordan, B.A.: Metallurgical observations on some metallic surgical implants which failed in vivo. Journal of Biomedical Materials Research 6, 33 (1972)
2. Becker, H., Schaller, G., Schmid, H.J., Zwicker, U.: Werkstoffprobleme bei Hüftgelenkimplantaten. Fachberichte der Deutschen Gesellschaft für Biomedizinische Technik 2, 35 (1973)
3. Williams, D.F., Meachim, G.: A combined metallurgical and histological study of tissue-prosthesis interactions in orthopedic patients. Journal of Biomedical Materials Research 5, 1 (1974)
4. Coleman, R.F., Herrington, J., Scales, J.T.: Concentration of wear products in hair, blood, and urine after total hip replacement. British Medical Journal 1, 527 (1973)
5. Zeisler, R., Lux, F.: Investigations of the corrosive deposition of components of metal implants and of the behaviour of biological trace elements in metallosis tissue by means of instrumental multi-element activation analysis. Journal of Radioanalytical Chemistry 19, 289 (1974)
6. Winter, G.D.: Tissue reactions to metallic wear and corrosion products in human patients. Journal of Biomedical Materials Research Symposium 5, 11 (1974)
7. Willert, H.G., Semlitsch, M.: Kapselreaktionen auf Kunststoff und Metallabrieb. Technische Rundschau Sulzer 2, 1 (1975)
8. Contzen, H.: Abakteriello Osteomyelitis durch Metallose. Langenbecks Archiv für Chirurgie 334, 555 (1973)
9. Winter, G.D.: Prosthesis and tissue: the interface problem. Biomedical Engineering 21, 390 (1973)
10. Evans, E.M., Freeman, M.A.R., Miller, A.J., Vernon-Roberts, B.: Metal sensitivity as a cause of bone necrosis and loosening of the prosthesis in total joint replacement. The Journal of Bone and Joint Surgery 56-B, 626 (1974)
11. Zitter, H.: Schadensfälle bei osteosynthetischen Implantaten und ihre Ursachen. Werkstoffe und Korrosion 22, 598 (1971)
12. Fäßler, K., Sinn, R., Spähn, H.: Zum Versagen metallischer Implantate infolge korrosiver und mechanisch korrosiver Einwirkungen. Biomedizinische Technik 18, 176 (1973)
13. Kaesche, H.: Die Korrosion der Metalle, Berlin-Heidelberg-New York: Springer-Verlag 1966
14. Herbsleb, G.: Einfluß der Oberflächenbeschaffenheit auf die Beständigkeit nichtrostender, austenitischer Chrom-Nickel-Stähle gegen transkristalline Spannungsrißkorrosion. Werkstoffe und Korrosion 24, 867 (1973)
15. Reutler, R.M., Greene, N.D.: Corrosion of surface defects in fine wires. Journal of Biomedical Materials Research 9, 597 (1975)
16. Bapna, M.S., Lautenschlager, E.P., Moser, J.B.: The influence of electrical potential and surface finish on the fatigue life of surgical implant materials. Journal of Biomedical Materials Research 9, 611 (1975)

17. Süry, P.: Zum Korrosionsverhalten gegossener und geschmiedeter Implantat-Werkstoffe unter Berücksichtigung von Verbundkonstruktionen bei Gelenkendoprothesen. Technische Rundschau Sulzer 1, 1 (1974)

18. Thull, R., Schaldach, M.: Physikalisch-chemische Aspekte chirurgischer Metallimplantate. 23. Kongreß der Deutschen Gesellschaft für Kiefer- und Gesichtschirurgie, Basel 1973

19. Sherwin, M.P., Taylor, D.E., Waterhouse, R.B.: An electrochemical investigation of fretting corrosion in stainless steel. Corrosion Science 11, 419 (1971)

20. Rubin, B.T.: Kinetics of oxide film repair on titanium. Electroanalytical Chemistry and Interfacial Electrochemistry 58, 323 (1975)

21. Butman, G.M., Tseung, A.C.C.: The kinetics of the anodic formation of the passive film on stainless steel. Corrosion Science 12, 415 (1972)

22. Thull, R., Seidel, K., Baacke, M.: Problematik der mechanischen und elektrochemischen Belastungssimulation von Kniegelenkprothesen. 61. Tagung der Deutschen Gesellschaft für Orthopädie und Traumatologie, Saarbrücken 1974

23. Swanson, S.A.V., Freeman, M.A.R., Heath, J.C.: Laboratory test on total joint replacement prostheses. The Journal of Bone and Joint Surgery 55-B, 759 (1973)

MECHANICAL PROPERTIES OF METALLIC MATERIALS FOR LONGTERM USE IN HIGHLY STRESSED LOCOMOTOR SYSTEMS

H.U. Zwicker and H.J. Schmid

Prostheses for long-term use in the highly stressed locomotor system as artificial hip and knee joints may consist of ceramics, metal alloys, polymers or of compounds of these different materials. Because ceramics and polymers are the subject of two articles in this book written by Sauer and Hulbert only alloys will be described in the following paper.

The selection of alloys for implants involves such factors as compatibility of the materials with the human body, friction and wear, and mechanical properties. Operational tests and studies on friction and wear have been discussed in detail in another paper (1). In highly stressed locomotor systems, only materials with mechanical properties which can resist the high stresses involved can be used. The alloys considered in this paper are presently in use or are such materials as are recommended for this application and are yet to be tested. Cobalt-base casting alloys and type 316 stainless steel will be discussed. These materials are commonly used. In addition a cobalt-based alloy and the well-known titanium alloy containing 6 % aluminium and 4 % vanadium used in aircraft industry will be described. These four alloys are believed to have the necessary high fatigue strength to withstand the numerous stress cycles the hip and knee prostheses have to sustain during service. Fatigue failures, for example of the femoral stems of total hip prostheses have often occurred, and are described in other publications (1,2), and in the chapter written by Weightman. Fig. 1 shows a hip prosthesis which has broken twice after five years of service.

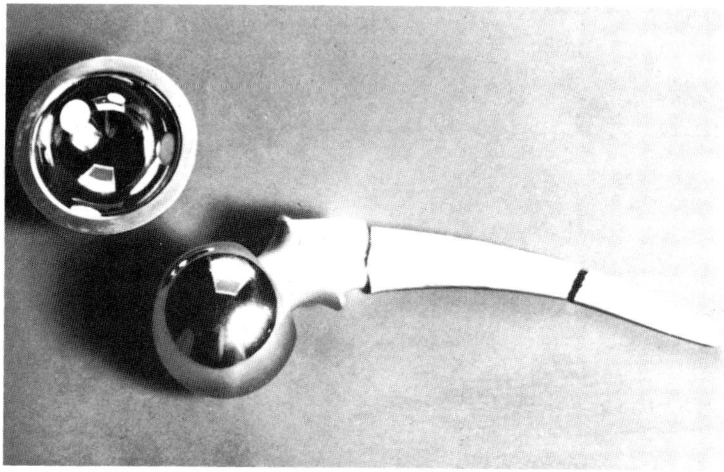

Fig. 1 Hip prosthesis broken into three parts in a human body

The toxicity of the individual metallic components of an alloy may be considered of secondary importance. But even so-called non-corrosive alloys release small quantities of ions into the surrounding tissue. In addition, friction between a metallic implant and the adjacent bone may occur since there is a great difference in the elastic moduli of the bone cement and the alloys. Filler material in bone cement such as zirconium-oxide can be very hard and may wear away metallic particles from the implanted stem of a hip prosthesis. Therefore one must consider the influence of these materials in the human body where long service is required.

SELECTION OF MATERIALS

All metallic materials used in hip or knee prostheses are alloys. Most of the alloys used for long-term applications in highly stressed locomotor systems have been developed for other applications. For example cobalt-based alloys were developed for high temperature application such as turbine blades in aircraft and other industries. The alloys have to be matched to the problems arising from compatibility with the human body. These include wear resistance under abrasive conditions and the high stresses which may occur during their continued use in the surrounding physiological solution containing sodium chloride and other substances that promote pitting and stress corrosion. Experiments on the toxicity of metal ions were made on rabbit fibrocytes (3) and chicken femurs (4). The results of these experiments with 10^{-5} and 10^{-3} molar sodium chloride solutions and pure metals used as components of the alloys described in this article are summarized in Table 1. It can be seen that besides aluminium, iron, and titanium, all

Table 1 Toxicity of elements of alloys

Toxicity of elements of metallic alloys	Rabbit fibrocytes Metal	Rabbit fibrocytes Cl-ion 10^{-5}m	Chicken femurs Cl-ion 10^{-3} m	Histology of rabbit tissue
Aluminium (Al)	0	n.i.	0	enclosed
Chromium (Cr)	0	+	+	n.i.
Cobalt (Co)	++	++	++	toxic
Copper (Cu)	++	++	n.i.	toxic
Iron (Fe)	0	0	0	enclosed
Nickel (Ni)	+	++	++	toxic
Molybdenum (Mo)	0	n.i.	n.i.	enclosed
Titanium (Ti)	0	n.i.	0	vital
Vanadium (V)	n.i.	n.i.	++	toxic

Effect on the growth of rabbit fibrocytes or chicken femurs in tissue culture

n.i. — not investigated,
0 — no inhibition,
\+ — slight inhibition,
++ — strong inhibition

these metals are more or less toxic. Table 2 shows the composition of the alloys investigated (5-7) in this work. All of these alloys contain toxic constituents. It seems that, up till now, there is no metallic material available which is free from toxic elements, and which might be used as non-toxic material for hip or knee prostheses. Tests with implants of CoCrMo-, FeCrNiMo- alloys and titanium in the back muscles of New Zealand White Rabbits have also shown that only titanium has properties suitable for surgical implants in human subjects (8).

All external stresses cause a strain on the metallic implanted materials, the degree of which depends on the mechanical properties of the material. A given not too high, external stress on bone originates a more than tenfold strain than on one of the metallic materials mentioned above. Table 3 shows values of the densities and elastic moduli of bone, bone cement (polymethylmethacrylate) and of high-density polyethylene usually used for the hip cups. The elastic modulus of this latter material is even less than that of bone and therefore it has a higher damping capacity and absorbes shock waves easier than bone. The elastic moduli of the metallic materials used or proposed for hip- or knee-prostheses are summarized in Table 4. The titanium alloy containing 6 % aluminium and 4 % vanadium has the lowest elastic modulus and the lowest density. Abrasive wear of these materials against polyethylene is in all cases about 0.14 mm/year (7,9).

Table 2 Composition of alloys

Ele-ments	Castings CoCrMo	Wrought materials (forgings) CoNiCrMoTi	FeCrNiMo (316L)	TiAlV
Al	—	—	—	6 w/o
C	0.25 w/o	< 0.025 w/o	0.07 w/o (<0.03 w/o)	< 0.08 w/o
Cr	28 w/o	19 w/o	19 w/o	—
Co	balance	balance	3 w/o	—
Cu	—	—	< 0.1 w/o	—
Fe	< 1 w/o	< 1 w/o	balance	< 0.25 w/o
Ni	< 2.5 w/o	35 w/o	15 w/o	—
Mn	< 1 w/o	< 0.15 w/o	< 2 w/o	—
Mo	6 w/o	9.5 w/o	3 w/o	—
Si	< 1 w/o	< 0.15 w/o	< 0.75 w/o	—
Ti	—	0.8 w/o	—	balance
V	—	—	—	4 w/o

Table 3 Values of elastic modulus and density of bone, bone cement and high density polyethylene

Elastic (tensile) modulus	Bone	Bone cement polymethyl-methacrylate	Hip cup high density polyethylene
N/mm^2	$4.9 \cdot 10^3$-$9 \cdot 10^3$	$3 \cdot 10^3$	$0.5 \cdot 10^3$
PSI	$711 \cdot 10^3$-$1422 \cdot 10^3$	$435 \cdot 10^3$	$72.5 \cdot 10^3$
Kp/mm^2	$0.5 \cdot 10^3$-$1 \cdot 10^3$	306	51
Density g/cm^3	~ 1	~ 1	0.95-0.97

Table 4 Values of density, elastic modulus and abrasive wear of alloys proposed for use in hip prostheses (7,9)

Alloy type	Density g/cm^3	Elastic modulus (stiffness) $N/mm^2 \cdot 10^3$	PSI $\cdot 10^3$	$Kp/mm^2 \cdot 10^3$	Abrasive wear metallic alloy/PE mm/year
CoCrMo	8.0	200	29150	20.5	~ 0.14
CoNiCrMo	8.2	225	32700	23.0	~ 0.14
FeCrNiMo	7.8	200	29150	20.5	~ 0.14
TiAlV	4.4	118	17050	12.0	~ 0.14

If the stress on a material overcomes the limit of elasticity, plastic deformation occurs. The yield strength shortened with ($\sigma_{0.2}$) is the amount of force necessary for a plastic deformation of 0.2 % measured in a coaxial testing procedure. The results of such tests on the metallic materials for hip and knee prostheses are shown in Table 5. In addition, the results of fatigue tests and hardness measurements are presented (7,10). These tests are conducted on a rotating sample on the end of which different loads are placed to cause stresses. The sample has to withstand 10^7 rotations (fatigue strength, σ_{bw}). At higher stresses the samples will break at a number of rotations which is less than 10^7. The results of these investigations show that the fatigue strength does not correspond to the yield strength. The quotient, yield strength/fatigue strength, of the various materials may differ considerably. The stainless steel type 316 which is relatively soft and which has the lowest value of hardness, can increase its strength by deformation processes during the fatigue test and therefore has a relatively high fatigue strength, which is not much less than the yield strength. The toughness (Table 5), defined as elongation of a coaxial stressed sample after breaking, therefore manifests the highest value in this case.

Fig. 2 shows the stress-strain curves of three of the metallic materials considered in this paper and the corresponding micrographs of the microstructure in the unstressed condition. The micrographs of the casting of the CoCrMo-alloy, of the annealed stainless steel

Table 5 Yield and fatigue strength of different alloys proposed for use in hip prostheses (7,10)

Alloy type	Yield strength $\sigma_{0.2}$ N/mm^2	PSI	Kp/mm^2	Fatigue strength σ_{bw} N/mm^2	PSI	Kp/mm^2
CoCrMo	441	63990	45	196	28440	20
CoNiCrMo	637	92430	65	592	76790	54
FeCrNiMo	284	41240	29	245	35550	25
TiAlV	794	115180	81	392	56880	40

Alloy type	Toughness %	Hardness V.P.N.
CoCrMo	8	300
CoNiCrMo	35	300
FeCrNiMo	63	165
TiAlV	10	300

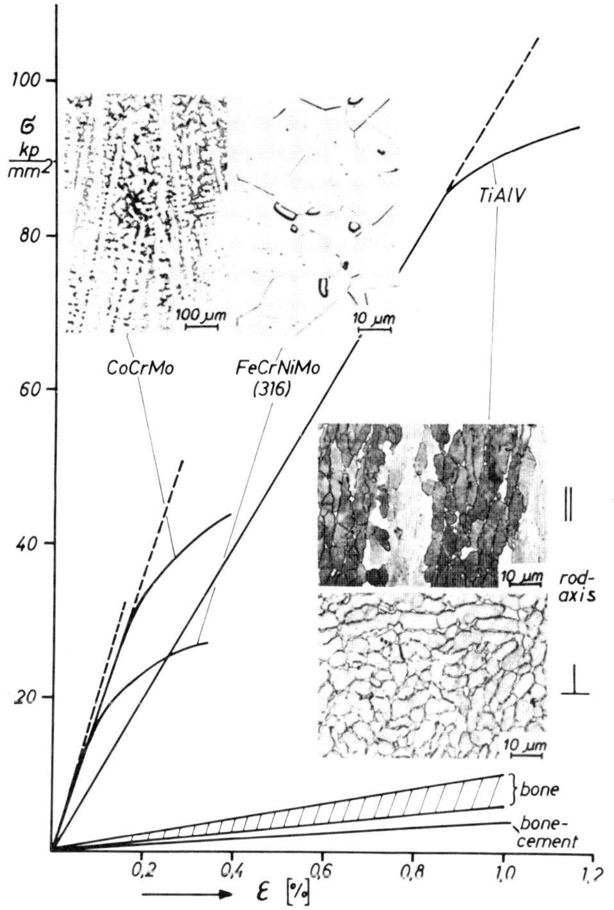

Fig. 2 Stress-strain relation for different materials and micrographs of the alloys

type 316 and of the wrought titanium alloy show at least two phases. In the CoCrMo-alloy the phases are cobalt solid solution and carbides, and in the type 316 steel mainly austenite with little δ-ferrite. In the titanium alloy the main part of the alloy consists of an α-phase and of a second phase (β). The alloy is therefore an $\alpha + \beta$ -alloy. This material was delivered as a forged rod of 65 mm in diameter.

To determine whether the orientation of the samples with respect to the rod axis influences the fatigue strength, samples with different angles to the rod axis were prepared. As the diameter of the rod was only 65 mm, 10 cm long rotating fatigue samples could not be prepared. For this reason smaller (30 mm long) push-pull samples (fatigue-strength σ ZD) were investigated. The minimum stress was + 5 Kp/mm^2. Maximum stresses (σ_0) of these differently orientated samples are presented in Fig. 3, together with results obtained in samples with the same shape from hip prostheses castings of CoCrMo-alloy. The scatter within the different directions in TiAlV-alloy is small, while the samples of the CoCrMo-castings manifest a much broader scatter and a continuous

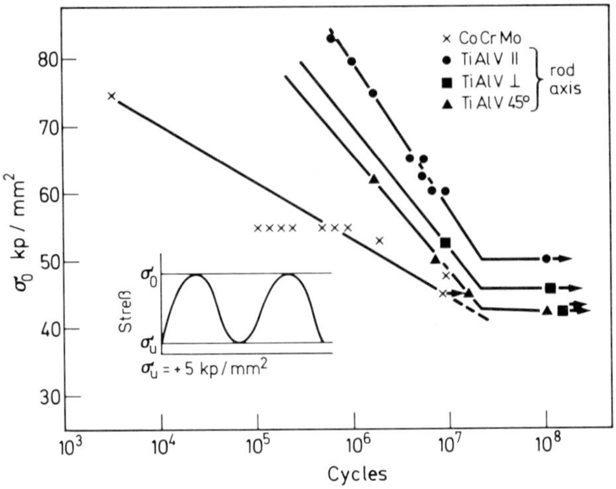

Fig. 3
Fatigue measurements of cast CoCrMo- and wrought TiAlV-alloy

decrease of maximum load σ_0 with increasing number of cycles. In constrast to the cast CoNiCrMo-alloy the wrought TiAlV-alloy shows a real fatigue limit. From Table 5 one can suppose that a real fatigue limit might be observed in wrought CoCrMo-alloy also.

EVALUATION OF STRESSES IN HIP PROSTHESES

As hip prostheses are more advanced than knee prostheses only hip prostheses were investigated. Initial investigations were done on calculation of the forces which may result on failure of these prostheses. In vivo measurements of these forces with patients having a body weight of 75 and 44 Kp are shown in Fig. 4 (11). The force on the sole (2 cm plastic) was also measured. Our measurement of these forces on the sole at different speeds in walking or running and going upstairs and downstairs are shown in Fig. 5. The forces estimated from these experiments on the hip prostheses are summarized in Table 6. This table shows that loads up to eight times the body weight may occur in the vertical direction on going downstairs with 21 cm high steps (1). These values are in good agreement with those reported in the chapter written by Paul in this book. A maximum load of 800 Kp was proposed and used for a simulation testing procedure for hip prostheses.

PROCEDURE FOR LONG–TERM TESTING OF HIP PROSTHESES

To simulate the forces which a hip prosthesis has to withstand, one must diminish the time for testing. Therefore the time for one walking step was diminished to 0.3 sec. In this procedure, testing for two weeks corresponds to about ten years service in the human body. As one may assume that the stem might become loose in the upper part

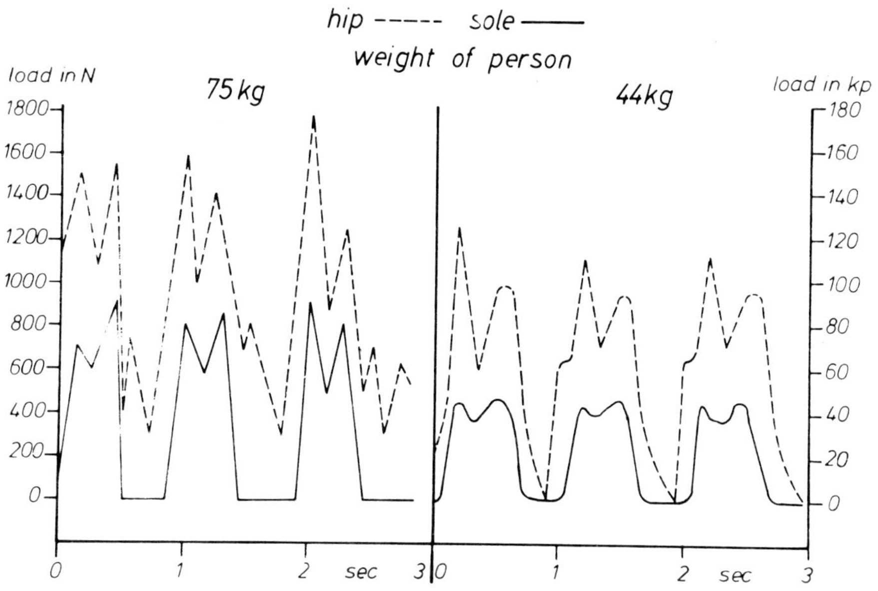

Fig. 4 In vivo measurements of load in hip and sole for persons weighing 75 and 44 Kp respectively; speed of walking: 1.3 m/sec (9)

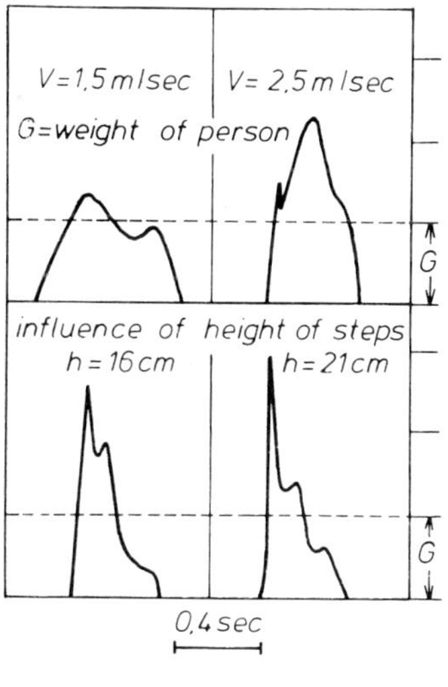

Fig. 5
Load history for simulation of forces in hip prostheses

after some time in service, only the lower half of the stem was fixed. An aqueous solution of sodium chloride (0.9 % by weight) maintained at 39 °C, was used to simulate the surrounding tissue. The strain on the stem was measured by strain gauges. Fig. 6 shows the arrangement of a hip prosthesis and the apparatus used for testing in a servo-hydraulic system with a prosthesis which was broken during fatigue test. The force was corrected by a computer system of the PTP 8 type. The deformation of the stem with

Table 6 Loads on hip prostheses calculated while walking, running and descending steps of different heights

Motion	Max. sole pressure load (measured)	Max. load on prosthesis (calculated)
Walking v = 1.5 m/sec	1.3 G	2 . . . 3 G
Running v = 2.5 m/sec	2.2 G	3 . . . 5 G
Descending a step of 16 cm in height	2.0 G	3 . . . 5 G
Descending a step of 21 cm in height	3.5 G	6 . . . 8 G

G = body weight

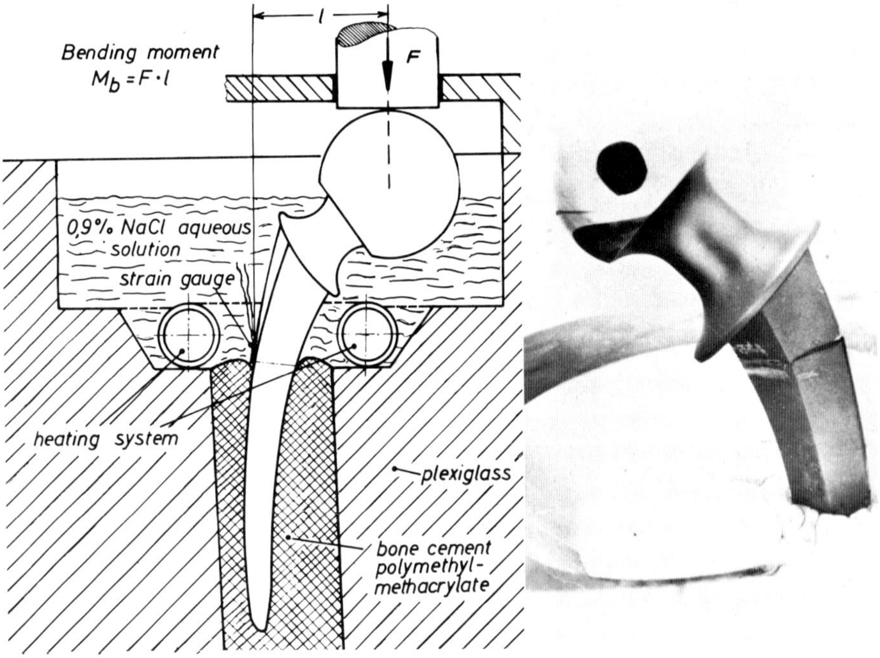

Fig. 6 Fixation of hip prostheses for low cycle fatigue measurements in 0.9 % by weight aqueous NaCl-solution at 39 °C

time was plotted electronically. The whole arrangement – the testing machine, the computer, the writing machine and oscillograph for supervising the strain gauges – is shown in Fig. 7. The servohydraulic machine was located in an adjoining room. The bending moment is calculated from the distance between the prosthesis (l) and the force imposed (F).

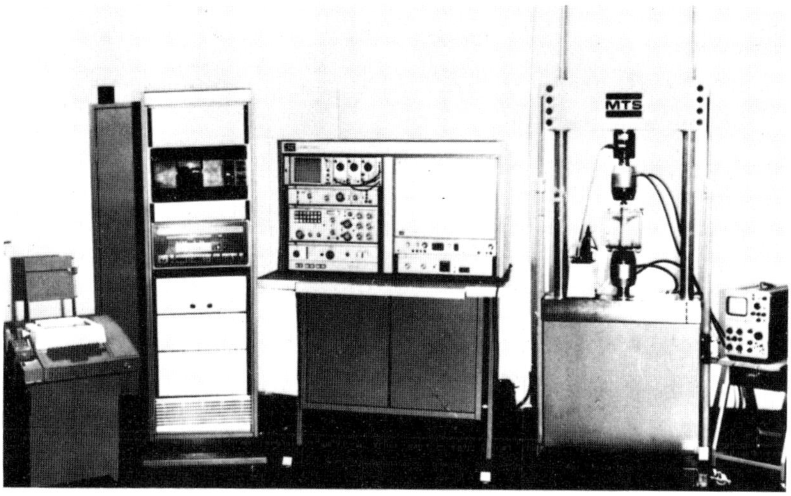

Fig. 7 Testing apparatus for low cycle fatigue testing of hip prostheses

RESULTS OF LONG–TERM TESTS

Fig. 8 summarizes the results obtained on different materials. The maximum load of one fatigue cycle was between 300 and 800 Kp. The material Type 1 (as cast condition) shows a broad scattering of the results in all different load cycles. Two prostheses broke

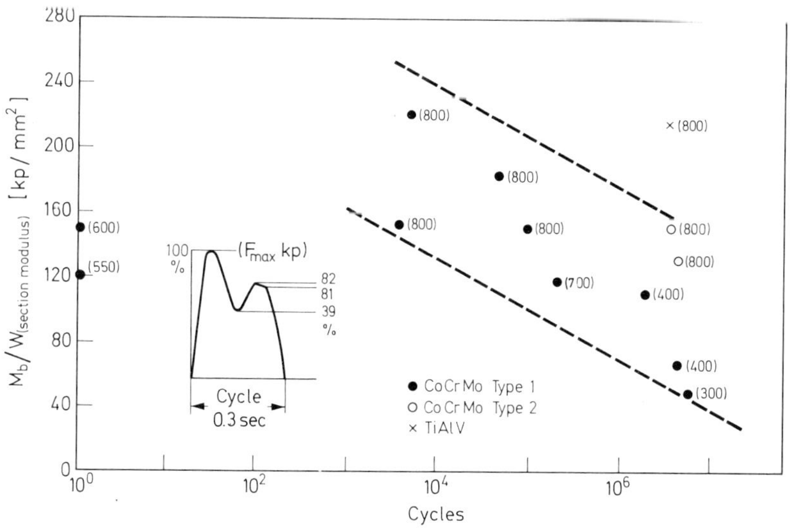

Fig. 8 Fatigue strength of hip prostheses made from cobalt-base alloy (as cast, type 1; annealed, type 2) and TiAlV-alloy

after the first cycle, one under a maximum load of 600 Kp, and the other under a maximum load of 550 Kp. The material Type 2 (annealed at ~1200 °C) with a greater proportion of dissolved carbides manifests a higher fatigue strength than Type 1 material in the two prostheses investigated. The highest fatigue strength of all the prostheses investigated was shown by the TiAlV-alloy. With a maximum load of 800 Kp it withstands $3.6 \cdot 10^6$ cycles. Stainless steel type 316 does not withstand the high stresses and shows deformation. The wrought CoNiCrMo-alloy has not yet been investigated.

MICROSTRUCTURE AND FATIGUE STRENGTH

The low fatigue strength of the castings has its origin in the microstructure, in the spaces and in the inclusions. If these materials are re-melted in an electric arc under an inert atmosphere, for example argon, the silicate impurities coagulate. In Fig. 9 coagulated silicates on a regulus of CoCrMo-alloy can be seen. The glassy material consists of aluminium-calcium-silicates. Fig. 10 shows the macro- and microstructure of a CoCrMo-casting. There are large plates of cobalt-rich primary crystals surrounded by a eutectic structure. Cracks may start on silicate inclusions, spaces or on the weakest part of the eutectic structure near the surface. Fig. 11 shows a photograph of the crack initiation on the fracture surface of a prosthesis that broke in a human body. The prostheses tested in the fatigue testing apparatus showed the same surface. The migration of the cracks into the prosthesis can be seen in Fig. 12. The crack migrates along the eutectic struc-

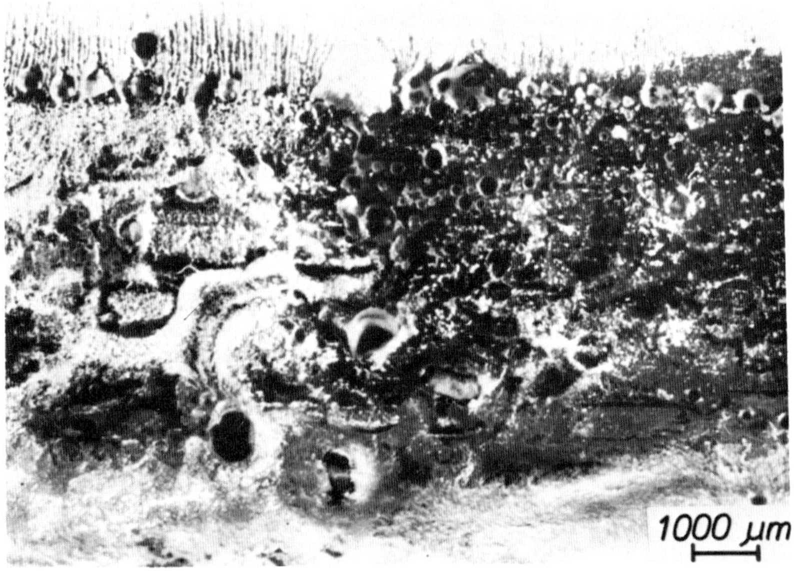

Fig. 9 Aluminium-calcium-silicates on CoCrMo-alloys melted under an argon-arc

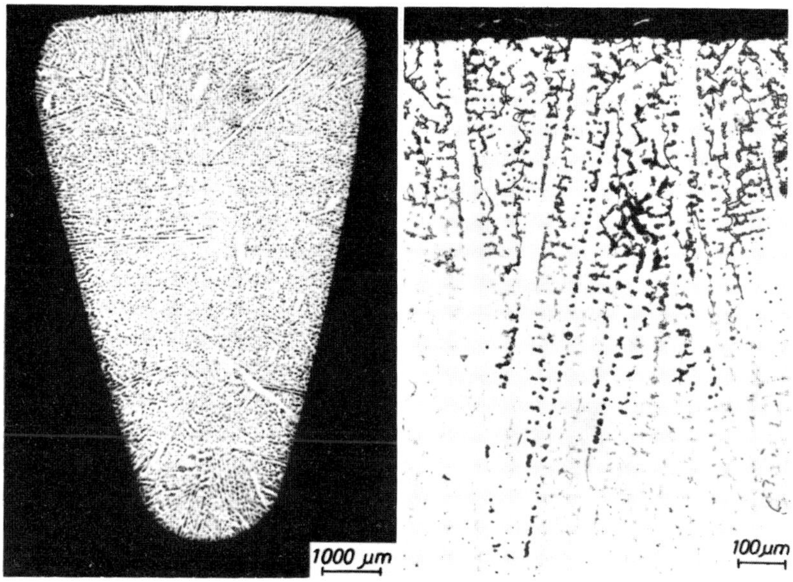

Fig. 10 Macro- and microstructure of a prosthesis casting of CoCrMo-alloy

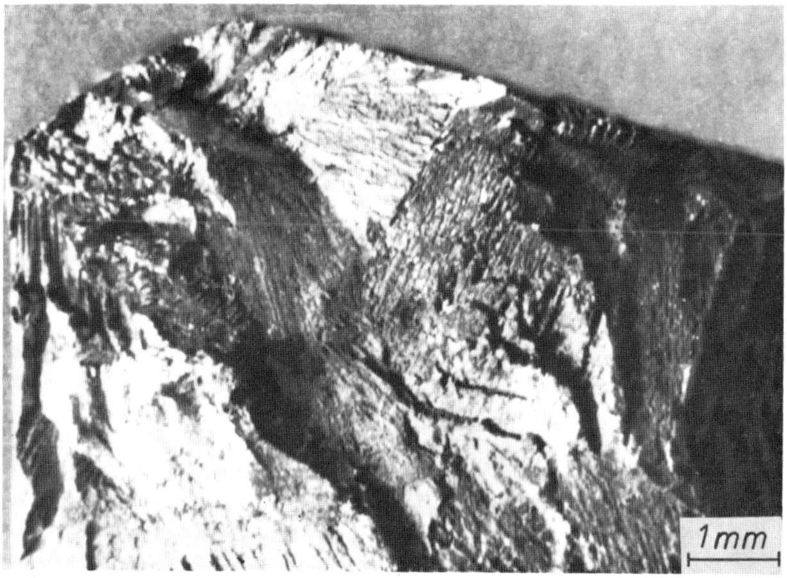

Fig. 11 Micrograph of the surface of fracture of a hip prosthesis broken in a human body. Fracture occured after an initiating crack

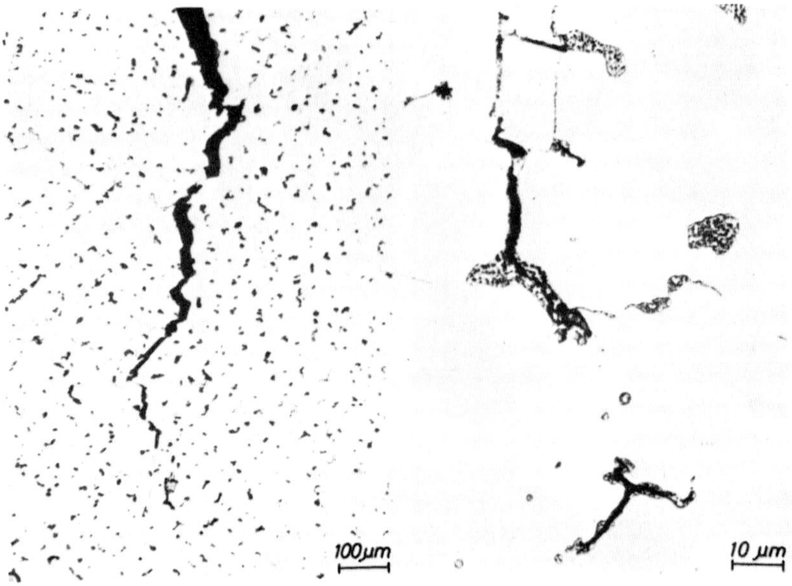

Fig. 12 Migration of a crack in a cast prosthesis of CoCrMo-alloy

ture. In these areas, the amount of the alloying elements molybdenum and chromium increases in the form of carbides. The content of cobalt and of other elements decreases, as can be seen from the microprobe analysis in Fig. 13. As has been shown by other investigations (2) the crystallitic areas of similar orientation are visible in the castings. Fig. 14 shows the whole crack area of such a casting and Fig. 15 the crack area of the TiAlV-alloy. The scanning microscope investigation shows, in the case of the casting, much smoother areas of fracture than in the TiAlV-alloy. At the moment we do not know whether hydrogen may be involved in the migration of cracks in the TiAlV-alloy.

SUMMARY AND DISCUSSION

To avoid any failures of prostheses during service in high stressed locomotor systems we may discuss the problems listed in Fig. 16. The easiest way to improve the strength of a prosthesis is to increase its dimensions. As the diameter of the hole in the femur is limited, the maximum diameter of the prosthesis must be fixed on this diameter. Fig. 17 shows a radiograph of hip joints. In an initial operation, a prosthesis with a short stem was inserted into one hip joint. Later, in a second operation, a thicker and longer prosthesis was inserted into the other hip joint. The danger of cracking is much greater in the short stem than in the long stem, which is stressed by bending forces to a much lower degree than the short prosthesis. Fig. 18 shows prostheses with long stems inserted in both hip joints. As has been mentioned in the chapter written by Beck in this book fixation for a correct position is easier in long stem prostheses than in short stem prostheses.

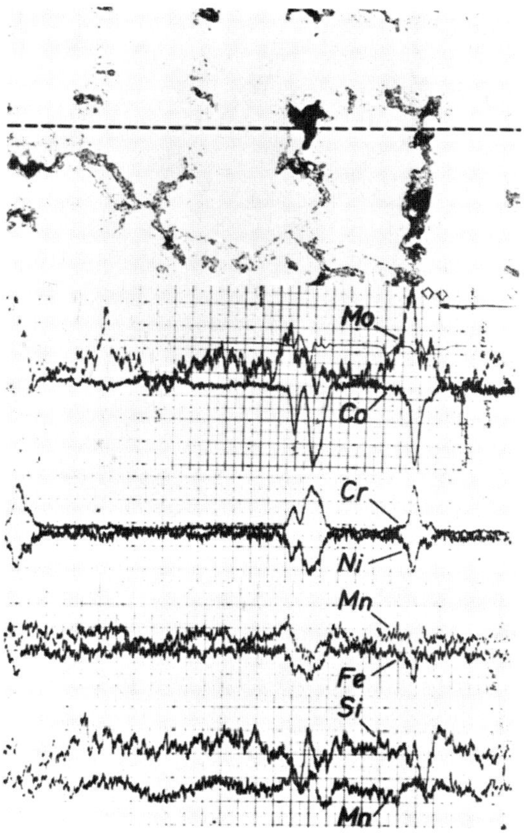

Fig. 13
Microprobe analysis of crack areas

In castings it is not possible to estimate the critical stresses which are at a maximum near the surface, because the microstructure, spaces and inclusions can increase these stresses to an indefinite level. Therefore, wrought material is superior in fatigue strength to material in the cast or cast and annealed condition. Usually annealing improves the fatigue strength of the castings, because microstresses for example originated by carbides which occur in the microstructure can at least partially be eliminated. This is not possible with spaces and inclusions.

Cracking always starts at the weakest point in or near the surface. Therefore an imperfect surface condition may favour the commencement of cracks. If the prostheses are implanted with bone cement this material may also start to crack. The stress concentration in these areas will increase and cracking may also start in the metallic material of the prostheses. For stainless steel and perhaps also for titanium alloys crevice corrosion may occur in areas in which there is no, or only a very small, exchange of ions into other areas.

From the materials science point of view, metallic titanium alloys could help to increase the fatigue strength of the prosthesis stem. Beyond this light weight and high damping capacity are additional properties of this material required by the clinicians for an applicable implant. The development of alloys with non toxic additions would be of

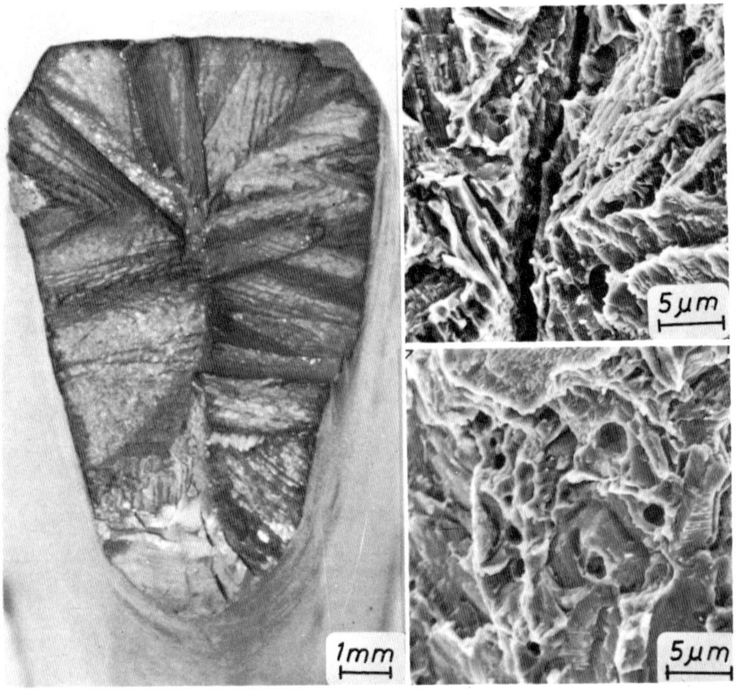

Fig. 14 Photograph of the surface of a cast CoCrMo hip prosthesis, broken in a human body, and scanning micrographs of different areas

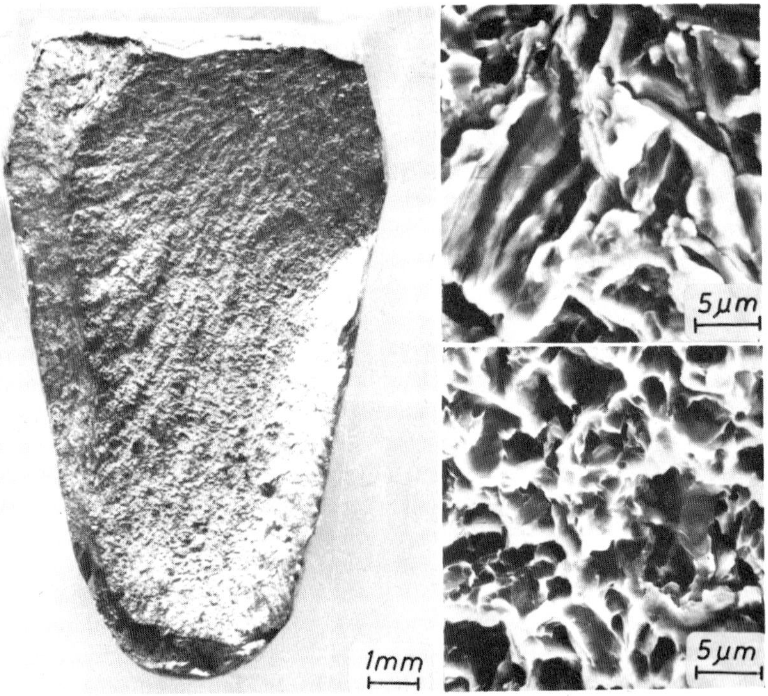

Fig. 15 Photograph of the surface of fracture of a TiAlV hip prosthesis, broken in a testing machine after $3.5 \cdot 10^6$ cycles (0-800-266-656-648-0 Kp) in physiol. NaCl-solution, 39 °C, and scanning micrographs of different areas

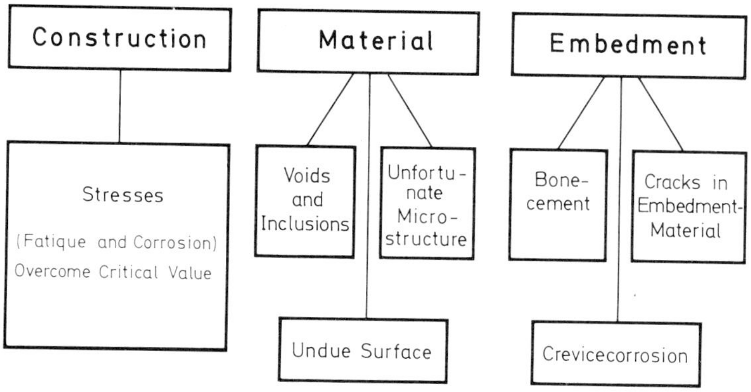

Fig. 16 Disposition of failure possibilities in highly stressed locomotor systems

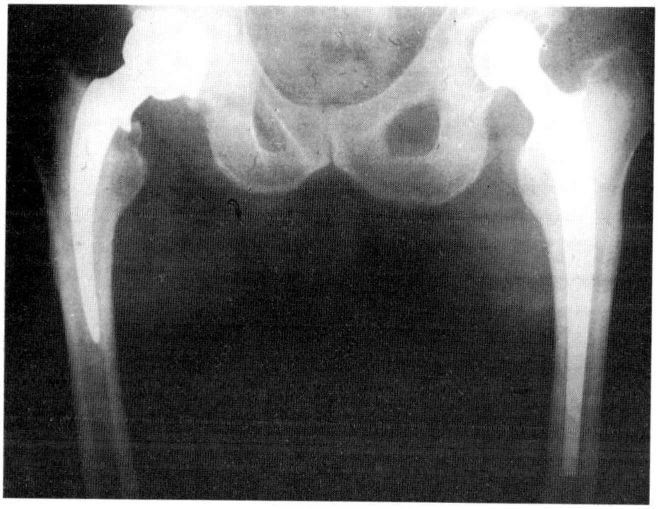

Fig. 17 Radiograph of short and long stem hip prostheses

importance. It seems that in the USSR such prostheses with a stem made from titanium alloys and a head made from CoCrMo-alloy are already in service. Such a prosthesis has been discussed in the chapter by Friedebold and Kölbel in this book. The most serious defect of these types for long-term use is the abrasive wear of the cups which are made from high-density polyethylene. The very high damping capacity of this materials permits it to propagate the shock waves to a much lower degree than material made from oxide ceramics. On the other hand, the wear resistance of a head and a cup made from oxide ceramics is far superior to the wear-resistance shown by all materials. The compatibility of ceramic oxide to the human body is as good as that of titanium. Some problems may be involved due to hard particles in the surface of oxide ceramics in moving contact with the tissue. Compounds of different materials may also help to overcome the difficulties involved in long-term service of prostheses in highly stressed locomotor systems.

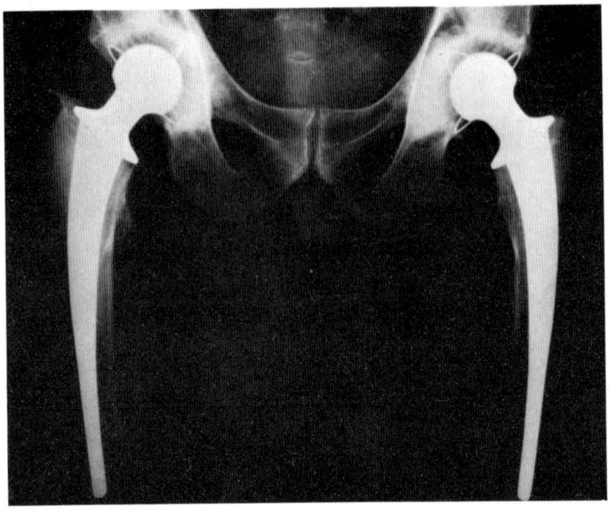

Fig. 18
Radiograph of a pair of long stem hip prostheses

REFERENCES

1. Becker, H. et.al.: Werkstoffprobleme bei Hüftgelenkimplantaten. Fachberichte der Jahrestagung der Deutschen Gesellschaft für Biomedizinische Technik, Erlangen 2, 35 (1973)
2. Semlitsch, M. et.al.: Bruchuntersuchungen an gegossenen und geschmiedeten Kobaltbasis-Legierungen mit dem Rasterelektronen-Mikroskop und Verhütungsmaßnahmen gegen Ermüdungsbrüche an Hüftgelenkendoprothesen. Beitr. elektronenmikroskop.Direktabb.Oberfl. 6, 263 (1973)
3. Hullinger, L. et.al.: Einfluß einiger reiner Metalle und Legierungen auf das Wachstum von Kaninchenfibrozyten in Gewebekulturen. Zeitschrift für die gesamte experimentelle Medizin 144, 145 (1967)
4. Steinemann, S. et.al.: Research Conference on Biomaterials, Tilton 1972 and 23. Kongress der Deutschen Gesellschaft für Kiefer- und Gesichtschirurgie, Basel 1973
5. Frank, E., Zitter, H.: Metallische Implantate in der Knochenchirurgie, Wien: Springer Verlag 1971
6. Williams, D.F., Roaf, R.: Implants in Surgery, London: W.B. Saunders Comp. Ltd. 1973
7. Semlitsch, M.: Technischer Fortschritt bei künstlichen Hüftgelenken. Technische Rundschau Sulzer 4 (1974)
8. Laing, P.G., Ferguson, A.B., Hodge, E.S.: Tissue reaction in rabbit muscle exposed to metallic implants. Journal of Biomedical Materials Research 1, 135 (1967)
9. Miller, D.A., Ainsworth, R.D. et.al.: A comparative evaluation of the wear of ultra-high molecular weight polyethylene abraded by Ti-6Al-4V, Wear, 28, 207 (1974)
10. Zwicker, U.: Die Systeme Ti-Al-Cr und Ti-Al-V und die technischen Titanlegierungen TiCr5A13 und TiAl6V4. Zeitschrift für Metallkunde 47, 535 (1956)
11. Rydell, N.: Studies on anatomy and function of bone and joints, Berlin-Heidelberg-New York: Springer-Verlag 1966

THE USE OF POLYMERS IN HIGH LOAD BEARING JOINTS IN THE LOCOMOTOR SYSTEM

B.W. Sauer, J.J. Klawitter, A.M. Weinstein, and M. Spector

Polymeric materials have been widely used as soft tissue and non-weight bearing implants for a number of years. However, the successful use of polymeric materials in high load bearing joints is a much more recent development. The prosthetic replacement of the major joints of the lower extremity, the hip and knee, imposes very severe environmental conditions on the implant materials. In addition to the hostile chemical environment, hip and knee joint prostheses are exposed to abrasive forces and to fatigue-producing cyclic loading and intermittent peak loads amounting to several times the normal body weight. For these reasons some polymers which were found to have acceptable biocompatibility in non-stressed applications were found to be quite unacceptable when used in areas of high load bearing due to their structural instability and poor abrasion resistance.

Although not the first use of polymeric materials in high load bearing joints, the introduction of the acrylic femoral head prosthesis by the Judet brothers in 1946 marked the first significant clinical usage of polymeric materials in this area. The original Judet prosthesis resembled a large round-headed rivet and was designed to be inserted in the medullary canal of the neck of the femur at an angle of 45° to the long axis of the femur. The Judets based their choice of materials on the reported biocompatibility of the acrylics in soft tissue applications and on rather limited mechanical testing. In 1950 they reported stem fractures in twelve of their earlier patients and consequently reinforced their prosthesis with a steel rod. Although the prosthesis appears to have performed satisfactorily in the hands of the Judets, continued problems with breakage, excessive wear, and loosening led to the abandonment of the prosthesis.

In an attempt to solve some of the problems with the Judet prosthesis other investigators reworked the stem configuration converting it from a transfixing type stem to an intramedullary stem but retained the acrylic femoral head. These prostheses fared no better than the original Judet design and were eventually abandoned.

Heck and Chandler (5) and Levy et al. (10) conducted studies using acrylic and Nylon Judet type prostheses. They reported fractures and extensive wear in the acrylic prostheses but only minimal tissue response to wear particles. On the other hand no fractures were reported for the Nylon prostheses but there was extensive wear and deformation. The tissue reaction to Nylon wear particles was more severe than that seen with acrylic wear particles. Levy et al. concluded that Nylon was unsuitable for use in the Judet prosthesis.

Scales (1957) after evaluating Nylon hip cup prostheses concluded that Nylon was unsuitable for any type of hip prosthesis exposed to abrasion by bone or cartilage. He reported that Nylon abrasion particles produced a histiocytic type tissue reaction which lead to the destruction of bone. In addition to the problem of wear and abrasion particles Nylon readily absorbs water, with a resultant dimensional instability and loss of mechanical properties. For these reasons Nylon except in the form of suture material has been abandoned as an implant material. Based on the poor, if not disastrous, results with acrylic and Nylon prostheses, most surgeons turned to all-metal prostheses.

There was a renewed interest in polymeric materials following Charnley's introduction of the "low friction" arthroplasty in 1959 (1). The prosthesis was developed in an attempt to reduce the friction between the femoral and acetabular components which was felt to be partially responsible for the loosening seen in all-metal total hips. The prosthesis consisted of a stainless steel femoral component and a Fluon (polytetrafluoroethylene, PTFE) acetabular component, both of which were held in place by a polymethylmethacrylate (PMMA) bone cement.

The first use of an acrylic bone cement was reported by Haboush (4). In 1951 he used a self-curing dental acrylic to cement a metallic femoral head replacement prosthesis and acetabular cup in place. Wiltse et al. (16) investigated the possible use of self-curing acrylic cement in orthopaedic surgery. They reported that there were no undesirable effects on the liver and kidney when the cement was allowed to cure in situ. Interestingly enough they reported that initially the cement was in contact with bone, but was later separated by a layer of hemopoietic tissue.

The early results of the "low friction" arthroplasty were very encouraging, with dramatic reductions in pain reported along with improved functionality. However, somewhat later Charnley (3) reported that in the arthroplasties performed between 1958 and 1962 in which Fluon cups were used, there was unacceptable wear and tissue irritation. Leidholt and Gorman (9) carried out experiments in dogs using total hip prostheses having either stainless steel femoral heads and Teflon (PTFE) cups, Teflon heads and stainless steel cups, or Teflon heads and Teflon cups. They reported good early results but progressive loss of function with time. On examination the Teflon components were found to be badly worn and there was a marked inflammatory response in the synovial and capsular tissue. They also reported their findings following the removal of a total prosthesis consisting of a Moore prosthesis and a Teflon cup 15 months after implantation. The clinical history and gross and microscopic findings correlated well with those reported in their experimental study. On the basis of their findings they concluded that "Teflon should not be used in any part of a prosthesis in weight-bearing joints".

Following the failure of the Fluon arthroplasties Charnley made the fortuitous choice of high density polyethylene (RCH 1000) as a replacement material to be used in the acetabular cups. As it turned out, high density polyethylene was much more resistant to abrasion under high loads than was Teflon and, more important, the polyethylene wear particles were well tolerated by the body when compared to those of Teflon.

Weber (15) designed a trunnion bearing prosthesis with a polymeric ball articulating with a metal trunnion and acetabular cup. Delrin, a polyacetal, was used in the first few prostheses which were implanted in 1968. In as short a time as 6 to 24 months, gross dimensional changes were noted due to its lack of resistance to "body chemicals" (14). In later trunnion bearing prostheses a series of different polyesters both plain and irradiated were used as the femoral head. Although the initial results were good, problems developed later, the details of which are discussed in a preceding article by Weber, and the use of these materials was discontinued.

CURRENT STATUS OF POLYMERIC BEARING SURFACES

At the present time high density/ultra high molecular weight polyethylene (RCH 1000, Hyfax 1900), is the accepted polymer for use as a bearing surface in total joint prostheses. It is used in a wide variety of applications ranging from simple bearing surfaces such as washers and sleeves for metallic hinge prostheses, to rather complex bearing surfaces and structural components. Although these polyethylenes have good wear characteristics, the wear rate, 0.1–0.2 mm/yr., must be taken into account when designing prosthetic components. However, at this stage of the development of total joint prostheses, wear of the polyethylene bearing surface has not been a significant clinical problem since failure by infection or loosening has preceded "wearing out" of the bearing surfaces. It is however important to continue the search for improved bearing materials since future developments in the area of prosthesis fixation and infection control will eventually lead to prolonged implant residence times. It must be remembered if we are to avoid the costly mistakes made in the past with acrylic, Nylon, and Teflon bearing surfaces, it will be necessary to institute an intensive multidisciplinary program to investigate all aspects of new candidate materials and not merely on laboratory wear measurements and bulk biocompatibility measurements alone. Biocompatibility in loco must be the prime consideration.

CURRENT STATUS OF PROSTHESIS FIXATION WITH POLYMERIC MATERIALS

By far the most commonly used polymer in weight bearing joints is the self-curing PMMA luting agent or bone cement. This material is used almost universally to provide a firm fixation of both metallic and polymeric prosthetic components to the skeleton.

Since the various aspects and problems associated with the use of self-curing PMMA are the subject of other articles in this book it would be inappropriate for a detailed discussion of this material at this time. However, in an effort to provide continuity with the material to follow on alternate methods of prosthesis fixation, a few general comments are in order.

When rigid metallic prostheses are fixed to bone by simple mechanical means such as screws or impaction there is a resulting mismatch of elastic moduli at the fixation interface. Many investigators feel that this mismatch of material properties at the fixation interface is responsible for loosening of the prosthesis. Charnley (2) felt that it was not so much the modulus mismatch but more importantly the failure to distribute the load uniformly over the bone. He felt that even if the prosthesis was made of a material having an identical modulus, e.g. bone, the bond would still fail if the load was concentrated on a very small area of the living bone of the host. When used properly the self-curing PMMA provides a uniform distribution of loads over the host bone and in addition interposes a material having a modulus of elasticity closer to that of bone than the rigid metallic components. The markedly improved results seen in implant arthroplasty of load bearing joints since the advent of PMMA luting agents are impressive. However, the use of self-curing PMMA is not without its problems. The success of PMMA fixed prostheses is highly dependent upon the skill of the surgeon. Technical errors such as poor mixing of the monomer and polymer, entrapment of air or fluids within the polymerizing mass, insertion of the cement mass prematurely or belatedly, inadequate filling of the medullary canal, and malposition of the prostheses all have a very definite influence on the outcome of the surgery. In addition to these technical problems, the question of long term local and systemic effects of methacrylate monomer and the local thermal damage produced by the polymerizing cement mass have caused investigators to search for improved luting agents or alternate methods of prosthesis fixation.

Mathys (11) developed a series of prostheses designed to be implanted without bone cement. These prostheses were fabricated from an acetal resin and were designed to more closely approximate the elastic modulus of bone. In addition, the surface of the implants contained macro-irregularities in order to provide an interdigitating surface for newly forming bone. Initial stabilization of the implants is provided by screw fixation. The current status of these "Isoelastic Joints" is presented in another article in this book.

A number of investigators have been examining the concept of bone growth into microporous materials as a means of prosthesis fixation. The general concept of bone growth into porous structures is discussed in another article by Klawitter. There are currently two porous polymeric systems which are being evaluated as interfacial materials for orthopaedic prostheses. Both of these systems are based on the application of porous polymeric coatings on polymeric or metallic prostheses.

Homsy et al. (7) developed a porous low modulus interfacial system using PTFE and pyrolytic graphite fibers. The resultant porous polymer, Proplast, ranges in pore volume from 70 to 90 percent and has a pore size range from 100 μm to 500 μm with dendritic pore interconnections greater than 200 μm. The mechanical properties of Proplast are shown in Table 1. Homsy, as did Charnley and others, reasoned that an interfacial material which was much less rigid than the metals used in orthopaedic implants would reduce the trauma to the surrounding bone. However, his theory differed from that of the other investigators, including our own, in that he felt the modulus of elasticity of the interfacial material should approximate that of granulation and fibrous tissue rather than cortical bone.

Table 1 Selected mechanical properties of three polymeric interfacial materials as compared to bone and a Co-Cr alloy

Material	Elastic modulus (MN/m^2)	Ultimate tensile strength (MN/m^2)
Co-Cr (cast alloy)	2.0×10^5	690
Bone (cortical)	1.7×10^4	100
PMMA (bone cement)	2.1×10^3	20
Bone (cancellous)	690	–
PHDPE (200 μm)	125	5
Proplast	4	1

Initial tissue ingrowth studies were conducted using 6.54 mm diameter specimens implanted in the lateral cortex of canine femora (6). They reported that loose immature collagen developed throughout the implant during the third, fourth, and fifth weeks with the formation of dense collagen beginning at the periphery of the implants and extending centrally with increasing time. No mention was made of bone ingrowth. In later studies (7) Proplast was evaluated as an interfacial material for canine femoral head prostheses in the form of a 1,000 μm thick coating. They reported that by 10 weeks the coating was thoroughly infiltrated with dense mature collagen and bone was reported in sections made after 15 months of implantation. Rotational stress to displace a 16 month specimen was reported to be 0.6 MN/m^2.

Based on their experimental work clinical investigations were begun in a number of areas including femoral head prostheses. The results of the femoral head arthroplasties are reported to be very encouraging after two years in service.

We are currently evaluating another polymeric interfacial material in our laboratories. This material is fabricated from porous high density polyethylene (PHDPE) (*Biopor, Porex Materials Corporation, 7380-A Bohannon Road, Fairburn, Georgia 30213 USA). It can be made in a wide range of pore sizes but for our ingrowth studies we are using a material having a mean pore diameter of approximately 200 μm with a 40 to 50 % porosity (Fig. 1). Some selected mechanical properties of polyethylene are shown in Table 1. It should be pointed out that although the modulus of elasticity is significantly greater than that of Proplast it can still be considered a low modulus material when compared to bone and metals. We would prefer to consider it as an intermediate modulus material having a sufficient flexibility to greatly reduce stress concentration and yet possessing enough rigidity to maintain pore structure integrity under load conditions. In contrast to Homsy, we prefer to insert the prostheses using moderate pressure, i.e., mild impaction, to ensure optimum bone contact for initial stabilization and to facilitate early bone ingrowth.

Early ingrowth and biocompatibility studies (13) performed on PHDPE showed it to be well tolerated by the body and to accept rapid bone ingrowth. Sections taken from 6.54 mm specimens which were surgically implanted in the lateral cortex of canine femora showed that ingrown bone had completely penetrated the implant by four weeks (Fig. 2). Histologic examination of the sections showed well developed bone deep within the implants (Fig. 3). In a later study we examined the ingrowth kinetics during the

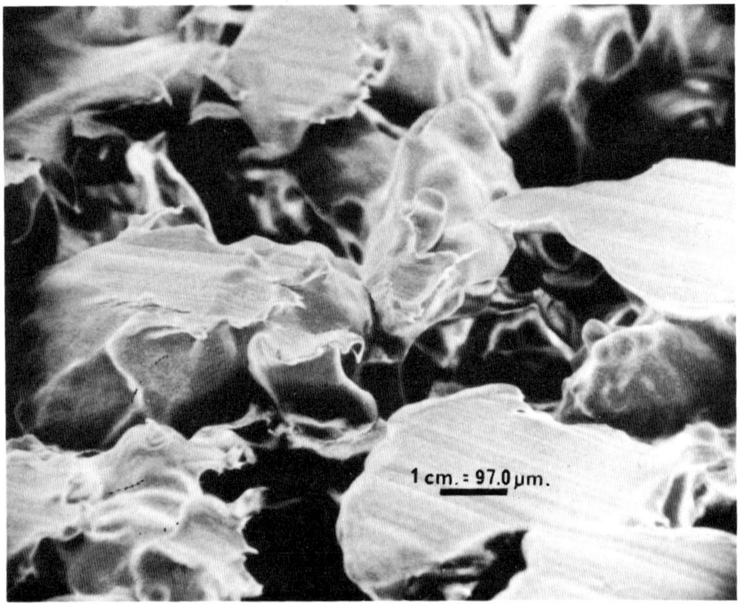

Fig. 1 Scanning electron micrograph of the cut surface of 200 μm PHDPE

early post implant phase (12). Implants 4 mm in diameter were surgically implanted in the lateral cortex of canine femora. These implants were subsequently removed by biopsy

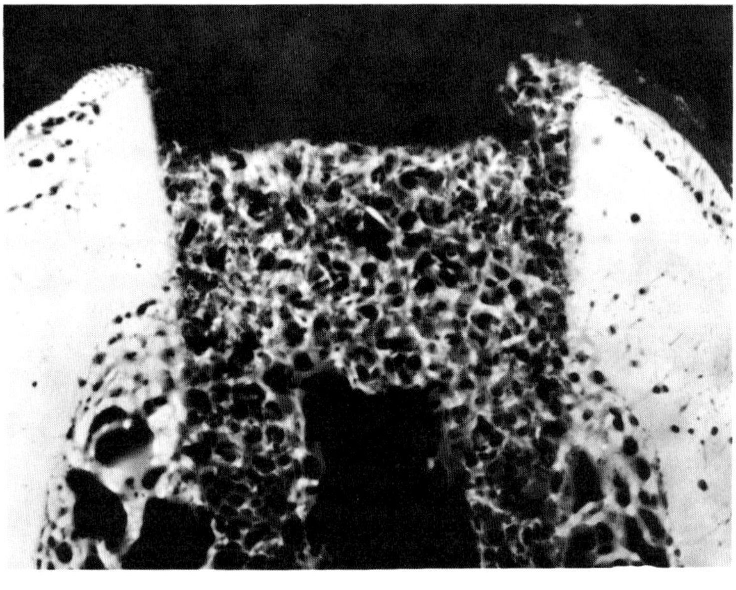

Fig. 2 Complete penetration of a 6.54 mm diameter pellet of 100 μm PHDPE at 4 weeks

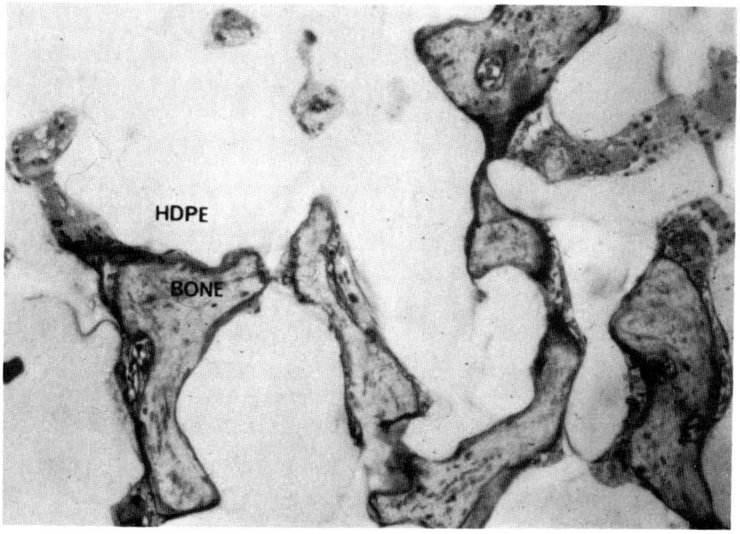

Fig. 3 Undecalcified histologic section taken from a pellet of 100 µm PHDPE showing mineralized bone deep within the implant at 4 weeks

at one, two, three, and eight weeks. Microradiographs (Fig. 4) made from these specimens showed that at two weeks there was complete bridging of the implant in the endosteal region. Examination of the three week specimen revealed that at this time the implant was almost completely filled with ingrown bone. Examination of the eight week specimen revealed extensive remodeling of the ingrown bone in the cortical region. The thickening of the bone spicules in this area suggests that the relatively low modulus of the PHDPE may provide for stress transmission from the cortex to the bone spicules in the cortical region of the implant.

The next phase in our evaluation of PHDPE was to examine the mechanical properties of the bone/implant interface. For this study we used unloaded intramedullary implants consisting of stainless steel rods with a 3 mm thick coating of PHDPE. The implants were surgically implanted in the medullary canal of canine femora. After implant periods of two, four, eight, and sixteen weeks the implants were subjected to pull out tests. The results of these tests are shown in Table 2. Histologic examination of the retrieved implants showed an increasing amount of bone ingrowth which corresponded with the increasing interfacial strength. Histologic examination also revealed that failure occurred both in the PHDPE and the ingrown bone spicules.

Our evaluation of PHDPE under true loaded conditions has been rather limited. We have had, however, an opportunity to examine a one year biopsy specimen taken from a canine femoral head prosthesis. The coated hip is shown in Fig. 5. Using a hollow biopsy burr, a bone/PHDPE biopsy was taken from the mid-shaft region, fractured, and examined using scanning electron microscopy (Fig. 6). Fig. 7 shows the complex nature of the fracture surface of the cortical bone. It can be readily seen that there is a fracturing of bone spicules as well as a pulling-out and tearing of HDPE. Since HDPE spicules are

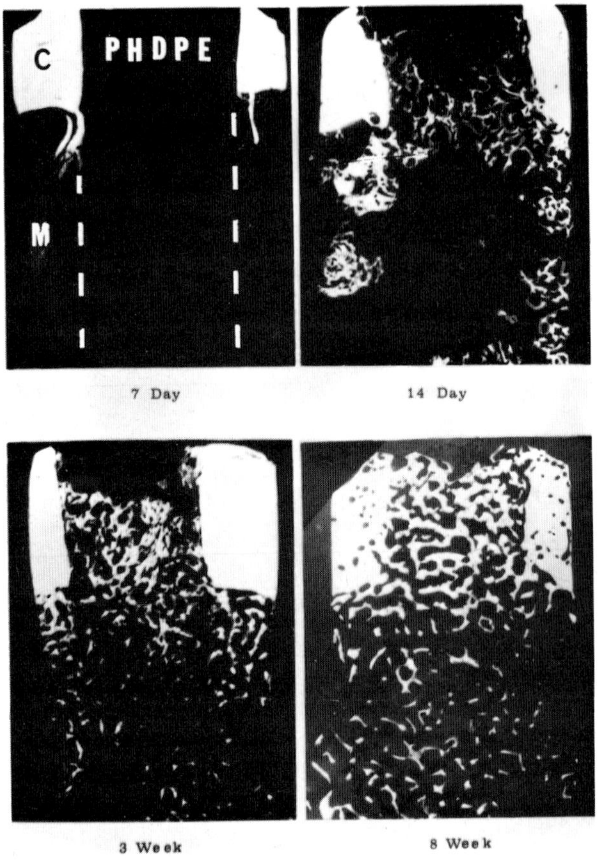

Fig. 4
Bone spicule development within 4 mm diameter PHDPE pellets removed at one, two, three, and eight weeks. Note enlargement of the spicules in the cortical region of the eight week implant

Table 2 Pull-out strength vs. duration of implantation for PHDPE coated femoral intramedullary stem

Implant residence time (weeks)	Pull-out strength (MN/m^2)
2	0.25
4	0.69
8	0.95
16	0.80 bone fractured

present in the bone side of the fracture interface it can be said that fracture occurred not through the original bone/PHDPE interface but deeper in the porous coating itself.

Based on the results of our in vitro and animal experiments, we elected to initiate limited clinical trials using PHDPE as an interfacial material for prosthesis fixation. Our first studies involved the use of PHDPE to fabricate caps for controlling bone overgrowth in the juvenile amputee (12). Although the caps do not represent a true weight bearing prosthesis they did provide us with a model system stabilization by bone ingrowth with

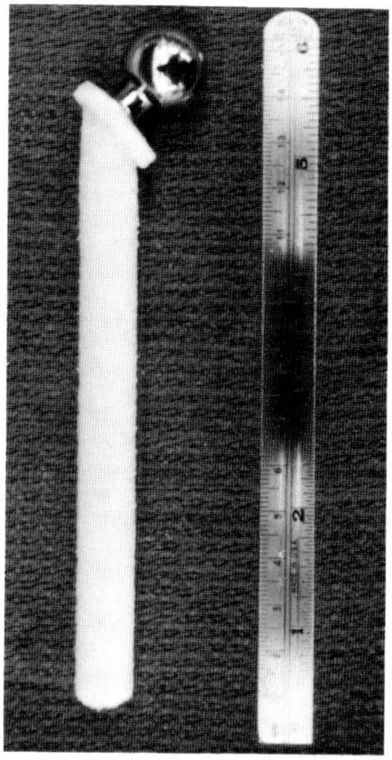

Fig. 5
PHDPE coated canine hip prosthesis

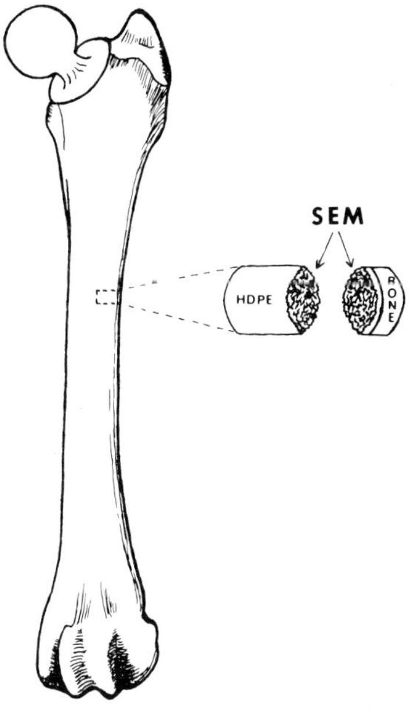

Fig. 6
Canine femur showing the location of the biopsy specimen in Fig. 7

little risk to the patient. The caps consist of a porous intramedullary stem and pericortical cuff joined at one end. In the early caps medical grade Silastic adhesive was used to seal the pores in the closed end. In our most recent model the pores in the closed end are sealed with non-porous HDPE (Fig. 8). The implants have been well tolerated with no evidence of loosening (Fig. 9). The status of our first six implants is shown in Table 3. The caps are currently manufactured (* Biopor, Porex Materials Corporation) in five sizes with stem diameters of 5, 7, 9, 11, and 13 mm.

Our clinical trials to date with true prostheses have been limited to a few select patients who for various reasons were not suitable for more routine procedures. Our first patient

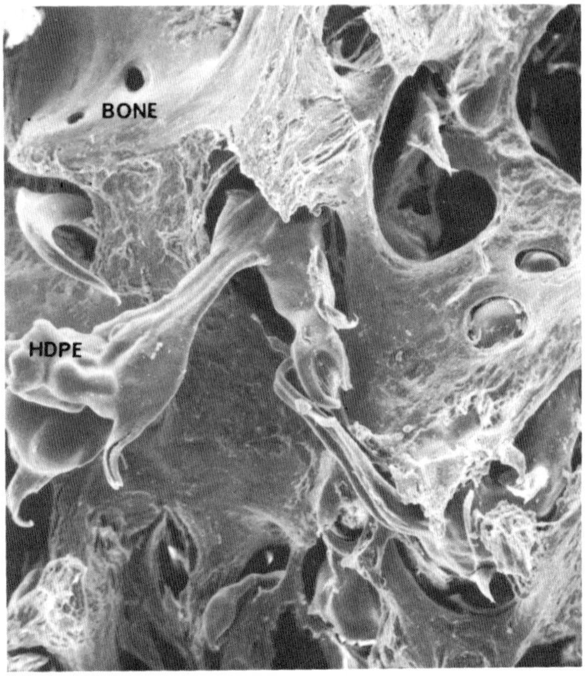

Fig. 7
Scanning electron micrograph of the fracture surface of a one year bone/PHDPE biopsy specimen taken from a weight bearing prosthesis

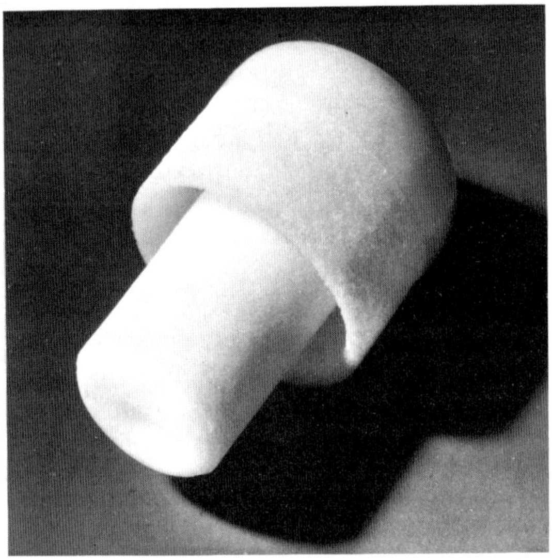

Fig. 8
PHDPE bone cap for controlling bone overgrowth in the juvenile amputee

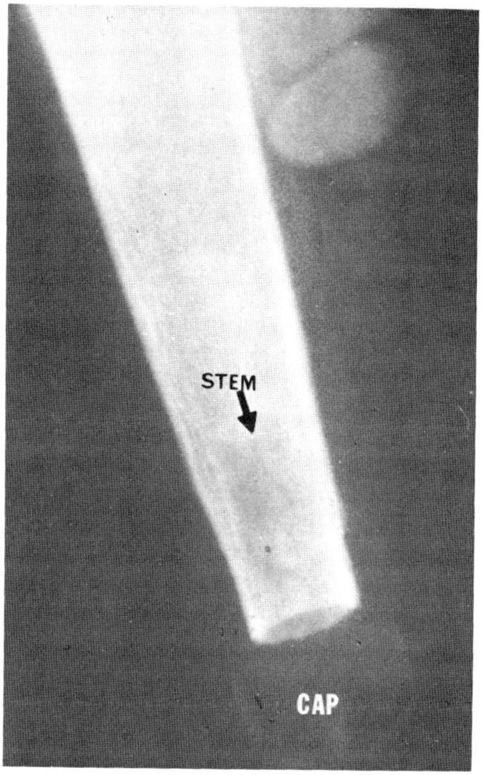

Fig. 9
Roentgenogram showing a bone cap two years after insertion

Table 3 Current status of bone overgrowth caps in six patients

Patient	Cap type	Site	Duration (months) as of Nov. 75	Results	Complications
CC	HDPE/Silastic	femur	27	no recurrence	breakdown of Silastic
SP	HDPE/Silastic	humerus	24	no recurrence	none
RW	HDPE/Silastic	tibia	23	no recurrence	none
KY	HDPE	tibia	20	no recurrence	none
MH	HDPE	tibia	15	no recurrence	infection – cleared cap still in place
LW	HDPE	tibia	12	no recurrence	none

required surgical revision of the elbow due to repeated trauma. The prosthesis (Fig. 10) was inserted in October of 1974. Six months later it became necessary to remove the prosthesis due to infection secondary to a traumatic episode involving the elbow joint. Upon examination of the prosthesis, bone ingrowth, as expected, was found only in a few isolated areas not associated with the infectious process.

Our remaining two clinical cases required partial femoral prostheses following the resec-
cepted standards in their respective roles as bearing surfaces and interfacial materials.

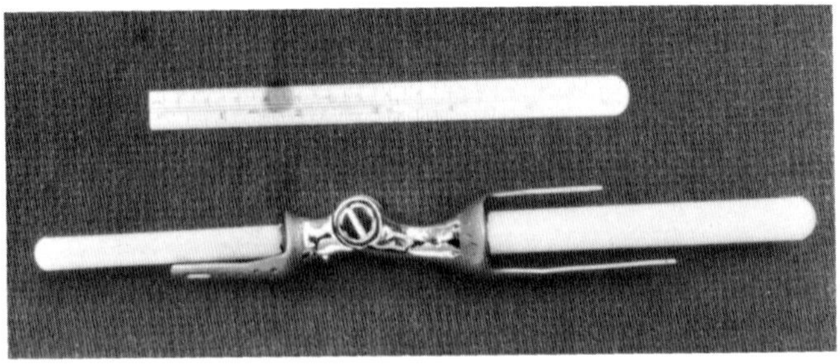

Fig. 10 PHDPE coated total elbow prosthesis

tion of giant cell tumors. In one patient the tumor involved the proximal femur and in the other partial condylar replacement was necessary. The prostheses are shown in Figs. 11 and 12. Although at present only short term results (approx. 6 months) are available, the patients continue to function satisfactorily with no evidence of loosening of the prostheses.

Although we do not anticipate expansion of our clinical trials to include routine hip and knee arthroplasties until more information is available on the performance of PHDPE in loco, we are presently examining prototype prostheses (Fig. 13).

CONCLUSION

At present polymeric materials are used extensively in load bearing joints. Both high density/ultra high molecular weight polyethylene and acrylic bone cement are the ac-

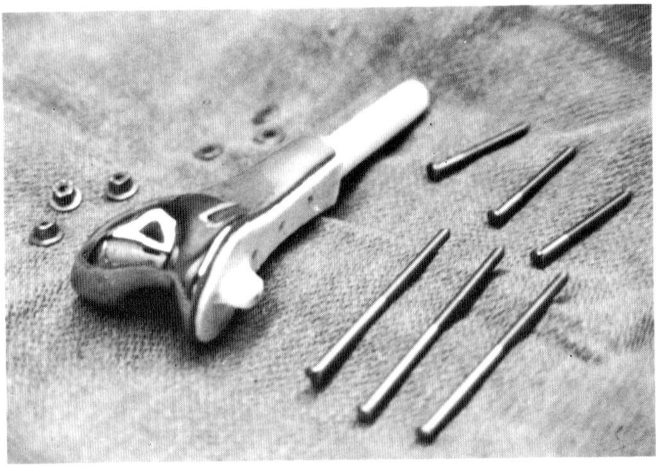

Fig. 11 PHDPE coated femoral condyle replacement prosthesis

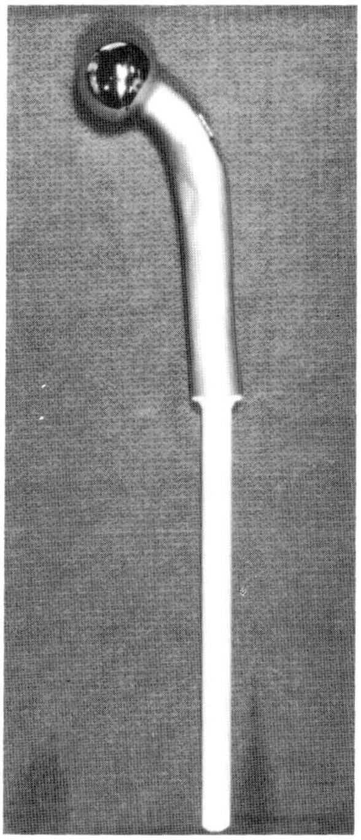

Fig. 12
PHDPE coated proximal femur prosthesis

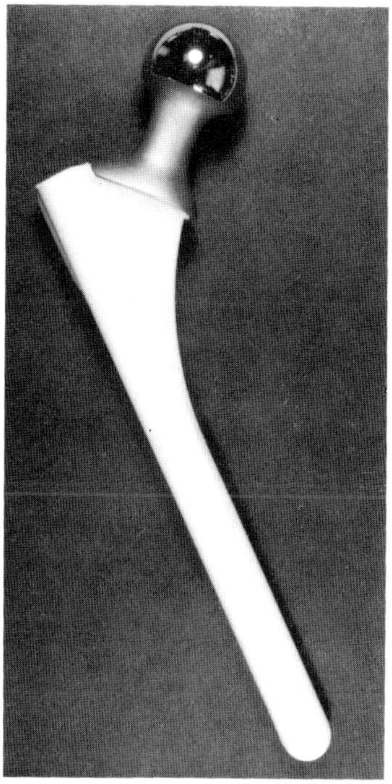

Fig. 13
PHDPE coated Austin Moore type hip prosthesis

This is not to say that better materials will not be available in the future. Our present philosophy should be one of cautious optimism. We should continue to optimize designs using our existing polymeric materials and at the same time continue the search for improved materials. We should, however, always keep in mind the mistakes of the past and avoid plunging into widespread clinical usage of a material or design before it has undergone exhaustive laboratory testing.

REFERENCES

1. Charnley, J.: The lubrication of animal joints. New Scientist 6, 60 (1959)
2. Charnley, J.: Total prosthetic replacement of the hip. Physiotherapy 53, 407 (1967)
3. Charnley, J.: Fluon as a bearing material. Journal of Bone and Joint Surgery 45 B, 622 (1963)
4. Haboush, E.J.: A new operation for arthroplasty of the hip based on biomechanics, photoelasticity, fast-setting dental acrylic, and other considerations. Bulletin of the Hospital for Joint Diseases 14, 242 (1953)
5. Heck, C.V. and Chandler, F.A.: Material failures in hip prostheses. Journal of Bone and Joint Surgery 36 A, 1059 (1954)

6. Homsy, C.A., Cain, T.E., Anderson, M.S. and King, J.W.: Dynamic stabilization of implanted prostheses. Journal of Bone and Joint Surgery 52 A, 604 (1970)

7. Homsy, C.A., Cain, T.E., Kessler, F.B., Anderson, M.S. and King, J.W.: Porous implant system for prosthesis stabilization. Clinical Orthopaedics and Related Research 89, 220 (1972)

8. Judet, J., Judet, R.: The use of an artificial femoral head for arthroplasty of the hip joint. Journal of Bone and Joint Surgery 32 B, 166 (1950)

9. Leidholt, J.D., and Gorman, H.A.: Teflon hip prosthesis in dogs. Journal of Bone and Joint Surgery 47 A, 1414 (1965)

10. Levy, L.J., Lipscomb, C.P. and McDonald, H.C.: Complications of Judet Arthroplasty due to foreign-body reaction to Nylon prostheses. Journal of Bone and Joint Surgery 36 A, 1175 (1954)

11. Mathys, R.: Current use of plastics in artificial joints, 6th Mainz Traumatology Symposium (1973)

12. Sauer, B.W., Spector, M. and Flemming, W.R.: Ingrowth kinetics of bone in porous high density polyethylene. Proceedings of 28th Annual Conference of Engineering in Medicine and Biology, New Orleans, 38 (1975)

13. Sauer, B.W., Weinstein, A.M., Klawitter, J.J., Hulbert, S.F., Leonard, R.B. and Bagwell, J.G.: The role of porous polymeric materials in prosthesis attachment. Journal of Biomedical Materials Research Symposium 5, 145 (1974)

14. Semlitsch, M.: Artificial Joint Material Development, Engineering in Medicine 2, 89 (1973)

15. Weber, B.G.: Total hip replacement with rotationendoprosthesis. Clinical Orthopaedics and Related Research 72, 79 (1970)

16. Wiltse, L.L., Hall, R.H. and Stenehjem, J.C.: Experimental studies regarding the possible use of a self-curing acrylic in orthopaedic surgery. Journal of Bone and Joint Surgery 39 A, 961 (1957)

CERAMICS AS A NEW APPROACH TO THE IMPROVEMENT OF ARTIFICIAL JOINTS

S.F. Hulbert and J.J. Klawitter

Orthopaedic prosthetic devices currently used are held in place by one of three methods:

1. the impaction of the prosthesis into bone,
2. direct mechanical fixation such as with screws, pins, nails, etc.
3. polymethylmethacrylate polymerization in situ used as a luting agent or a filler between the prosthesis and bone.

None of these methods is entirely satisfactory for permanent attachment of a load-bearing prosthesis to the skeletal system.

Devices impacted into bone are held in place by residual compressive stresses and depend upon a favorable anatomical situation – i.e., the impaction of the stem of the femoral hip prosthesis into the marrow cavity of the femur. Typically, the areas of contact between the prosthesis and the bone are localized, resulting in stress concentrations, pressure necrosis, and eventual loosening of the device (1,2).

The conventional means of skeletal attachment – screws, pins, nails, etc. – have proven very successful in temporary stabilizing of fracture fragments during the healing process. They have been found to be unsuccessful, however, in anchoring load-bearing skeletal prostheses for the long-term. Here again, stress concentrations at isolated points of attachment often lead to unacceptable stress levels, pressure necrosis of bone, prosthetic material failure, and eventual loosening of the device (1).

The use of polymethylmethacrylate as a filler or luting agent (the socalled cementing approach) between the prosthesis and bone eliminates major areas of stress concentration and initially secures the prosthesis firmly in place (2-8). The use of acrylic fillers for prosthesis stabilization is a major step forward in joint replacement technology. However, there are several problems associated with its use. In human application, the use of the acrylic filler has been blamed for eighteen reported cases of cardiac arrest following the introduction of the cement into the femur (9). Emboli of air, fat, and bone marrow in the lungs, pelvic veins, coronary arteries, kidney, and brain were found during autopsy. It is well documented clinically that a blood pressure drop is often encountered when the acrylic filler is introduced into the intermedullary cavity. Methylmethacrylate has been observed in the central circulation of canines within a few seconds after insertion of the filler into the medullary cavity (10). The use of the acrylic filler has been shown to cause pulmonary hemorrhagic lesions in laboratory animals. The temperature at the interface between the bone and the filler has been reported to peak at approximately 80 ^{o}C during the polymerization of the acrylic filler. This results in coagulative necrosis adjacent to the implant by the first day post-operatively, with the establishment of a fibrous pseudomembrane by the second day post-operatively. A laboratory animal investigation has demonstrated that the fibrous membrane is still present one year post-operatively and appears to increase in thickness with time (11). Another problem with the acrylic stabilization of joint prostheses has been the manifestation of late infection (12).

The problems of skeletal attachment have stimulated biomaterials researchers to examine high-strength, grooved, undulating, porous, etc., materials designed to accept tissue ingrowth as a means of attaching load-bearing devices to the skeletal system. In this application, the inert porous material provides a scaffold into which tissue will grow and in this manner anchor the porous body to the living tissue. This "self-locking" property is extremely important in prosthesis design since it can be used to distribute mechanical loads over a large area and thus reduce excessive localized stresses.

Porous ceramic (13), metallic (14), and polymeric (15) materials are all being considered for use in joint prosthesis stabilization via tissue ingrowth into surface undulations. However, there are a number of factors which suggest that ceramics will be the material of choice. Ceramic materials are characteristically very inert, high-strength, abrasion-resistant compounds which possess a well-documented history as materials of choice for applications in highly-corrosive environments (16). The increased surface area associated with undulating surfaces compared with non-porous materials and the fact that living tissue must exist within the grooves and in intimate contact with artificial materials points directly to the necessity of choosing a material which is as chemically inert and as non-toxic as possible. Ceramics may be composed of ions commonly found in the physiological environment (calcium, potassium, magnesium, sodium, etc.) and of ions showing limited toxicity to body tissue (aluminum and titanium) (17). Thus, even in those cases where ceramics may undergo limited long-term degradation the constituent ion concentration in adjacent tissue may be easily controlled by the body's natural regulatory mechanisms.

The compatibility of alumina, titania, zirconia, zircon, mullite, spinel, calcium titanate, calcium zirconate, and anorthite with bone and soft tissue has been well documented (18-23). In addition to the above oxide ceramics, vitreous carbon (24-25) and LTI carbon (26) have been shown to be extremely inert in the physiological environment.

Another concept being investigated for the stabilization of joint prostheses is the direct chemical bonding of the implant material to bone. The most promising materials to date are the so-called "bioglasses". It has been demonstrated that by controlling the chemical composition of certain sodium-calcium-phosphate-silicate glasses, one can develop a chemical bond between the glass and bone (27). The mechanism for the development of this bone is postulated to be the production of an amorphous ion surface gel on the bioglass similar to the substance comprising the "cement line" in mature bone. Collagen fiber produced by the osteoblasts becomes attached to the bonding layer and mineralization occurs on the collagen fibers yielding crystals bridging between the implant surface and mature bone.

A second major problem in addition to long-term stabilization of joint prostheses is tissue reaction to wear debris, corrosion, degradation, and hydration products (28).

High alumina ceramic joint prostheses have been demonstrated to be more wear-resistant than metal to metal or metal to polymer prostheses (29). The ceramic wear particles are also more easily tolerated by the physiological environment than metallic or polymeric wear debris (29).

Five ceramic hip prostheses are presently being clinically tested. Boutin (30) and his associates are testing a prosthesis where the acetabular component and the femoral head are made out of a high-alumina ceramic. The intermedullary stem component is metallic. The major factors in the design are elimination of the acrylic filler in the stabilization of the acetabular component by use of direct stabilization via tissue ingrowth and the minimizing of wear debris by use of a ceramic to ceramic bearing surface. Boutin and his associates have implanted more than 1,000 ceramic prostheses to date. Mittelmeier (31) and his associates have clinically tested a similar prosthesis with the added advantage that the femoral stem has an undulating metallic surface, thus eliminating the need for "cementing" the femoral component. Jentschura (32,33) and his associates are testing a total high-alumina ceramic hip prosthesis. The acetabular component is stabilization via tissue ingrowth and the femoral component is stabilized via direct chemical bonding. A "bioglass" coating is placed on the alumina stem. Paltrinieri (34) and his associates are testing a prosthesis where the femoral stem has a plasma-sprayed coating of alumina. The undulating surface allows for stabilization via tissue ingrowth.

Zeibig (35-37) and associates have developed and clinically tested a number of alumina orthopaedic appliances where stabilization of the prosthesis is accomplished by tissue ingrowth into a conical sleeve. The design change from a "stem" to a "sleeve" takes advantage of the high compressive strength of ceramics and minimizes the problem of low bending strength.

There have been two comparative studies of tissue ingrowth, impaction, and cementation for fixation of hip prostheses in animals (11,38). In both studies it was found that tissue ingrowth provided significantly better fixation and thus better implant performance than using cementation or impaction.

To date, there have been no reported clinical trials of the use of ceramics in knee prostheses. However, the application of a porous aluminum oxide ceramic to achieve load bearing fixation of a tibial plateau prosthesis has been demonstrated in swine (39).

Graves and co-workers (40,41) have investigated extensively the feasibility of employing resorbable ceramic oxide compositions as synthetic segmental bone grafts. There are several potential advantages to using a resorbable (bio-degradable) ceramic as an implant material. The most important is that the deleterious long-term effect of stress-concentration at the interface of dissimilar materials is avoided by the eventual total resorption and replacement of the ceramic by bone. The two most promising resorbable systems studied to date are calcium-phosphate and the calcium-aluminate system.

Alumina, vitreous carbon, and LTI carbon are all more chemically inert in the physiological environment than any of the present metallic or polymeric implants. Alumina has the advantage of high strength and ultra-high wear resistance. Another advantage of alumina is that advanced technology is readily available and widely distributed for producing precision orthopaedic appliances. Alumina also lends itself to a wide variety of designs. The excellent mechanical properties of alumina suggest that even though there are many other ceramics with excellent biocompatibility, it will be the major ceramic used in joint prostheses.

The carbon materials have the additional advantage of having a modulus of elasticity approximately equal to that of cortical bone. LTI carbon has a flexural strength approximately three times that of vitreous carbon, and thus is more suited to serve as a structurally loaded implant than vitreous carbon. LTI carbon has an outstanding static and cyclic fatigue resistance in the physiological environments (42). All oxide ceramics tested to date have been found to be thrombogenic (43), while LTI carbon is very non-thrombogenic (26). LTI carbon is now the material of choice in most heart valves, and more than 100,000 LTI carbon parts have been delivered for clinical use. LTI carbon also has one of the best performance records to date of any material tested as a transcutaneous implant. Applications of LTI carbon transcutaneous leads in humans include those for direct skeletal attachment of prosthetic limbs and lead-throughs in humans include those for direct skeletal attachment of prosthetic limbs and lead-throughs for electrical stimulation of the nervous system (44). The data available suggests that in the future LTI carbon will be the material of choice in orthopaedic implants requiring transcutaneous leads.

The potential of carbon, ceramic, or bioglass coatings on metal implants is an interesting possibility. It has been documented that the biocompatibility can be improved using carbon or ceramic coatings (45). The use of carbon coatings would be particularly useful if a non-thrombogenic surface is required. It has also been documented that bioglass coatings can lead to improved stability of metal implants (46). However, the question of wear resistance and/or scratch resistance of coatings of metallic implants is a serious one. Any disruption of the coating would lead to an aggravated corrosive situation as a result of the setting up of a concentration cell. The potential use of ceramic coatings on metal implants needs considerably more laboratory study and evaluation in laboratory animals. The use of bioglass coatings on crystalline ceramics is not subject to the same limitations as coatings on metals, and thus will probably play a significant role in future implant design.

In summary, the results from ongoing clinical evaluations and several investigations involving laboratory animals suggest that in the future ceramics will play a major role in improved joint prosthesis design.

REFERENCES

1. Hirsch, C.: Clinical problems in total hip replacements. Journal of Biomedical Materials Research Symposium No. 5, 227 (1974)
2. Charnley, J.: A biochemical analysis of the use of cement to anchor the femoral head prosthesis. Journal of Bone and Joint Surgery 47 B, 354 (1965)

3. Charnley, J., Kettlewell, J.: The elimination of slip between prosthesis and femur. Journal of Bone and Joint Surgery 47 B, 55 (1965)

4. Charnley, J., Follacci, F.M., Hammond, B.T.: The long term reaction of bone to self-curing acrylic cement. Journal of Bone and Joint Surgery 50 B, 822 (1968)

5. Charnley, J.: Anchorage of the femoral head prosthesis to the shaft of the femur. Journal of Bone and Joint Surgery 42 B, 28 (1960)

6. Charnley, J.: The long term results of low-friction arthroplasty performed as primary intervention. Journal of Bone and Joint Surgery 54-B, 61 (1972)

7. Charnley, J., Follacci, F.M: A comparison of the results of femoral head prosthesis with and without cement. Clinical Orthopaedics and Related Research 62, 156 (1969)

8. Amstutz, H.C., Lurie, L., Pollough, P.: Skeletal fixation with self-curing polymethyl methacrylate. Clinical Orthopaedics and Related Research 65, 163 (1972)

9. Kepes, E.R., Underwood, P.S., Becsey, L.: Intraoperative death associated with acrylic bone cement. Journal of the American Medical Association 222, 59 (1972)

10. Homsy, C.A., Tullos, H.S., King, J.W.: Evaluation of rapid-cure acrylic compound for prosthesis stabilization. Clinical Orthopaedics and Related Research 67, 169 (1969)

11. Hulbert, S.F., Richbourg, H.L., Klawitter, J.J., and Sauer, B.W.: Evaluation of a metal-ceramic composite hip prosthesis. Journal of Biomedical Materials Research Symposium No. 6, 189 (1975)

12. Charnley, J.: Acrylic cement in orthopaedic surgery. Edinburgh and London: E & S Livingstone, pp. 108-114 (1970)

13. Klawitter, J.J., Hulbert, S.F.: Application of porous ceramics for attachment of load bearing internal orthopedic appliances. Journal of Biomaterials Research 5, 161 (1971)

14. Galante, J., Rostoker, W., Lueck, R., Ray, R.D.: Sintered fiber metal composites as a basis for attachment of implants to bone. Journal of Bone and Joint Surgery 53 A, (1971)

15. Taylor, D.F., Smith, F.B.: Porous methylmethacrylate as an implant material. Journal of Biomedical Materials Research Symposium No. 2, 467 (1972)

16. Kriegel, W.W., Palmour, L., (editors): Ceramics in severe environments. New York: Plenum Press 1971

17. Ferguson, A.B., Laing, P.G., Hodge, E.S.: The ionization of metal implants in the living tissues. Journal of Bone and Joint Surgery 42 A, 77 (1960)

18. Hulbert, S.F., Cooke, F.W., Klawitter, J.J., Leonard, R.B., Sauer, B.W., Moyle, D.D.: Attachment of prostheses to the musculo-skeletal system by tissue ingrowth and mechanical interlocking. Journal of Biomedical Materials Research Symposium No. 4, 1 (1973)

19. Hulbert, S.F., Matthews, J.R., Klawitter, J.J., Sauer, B.W., Leonard, R.B.: Effect of stress on tissue ingrowth into porous aluminum oxide. Journal of Biomedical Materials Research Symposium No. 5, 85 (1974)

20. Richardson, W.C., Klawitter, J.J., Sauer, B.W., Pruitt, J.R. Hulbert, S.F.: Soft tissue response to four dense ceramic materials and two clinically used biomaterials. Journal of Biomedical Materials Research Symposium No. 6, 73 (1975)

21. Hulbert, S.F., Morrison, S.J., Klawitter, J.J.: Tissue reaction to three ceramics of porous and non-porous structures. Journal of Biomedical Materials Research 6, 347 (1972)

22. Hulbert, S.F., Bowman, L.S., Klawitter, J.J., Sauer, B.W., Leonard, R.B.: Characterization of tissue growth into pellets and partial sections of porous porcelain and titania implanted in bone. In: V.D. Frechette, W.C. LaCourse, V.L. Burdick, edit., Surfaces and interfaces of glass and ceramics, New York: Plenum Publishing Corporation 1974, pp. 283-298

23. Hulbert, S.F., Klawitter, J.J., and Leonard, R.B.: Use of porous ceramics as surgical implants. Reprinted from Medical Engineering, C.D. Ray, edit., Chicago: Year Book Medical Publishers Inc. 1974, pp. 1139-1145

24. Dumas, M. and Myers, H.M.: The vitreous carbon tooth root replacement system: A surgical discipline. International Journal of Oral Surgery 3, 1 (1974)

25. Grenoble, D.E., Kim, R.L., Voss, R., Melrose, R.S., Wollschlager, G., Knoell, A.C., Gupta, K.K.: Development and testing of a vitreous carbon dental implant. Proceedings of the 18th National SAMPE Symposium, April, 276 (1973)

26. Bruck, S.D., Rabin, S., Ferguson, R.J.: Evaluation of biocompatible materials. Biomaterials, Medical Devices and Artificial Organs 1 (1), 191 (1973)

27. Hench, L.L., Paschall, H.A.: Histochemical responses at a biomaterial's interface. Journal of Biomedical Materials Research Symposium No. 5, 49 (1974)

28. Winter, G.D.: Tissue reactions to metallic wear and corrosion products in human patients. Journal of Biomedical Materials Research Symposium No. 5, 11 (1974)

29. Griss, P., Krempien, B., Von Andrian-Werburg, H., Heimke, G., Fleiner, R., Diehm, T.: Experimental analysis of ceramic-tissue interactions. A morphologic, fluorescenceoptic, and radiographic study on dense alumina oxide ceramic in various animals. Journal of Biomedical Materials Research Symposium No. 5, 39 (1974)

30. Boutin, P.: Les prostheses totales de la hanche en alumine. Revue de Chirurgie Orthopedique 60 (3), 233 (1974)

31. Mittelmeier, H.: Zementlose Verankerung von Endoprothesen nach dem Tragrippenprinzip. Zeitschrift für Orthopädie 112, 27 (1974)

32. Jentschura, X., Griss, P., Heimke, G., Greenspan, D., Hench, L.L., Krempian, B.: In-vivo evaluation of bioglass coated alumina hip prostheses. Paper presented at the 7th International Biomaterials Symposium, Clemson University, Clemson, SC, April 1975

33. Griss, P., Heimke, G., Von Andrian-Werburg, H., Krempian, B., Reipa, S., Lauterbach, H., Hartung, H.: Morphological and biomechanical aspects of Al_2O_3 ceramic joint replacement. Experimental results and design considerations for human endoprostheses. Journal of Biomedical Materials Research Symposium No. 6, 177 (1975)

34. Paltrinieri, M., Cini, L., Pizzoferrato, A., Sandrolini, S., Trentani, C., Zolezzi, C.: Impianto senza cemento di artroprotesi d'anca con riporto superficiale di allumina. La Chirurgia degli Organi di Movimento 57, 1 (1975)

35. Engelhardt, A., Salzer, M., Zeibig, A., Locke: Experiences with Al_2O_3 implantations in humans to bridge resection defects. Journal of Biomedical Materials Research Symposium No. 6, 227 (1975)

36. Salzer, M., Locke, H., Zweymuller, K., Plenk, H., Punzet, G., Zeibig, A.: Further experimental and clinical experiences on endoprostheses made of alumina. Paper presented at the 7th International Biomaterials Symposium, Clemson University, Clemson, SC April 1975

37. Locke, H., Stärk, N., Zeibig, A.: Anchoring implants to bone using conical sleeves. Paper presented at the 7th International Biomaterials Symposium, Clemson University, Clemson, SC, April 1975

38. Nunamaker, D.N., Black, J., Tronzo, R.G.: A comparison of biological ingrowth and cementation for fixation of the total hip prosthesis. Paper presented at the 7th International Biomaterials Symposium, Clemson University, Clemson, SC, April 1975

39. Klawitter, J.J., Bhatti, N.A.: Study of the application of a porous aluminum oxide ceramic to achieve load bearing fixation of tibial plateau implants in swine. Paper presented at the 6th International Biomaterials Symposium, Clemson University, Clemson, SC, April 1975

40. Graves, G.A., Villanueva, A.R.: The influence of compositional variations on bone ingrowth of implanted porous calcium aluminate ceramics. Journal of Biomedical Materials Research Symposium No. 6, 17 (1975)

41. Graves, G.A., Hentrich, R.L.: Resorbable ceramic implants. Journal of Biomedical Materials Research Symposium No. 2 (Part 1), 91 (1972)

42. Kaae, J.L.: The mechanical properties of glassy and isotropic pyrolytic carbons. Journal of Biomedical Materials Research 6, 279 (1972)

43. Hulbert, S.F., King, F.M., Klawitter, J.J.: Initial surface interaction of blood and blood components with Al_2O_3 and TiO_2. Journal of Biomedical Materials Research Symposium No. 2 (Part 1), 68 (1972)

44. Mooney, V., Predecki, P.K., Renning, J., Gray, J.: Skeletal extension of limb prosthetic attachments – problems in tissue reaction. Journal of Biomedical Materials Research Symposium No. 2 (Part 1), 143 (1972)

45. Hulbert, S.F., Klawitter, J.J., Fain, C.C., Sauer, B.W., Cueman, G.F.: Evaluation of chemical vapor deposition coatings of TiO_2 on orthopedic implants. Paper presented at the 1973 Materials Engineering Congress, Chicago, IL, October 4 (1973)

46. Piotrowski, G., Hench, L.L., Allen, W.C., Miller, G.J.: Mechanical studies of the bone bioglass interfacial bond. Journal of Biomedical Materials Research Symposium No. 6, 47 (1975)

THE POLYMERIZATION OF SELF–CURING ACRYLIC CEMENTS AND PROBLEMS DUE TO THE CEMENT ANCHORAGE OF JOINT PROSTHESES

H.U. Debrunner, A. Wettstein, and P. Hofer

The idea of using a cement to anchor endoprostheses in bone first occurred to Gluck in 1890 (5). He employed a mixture of colophonium, powdered pumice and gypsum to fix his ivory endoprostheses.

Acrylic acid has been known since 1843. In 1901 Rohm was working on methylmethacrylic resins (9). In 1928 a German patent described a new synthetic material of high-polymer methylmethacrylate, which was soon marketed on an industrial scale by various producers under the names Plexiglas, Perspex, Lucite etc. Already by 1930 artificial teeth and dentures were being made from this material. It was discovered that a mixture of polymer powder and monomer was self-curing at low temperature, and this accordingly found application in medicine. This new self-curing synthetic material became familiar in dentistry under the names Paladon/Polapont.

After 1940 the new material was also employed in surgery, for filling in bone defects in the skull, stabilizing the cervical vertebrae etc.

In 1951 Kiaer and Jansen reported on the use of self-curing acrylic cement in hip surgery (13), and in the same year Haboušh (6) employed this cement to fix a total hip joint prosthesis. These were probably the first workers to use acrylic cement in hip operations.

After Spealman's report on the toxicity of the monomeric methylmethacrylate in 1945 (20), experimental investigations on the compatibility of the new cements were published, inter alia, by Henrichsen and collaborators in 1953 (7) and by Wiltse and collaborators in 1957 (22). The good biocompatibility of commercial Plexiglas, which was produced on an industrial scale and became the primary material for the production of endoprostheses (e.g. by Judet), was confirmed by numerous investigations (4).

In 1958 Charnley began anchoring his endoprostheses in the bone with self-curing acrylic cement. Through his publications this procedure achieved international recognition, and more and more "bone cements" appeared on the market.

In 1962 M.E. Müller (15) reported on 60 total Charnley prostheses that had been cemented with "Palacos" without complications.

Soon, however, it became clear that self-curing acrylic cement had short-comings as well as considerable advantages. Thus while the problem of anchoring the prosthesis during the operation is largely solved, experience is increasingly teaching us that the fixation of endoprostheses is a problem of force transmission between foreign body and living bone, which has still to be solved biomechanically with long-term reliability. The interface problem between foreign body and living bone has been shifted by cement fixation from the endoprosthesis/bone interface to the cement/bone interface. Consequently more attempts are being made again to anchor endoprostheses without cement, and the question arises as to whether better long-term results might not be achieved with other cements. If the extensive literature is examined, it will be noticed that very little is known about the processes and changes in the cement itself, which take place during the polymerization and curing of the self-curing acrylic cements. But a knowledge of what happens here is crucial to the handling during the operation. Equally, it is impossible to select the right cement unless the various properties of the commercial products are known.

Today, four main commercially available self-curing acrylic cements are employed for fixing endoprostheses, all of them with the same basic formula of solid bead polymer and liquid monomeric methylmethacrylate:

1. CMW Bone Cement (CMW Laboratories Ltd., Marton, Blackpool)
2. Palacos R (Kulzer & Co. GmbH, Bad Homburg v.d.H.)
3. Simplex (North Hill Plastics Ltd., London)
4. Sulfix-6 (Sulzer Brothers Limited, Winterthur)

These cements differ from one another in the way their polymerization proceeds.

THE POLYMERIZATION OF METHACRYLATE (MMA) TO POLYMETHYLMETHACRYLATE (PMMA)

Methacrylate esters polymerize under certain conditions to polymethacrylate. We are interested primarily in methylmethacrylate ester (MMA), which solidifies into a glassy translucent mass upon polymerizing into polymethacrylate (PMMA); this is marketed under the names Plexiglas, Acrylglas etc. (Fig. 1).

Monomer methacrylate ester (MMA) is a colourless liquid having a molecular weight of 100 with a characteristic pungent smell, density $\rho = 0.94$ g/cm^2 and boiling point 100 ^{o}C (Table 1). To prevent spontaneous polymerization MMA is sold with an inhibitor

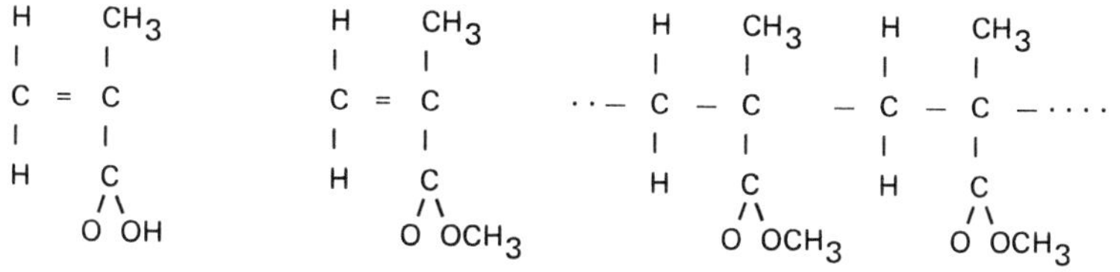

Methacrylic acid — Methylmethacrylate (MMA) — Polymethylmethacrylate (PMMA)

Fig. 1 Chemical structure of MMA and PMMA

Table 1 Some of the physical properties of MMA and PMMA

MMA:	Molecular weight	=	100
	Boiling point	=	100 °C
	Heat of polymerization	=	13.28 Kcal/mole
	(MMA/PMMA)	=	132.8 cal/g
		=	124.8 cal/ccm
	Density	=	0.94 g/cm^3
PMMA:	Density	=	1.18 g/cm^3
	Specific heat	=	0.35 cal/g per °C

or stabilizer added (usually hydroquinone). Polymerization is triggered and assisted by hardeners (catalysts). Dibenzoyl peroxide is mainly used as a catalyst today. Polymerization means the linking of the MMA molecules into long chains of PMMA. In the process the clear liquid first turns viscous and sticky, then gel-like, and finally solidifies to polymethylmethacrylate (PMMA). The polymerized PMMA has a density of $\rho = 1.18$ g/cm^3, retains its shape stability up to 90-100 °C, and is colourless, hard and transparent if no fillers are used. The polymerization takes place faster at higher temperatures than at room temperature.

The forming of molecule chains is accompanied by the release of heat, with a heat of polymerization of 13.28 Kcal/mole or 132.8 cal/g. With the release of the heat of polymerization the temperature of the polymerizing substance is raised, accelerating polymerization in turn. Without dissipation of heat the MMA would be heated to some 300 °C. If good heat dissipation is ensured (thin cement layer, good contact with a layer of high conductivity) and if the rate of polymerization can be kept low, the temperature rise is less marked.

It has been shown that the progress of the polymerization of MMA into PMMA can be best characterized by the temperature curve within the cement. In a first approximation it can be assumed that the rate of polymerization is proportional to the rate of temperature change (°C/min) (Fig. 2).

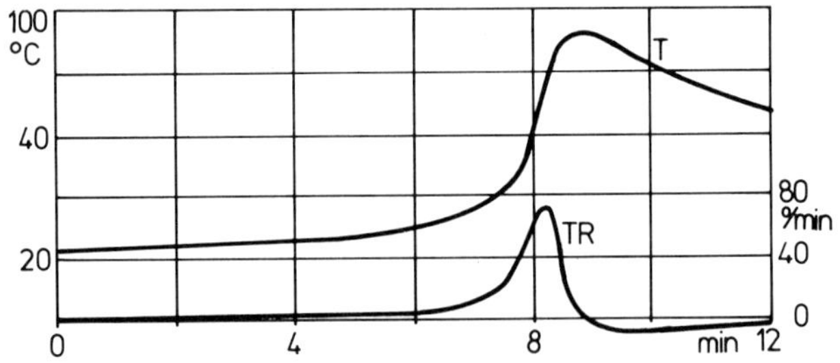

Fig. 2 Temperature curves for the polymerization of an acrylic cement.
Above: temperature T.
Below: rate of temperature change TR, paralleling the rate of polymerization

At low temperatures (room temperature) polymerization is not quite complete. The degree of polymerization indicates how much of the original substance has been polymerized. The monomer content still remaining is termed the residual monomer content (in %). Under high pressure and high temperature it is possible to achieve a very low residual monomer content. In the case of polymerization without increased pressure and at low temperature, a residual monomer content of 1-4 % will persist even over long periods of observation.

SELF–CURING ACRYLIC CEMENTS (BONE CEMENTS)

The term "cement" is taken to mean paste-like substances which set to form a hard mass and which in their soft state can be applied so as to join other bodies together and fill out hollow spaces.

Pure MMA is unsuitable for use as bone cement. By mixing 2 parts of bead polymer (small globules of PMMA measuring 5 to 130 microns in diameter) with 1 part liquid MMA, a pasty cement curing at low temperatures is obtained (Tables 2, 3). The liquid MMA fills out the interspaces between the polymer globules, cementing the individual

Table 2 General composition of bone cements

Liquid (16-18.8 g):		
Methylmethacrylate (MMA) or		
Any butyl methacrylate	(monomer)	
Hydroquinone or amine	(stabilizer)	approx. 2 %
Powder (40 g):		
Bead polymerizate (PMMA)	(polymer)	90-100 %
Dibenzoyl peroxide	(catalyst)	
Barium sulphate or	(contrast medium)	5-10 %
Zirconium oxide	(contrast medium)	10 %

Table 3 Terminology according to DIN 16945/6

Reaction resins are liquid or liquefiable resins which cure by polyaddition or polymerization, either by themselves or aided by reagents (hardeners, accelerators etc.) without separation of volatile components.

Methacrylate resins are reaction resins consisting of a polymerizable mixture of polymeric and monomeric methacrylate esters.

Reaction resin compounds are mixtures of a reaction resin and the necessary reagents (hardener, accelerator etc.) with or without fillers, ready for working.

Casting resin moulded plastics are cured substances from reaction resin compounds, which become moulded parts after pouring into moulds and hardening of the reaction resin compound.

beads into a solid mass after curing. PMMA dissolves slightly in MMA, so that during the mixing process the surface of the polymer globules is softened somewhat and partially dissolved (Figs. 3, 4). Consequently, during polymerization the globules and the monomer between them melt into a homogeneous mass (Fig. 5). Results of this mixing are:

a. the reaction mixture can be handled as a paste,
b. the maximum temperature can be kept low (less heat of polymerization), and
c. the shrinkage due to polymerization is less than with pure MMA.

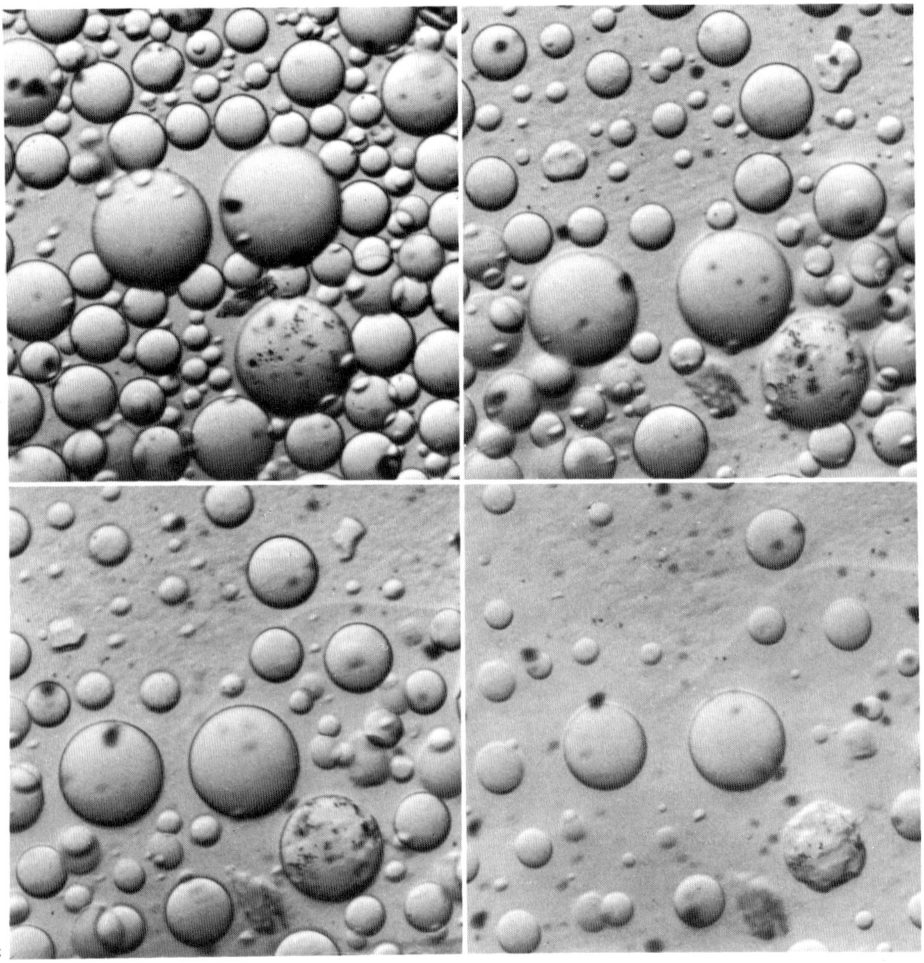

a b c d

Fig. 3a-d Partial solution of polymer globules in monomer (without benzoyl peroxide). Note the partial dissolution on the surface of the globule in the lower part of the picture (x 300)

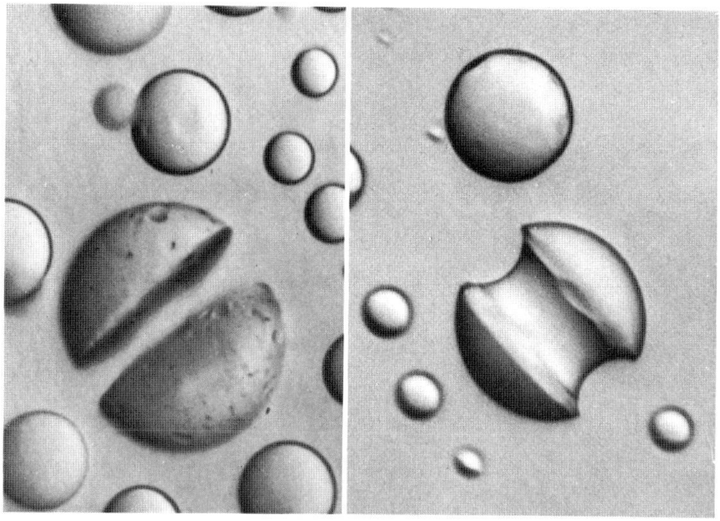

Fig. 4 Equatorial dissolution of polymer globules in monomer (x 400)

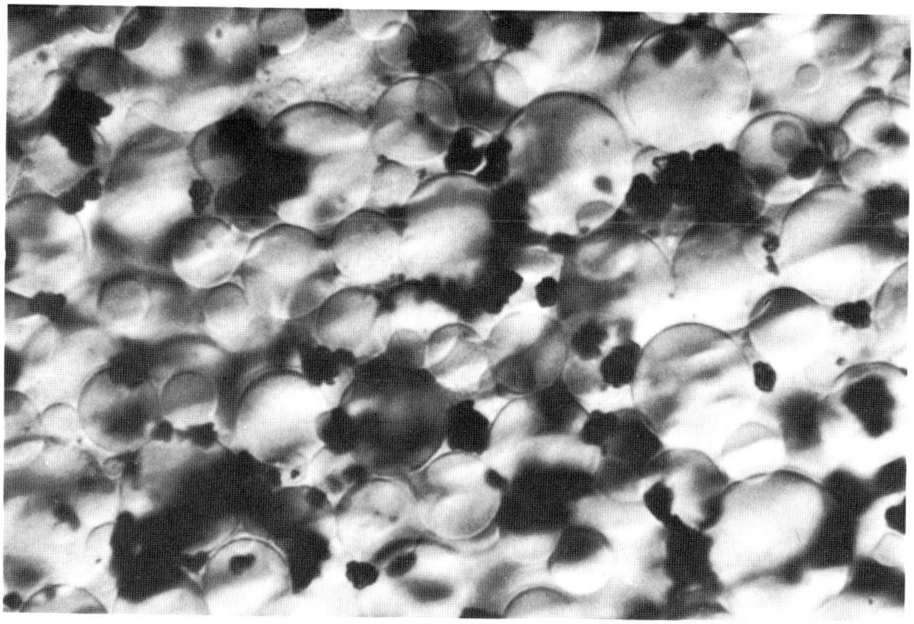

Fig. 5 Polymerization of Sulfix-6 under the microscope (x 400).

a. 8.5 min., polymer globules sharply defined, interspaces filled with monomer. Black: Contrast medium

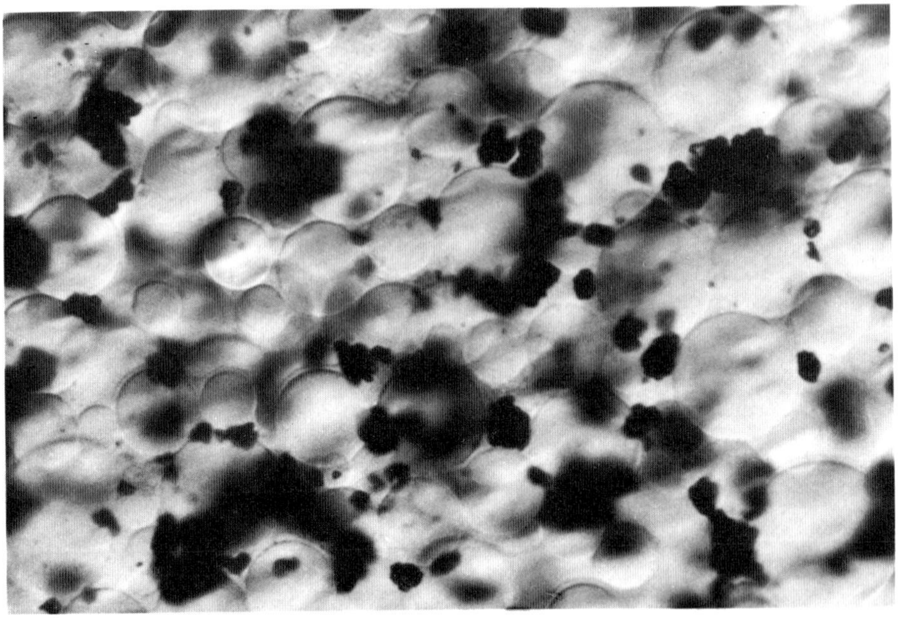

Fig. 5b 9 min., with progressive polymerization the index of refraction of polymer globules and monomer becomes more equal, and the contours disappear

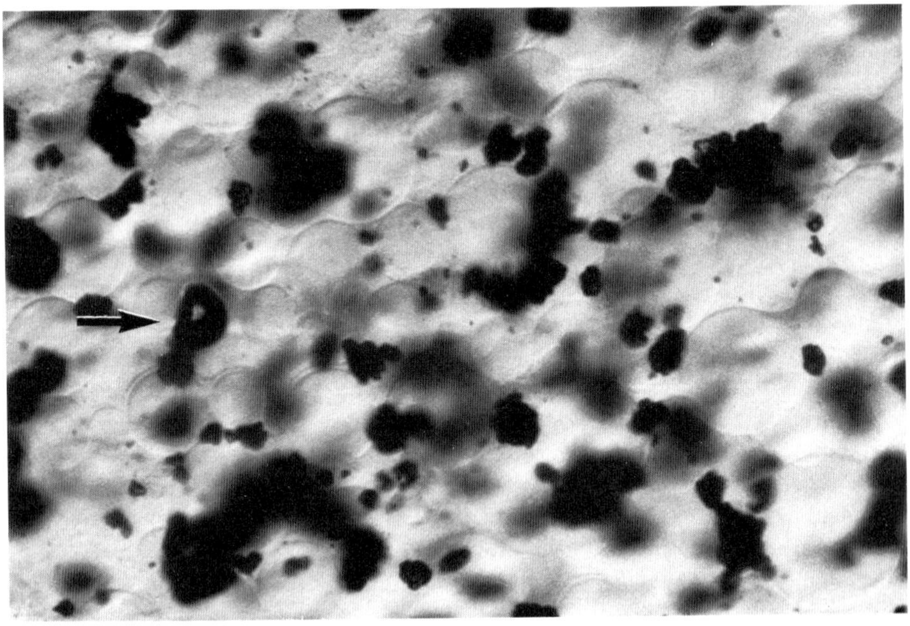

Fig. 5c 9.5 min., a new bubble is appearing (→). It will attain its ultimate size in 3/4 minute (pore formation)

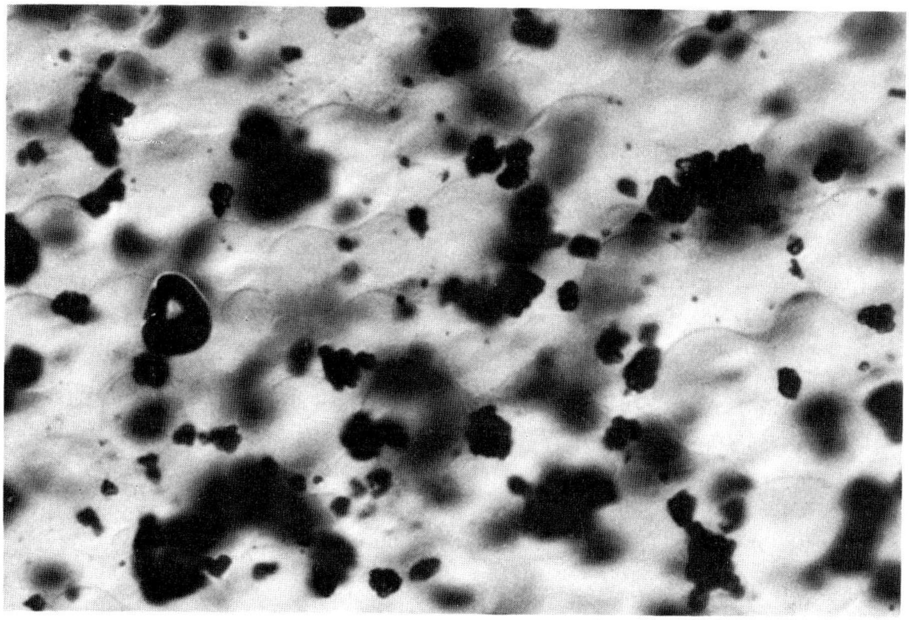

Fig. 5d 10 min.

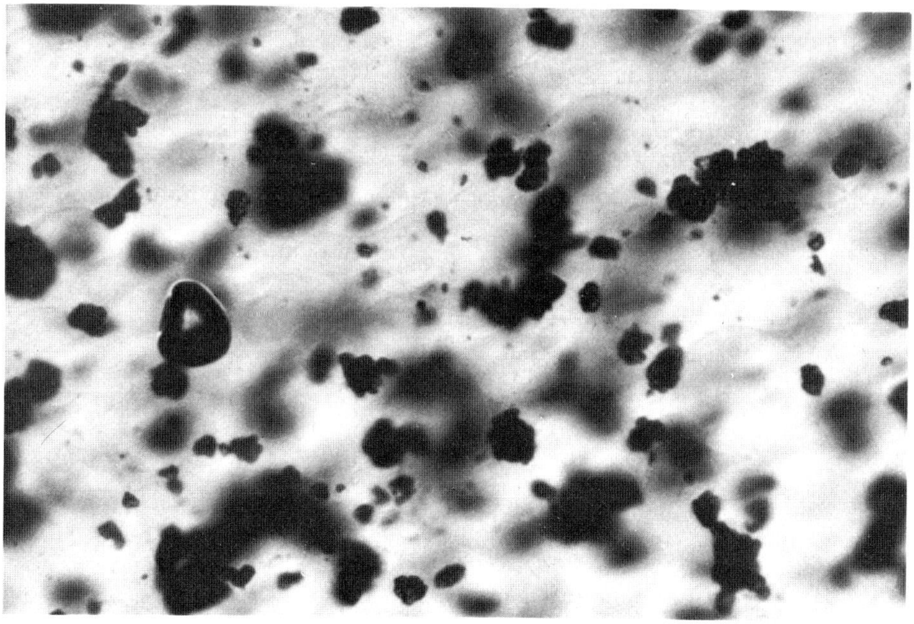

Fig. 5e 10.5 min.

For the bone cements too the progress of polymerization is best illustrated by the temperature curve or rate of temperature change within the cement. The heat liberated by polymerization of the MMA component heats the cement mixture progressively as the polymerization proceeds. In the mixing phase the rate of temperature increase is small, but towards the end of the processing time it quickens, reaching its maximum during the cure.

The maximum temperatures reached in the cement, and the curing time depend, among other things, on the mixing ratio, initial temperature, layer thickness and dissipation of heat to the environment.

CURING THE CEMENT MIXTURE AND TEMPERATURE BEHAVIOUR

Bone cements are marketed in suitably weighed quantities and in sterile condition. Mixing the liquid with the powder is done in a mixing bowl, using a spatula. For practical reasons we divide the curing process into the mixing time, handling time and the actual curing time, designating the beginning of the handling time V_A and its end V_E. The mixing, handling and curing phases merge into one another without sharp divisions (Fig. 6).

MIXING PHASE

At first the mixture has a somewhat granular feel, but after 1/2-2 1/2 minutes in the case of Sulfix-6 a sticky, easy-flowing mass results. With CMW the granular phase is less marked. Palacos R becomes less liquid than Sulfix-6, the granular phase passing quickly into the sticky phase. With Simplex the mixture remains very dry at first, then it liquefies and assumes a medium consistency. For filling the cement syringe the relatively long granular phase of Sulfix-6, during which the cement has a pretty low viscosity, is an advantage.

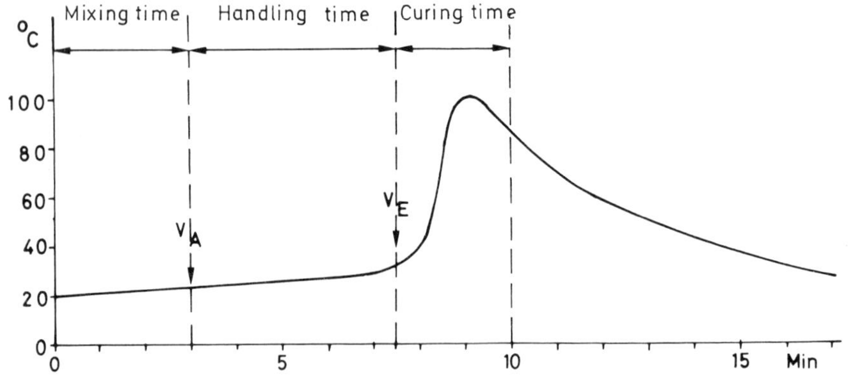

Fig. 6 Phases in the curing of acrylic cement. V_A = beginning, V_E = end of handling time. With Sulfix-6 the mixing time is divided into mixing and standing times

For a cement like Sulfix-6 the mixing time is very short and the mixture can stand for a few minutes (standing time). Air bubbles introduced by mixing with the spatula are voided visibly, producing a cement with less porosity than the other cements.

During the second part of the mixing phase the cement mixture flows more or less well. When touched it sticks to the finger and long, fine threads can be drawn.

When the finger can be removed cleanly, without any material adhering, the phase is termed (V_A). This point signifies the begin of the working time or handling phase.

HANDLING PHASE

A phase now follows, during which the doughy mass no longer sticks to the glove and can be moulded easily. In this state the cement is most suitable for filling into bone cavities and plastic deformation easily occurs. The temperature rises slowly by a few ^oC. The cement becomes increasingly stiff and offers more resistance to the finger moulding it. At the same time a certain elasticity becomes noticeable in the cement: the folds kneaded into it no longer disappear completely. Moreover small folds appear in the surface of the cement during deformation, indicating surface consolidation. When this stage is reached the cement has more or less attained body temperature.

CURING PHASE

The temperature now rises rapidly to a maximum, while the cement hardens quickly and can no longer be moulded. Curing is largely concluded about 1 minute after reaching maximum temperature (Table 4). From this time on the cement undergoes no further changes.

DEFINITIONS OF THE INDIVIDUAL PHASES

The ISO (International Standardization Organization) has issued standards characterizing the properties of plastics. They are largely in line with the corresponding DIN standards. For the standardization of bone cements a draft proposal was drawn up in 1975. It also defines the various curing phases (Table 5).

The transition from mixing phase to handling phase, designated V_A (commencement of handling time) is reached when threads can no longer be drawn with the finger or a glass rod. It is important that this test should be applied to material from the middle of the cement, and not just to the surface of the mix, which often dries out somewhat.

The ISO draft proposal defines the end of the handling phase as the moment when the temperature of the cement reaches half of the total temperature rise. This moment coincides roughly with the steepest rate of temperature rise. According to our experience deformation is still possible at this moment, but the mass hardens only a few seconds later and can no longer be moulded. For this reason we have taken the end of the handling

Table 4 Heat balance during the curing of an acrylic cement

20 ccm monomer (18.8 g) + 40 g bead polymer

Heat of polymerization	= 132.8 cal/g MMA
Specific heat PMMA	= 0.35 cal/^{o}C

Heating without outward loss of heat:

Heat released	= 18.8 · 132.8 cal = 2496 cal
Heating from 58.8 g PMMA	$= \frac{2496}{0.35 \cdot 58.8} = 121.3\ ^{o}C$

Estimated heat emission for a half-value period of 1 1/2 minutes:
Cement quantity used:

a. for the socket approx. 30 g with a surface of approx. 55 cm^2
Heat generated $\simeq$1200 cal

Heat emission $\frac{600\ cal}{55\ cm^2 \cdot 1.5\ min} \simeq 7\ cal/cm^2$ per min

b. for the femur prosthesis approx. 45 g, surface approx. 70 cm^2
Heat generated $\simeq$1800 cal

Heat emission $\frac{900}{70 \cdot 1.5} \simeq 8.5\ cal/cm^2$ per min

Table 5 Testing of methacrylate resin compounds (DIN 16945)

Temperature rise Determination of the maximum temperature and the time taken for the temperature rise during the curing of reaction resin compounds from methacrylate resins (DIN 16945). According to ISO/R 584-1967 the rate of increase for the temperature rise during the cure is also determined
Setting time The setting time states when and at what temperature the reaction mass gels The setting time is defined as the interval from the start of the test to the time at which the reaction resin compound passes from the liquid into the gelled state
Total volume contraction The total shrinkage is calculated from the density of the reaction resin compound at 20 ^{o}C and the density of the reaction resin moulding at 20 ^{o}C

time V_E, which is important in practice, to be the moment when the cement offers more resistance to the moulding finger, becoming somewhat elastic (especially marked with Palacos R) so that folds can no longer be kneaded out. We have established that in vitro, V_E coincides fairly exactly with the time at which the cement mixture reaches a temperature of 32-34 ^{o}C, i.e. at the lower kink in the steeply rising temperature curve. Consequently our V_E is about 1 minute before the end of handling according to the draft ISO proposal. As a rough rule derived from our experience, the cement passes into the curing phase when it exceeds normal body temperature, after which it should no longer be moulded.

DEPENDENCE OF CURE BEHAVIOUR ON STARTING TEMPERATURE, LAYER THICKNESS AND MIXING RATIO

In order to analyze the curing of these cements we have carried out model tests, allowing the various factors of influence to be examined separately. Small dishes of aluminium or Teflon were employed, 40 mm in diameter and 10 mm high, into which the freshly mixed cement was poured. A thermocouple was introduced centrally into the cement mass. If necessary the dish with the cement was cooled in water.

With higher starting (i.e. room) temperatures polymerization is shortened, and with it the handling time. The commercial bone cements may be classified as follows:

Palacos:	V_A begins earliest, V_E in 2nd place
CMW:	V_A begins somewhat later, V_E in 1st place
Simplex:	V_A begins in 3rd place, V_E in 4th place
Sulfix-6:	V_A begins latest, V_E in 3rd place

The maximum temperature of the cements is likewise governed by the room or starting temperature. In our model tests it rose about 2.5 °C for every 1 °C increase in the room temperature (Fig. 7).

The maximum temperature also depends on the thickness of the cement layer. The thicker the layer, the higher the temperature attained and the shorter the polymerization time (Fig. 8).

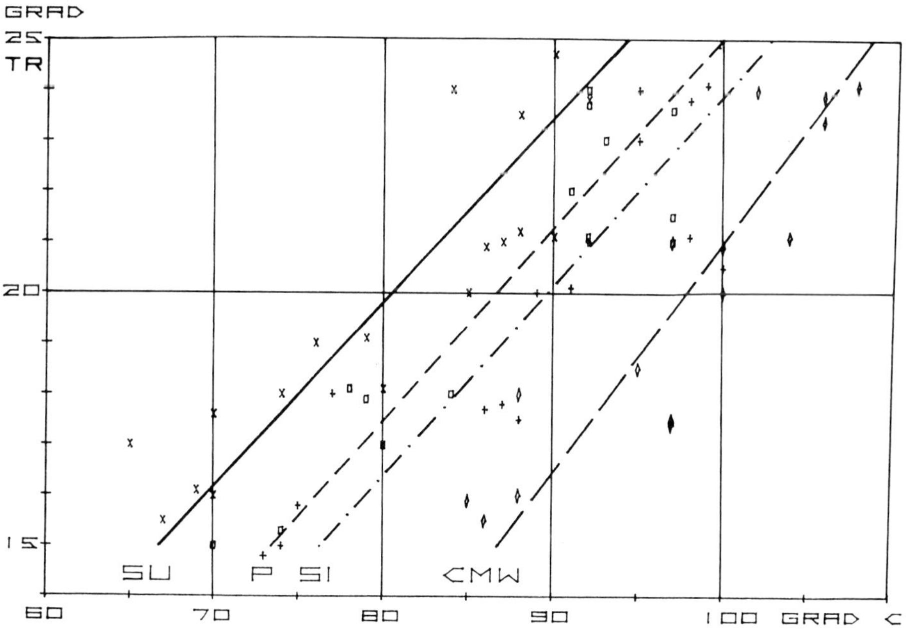

Fig. 7 Maximum temperatures T reached at various room temperatures TR, for Sulfix-6 (SU), Palacos (P), Simplex (SI) and CMW (CMW)

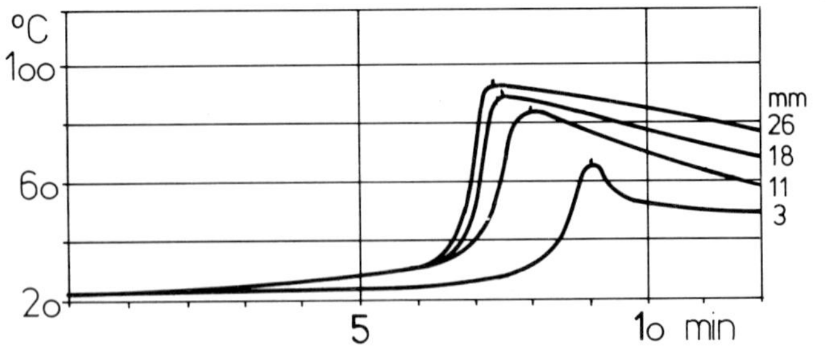

Fig. 8a Dependence of maximum temperature and rate of polymerization on the layer thickness (right-hand scale) with Sulfix-6

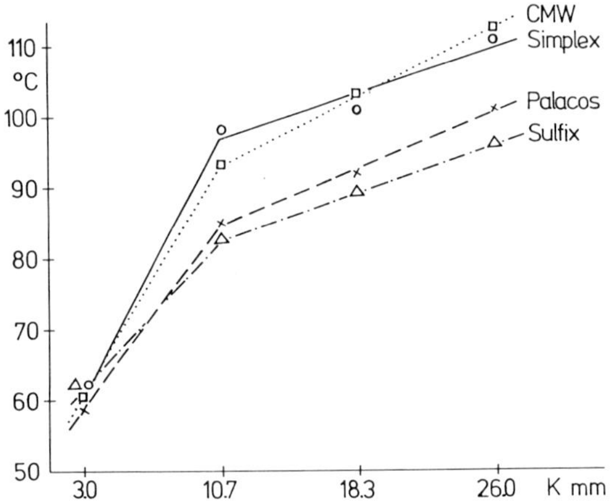

Fig. 8b
Dependence of maximum temperature on layer thickness K

In addition, the polymerization time and the maximum temperature can be influenced by varying the mixing ratio of powder and liquid. A great deal of liquid with the same amount of powder gives longer polymerization and higher maximum temperatures, while little liquid results in speedier polymerization and lower maximum temperatures (Fig. 9).

These differences are also of practical consequence when cementing-in endoprostheses. As a general rule the thickness of the layer between prosthesis and bone is not uniform. Thick layers set faster than thin ones, and generate higher maximum temperatures. Differences in the layer thickness are probably even capable of setting up undesirable stresses in the cement.

It should be pointed out that the finished cement mixture was left to itself in our model sets. In surgical applications the cement is often kneaded in the hand, so that the surface is constantly renewed and its temperature raised in places, with the result that polymerization is accelerated locally. It is advisable to refrain from kneading the cement to obtain a homogeneous mass.

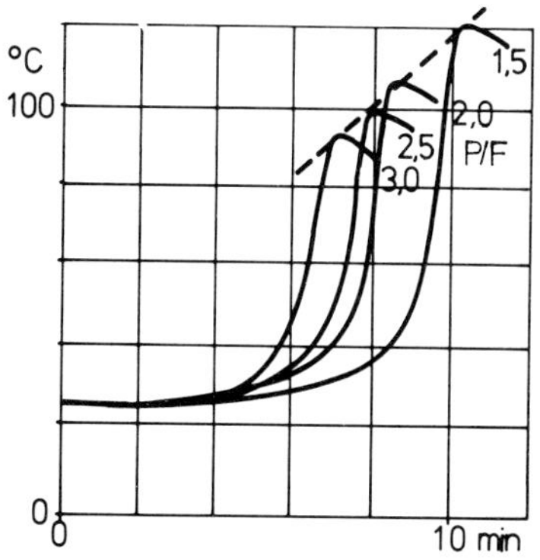

Fig. 9
Dependence of maximum temperature and rate of polymerization on the mixing ratio P/F (bead polymer/liquid) according to Meyer et al. (14)

ALTERATION OF THE PHYSICAL PROPERTIES DURING POLYMERIZATION

During the polymerization process the physical properties of the cement mixture change in obedience to certain laws. The most obvious change is the increase in consistency from the pourable liquid state to a plastic paste and then to a hard-elastic form. Quantitative and hence comparable determination of the consistency is difficult, because the viscous-plastic-elastic range is very wide and is passed through in a few minutes. Dynamic testing methods are needed above all, and these call for fundamentally different measuring facilities in each phase (liquid-paste-solid). There are however some simpler investigation methods, and these are set out below.

CONSISTENCY OF THE CEMENT MIXTURE

The consistency of the cement mix can be determined indirectly within the required range by the following means:

1. Penetrometer test: With the penetrometer the penetration depth of a metal rod subjected to a certain force during a certain time is measured at intervals of 30 seconds. The penetrometer curves reveal a more or less straight line during the handling time. Once the cement is hard, the metal rod no longer sinks (Fig. 10) (23, 24).
2. Extrusion test: When the cement mix is expelled from the cement syringe, it comes out in a string which flattens under its own weight. By measuring the final width of the string it is possible to judge the consistency and the change in it (Fig. 11).
3. Vibration tests: The mechanical resistance opposing a deformation can be recorded continuously by exposing the cement to an oscillating punch. Vibration investigations of this kind are being performed in our laboratory. Among other things we have measured the transadmittance, i.e. the transmission of mechanical vibrations through the hardening cement, and very interesting curves have been recorded. However, although the frequency-dependence of the transadmittance does yield curves which correlate very closely to the handling time, no unified results are obtained for the

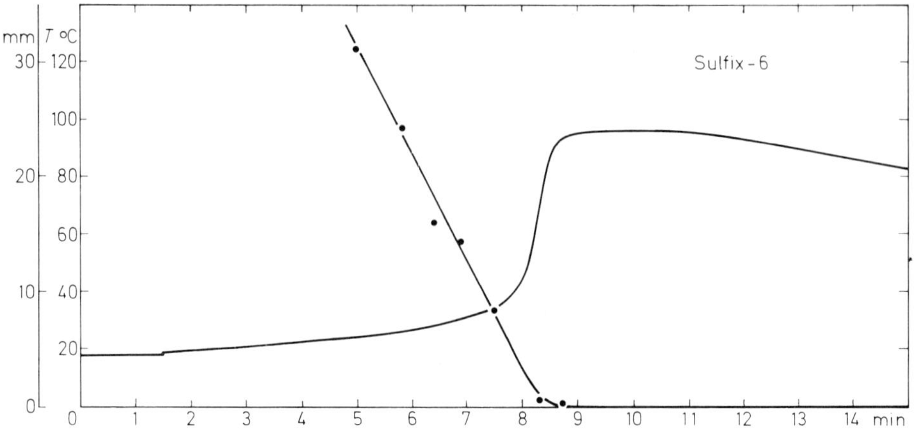

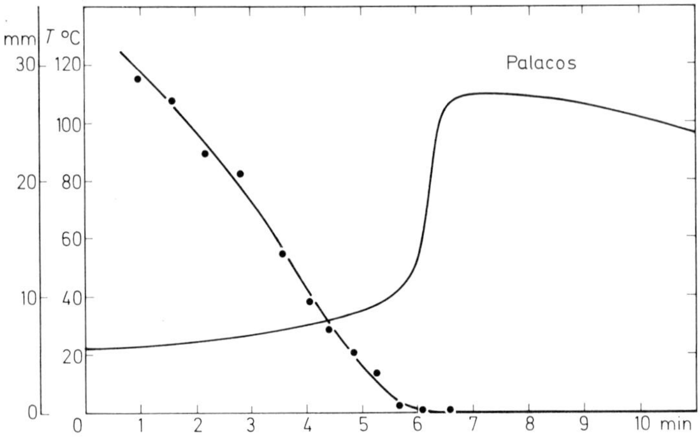

Fig. 10a,b Penetrometer values (penetration depth) as a function of the cement temperature with various cements

various commercial cement mixtures. At 750 Hz the minimum and maximum transadmittance agrees well with V_A and V_E for Simplex and Palacos K, but not for CMW and Sulfix-6. By adopting different measuring frequencies it is possible to obtain better agreement of the curves with V_A and V_E for these two latter cements also (Fig. 12).

4. The modulus of shear or its reciprocal (compliance) may also be measured to characterize the change in consistency. For this the acceleration of a cylinder plunging into the cement is measured, maintaining constant vibration force. The amount of acceleration and the phase shift between force and acceleration can be recorded continuously, providing a measure for the consolidation of the cement (Fig. 13).

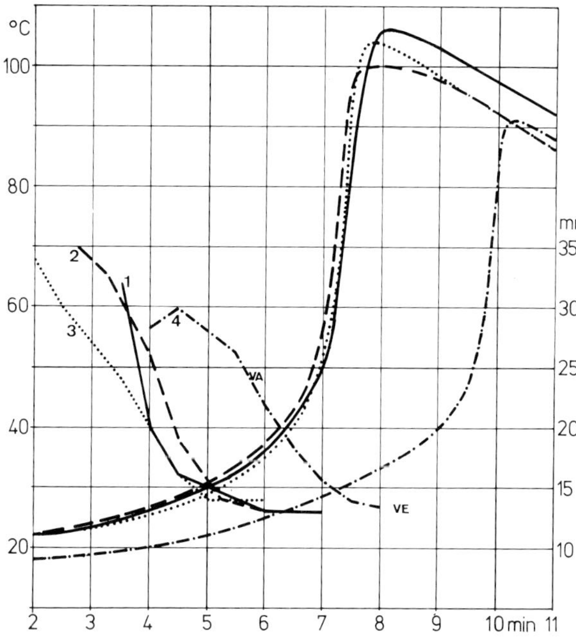

Fig. 11a
Width of the extruded string (right-hand scale) and temperature curve for three samples of Sulfix-6

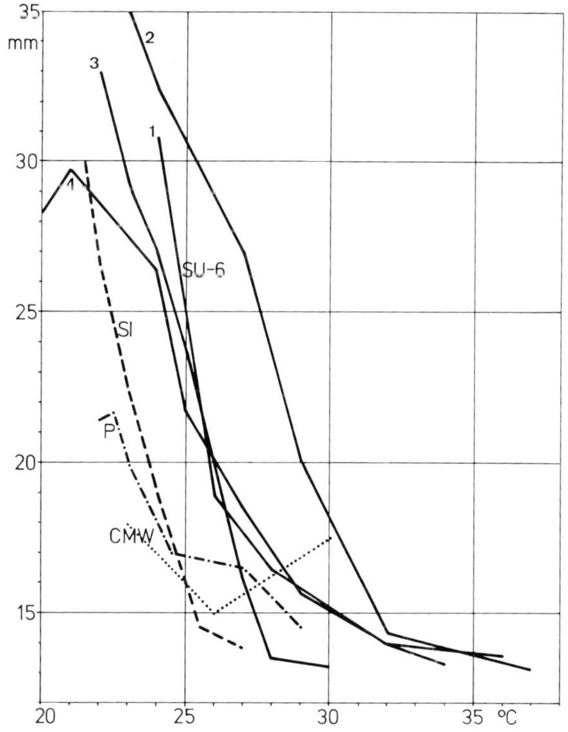

Fig. 11b
Width of the extruded string of acrylic cements

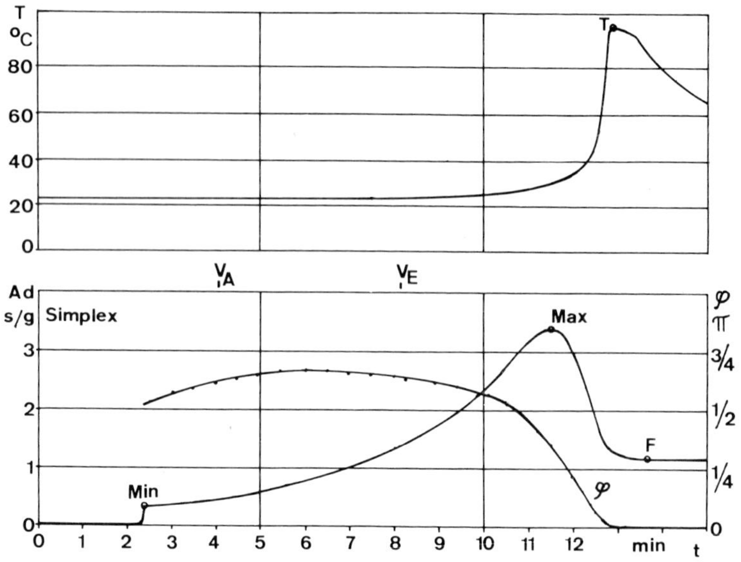

Fig. 12 Transadmittance and phase angle for Palacos-K

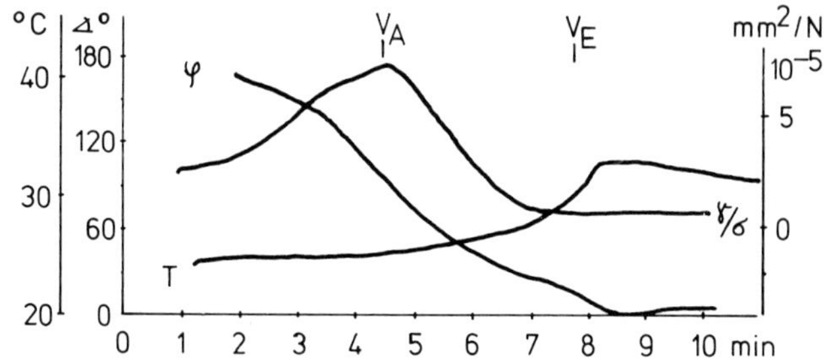

Fig. 13 Shear modulus calculation. γ/σ and phase angle as a function of time in the polymerization of Sulfix-6. T = cement temperature

VOLUME AND DENSITY CHANGE DURING POLYMERIZATION, POROSITY

Through the polymerization of MMA to PMMA, the density ρ rises from 0.94 g/cm^3 for MMA to 1.18 g/cm^3 for PMMA. Since the weight G remains unchanged, the volume V alters according to $V = G/\rho$. The reduction in volume due to polymerization is 25.53 % (referred to the end product) for pure MMA, i.e. the volume of the PMMA is only 79.66 % that of the MMA.

If bead polymer is mixed with liquid MMA in a ratio of 40 g PMMA : 20 cm^3 MMA, the initial mixture has a density of 1.09 g/cm^3. Polymerization shrinkage will then still amount to 7.6 %. Further reduction of the MMA content to 16 g gives a polymerization shrinkage of 6.78 %, because only the MMA part changes its density. Additions of 10-20 % $BaSO_4$ or ZrO_2 will raise the shrinkage again by about 0.4 % (Table 6).

Table 6 Loss of volume in the polymerization of MMA (a) and acrylic cements of various compositions (b, c, d),

$\Delta V = 100 \cdot (\rho_E - \rho_A) / \rho_E$

ρ_A = initial density

ρ_E = final density

		ρ_A	ρ_E	ΔV (%)
a) MMA →	PMMA	0.94	1.18	-20.34
b) 20 cm^3 MMA + 40 g PMMA →	58.8 g PMMA	1.09	1.18	- 7.63
c) 16 g MMA + 40 g PMMA →	56 g PMMA	1.10	1.18	- 6.78
d) 16 g MMA + 36 g PMMA + 4 g ZrO_2 →	56 g (PMMA + ZrO_2)	1.16	1.125	- 7.20

It will be seen in all tests that the shrinkage is greatest during the curing phase. It is small during the mixing and handling phases, and it provides an indication for the end of polymerization after the curing phase (Fig. 14).

In theory the cured cement with contrast medium ought to show a density of about 1.25 g/cm^3 (e.g. Sulfix-6), without contrast medium 1.18 g/cm^3. However values of ρ from 1.04 to 1.21 g/cm^3 are ascertained on bone cements cured in the usual way. The reduced density is explained by the presence of small cavities (pores) occurring regularly, attaining diameters up to 2-3 mm. Owing to this porosity, while the weight of material corresponds to the original input weight, the final volume includes the pores as well as the material volume. The total density of the cured cement is thus:

$$\rho_G = \frac{m_z}{Vol_z + Vol_p}$$

where ρ_G = total density
m_z = mass of the cement
Vol_z = volume of the cement mass
Vol_p = volume of the pores

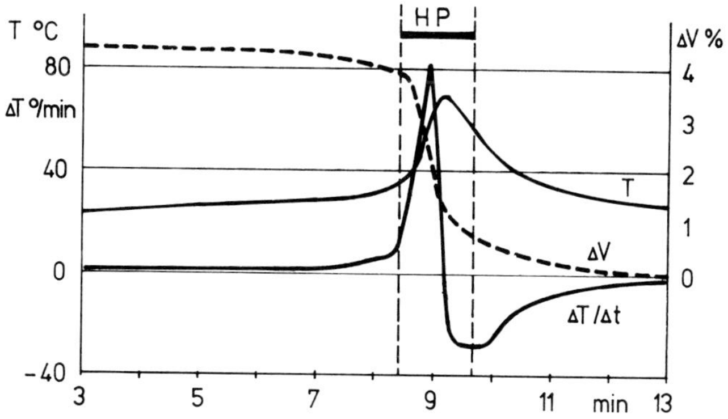

Fig. 14a Volume contraction ΔV and rate of temperature change $\Delta T / \Delta t$. T = cement temperature. HP = curing time

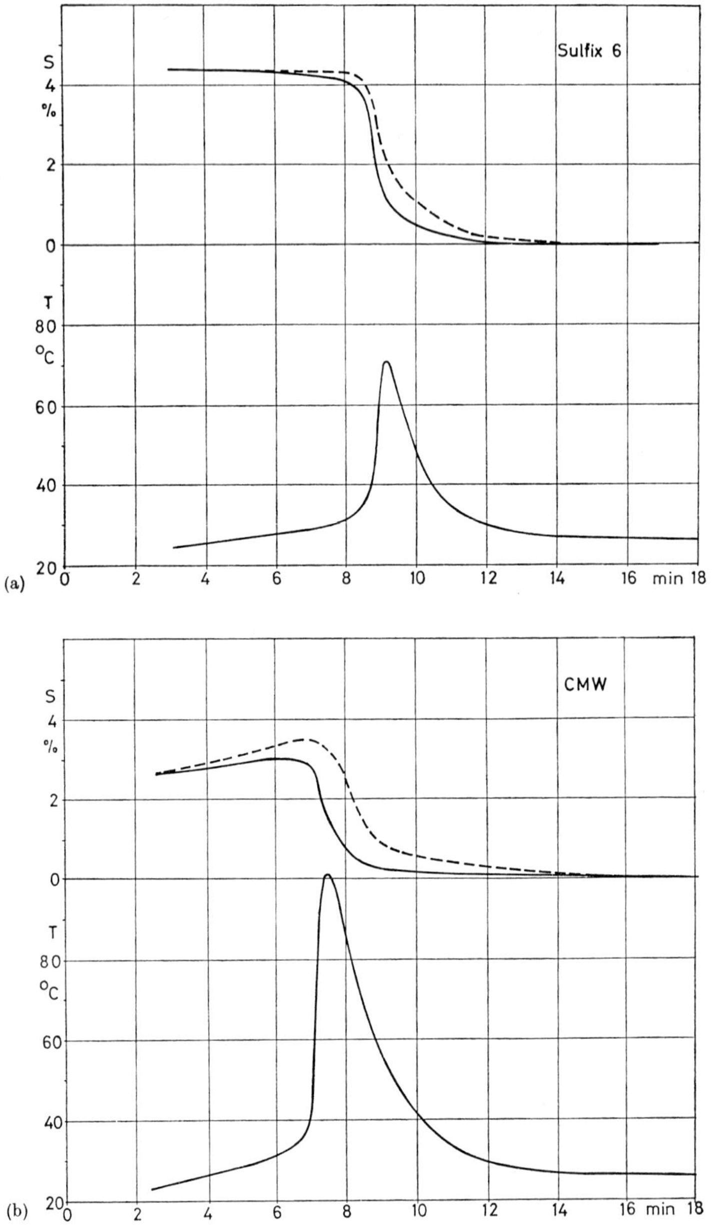

Fig. 14b Volume contraction of Sulfix-6 and CMW during curing.

Upper curves: contraction as percentage of final volume (— pure polymerization shrinkage, - - - total shrinkage). The difference is accounted for by thermal expansion contraction.

Lower curves: temperature

Charnley and other investigators discovered in tests that under certain conditions an expansion of the cement by 1-3 % may be observed instead of a shrinkage. This can be explained only by the appearance of fresh pores or enlargement of the original pores in the course of curing.

The question that now arises is: how do the pores occur in the cement? There are two possibilities:

a. Small air inclusions are stirred into the cement paste during mixing, and expand under the effect of heat, and
b. the heating of the cement causes monomer MMA to evaporate in micro-areas, forming small cavities in the setting mass (Fig. 15). Since the cement becomes solid at the highest temperature reached, these cavities do not collapse afterwards but increase the total volume.

Though both phenomena are involved in the formation of pores, the creation of fresh cavities is probably more important for the reduction of shrinkage. Air bubbles are generally bigger and form cavities which are easily visible. Large pores impair the strength more than small ones. When the cement is cured under high pressure (above 2 Kp/cm^2) it is possible to obtain clear, transparent cement samples which seldom reveal any air inclusion.

When Sulfix-6 is polymerized under slight overpressure, already at 1.5 Kp/cm^2 only odd air bubbles can be detected in the otherwise homogeneous and transparent cement. The other cements need a higher pressure to inhibit the formation of pores (e.g. about 2 Kp/cm^2 for CMW).

Porosity is characterized by three parameters: degree of porosity, pore size and number of pores per unit volume:

1. The degree of porosity P indicates the percentage of the cured cement by volume occupied by pores. This percentage is determined by the spot counting method (Weibel) on the cement section after dyeing the pores selectively.
2. The pore size in a given cement does not depend on the maximum temperature. About 95 % of the pores have a diameter of less than 300 μm, with a mean of 140-240 μm. Only 5 % exceed 300 μm in diameter (Figs. 16, 17).
3. The number of pores per unit volume A_v does depend on the maximum temperature.

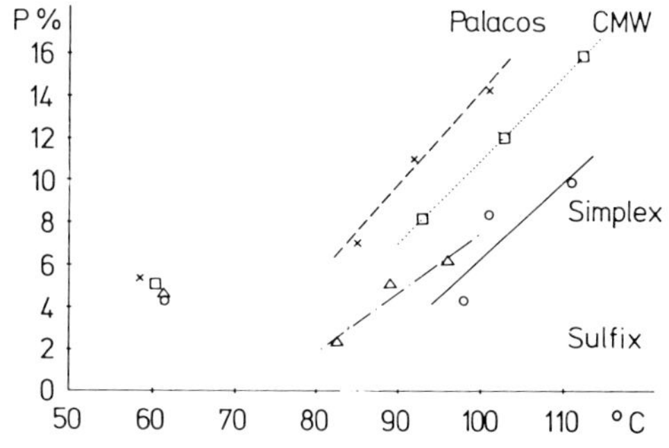

Fig. 15
Degree of porosity P versus maximum temperature for four bone cements

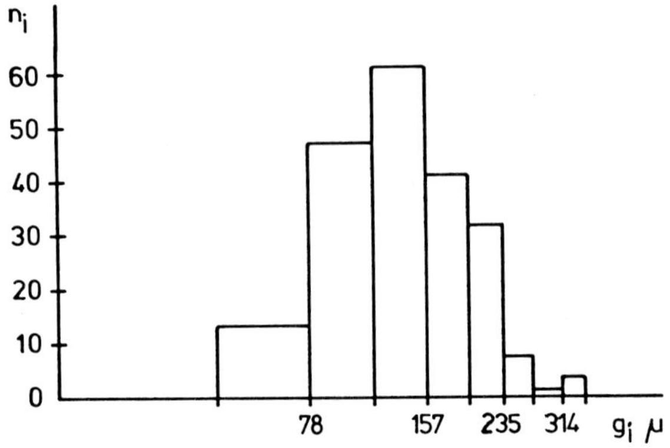

Fig. 16
Pore size distribution in CMW
(maximum temperature 103 °C)

At T_{max} = 60 °C, depending upon the cement, A_v amounts to 4-16/mm^3, but at 100 °C it is 33/mm^3 (Fig. 18).

From these tests it is clear that one part of the porosity consists of newly formed pores, resulting from the evaporation of liquid monomer in micro-areas, while the other part consists of air bubbles stirred in, which also contribute to the porosity expansion. This view is supported by the fact that the porosity can be influenced experimentally by certain measures. Adding alcohol (boiling point 78 °C) to Sulfix-6 for example gives much higher porosity in this cement, while polymerization under relatively small overpressure gives rise to a clear, transparent cement in which only few air bubbles are included.

The same results have been observed with the other cements, except that much more air bubbles are included in these than in Sulfix-6.

Depending on the cement mixture, only 7-9 % porosity is sufficient to offset the polymerization shrinkage so that the cured cement has the same density as the original mix (Fig. 19). Investigations by de Wijn et al. (21) reveal that, with the usual porosity, the bending and compressive strengths of acrylic cements drop to nearly half the values of compact cement. Our own tests confirm this loss of strength through increased porosity in the case of torsional strength. It is therefore not advisable to attempt expansion of the curing cement through increased porosity because the good mechanical properties of the cement will suffer as a result.

Superimposed upon these two volume changes during the cure, however, is another phenomenon: thermal expansion and contraction. Acrylic cements have a coefficient of thermal expansion of about $220 \cdot 10^{-6}$. When the soft cement mix becomes heated as a result of polymerization, the mixture expands and sets. Upon cooling, the cement shrinks in proportion to the temperature drop. During cooling from 67 °C down to body temperature, this thermal contraction amounts to 0.68 % by volume, or 4.5 μm with a cement thickness of 2 mm (Tables 7, 8, 9). Because this thermal contraction begins after curing, it is not possible to obtain a better anchorage by pressing the endoprosthesis in during curing — as our exhaustive tests have demonstrated.

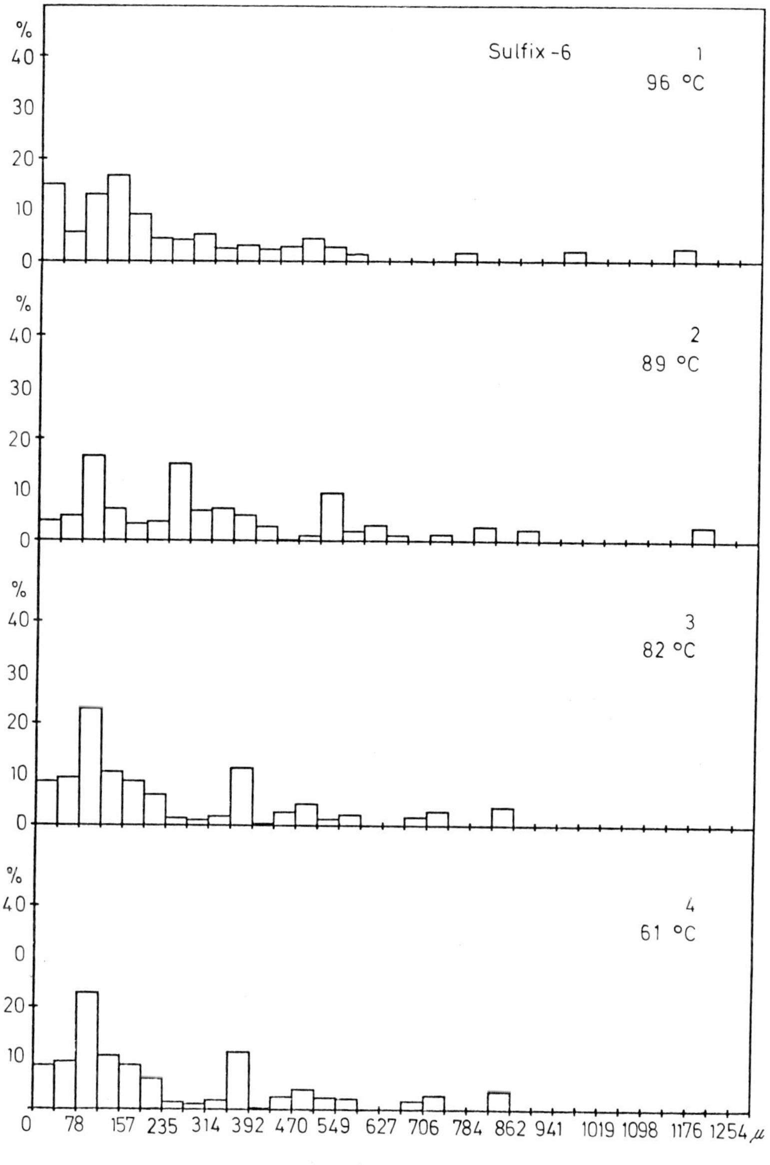

Fig. 17 Mean pore size for Sulfix-6 at various maximum temperatures

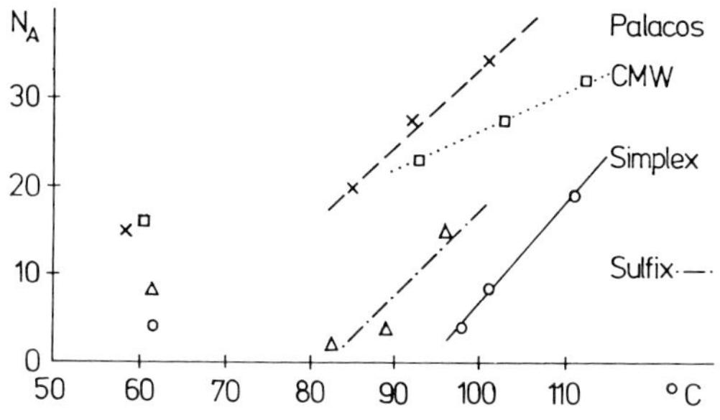

Fig. 18
Number of pores per mm^3 versus maximum temperature

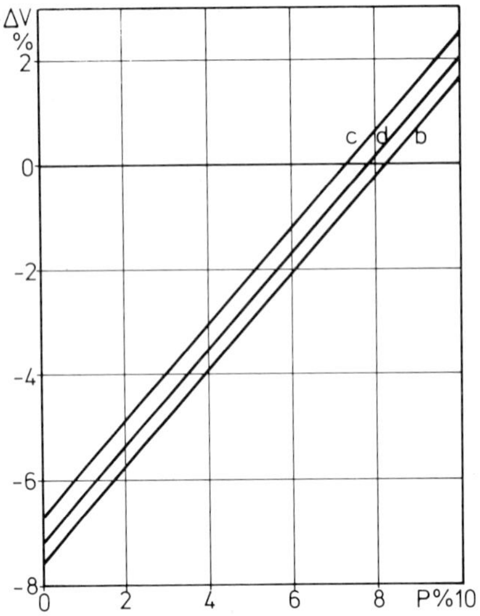

Fig. 19
Influence of degree of porosity P on total shrinkage Δ V (b, c, d as in Table 6)

Table 7 Thermal expansion/contraction ΔV of acrylic cements with various temperature differences Δt.

$\Delta V = V_o \cdot \beta \cdot \Delta t$

V_o = initial volume

β = coefficient of thermal expansion = $227 \cdot 10^{-6}$

Δt	=	20 °C	ΔV	=	0.45 %
		30 °C			0.68 %
		40 °C			0.91 %
		50 °C			1.14 %
		60 °C			1.36 %

Table 8 Total contraction and thermal contraction with different degrees of porosity and temperature differences

	Porosity %	Max. temp. T_{max}	Final temp. T_E	Contraction total %	Contraction thermal only %
a)	2	57 °C	37 °C	-5.3	-0.5
b)	4	67 °C	37 °C	-3.9	00.7
c)	6	77 °C	37 °C	-2.1	-0.9
d)	8	87 °C	37 °C	+0.7	-1.1

Table 9 Linear contraction Δl of cement per mm with different volume contractions ΔV

ΔV	=	1 %	Δl	=	3.3 µm
		2 %			6.6 µm
		3 %			10.0 µm
		4 %			13.3 µm
		5 %			16.6 µm

RELEASE OF MMA DURING POLYMERIZATION

At room temperature MMA evaporates at a rate of 0.66 mg/cm^2 per minute. It is picked up by the air from the cement mix too (MMA and PMMA). We ascertained an evaporation loss of 0.5 mg/cm^2 per minute during the mixing and handling phases. This rises briefly to 2.3-3.6 mg/cm^2 per minute when the cement temperature reaches its maximum, dropping two minutes later to unmeasurable values (Fig. 20).

Owing to this evaporation a consolidated skin forms on the surface of the mixture and quickly loses its stickiness. For the experimental determination of the handling time the formation of a surface skin is a disadvantage, because thread-drawing ceases on the surface before the corresponding consistency is attained below.

It must be assumed that the release of monomer from the mixture surface takes place on the same scale within the living tissue also. The stem of a standard femur prosthesis (Type Müller-Charnley) has a surface of 42 cm^2, so that a cement surface of about 70 cm^2 must be reckoned with in the femur. If this surface gives off 2 mg/cm^2 during the cure lasting 1 minute, this means that 140 mg of monomer pass into the tissues; part of this may get into the bloodstream and then produce a pharmacological effect (e.g. increased respiratory rate). According to Kutzman and Ohnsorge the LD_{50} for mice is 300 mg/Kg body weight, while Homsy states that 125 mg/100 ml in the blood of dogs is fatal (10). A quantity of 2.4 mg/Kg MMA may induce an alteration in the respiratory rate of mice, so that a pharmacological action must be expected in some cases when an endoprosthesis is introduced into the femur.

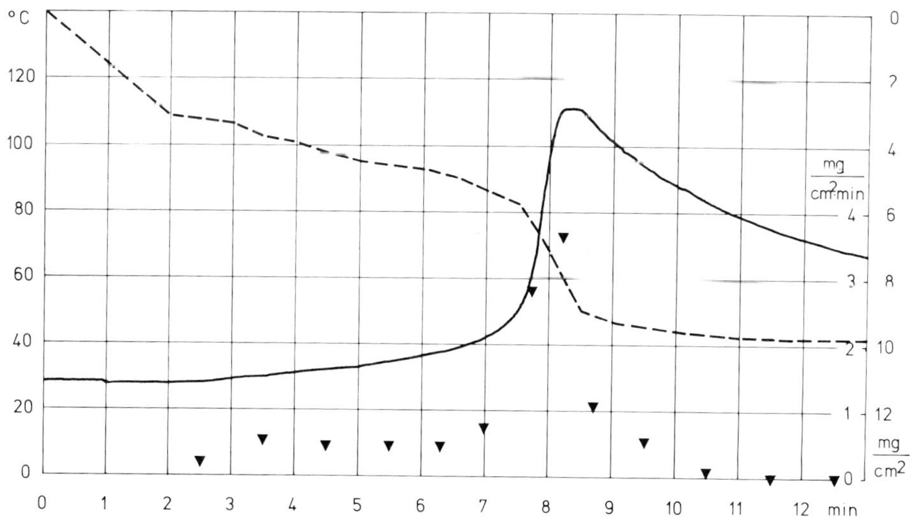

Fig. 20 Evaporation of monomer from the surface of a setting cement. Solid curve = cement temperature. Broken curve = total monomer release in mg per cm^2 (right-hand scale). ▼ = evaporation in mg/cm^2 per minute

Willert and Semlitsch have introduced curing cement into tissue medium 3-4 minutes after the start of mixing, and they discovered that 0.25-2.6 % monomer is given up to the tissue before the cement cures. With 40 g cement containing about 12 g monomer, this represents a quantity of 30 to 312 mg. From this it will be seen that our estimation agrees well with the measured quantities in the order of magnitude (17).

TIMING OF THE CURING PHASE

All observations serve to indicate that polymerization proceeds slowly at first after mixing, with the main polymerization phase commencing shortly before the maximum temperature is reached. On the temperature curve the main polymerization phase is easy to fix, because the steepest rate of temperature change occurs there (Figs. 2 and 14a). During the main polymerization phase, which lasts about 1 minute, the greatest changes are observed in the cement:

- the cement becomes hard,
- polymerization shrinkage reaches its maximum, and
- release of monomer to the environment reaches its maximum.

During the main polymerization phase the outer shape of the cement becomes fixed. Stresses introduced into the material structure by external deformation (pressing, kneading, movement of the endoprosthesis etc.) are fixed due to solidification.

ANCHORING ENDOPROSTHESES IN CEMENT

Endoprostheses are made of plastics or metal. The acrylic cements do not adhere very firmly either to the usual plastics or to metals. Accordingly firm fixation of the endoprosthesis in the cement can be achieved only by mechanical keying. For the stem of the femoral head prosthesis this keying is relatively easy to provide. Prosthesis metals have a coefficient of cubical expansion some 3 times lower than that of acrylic cement. Consequently during thermal contraction the prosthesis stem surrounded by cement shrinks less than the cement, so that the latter tightens its grip. Moreover the mechanical loading of the femur endoprosthesis is such that the latter is pressed into the cement sheath.

Anchoring the acetabulum of polyethylene is much more problematical. The bone cement does not adhere very well to the material of the socket. The coefficient of friction between cement and polyethylene is between 0.08-0.17, depending on the smoothness of the surface. To rotate a smooth socket cemented-in in vitro in the cement, without grooves, a torque of 30 Kp·cm or a tangential force of 19 Kp acting on the edge of the endoprosthesis is sufficient. This is possible only because the surrounding cement is pressed against the plastics socket at a radial force of about 4 Kp/cm^2. Our own tests disclosed that cements pressed against smooth polyethylene or Protasul during the handling phase give an adhesion which resists a load of 0.2-1 N/mm^2 or 2-10 Kp/mm^2 for tangential forces. To overcome this adhesive bond a torque of some 400-500 Kp·cm would be needed in theory for the socket described. This is much more than we were able to measure in the test. When the cement and endoprosthesis cool down, mechanical stresses occur at the interface due to the differing expansion coefficients. They overcome the adhesion, so that only the keying remains effective. Consequently the socket can be held in the cement only if its surface is provided with radial and circular grooves, which are pressed into the cement. These grooves then assure the necessary mechanical grip, which gives cohesion.

During the main curing phase the endoprosthesis must not be moved, otherwise the mechanical keying will suffer. For anchoring the socket endoprosthesis in the cement, a cement which is soft and non-elastic in the handling phase and does not shrink too little is favourable. If the acetabulum prosthesis is inserted when the cement is already hardening, it may happen that the cement no longer penetrates deeply enough into the surface grooves, so that the keying is inadequate.

ANCHORAGE BETWEEN CEMENT AND BONE

Between cement and bone tissue there is again no real adhesion. Here too the mechanical strength of the bond between the two materials derives from the keying action. To prepare the cement bed in the bone, part of the spongiosa is removed. This leaves an irregular surface, characterized by projecting, broken-off spongiosa ridges with marrow still located at the bottom of the recesses. By forcing in the endoprosthesis mechanically the cement is forced into these recesses and surrounds the spongiosa trabeculae (Fig. 21).

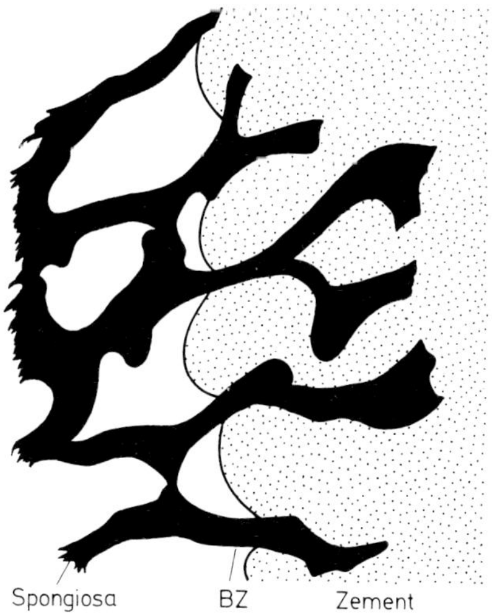

Fig. 21
The spongiosa trabeculae surrounded by the cement (dotted)

Owing to the shrinkage of the cement in curing and cooling, the more or less hardened cement may withdraw somewhat from the surrounding spongiosa, which may possibly improve the keying slightly.

The inside of the upper half of the femoral shaft is generally covered with a more or less marked spongiosa layer, which is formed by sheets of spongiosa running circularly. Here the anchorage is as good as in the spongiosa of the trochanter. Only where the cortex is exposed in the femur is keying no longer possible in the manner described. The cement does not hold on smooth bone surfaces and, owing to the shrinkage during cooling, the cement filling contracts somewhat, so that it fits only loosely inside a smooth bone tube.

The future of endoprosthesis anchorage depends on how the interface develops between the cement with the spongiosa trabeculae filled with it, and the living bone tissue. Shortly after introducing the cement a boundary layer 0.5 to 1 mm deep with oedema and necrosis of the bone marrow can be observed (Fig. 22). At the same time intensive formation of new bone commences, which after only a few days leads to the creation of a boundary layer running parallel with the surface of the foreign body and reaching it in places, though for the most part it is separated from it by a fine layer of connective tissue (Fig. 23). The spongiosa trabeculae keying with the cement retain their full mechanical efficiency even though the bone cells die off, and they may be expected to give sufficient mechanical hold generally until they are reinforced by the juxtaposition of new bone tissue (Fig. 24).

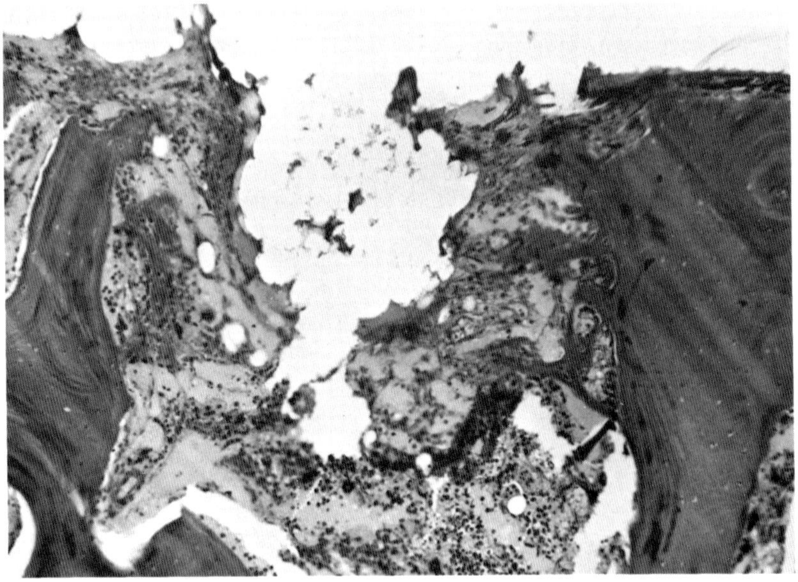

Fig. 22 Oedema in the layer adjacent to the cement (above, detached) after 8 days implantation in a dog (x 122)

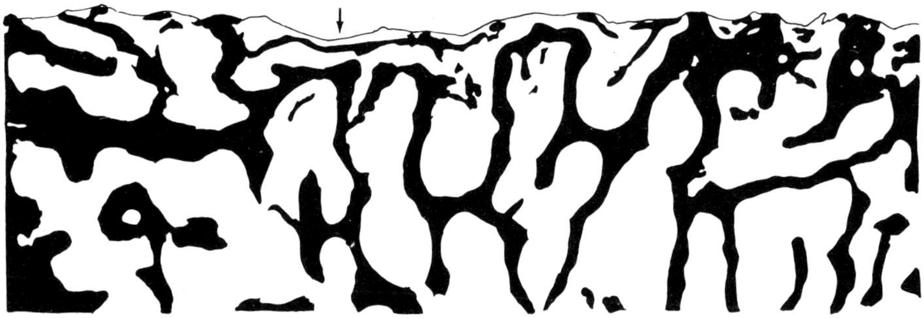

Fig. 23 Formation of a bone layer (↓) facing the bone, bone black, cement boundary above, after 18 days in a dog (x 58)

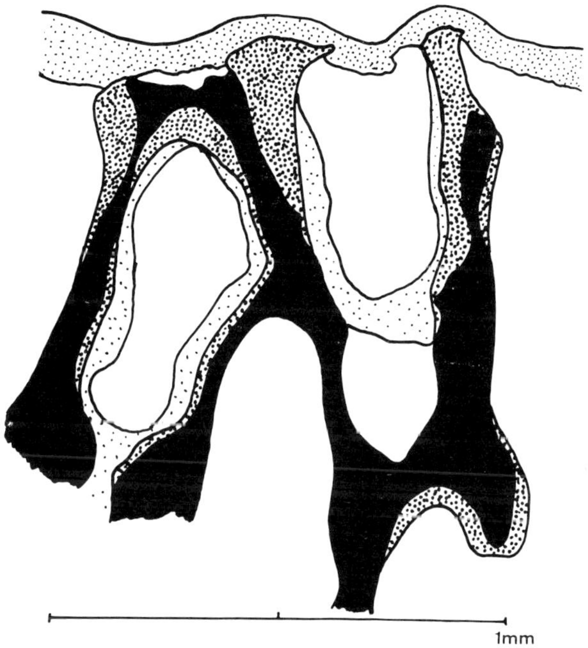

Fig. 24 Bone juxtaposition to support the cement.
Black: previous bone trabeculae.
Dotted areas: bone juxtaposition at various times, after 8 weeks in a dog (x 107)

However this bone building is accompanied at the same time by an accelerated breakdown of necrotic bone ridges. Of importance is that this breakdown must not proceed faster than the formation of new bone and that excessive mechanical loading is avoided during this reconstruction period, whose duration is as yet insufficiently known to us. Apart from continuous loading, in particular peak loads that might be applied play a major part.

It is very probable that not only for a short time after the implantation of cement but even after a period of years, local metabolic changes may still lead to alterations in the ratio of bone breakdown to new bone formation, and hence to detrimental effects. The best anchorage of the cement in the bone is provided by the restructuring of the fixing spongiosa, the principal role probably being played by the flat bone sheets connected to the spongiosa trabeculae keyed with the cement, which adhere firmly to excised pieces (Fig. 25).

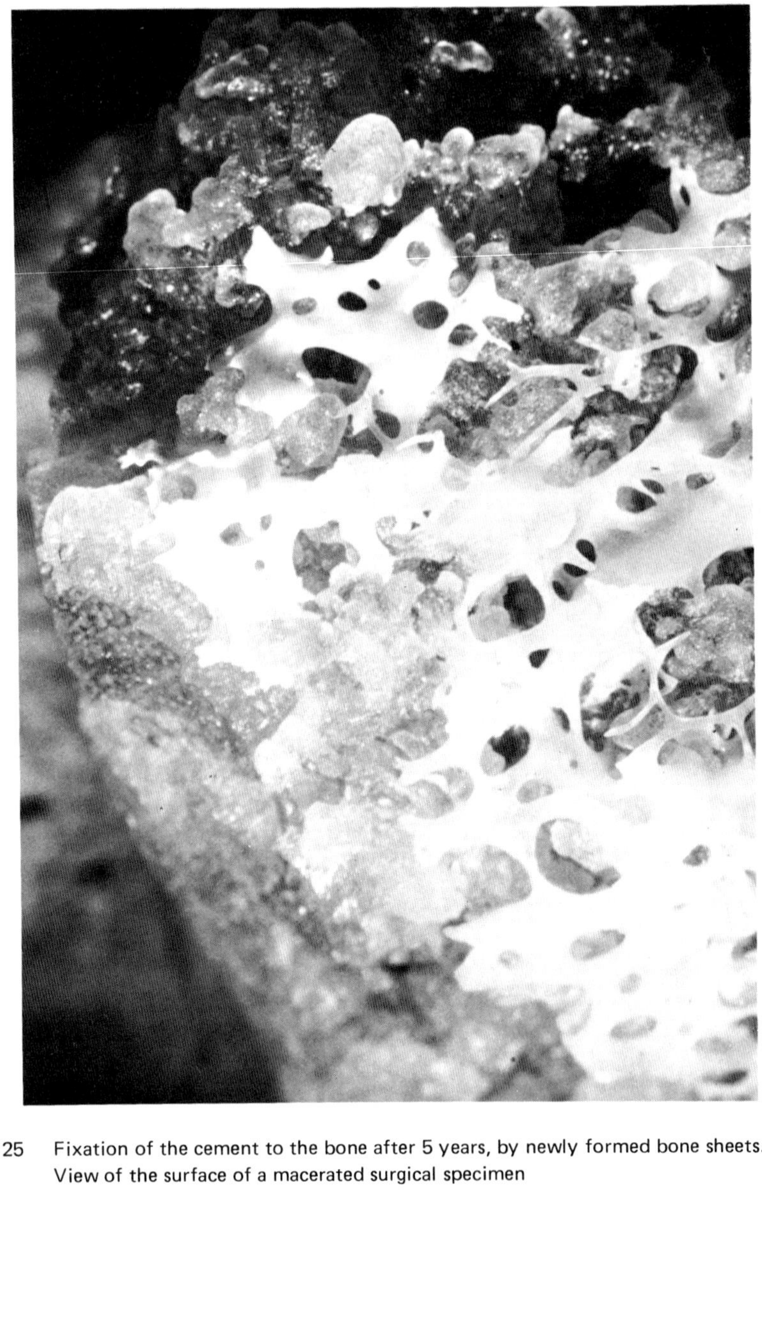

Fig. 25 Fixation of the cement to the bone after 5 years, by newly formed bone sheets. View of the surface of a macerated surgical specimen

REFERENCES

1. Bechtel, A., Willert, H.-G., Frech, H.A.: Bestimmung des Monomergehaltes von Methacryl-säure-methylester in Knochenmark, Fett und Blut nach dem Aushärten verschiedener "Knochenzemente". Chromatographia 6, 226 (1975)
2. Charnley, J.: Anchorage of the femoral head prosthesis to the shaft of the femur. Journal of Bone and Joint Surgery 42-B, 28 (1960)
3. Charnley, J.: Acrylic cement in orthopaedic surgery, Edinburgh and London: E. & S. Livingstone 1970
4. Debrunner, H.U.: Die Verträglichkeit von Polymethylmethakrylat. Zeitschrift für Orthopädie 83, 557 (1953)
5. Gluck, Th.: Referat über die durch das moderne chirurgische Experiment gewonnenen positiven Resultate, betreffend die Naht und den Ersatz von Defekten höherer Gewebe, sowie über die Verwertung resorbierbarer und lebendiger Tampons in der Chirurgie. Archiv für klinische Chirurgie 41, 187 (1890)
6. Haboush, E.J.: A new operation for arthroplasty of the hip. Bulletin of the Hospital for Joint Diseases 14, 242 (1953)
7. Henrichsen, E., Jansen, K., Krogh-Poulsen, W.: Experimental investigation of the tissue reaction to acrylic plastics. Acta Orthopaedica Scandinavica 22, 141 (1953)
8. Hofer, P.: Die Porosität von Knochenzementen, Dissertation at the Berne University 1975
9. Holland, Ch.J., Kim, K.C., Malik, M.I., Ritter, M.A.: A histologic and hemodynamic study of the toxic effects of monomeric methylmethacrylate. Clinical Orthopaedics 90, 262 (1973)
10. Homsy, Ch.A.: Implant stabilization. Orthopaedics Clinical N. Amer. 4, 295 (1973)
11. Judet, J.: Protheses en resine acrylic. Memoires de l'Academie de Chirurgie 73, 561 (1947)
12. Judet, J., Judet, R., Lafrange, J., Dunoyer, J.: Resection-reconstruction de la hanche, Paris: 1952
13. Kiaer, M.S.: Experimental investigation of the tissue reaction to acrylic plastics. Soc. intern. Chir. Orthop. 5 e Congres, Stockholm 1951, p. 534
14. Meyer, P.R.jr., Lautenschlager, E.P., Moore, B.K.: On the setting properties of acrylic bone cement. Journal of Bone and Joint Surgery 55-A, 149 (1973)
15. Müller, M.E.: Die Verwendung von Kunstharzen in der Knochenchirurgie. Archiv für orthopädische und Unfall-Chirurgie 54, 513 (1962)
16. Ohnsorge, J., Grötz, J.: Kurzzeitige und langzeitige Dimensionsänderung des aushärtenden Knochenzementes. Zeitschrift für Orthopädie 112, 975 (1974)
17. Semlitsch, M., Anliker, W., Willert, H.G.: Die Monomerabgabe von aushärtendem Knochen-zement in Abhängigkeit von der Verarbeitungstechnik. Sulzer Technische Mitteilung T 80/75, 1975
18. Smith, D.C., Bains, M.E.D.: The detection and estimation of residual monomer in polymethylmethacrylate. Journal of Dental Research 35, 16 (1956)
19. Smith, D.C.: Lutes, glues, cements and adhesives in medicine and dentistry. Biomedical Engineering 8, 108 (1973)
20. Spealman, C.R., Main, R.J., Haag, H.B., Larson, P.S.: Monomeric methylmethacrylate. Industr. Medicine 14, 292 (1945)
21. De Wijn, J.R., Sloof, T.J.J.H., Driessens, F.C.M.: Characterization of bone cements. Acta Orthopaedica Scandinavica 46, 38 (1975)

22. Wiltse, L.L., Hall, R.H., Stenehjem, J.C.: Experimental studies regarding the possible use of self-curing acrylic in orthopaedic surgery. Journal of Bone and Joint Surgery 39-A, 961 (1957)

23. Willert, H.G.: Die quantitative Bestimmung der Abgabe von monomerem Methylakrylat verschiedener Knochenzemente an das umgebende Gewebe während der Polymerisation. Battelle Information 18, 1-7 (1973)

24. Willert, H.G., Frech, H.A., Bechtel, A.: Measurements of the Quantity of Monomer Leaching out of Acrylic Bone Cement into Surrounding Tissues during the Process of Polymerization. Symposium Biomedical Applications of Polymers, Plenum Publishing Corporation (1973), pp. 121-133

PROBLEMS ASSOCIATED WITH THE CEMENT ANCHORAGE OF ARTIFICIAL JOINTS

H.-G. Willert and M. Semlitsch

In artificial joint replacement the parts of the endoprosthesis are fixed to the bone by means of the self-curing bone cement methylmethacrylate (MMA). Before implantation it is necessary to prepare a proper bed in the bone. For instance, in the proximal end of the femur, after removal of the femoral head, a channel must be made in the marrow cavity and some of the cancellous bone has to be removed; by this means the network of the bone trabeculae is cracked (Fig. 1). The cement dough, which is now pressed into the implant bed enters the marrow spaces under pressure, forming fingerlike protrusions.

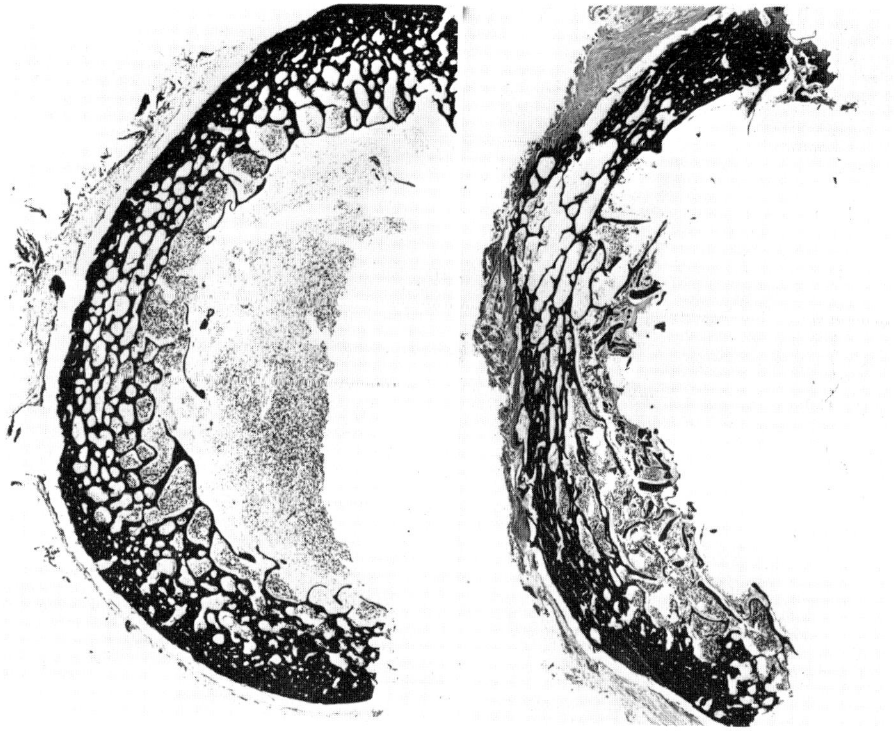

Fig. 1 Cross-sections through the shaft of the femur. Macrophotograph 8:1.
Left: Intact bone and bone marrow, no implant.
Right: Cracked spongiosa and opened marrow spaces 9 weeks after implantation of cement and prosthesis

The resulting interdigitation between bone and cement provides the fixation of the implant. The loadability of the bone is increased, as the load transmission from the prosthesis to the bone is more equally distributed than without using cement (2,3,5,20,22). The cement is fixed in the bone only mechanically by the irregular protrusions between the supporting bone pillars. A chemical bond between the tissue and bone cement does not occur.

The shape of the surface of the cured cement gives an idea of the quality of its fixation in the bone: An irregular surface indicates good fixation in the cancellous bone. A smooth surface indicates poor fixation in the compacta of sclerotic bone (Fig. 2).

In this article we look more closely at the problems associated with the cement anchorage of joint prosthesis.

Our discussion is based mainly on the results of our own investigations, which to date, have been published only in part (24-28).

The implantation of cement and endoprosthesis causes changes at the interface between cement and tissue as well as between prosthesis and bone cement. These changes are important because they may influence the durability of the implant's fixation.

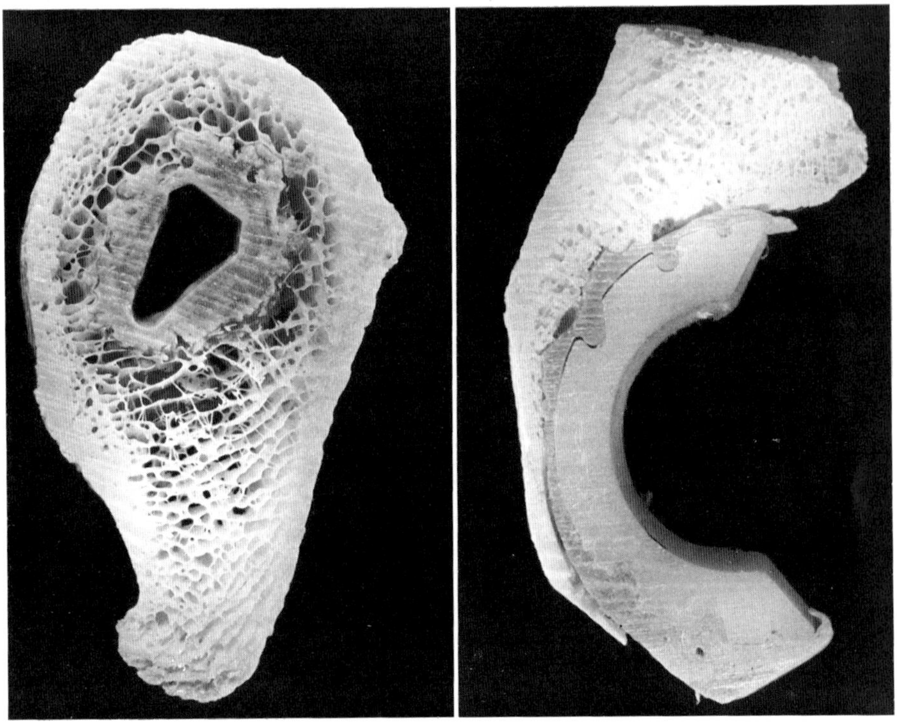

Fig. 2 Left: Good fixation of the bone cement in the cancellous bone of the proximal femur by multiple protrusions. Macrophotograph 3:1

Right: Poor fixation of the bone cement in the sclerotic and subchondral bone. Macrophotograph 2:1

TISSUE CHANGES

Actually this concerns the reaction of the tissue to the implanted cement and includes several overlapping processes (Table 1):

1. immediately after implantation of the bone cement the adjacent bone and bone marrow die, that is, tissue necrosis sets in;
2. the tissue develops a foreign body reaction against the foreign material; and
3. by remodeling the bone adapts to the changes in mechanical loading.

The necrosis of bone and bone marrow occurs within a layer, 3 mm deep, all around the implant (Fig. 3). Possible causes for the necrosis of the tissue are:

1. destruction of blood vessels
2. generation of heat by polymerization
3. toxicity of the monomer of the methylmethacrylate

All these influences become effective at the same time, namely at the moment of implantation.

The disconnected blood vessels lead to an interruption of the bloodflow within the proximal end of the femur: During preparation of the prosthetic bed in the femur, as a result of the removal of the femoral head and the contents of the marrow cavity, the intraosseous vessels of the upper end of the femur are damaged.

This applies to the descending metaphysial arteries, which are branches of the artery of the lateral femoral neck, as well as to the ascending branches of the nutritive artery (Fig. 4).

Table 1 The tissue reactions after implantation of cement and prosthesis

Bone and Bone-marrow			
After implantation	Due to	Result is	Surrounding tissue responds with
Immediately	preparation of implant bed	destruction of blood vessels tissue damage	death of tissue (necrosis)
	in situ polymerization of bone cement	generation of heat release of toxic monomer	
Early	insertion of the foreign material	irritation by the foreign body	foreign body reaction
Late	replacement of joint and skeletal parts by endoprosthesis	change of the mechanical load of the bone	adaptation of the bone by re-modeling (transformation)

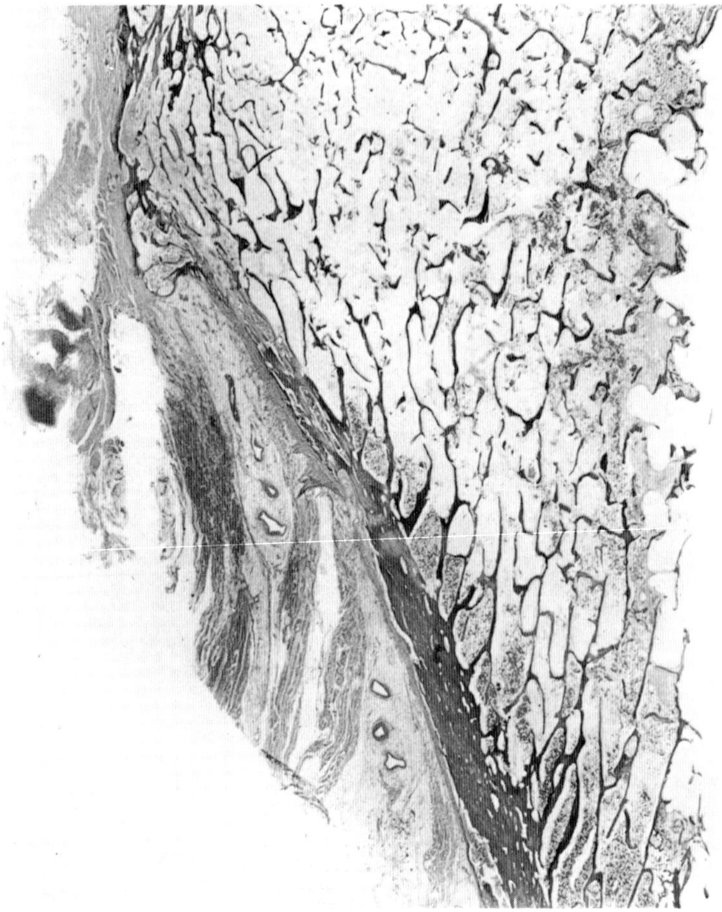

Fig. 3 Section through the greater trochanter of the femur, 10 weeks after implantation of a femoral head prosthesis. At the right edge irregular border between cancellous bone and cement. A layer of necrotic bone and bone marrow is adjacent to the cement. Macrophotograph 3:1

The heat generated during polymerization of the methylmethacrylate has been dealt with in more detail in another article in this book. Furthermore, the rise in temperature within the bone cement has been the subject of extensive studies published in recent literature (4,9,10,12,14,15,17,18,29).

On the other hand, information on the diffusion of the monomer into the surrounding tissue during the polymerization of the cement is still very scarce and incomplete.

For this reason we carried out several series of investigations to detect the amount of monomer leaching out of the cement:

We are justified in assuming that the greater part of the monomer evaporates from the cement during the process of polymerization. Therefore, samples of different types of

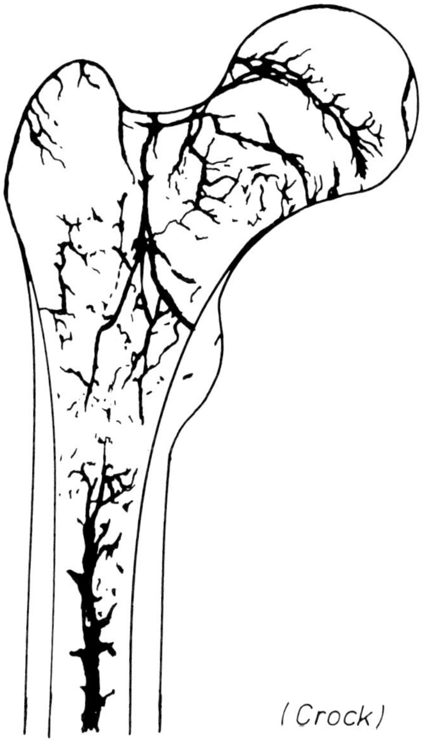

Fig. 4
Branches of the descending metaphysial arteries and of the ascending nutritive artery (1)

cement were placed in a test medium after previous polymerization to the same degree of consistence. Then the cement sample was allowed to polymerize completely within the medium.

In the first study, the test medium used was human bone marrow, which was removed from the femur during operation. Up to 60 hours after the cement samples (* CMW Bone Cement, Palacos-R, Sulfix 6) had hardened completely, we separated the bone marrow by centrifugation into three fractions (1. pure fat, 2. fibres, cells and fatty substances, 3. erythrocytes) and determined the content of monomer in each fraction quantitatively by gas chromatography.

We found that of the tissue components in particular the fat of the marrow extracts from the superficial layers of the cement the monomer which has not yet polymerized (26). The monomer attains a concentration in the tissue exceeding 0.01 % by weight and therefore reaches cytotoxic doses (11,13).

Similar results were obtained in a second study: Instead of bone marrow we used n-heptan as test medium. The amount of monomer leached out of the cement was determined by infrared-spectrophotometry (Fig. 5).

In both tests we found that Sulfix 6 evaporated the comparatively smallest quantity of the monomer. Also the introduction of this cement by syringe gave rise to no higher values.

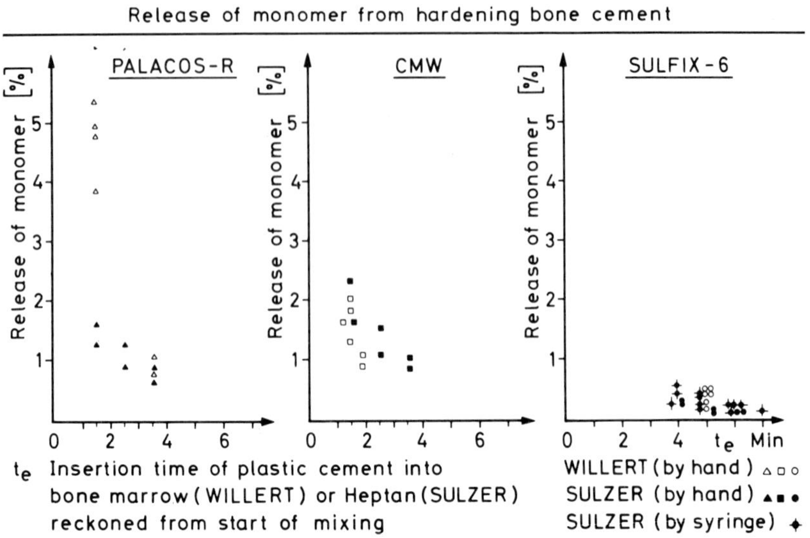

Fig. 5 Release of the monomer from different types of polymerizing bone cement

The tissue reaction to the detrimental influences mentioned above progresses through 3 phases (Fig. 6).

1. The post-operative tissue damage begins when the artificial joint is implanted, and covers the development of the first tissue reactions within the following 2-3 weeks.
2. In the second phase the repair of tissue damage occurs. It extends from the third week over several months and may even last a year or longer.

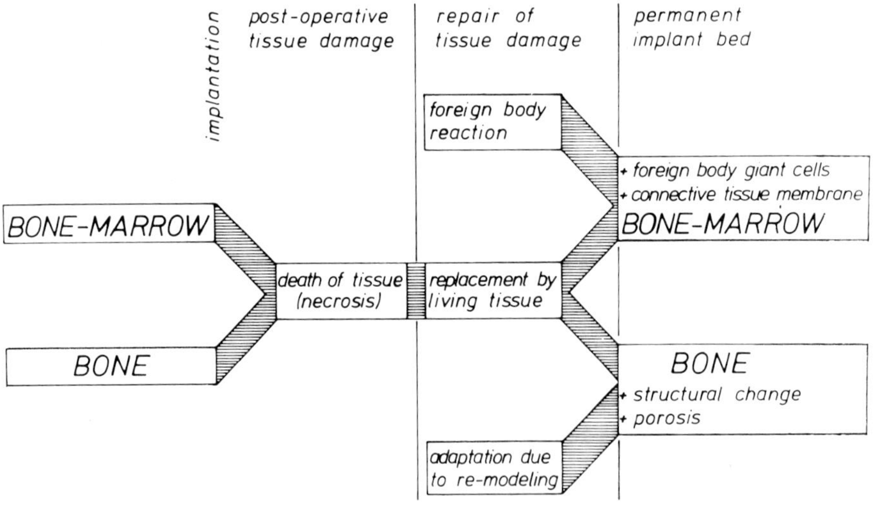

Fig. 6 Changes in tissue and bone structure after implantation of a prosthesis

3. The permanent implant bed is prepared after the tissue reaction has so far subsided that a certain balance between implant and bed is established. According to our examinations this stage is reached at the latest two years after the implantation.

The formation of necrosis during post-operative tissue damage morphologically resembles a bone infarct.

The necrotic area is demarcated from the intact tissue by a zone of hyperemia. After a short while an organization process starts from the vessels of the intact surroundings. First of all phagocytes remove the fat from the necrotic marrow, which process is called lipophagia. Thereafter fingers of connective tissue and capillaries invade the necrotic area. This process indicates the beginning of the repair of tissue damage. During this phase the damaged bone marrow is replaced by a reticulum of collagenous fibres and in the deeper parts of the marrow spaces hemopoietic bone marrow as well as fat marrow gradually reappears. At the contact surface to the acrylic cement the process of tissue regeneration is partly concealed by the foreign body reaction to the implant, recognized by the presence of foreign body giant cells.

In the course of marrow organization there begins a remodeling of the bone, during which dead bone is resorbed (Fig. 7) and at the same time new bone produced. The new bone is formed either as coarse fibrillar bone by metaplasia within the connective tissue, or as lamellar bone by accretion of new bone lamellae to the existing trabeculae.

After complete disappearance of tissue necrosis the repair of tissue damage, after 2 years at the latest, establishes the permanent implant bed. It is characterized by the persistance of a thin connective tissue membrane at the boundary with the bone cement. Its collagenous fibres are orientated parallel to the surface of the cement. The membrane covers

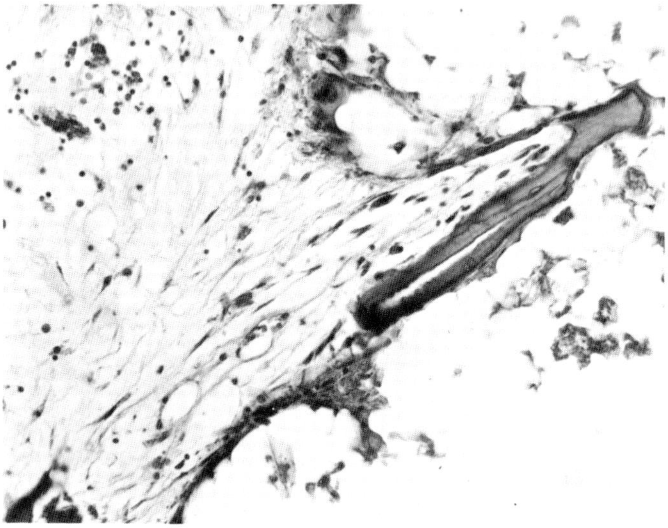

Fig. 7 Fibroosteoclastic resorption of a bone trabeculum adjacent to the acrylic cement, 11 weeks after implantation. Macrophotograph 200:1

the bone marrow and the bone (Fig. 8). The surface on the other side of the membrane facing the cement is occupied by multinucleate foreign body giant cells (Fig. 9). The marrow spaces beyond the connective tissue membrane contain regular hemopoietic bone marrow and fat cells in varying distribution (Fig. 10). The bone of the implant bed has, meanwhile, become virtually completely revitalized, although the remodeling processes are still going on.

The bone remodeling, which aims at a replacement of the dead by new, living bone tissue is now based on a reorientation, which adapts the architecture of the bone to the changes in mechanical stress.

This adaptation process is subjected to laws already formulated by Wolff (30) and further developed by Pauwels (19): The structure of the bone, that is arrangement, density and quantity of the bone tissue, correlates everywhere to the tensile and compressive stress. A change of the flux of force causes a corresponding change of the bone structure. This is known to take place as follows:

- by the remodeling of the cancellous architecture within the femoral neck after intertrochanteric displacement osteotomy,
- by the modification of the vertebral bodies in cases of scoliosis; here also adjust the trabeculae of the spongiosa into the direction of load,
- by the enlargement of the Haversian channels (Fig. 11) of the compact bone in cases of immobilization osteoporosis (23).

At the proximal end of the femur the stressing pattern changes fundamentally after insertion of the endoprosthesis: The tensile and compressive stress in the shaft is no longer transmitted from the femoral head through the neck into the shaft, but the load is now transferred from the cement implant to the shaft (Fig. 15). The result of this is a rearrangement of the trabeculae in a more parallel position to the cement surface, as well as a rarefication of the bone, that is, an osteoporosis (Fig. 12).

THE CHANGES AT THE SURFACE OF THE BONE CEMENT

During the insertion, the loss of the monomer by evaporation as well as the shift of the cement dough leads to a disturbance in the bond of the polymer particles (Table 2). There is too little or no interconnection between the particles so that these remain more or less isolated. Therefore, between the particles there appear spaces and clefts so that the structure looks like a wide-meshed texture (Fig. 13). Cells grow into the clefts and pores of the cement, so that the structure of the tissue then provides an exact copy of the finer structure of the cement surface (Figs. 8 and 9). Under the mechanical loading caused by micro-movements of the cement plug individual, or groups of particles, may be broken out of the bond and can then be found as fragments of polymethylmethacrylate (PMMA) in the connective tissue in the neighbourhood of the cement implant.

In the recent literature, another problem has been discussed: the degree of shrinkage during hardening of the cement.

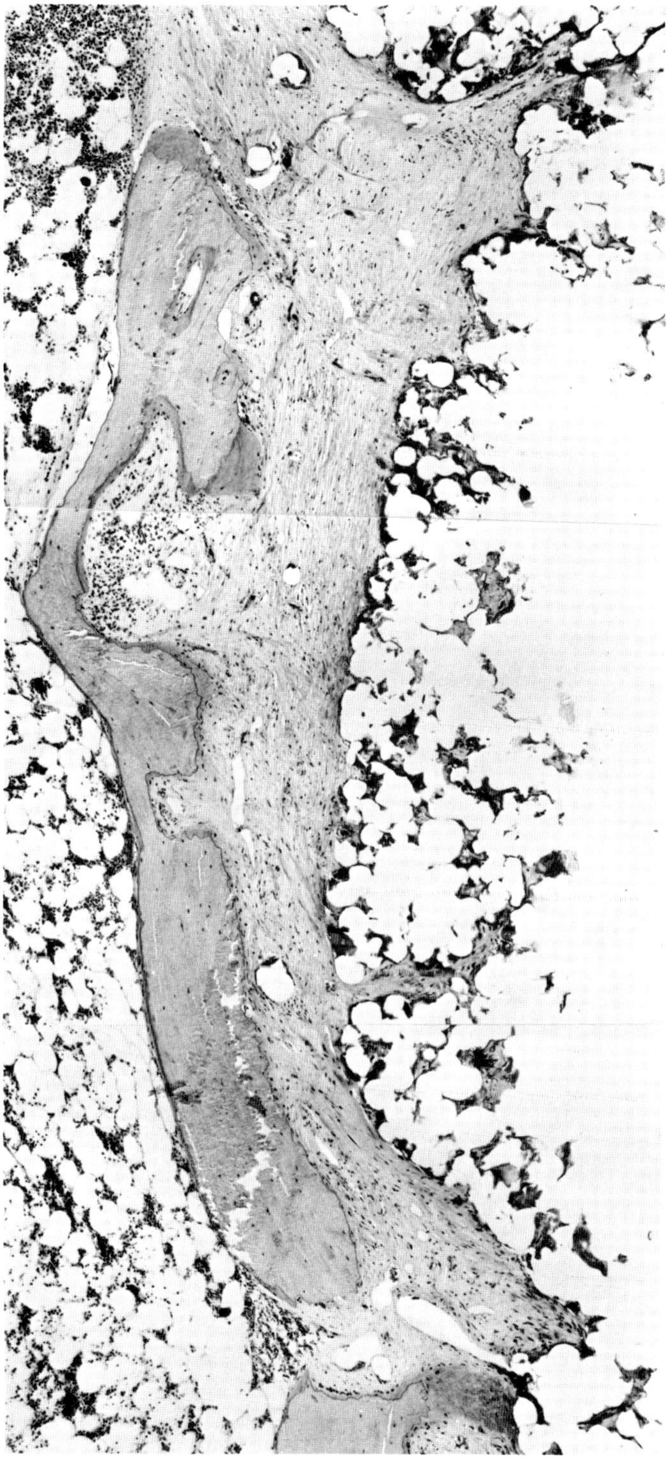

Fig. 8 Osseous abutment of the cement cage, 5 years after implantation. Tissue septa surround empty spaces where the cement was dissolved during preparation of the specimen. Macrophotograph 65:1

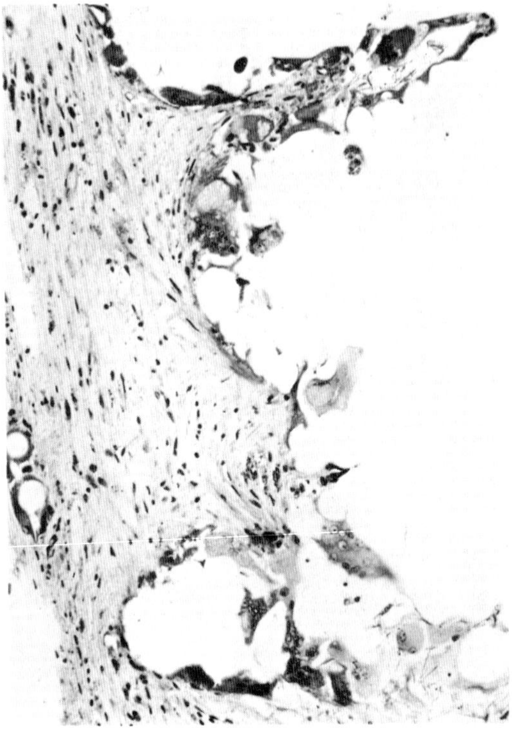

Fig. 9 Foreign body giant cells, lining the connective tissue membrane, 4 years after implantation of a femoral head prosthesis with bone cement. Macrophotograph 32:1

The measurements reported (4,6,8,16) show a shrinkage of up to 5 %. These values have been determined by volumetric measurements, starting at an early stage of polymerization. They represent a shrinkage in all three dimensions (Table 3). Schneider and Eulenberger (21) pointed out that a better approximation to the clinical application would be a measurement of the linear shrinkage. For the laboratory test they recommended the use of a steel tube. On the basis of this suggestion and the studies of de Wijn (7), we carried out the following experiments (Table 3, Fig. 14):

We put the cement dough (* CMW Bone Cement, Palacos-R, Simplex, Sulfix 6) into a steel tube and inserted a steel rod centrally half way up the cylinder. After hardening, the cement samples were taken out of the steel tube and immersed in a physiological salt solution at 37 °C for up to 64 days. The cement cylinders were measured after various time intervals at 6 points, 3 within and 3 beyond the position of the rod. The results of these measurements are as follows:

The part of the cement cylinder without rod shows a greater shrinkage than the part with rod. That means, the rod hinders the shrinkage of the cement. Furthermore, possibly owing to a better heat convection, the ends of the cylinder exhibit less shrinkage than the middle section. The four bone cements tested, differ markedly in the amount of shrinkage. Of these CMW Bone Cement shows the greatest, Sulfix 6 the smallest variations.

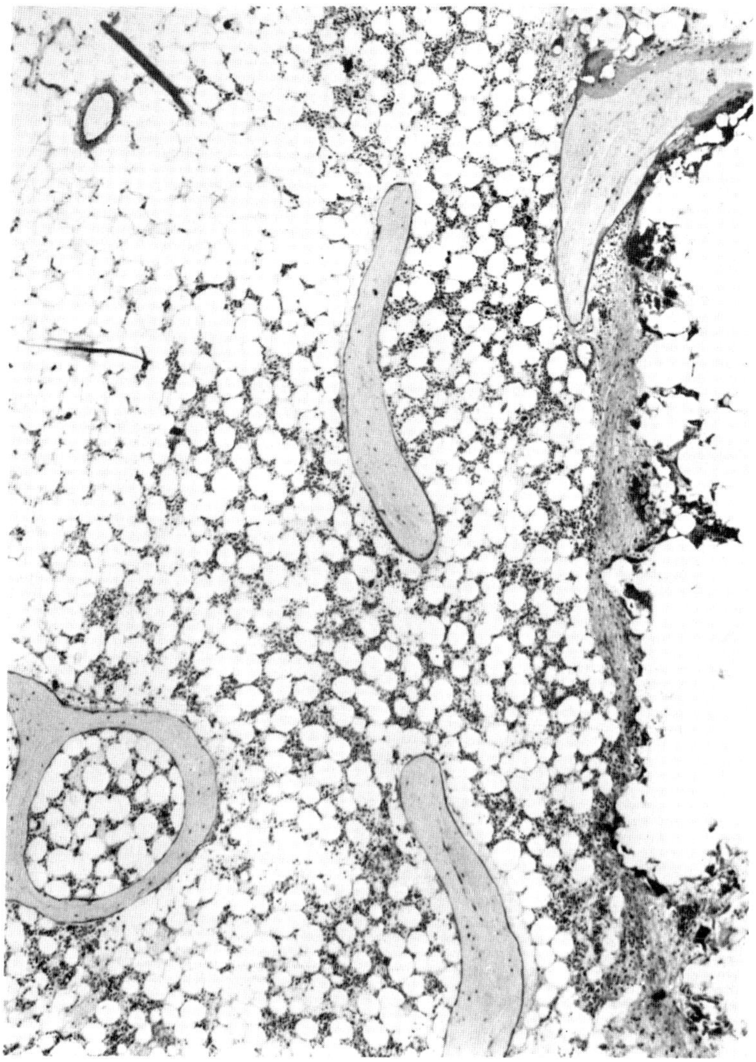

Fig. 10 Osseous abutment of the cement cage, 4 years after implantation. Hemopoietic bone marrow beyond the connective tissue membrane. Macrophotograph 32:1

The storage of the cement samples in salt solution results in a linear re-expansion of the specimens in the range of 0.2 to 0.3 % of the diameter. This means the shrinkage will be compensated to a certain extent by the subsequent swelling.

From our findings we conclude that the effects of shrinkage of the cement during hardening under clinical conditions are not as negative as one might have suspected.

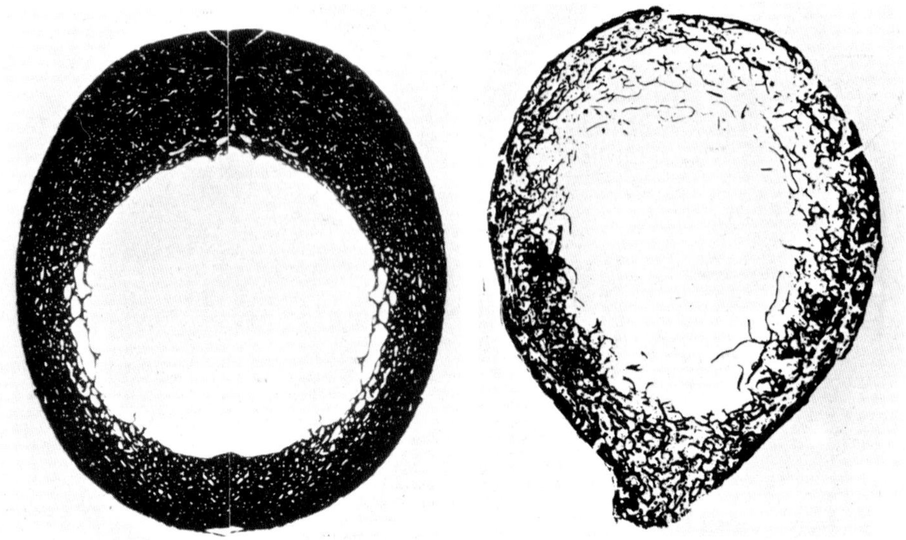

Fig. 11 Left: Cross-section through a shaft of a normal femur.
Right: Cross-section through a femur with severe osteoporosis due to inactivity.
Macrophotographs 2:1

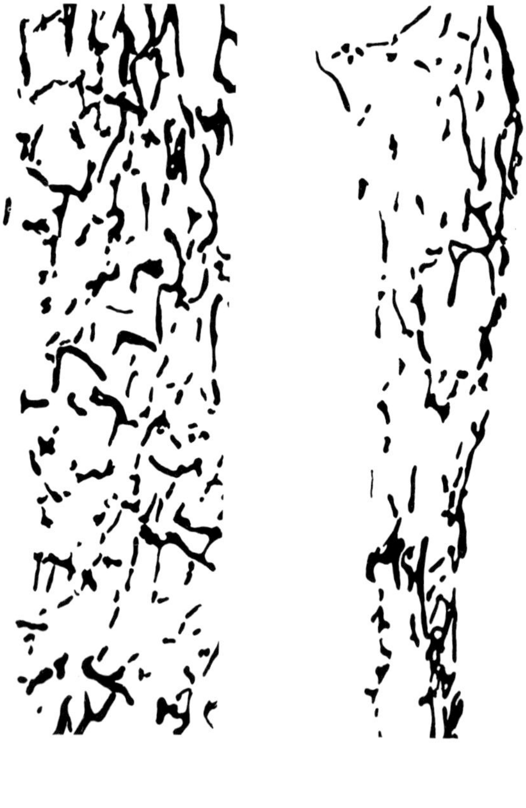

Fig. 12
The pattern of bone trabeculae has become completely transformed, as a result of remodeling and adaptation. Boundary to cement on the left. Drawings from Macrophotographs 20:1
Left: 11 weeks after implantation
Right: 4 years after implantation

Table 2 Changes at the surface of the bone cement after implantation

Bone Cement				
After implantation	Due to	Result is	Changes of the surface of the cement	
Immediately	contact with the tissue	evaporation of the monomer	disturbance of the superficial bond ⇒	mechanical weakening of the superficial structure
	introduction by force	formation of threads disarrangement and shift of the spheres		
Early	foreign body reaction of the tissue	cells growing around the cement surface	?	
Late	mechanical stress	micro movements of the cement plug	breaking of spheres of the bond ⇒	mechanical weakening of the anchorage

WHICH CONSEQUENCES RESULT FROM THE CHANGES OF THE IMPLANT BED AND THE BONE CEMENT IN PRACTICE?

Since the processes under discussion take place at the interface between tissue and cement, they are all in some way connected with the anchorage of the endoprosthetic parts (Fig. 6):

Apart from separating the tissue from the implant, the connective tissue membrane also has a favorable and desirable mechanical effect. Together with the giant cells and the adjacent bone marrow the membrane is able to damp minor movements of the implant (5), which are induced by the alternating loading and unloading between the rigid cement and the bone (Fig. 15). But if the micro-movements of the implant exceed the plasticity of the connective tissue layer, the result is damage to the tissue, which reacts with bleeding and exudation of fibrin.

This damage is then repaired by granulation tissue which organizes blood and fibrin and changes into a scar. The granulation tissue, on the other hand, is capable of resorbing the bone (Fig. 16), which leads to a diminution of bone anchors and a weakening of the mechanical cement fixation.

There is another mechanism of loosening of the implant, where the connective tissue membrane between bone and cement plays an important role (Fig. 17 and 18). We found that the membrane as well as the bone marrow adjacent to the implant can become involved in the foreign body reaction against wear products originating from the artificial joint surfaces. This happens, in particular when large amounts of particles were abraded and when the capsule around the joint is no longer capable of storing the particles and carrying them away. Then, within the connective tissue membrane between bone and cement, a foreign body granulation tissue develops which also induces a resorption of the adjacent bone (28).

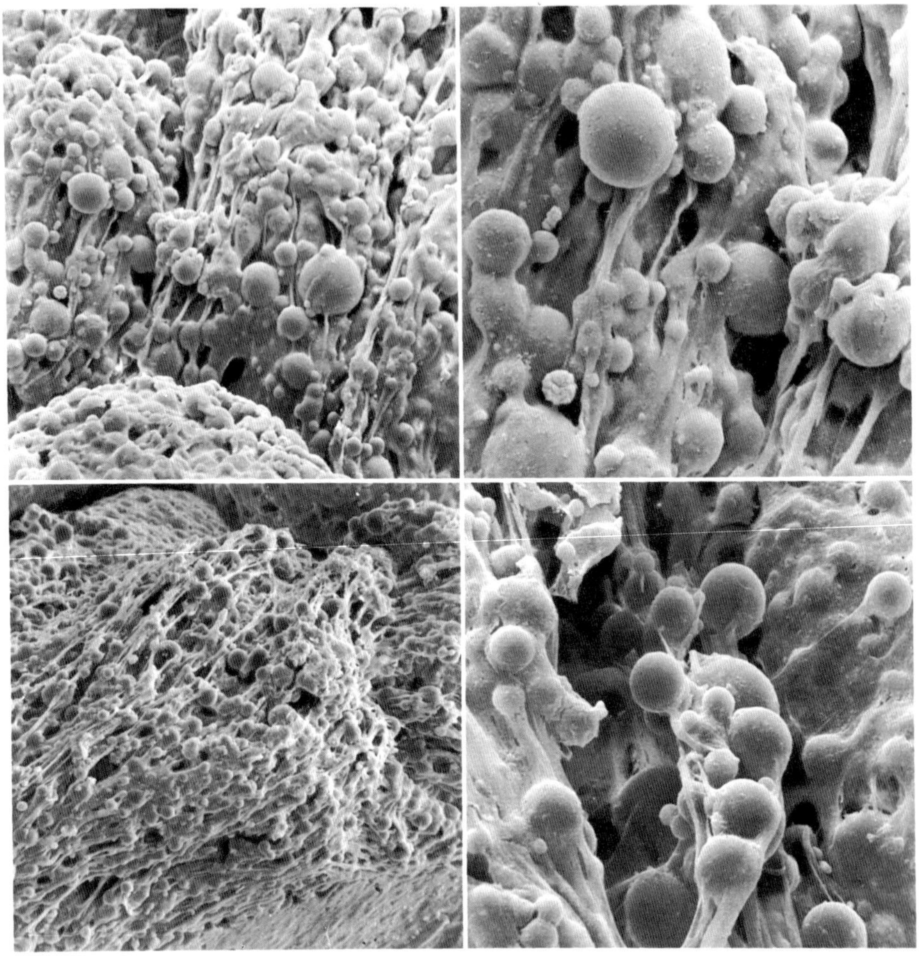

Fig. 13 Surfaces of bone cement pieces removed during re-operation. Particles are partly exposed and separated by gaps and clefts, partly connected and bridged by threads.
Scanning electron micrographs
Specimen 2 years 5 months after implantation
160:1 400:1
Specimen 5 months after implantation
80:1 290:1

The remodeling of the bone not only results in a re-orientation, but also in a diminution of the bone trabeculae (Fig. 12). First of all the necrotic trabeculae are concerned, that is, those which have had contact with the cement. In some of the old necrotic trabeculae resorption is not followed by a new formation of bone, but they are replaced by connective tissue (Fig. 7). Usually the newly formed trabeculae do not gain direct contact with the cement, but are separated by a connective tissue layer. But even if contact to the cement is established, the bone does not press so firmly against the implant as the cement was formerly pressed against the bone anchors at time of implantation.

Table 3 Shrinkage of different bone cements.
Above: Measurements of cubic shrinkage, reported in the literature.
Below: Linear shrinkage, measured by de Wijn and found in our own experiments

Cubic shrinkage (β) of bone cement (%) CMW	Palacos-R	Simplex	Sulfix-6	Method	References
3.00-5.00				A	1970—Charnley
0.85				Ba	1973—Hupfauer
2.18	2.41	1.80		Bb	
2.51				Bc	
2.20-2.50	2.20-2.50			C	1974—Ohnsorge
2.24-3.17	2.63-3.57	2.12-2.57	2.51	D	1974—Debrunner

$\beta = 3\alpha$
A = volumetric measuring method with cigar-shaped cement cylinders (66.2 g) in water
B = volumetric measuring method with cement balls (Ba...17.5 g/Bb...35 g/Bc...52.5 g) in water
C = buoyancy method with density measurement of cement bars (50x50x4 mm) in formamide
D = buoyancy method with density measurement of cement cylinders (39 mm diam.x 10 mm height) in water

Linear shrinkage (α) of bone cement (%) CMW	Palacos-R	Simplex	Sulfix-6	Method	References
0.33-0.41	0.35-0.38			E	1974—de Wijn
0.48-0.58	0.36 0.53	0.31-0.48	0.30-0.33	Fa	1975—Semlitsch
0.77-0.87	0.66-0.82	0.47-0.65	0.40-0.44	Fb	
0.19-0.33	0.12-0.17	0.12-0.27	0.04-0.06	Fap	
0.45-0.62	0.34-0.57	0.26-0.43	0.19-0.22	Fbp	

$\beta = 3\alpha$
E = linear shrinkage of cement cylinders in steel tube (i.d. 22 mm x 100 mm height) with central glass rod (10 mm diam.)
F = linear shrinkage of cement cylinders in steel tube (i.d. 20 mm x 100 mm height) with (Fa) and without (Fb) central steel rod (10 mm diam.) before and after 64-day exposure in 0.9 % physiological salt solution (Fap, Fbp)

All in all, the reduction and re-orientation of the bone trabeculae lead to a decrease in the mechanical fixation of the implant. The process of healing and repair at the implant bed does not result in an improvement in fixation of the implant. On the contrary the cement implant attains its greatest stability immediately after its implantation.

The bone carrying the prosthesis two years after the implantation is no longer the same as that into which the cement had been pressed at implantation.

The bone cement has by no means a compact surface everywhere, which we might expect having in mind specimens polymerized under laboratory conditions. Due to incomplete interconnection of the particles, the surface of the cement in the medullary space is rather disarranged and porous, so that a mechanical weakness of the cement can lead to the end of life of the anchorage.

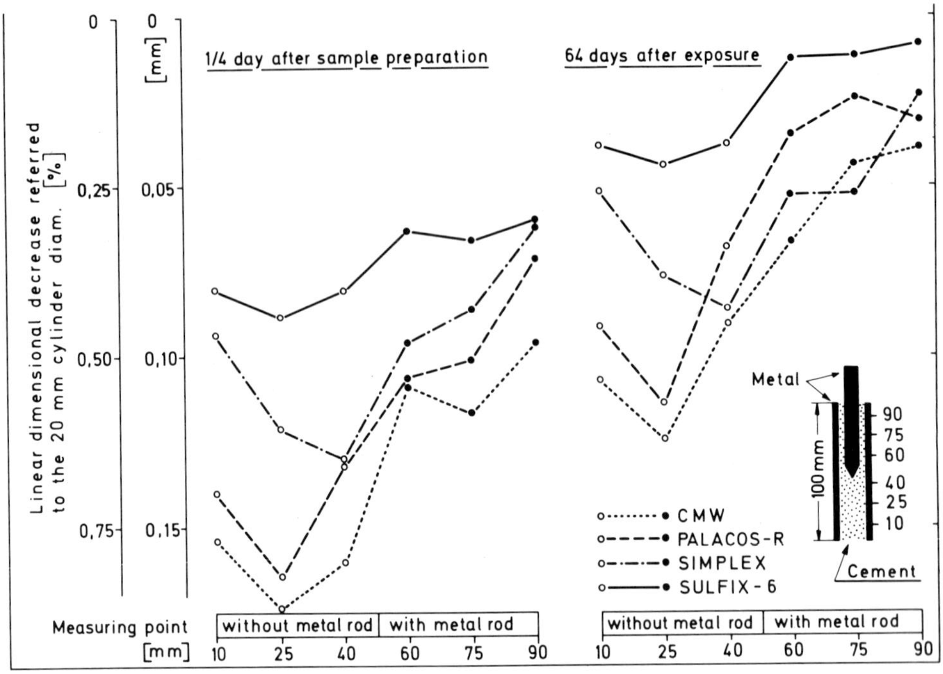

Fig. 14 Dimensional variation of bone cement 6 hours after preparation of the specimen and 64 days after exposure to 0.9 % salt solution at 37 °C

On the other hand, we feel that the shrinkage of the cement is not so important, since its linear dimension is relatively small and virtually completely compensated by the subsequent expansions.

All these processes, which result in a weakness of the cement anchorage, involve the danger of an implant loosening. However, the changes at the tissue and at the bone cement do not necessarily result in a loosening of the implant. This is proved by the fact that the majority of endoprostheses remain fully intact and highly functional for years without any recognizable change in their firm fixation. We know by clinical experience that, in the case of a well-cemented hip prosthesis the firmness of the anchorage, even after rebuilding of the bone bed, absolutely resists normal stressing.

Loosening is obviously only to be feared in the case of additional influences taking the form of an overstressing of the bony anchors or of the connective tissue membrane respectively. Such influences might be patient's overweight, extreme physical activity, wrong positioning and a high degree of friction of the artificial joint. Furthermore, in the case of poor technique with insufficient modeling or incomplete plugging of the implant bed, a concentration of the weight bearing in small areas of the bone results. Finally even an excessive production of wear particles from the joint surfaces can cause a loosening of the implant.

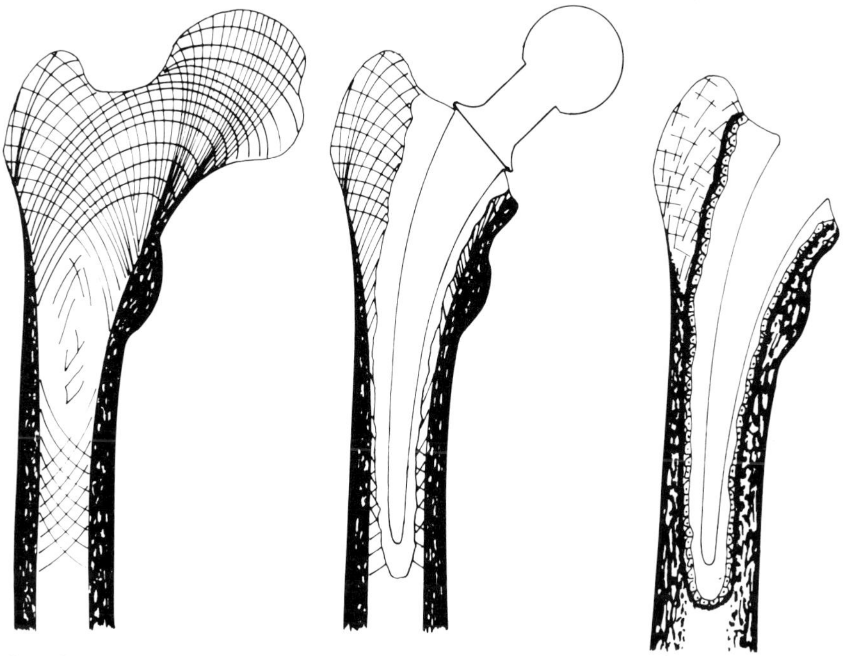

Fig. 15 Sketches of the proximal end of the femur.
Left: The cancellous bone is arranged in trabeculae which represent the direction of the tensile and compression forces (30).
Middle: Immediately after implantation of a femoral head prosthesis with bone cement (postoperative tissue damage).
Right: The permanent implant bed has been established: Bone and cement are separated by a connective tissue membrane. Additionally the surface of the bone cement is covered with foreign body giant cells. The bone has become porotic and adapted due to bone remodeling

Should a loosening of the prosthesis take place already in the first months after implantation, namely during the repair of tissue damage, we call this "early loosening". A reason for the early loosening might possibly be initial excessive removal of necrotic bone.

In the case of loosening long after the implantation when the permanent implant bed is established, we employ the term "late loosening". Here mechanical overstressing either of the connective tissue membrane or of the bone anchors, as well as the spreading of the foreign body reaction against wear particles to the connective tissue membrane may have resulted in a further resorption of bone and therefore in a further decrease of stability.

In any case, a loosening of the implant will progress and cannot be stopped. As soon as greater movements between the cement plug and the bony bed are possible, an increased surface abrasion of cement particles has to be considered.

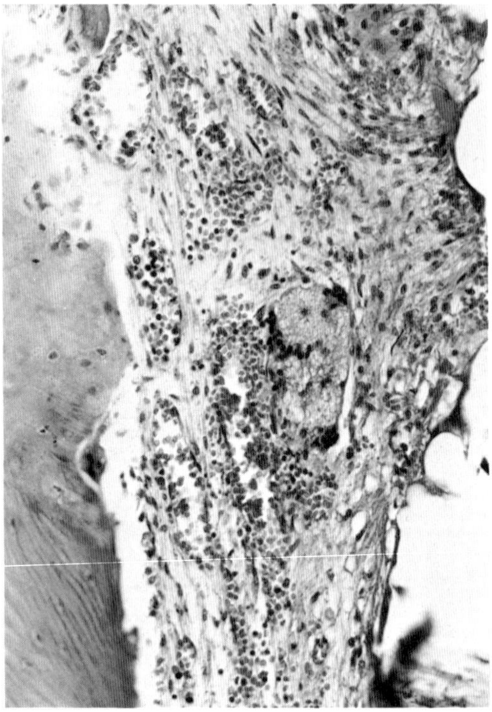

Fig. 16
Tissue membrane surrounding bone cement, empty space at the right edge, 4 years after implantation. The membrane shows hemorrhages and resorption of bone by osteoclasts, indicating mechanical stress and microtrauma. Macrophotograph 200:1

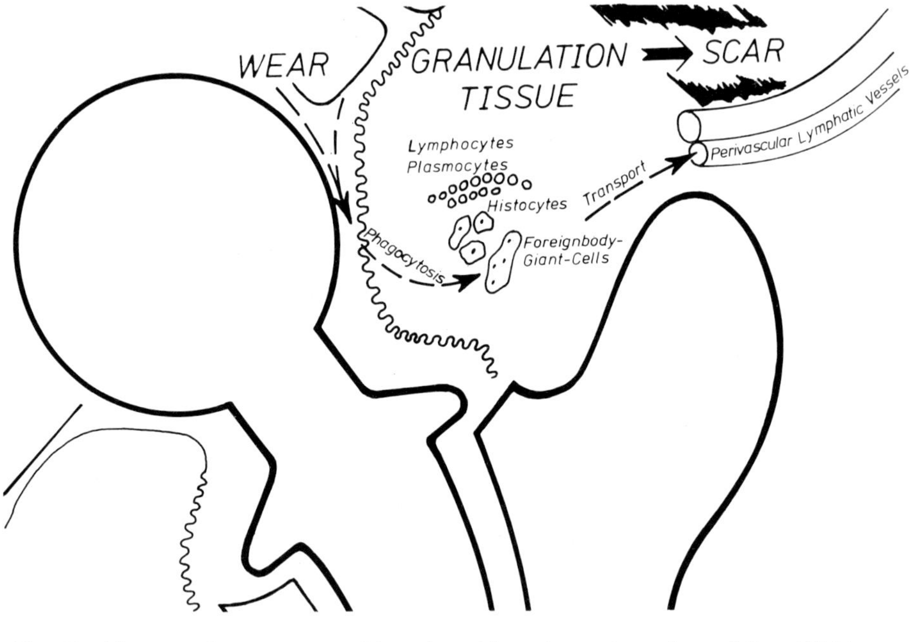

Fig. 17 Tissue reactions to wear particles, released from the moving surfaces of the artificial joint. Small amounts of foreign material can be carried away without difficulty and without overloading the tissue

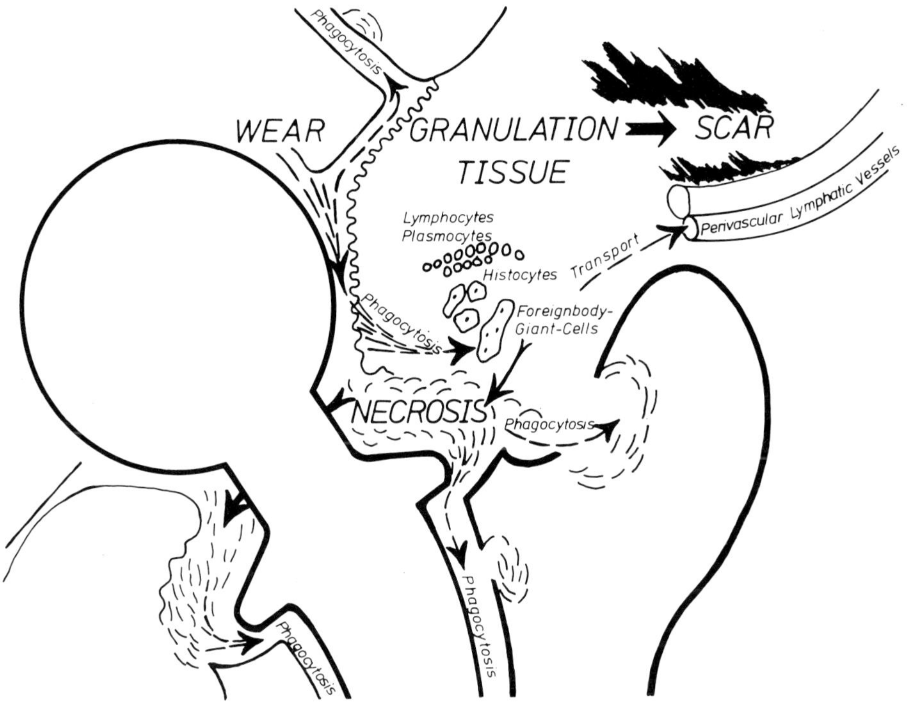

Fig. 18 Tissue reactions to an excessive release of wear particles. Granulation tissue within the articular capsule becomes necrotic. The bone marrow and the connective tissue membrane along the bone/cement interface is involved in the storage of particles and, as a result, in the foreign body reaction

Since the processes of resorption in the cancellous bone proceed more quickly than in the compact bone in the proximal femur, the cement loses its osseous abutment more excessive than in the distal part of the compact femur. Under loading a fracture of the proximal part of the cement cuff may first develop, possibly followed by a fatigue fracture of the prosthesis shaft (Fig. 19).

CONCLUSIONS REGARDING THE TECHNIQUE OF IMPLANTATION

1. The contact between cement and bone has to be as optimal as possible right from the moment of implantation. The cement must plug the implant bed completely. From the beginning the mechanical anchorage must be "overdimensioned" to such an extent that it holds the implant even after an atrophy of the osseous abutment.

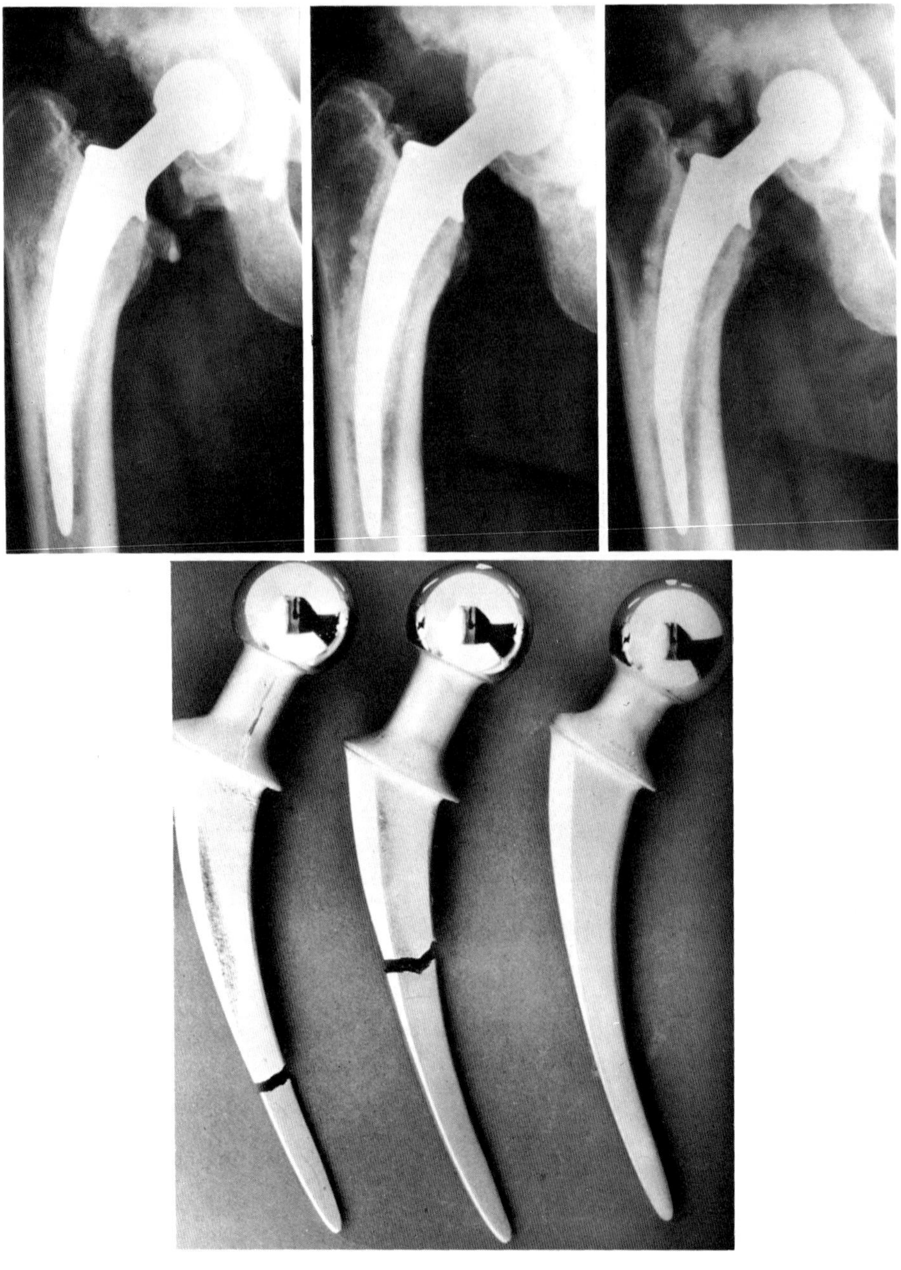

Fig. 19 Above: Consequences of faulty implantation technique. X-ray picture of a 63 years old man.

Left: 1 year 5 months after implantation. Cement does not extend to the distal tip of prosthesis. Loosening of the cement in the proximal end of the femur.

Middle: 1 year 6 months after implantation. Stem of the prosthesis is broken.

Right: 1 year 7 months after implantation. Dislocation of broken prosthesis fragments.

Below: Femoral prosthesis on the left is the one shown in the roentgenograms. For comparison, prostheses from other patients are shown. All three show polishing of the surface of the stem

2. The tissue damage in the implant bed should be as small as possible. For this reason careful preparation of the prosthetic bed is just as important as the right mixture ratio of the cement components and the right moment of implantation of the prosthesis into the femur.

3. Any overstressing of the mechanical anchorage must be avoided. It is therefore important that the prosthetic parts be cemented in the most optimal position, in order to ensure low friction of the artificial joint and to avoid shocks. Forced movements have to be avoided during post-operative exercises. Shock-absorbing heeled shoes reduce the mechanical loading on the anchorage during walking. Further aspects are reduction of overweight, moderate limitation of physical activity, and so on.

4. We should be aware that the production of wear particles from the joint surfaces may finally cause loosening of the implant. It is more likely that wear becomes a problem because it affects the fixation of the implant than because of wearing out of the parts of the prosthesis.

REFERENCES

1. Crock, H.V.: The blood supply of the lower limb bones in man. Edinburgh-London: Livingstone Ltd. 1967
2. Charnley, J.: The bonding of prostheses to bone by cement. Journal of Bone and Joint Surgery 46-B, 518 (1964)
3. Charnley, J.: Biomechanics in orthopaedic surgery. In: Biomechanics and Related Bio-Engineering Topics, Oxford-London-Frankfurt: Pergamon-Press 1965, pp. 99-110
4. Charnley, J.: Acrylic cement in orthopaedic surgery. Edinburgh-London: Livingstone Ltd. 1970
5. Charnley, J., Kettlewell, J.: The elimination of slip between prosthesis and femur. Journal of Bone and Joint Surgery 47-B, 56 (1965)
6. Debrunner, H.U.: Die Volumenanderungen von Knochenzementen während der Härtung. Archiv für orthopädische und Unfall-Chirurgie 81, 37 (1975)
7. De Wijn, J.R., Driessens, F.C., Slooff, Th.J.: Dimensional behavior of curing bone cement masses. Journal of Biomedical Materials Research Symposium 6, 99 (1975)
8. Hupfauer, W.: Volumenmessungen an Knochenzementen. Acta Traumatologica 3, 259 (1973)
9. Hupfauer, W.: In: O. Oest, K. Müller, W. Hupfauer, edit., Die Knochenzemente. Stuttgart: Ferd. Enke Verlag 1975, pp. 64-74
10. Lautenschlager, E.P., Moore, B.K., Schoenfeld, C.M.: Physical characteristics of setting of acrylic bone cement. Paper presented at the 5th Annual Biomaterials Symposium Clemson/S.C. (1973)
11. May, G.: Personal Communications (1973)
12. Meyer, P.R., Lautenschlager, E.P., Moore, B.K.: On the setting properties of acrylic bone cement. Journal of Bone and Joint Surgery 55-A, 149 (1973)
13. Mohr, H.J.: Pathologische Anatomie und kausale Genese der durch selbstpolymerisierendes Methacrylat hervorgerufenen Gewebsveränderungen. Zeitschrift für die gesamte experimentelle Medizin 130, 41 (1958)

14. Ohnsorge, J., Goebel, G.: Oberflächentemperaturen des abhärtenden Knochenzementes Palacos beim Verankern von Metallendoprothesen im Oberschenkelmarkraum. Archiv für orthopädische und Unfall-Chirurgie 67, 89 (1969)

15. Ohnsorge, J., Goebel, G.: Die Verwendung unterkühlter Metallendoprothesen in der Hüftchirurgie. Zeitschrift für Orthopädie 107, 683 (1970)

16. Ohnsorge, J., Groetz, J.: Kurzzeitige und langzeitige Dimensionsänderungen des aushärtenden Knochenzements. Zeitschrift für Orthopädie 112, 975 (1974)

17. Ohnsorge, J., Holm, R.: Änderungen der Spongiosafeinstruktur unter dem Einfluß des auspolymerisierenden Knochenzementes. Zeitschrift für Orthopädie 107, 405 (1970)

18. Ohnsorge, J., Kroesen, A.: Thermoelektrische Temperaturmessungen des abhärtenden Knochenzementes "Palacos". Zeitschrift für Orthopädie 106, 476 (1969)

19. Pauwels, F.: Gesammelte Abhandlungen zur funktionellen Anatomie des Bewegungsapparates, Berlin-Heidelberg-New York: Springer Verlag 1965

20. Scales, J.F.: Acrylic bone cement: Bond or plug. Journal of Bone and Joint Surgery 50-B, 698 (1968)

21. Schneider, R., Eulenberger, J.: Reoperationen von Hüftendoprothesen bei Instabilität, Prothesenfrakturen und Rekalzifizierung. Demonstrationsversuch der Schwindung von Knochenzement im Stahlzylinder. Presented on 6. Mainzer Unfall-Symposium (1973)

22. Slooff, Th.J.: The influence of the acrylic cement on the fixation of the hip endoprosthesis. Dissertation, Nijmegen: Thoben 1970

23. Willert, H.G.: Immobilisationsosteoporose. Langenbecks Archiv für klinische Chirurgie 315, 258 (1966)

24. Willert, H.G.: Tissue reactions around joint implants and bone cement. In: Arthroplasty of the Hip, Stuttgart: Georg Thieme Verlag 1973

25. Willert, H.G., Puls, P.: Die Reaktion des Knochens auf Knochenzement bei der Allo-Arthroplastik der Hüfte. Archiv für orthopädische und Unfall-Chirurgie 72, 33 (1972)

26. Willert, H.G., Frech, H.A., Bechtel, A.: Measurements of the quantity of monomer leaching out of acrylic bone cement into the surrounding tissues during the process of polymerization. In: H.P. Gregor, edit., Polymer Science and Technology, Biomedical Applications of Polymers, New York-London: Plenum Press, Vol. 7, pp. 121-133

27. Willert, H.G., Ludwig, J., Semlitsch, M.: Reaction of bone to methacrylate after hip arthroplasty. Journal of Bone and Joint Surgery 56-A, 1368 (1974)

28. Willert, H.G., Semlitsch, M.: Kapselreaktionen auf Kunststoff- und Metallabrieb bei Gelenkendoprothesen. Technische Rundschau Sulzer 2, 1 (1975)

29. Wiltse, L.L., Hall, R.H., Stenhjem, J.C.: Experimental studies regarding the possible use of selfcuring acrylic in orthopaedic surgery. Journal of Bone and Joint Surgery 39-A, 961 (1957)

30. Wolff, J.: Das Gesetz der Transformation der Knochen, Berlin: A. Hirschwald 1892

MECHANICAL PROPERTIES OF THE CEMENT/BONE BOND

R. Kölbel, G. Bergmann, and U. Boenick

It is to the introduction of acrylic bone cement by John Charnley, that we owe the breakthrough to routine total joint replacement. Charnley also gave us an initial analysis of the mechanics of fixation with cement — which still holds true — and an account of the morphological findings in post mortem specimens. Since fixation with cement has been such a success, we shall undertake to carry on with an analysis of its mechanics in order to proceed to even better solutions, possibly without acrylic cement.

As we now seem to know, the success of implant fixation depends largely on the mechanics of the interface and the reaction of living bone and not so much on the specific physical, chemical or mechanical properties of an otherwise inert material. In an analysis of interface mechanics, our first steps were tests to determine the mechanical properties of the cement/bone bond. The qualities of this bond form the basis for the bone remodeling process which leads to a functioning implant/bone interface.

MATERIALS AND METHODS

In hip and knee joint replacements the implants are anchored, at least partly, to cancellous bone, which, in the process of the operation, is devitalized to a certain extent and depth. We assume that during the initial phase of the implant fixation, that is, immediately after the operation, and from then on for several weeks, loads applied to implant and living bone are transmitted through and by a layer of dead bone. Hence we felt justified in applying in-vitro methods to determine the mechanical strength of the bond. There are two ways of testing this experimentally:

1. Simulation of a complete implant fixation in cadaveric bone and subjection to high loads in the physiological directions.
2. Simulation of an element of the zone of bonding and tests with normal and shearing forces.

We chose the second possibility because it gives us better control of the experiment and the interpretation of the results.

We cemented cancellous bone from femoral heads to blocks of PMMA, using Palacos bone cement (Fig. 1). Standardized test specimens for each of the tests were then produced on a lathe.

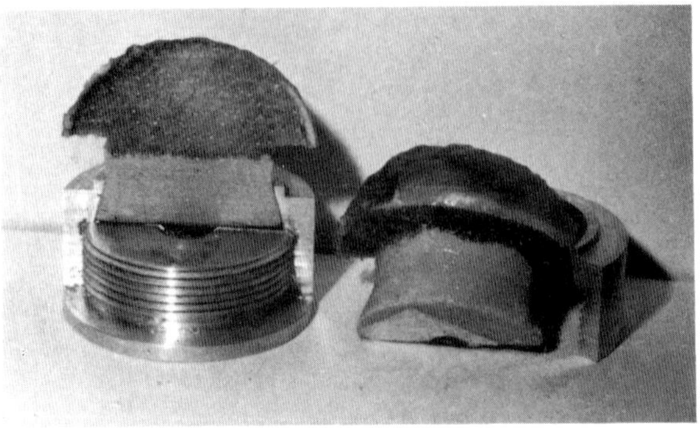

Fig. 1
Test specimen, femoral head and Palacos, for tensile test

In an initial series, specimens were subjected to static tensile loads (Fig. 2). 110 tests were performed on individual femoral heads from patients with osteoarthrosis and fracture of the neck of the femur. As can be seen in Table 1, the standard deviations were such that we did tests with pairs of test specimens manufactured from the same bone. Even so, the differences in the breaking loads of the "partners" of the same pair were considerable, although not as large as those for different pairs. On inspection (Fig. 3) of the fracture surfaces of all the specimens, we found that cancellous bone with normal and slightly hypertrophic trabeculae and interspaces large enough to allow deep penetration by cement gave better results than dense hypertrophic bone with narrow interspaces, or bone with wide interspaces but atrophic trabeculae. In almost all specimens with normal or wide interspaces, some bone was torn away with the cement block. In dense bone the separation occurred through fracture of cement plugs.

Static tests of shearing strength were done in two different experimental set-ups, in accordance with cases (a) and (b) in Fig. 4. In the first set-up we utilized cantilever type test specimens with a cylindrical cross-section (Fig. 5). These were subjected to a static shearing load, largely excluding bending moments. 57 test specimens were tested (Table 2).

In the second set-up we drilled cylindrical holes into the femoral head. A threaded bolt was cemented into this hole excluding the base in order to produce a cylindrical zone of bonding. A tensile force was applied to the bolt in order to produce a shearing force in the zone of bonding (Fig. 6). In this rig, which we also used for periodic testing, deformation was recorded against load: We found a non-linear behaviour, characteristic of viscoelastic materials (Fig. 7), and a creep curve which was linear on a double logarithmic scale. 19 specimens were tested (Table 2). Again we were impressed by the variation i.e. the standard deviations which are, however, common in biological materials. Differences in the results from the two different set-ups were highly significant for the fracture and cadavaric specimen groups. This is due to different arrangements of the cement/bone bond tested. The inspection of fracture surfaces showed more bone destruction than in the tensile tests in general and, specifically, even more so in specimens with higher breaking loads.

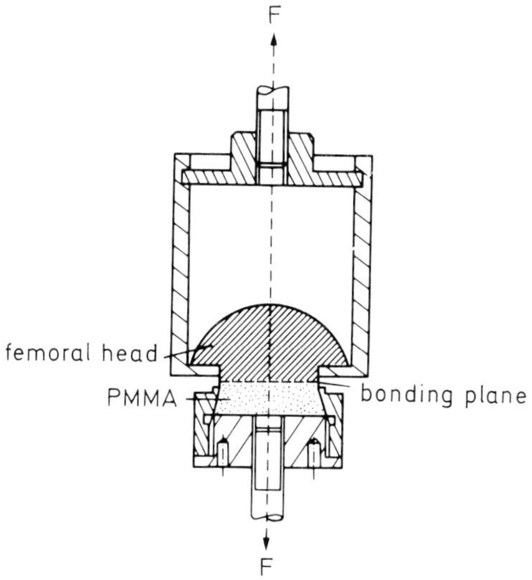

Fig. 2
Holding rig for tensile tests

Table 1 Average breaking load and average breaking stress, 110 tensile tests

	Static tensile strength	
	Load at failure	A.V. Breaking stress
Test specimens from femoral neck fractures	134.1 ± 65.5 Kgf	18.9 ± 9.2 Kgf/cm^2
Test specimens from osteoarthrosis	189 ± 83.3 Kgf	26.7 ± 11.8 Kgf/cm^2

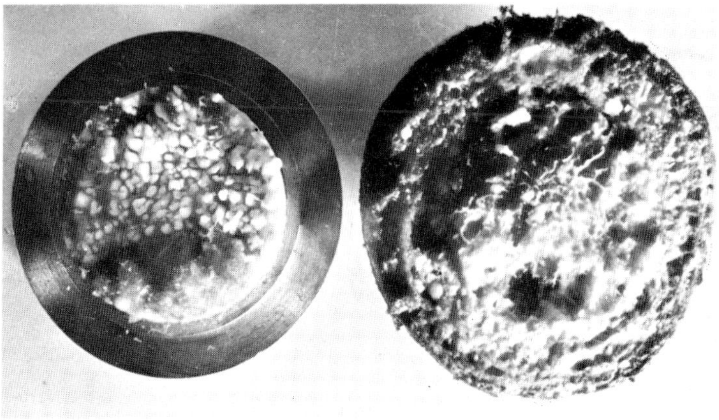

Fig. 3 Fracture surface after tensile test, area of bonding = 7.07 cm^2, breaking load 221 Kgf

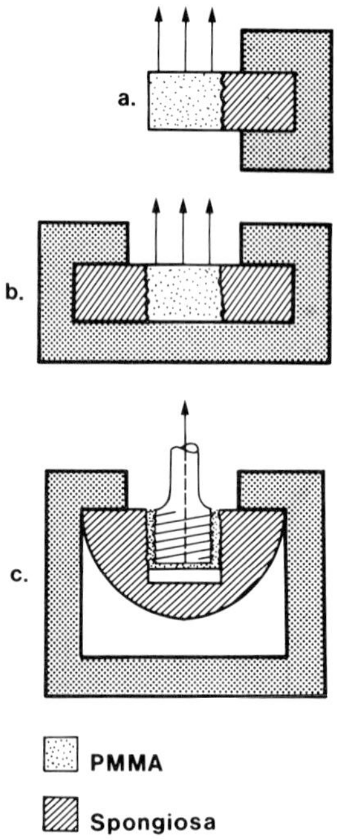

Fig. 4
Different arrangements for shear tests

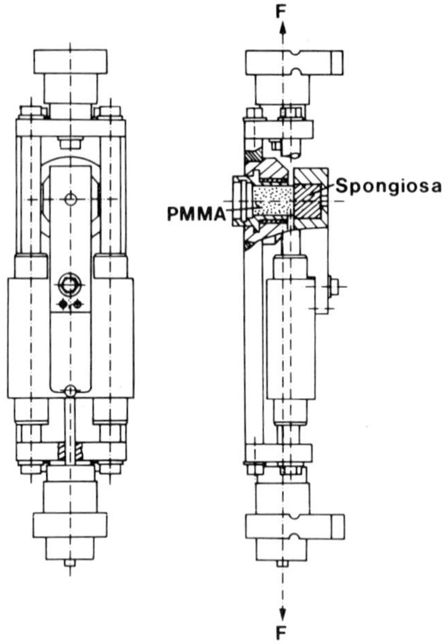

Fig. 5
Rig for static shear tests

We also did dynamic shear tests using the testing rig of Fig. 6 and a sinusoidal load characteristic (Fig. 8).

Table 2 Average results of static shear tests.
Set-up A: 57 tests using rig of Fig. 5
Set-up B: 19 tests using rig of Fig. 6

	Static shear strength (breaking stress)	
	Setup A	Setup B
Test specimens cadaveric and fracture	33.8 ± 5.6 Kgf/cm^2	54.6 ± 9.07 Kgf/cm^2
	$p < 0.0005$	
Test specimens osteoarthrosis	44.4 ± 15.5 Kgf/cm^2	60 ± 15.4 Kgf/cm^2
	$p < 0.1$	

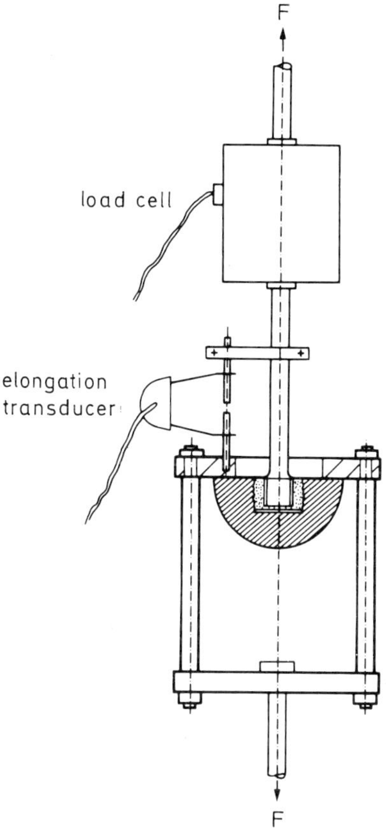

Fig. 6
Rig for static and cyclic shear tests

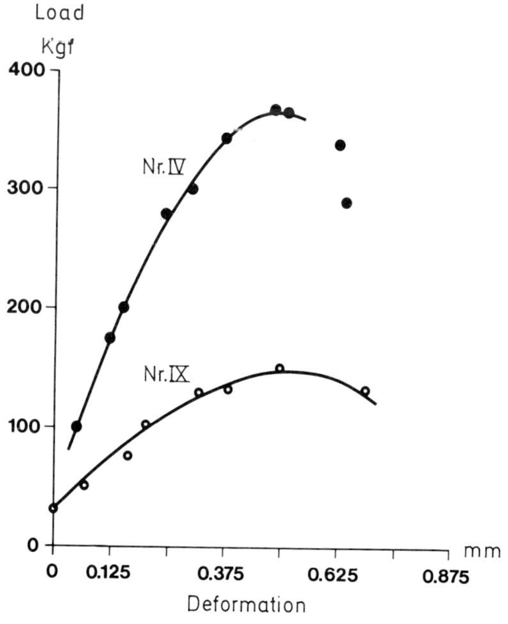

Fig. 7
Load deflection curves of shear tests;
load rate = 13 Kgf/sec,
cylindrical surface area = 5 cm^2.

Nr. IV: femoral head with coxarthrosis

Nr. IX: cadaveric specimen (normal senile)

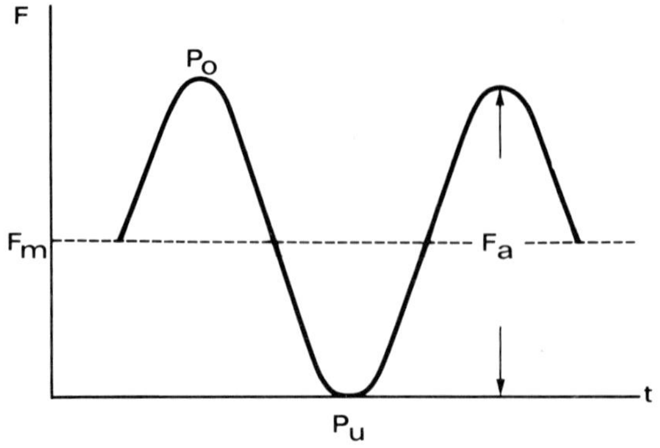

Fig. 8
Load characteristic for cyclic shear tests

16 specimens were subjected to cyclic loads. The cyclic load applied was referred to the static breaking load of a test specimen partner made of the same femoral head, or of the femoral head of the contralateral side. The load was therefore expressed in % of the static breaking load, F_{max} (Fig. 9). This to us looks something like a Wöhler-curve. It shows a trend towards higher numbers of load cycles before failure in specimens which were periodically loaded with around 50 % or less of the static breaking load.

Both after static and cyclic loading with this rig, a more or less complete cone of cancellous bone was torn out with the cement plug (Fig. 10). From the fracture surface it appeared that the fracture line or configuration was independent of trabecular orientation (Fig. 11). We are at present conducting cyclic tensile loading tests.

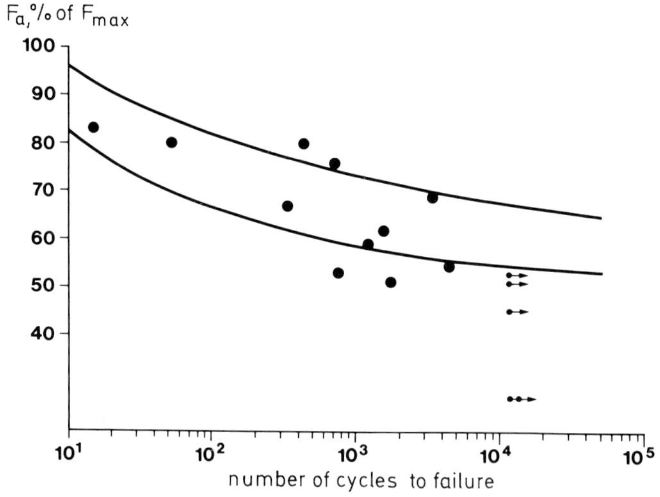

Fig. 9 Results of cyclic shear tests (f = 20/min)

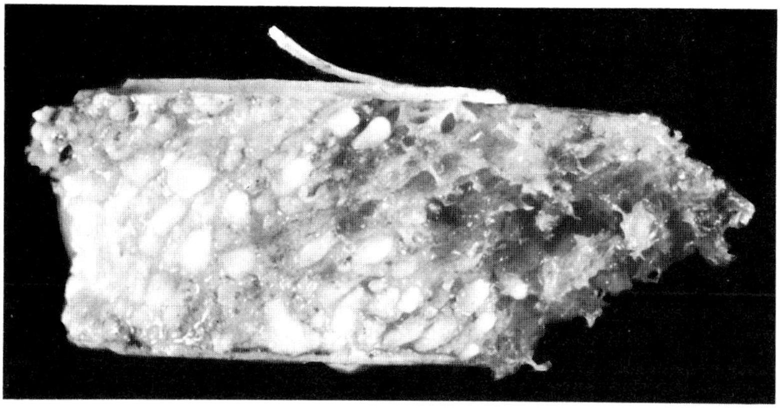

Fig. 10 Cement plug with adhering bone fragments, static shear test

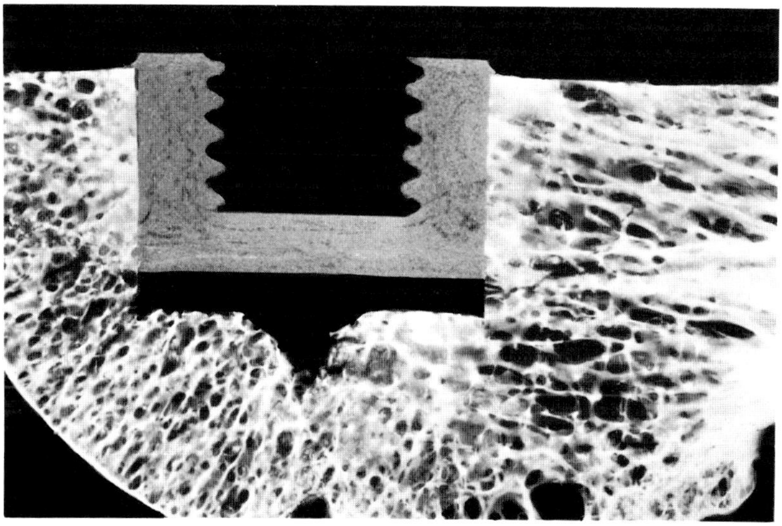

Fig. 11 Radiograph of 2 mm section through test specimen after static shear test; fracture line starts below base of cement plug

DISCUSSION

When working with biological material one has to realize that there are not only differences between the quality of bones from different individuals but also differences of quality within one and the same bone, depending on where and in which direction it is cut. We all know that a bone is an inhomogenous and anisotropic material. Moreover, bone is also anisotropic in a number of ways. This will make the calculation of the stresses in the fixation zone a very difficult proposition indeed.

Considering static shearing strength it is obvious that penetration of PMMA into the interspaces of cancellous bone produces a layer of two-phase material which is superior in strength to cancellous bone itself. In dense cancellous bone the penetration is inadequate, hence the weakest link of the chain is the cross-sectional area of the tiny cement spicules projecting into small bone interspaces. It is therefore logical to drill holes into very dense bone to allow adequate amounts of cement to penetrate.

Although we wished to compare our figures for several mechanical properties of the fresh bone/cement bond with loads or stresses occurring between implant and bone, we had difficulty finding useful figures in the literature.

For compressive stresses at the hip in the one-legged stance we measured 20 Kgf/cm^2 (6). This is for cartilage. We know that cancellous bone in this area is 2-6 times stronger (4). We may assume that the compressive strength of the bond is limited by the compressive strength of the bone.

With respect to shearing stresses, there are again no figures as yet available. We have therefore tried to imagine what stresses might occur between implant and bone and where (Fig. 12). The arrows parallel to the implant surface indicate shearing stresses. For the femoral component of a hip endoprosthesis we have calculated shearing stresses up to 5.25 Kgf/cm^2 in agreement with the findings of Charnley (2). Our values for critical shearing strength are greater than this by a factor of 10. Even for dynamic loads of the hip joint, shearing stresses would be well below 10 Kgf/cm^2.

From friction studies we know the order of magnitude of friction torques in artificial hip joint: 1-2 Kgf · m (1,7). These torques may produce shearing stresses in the zone of

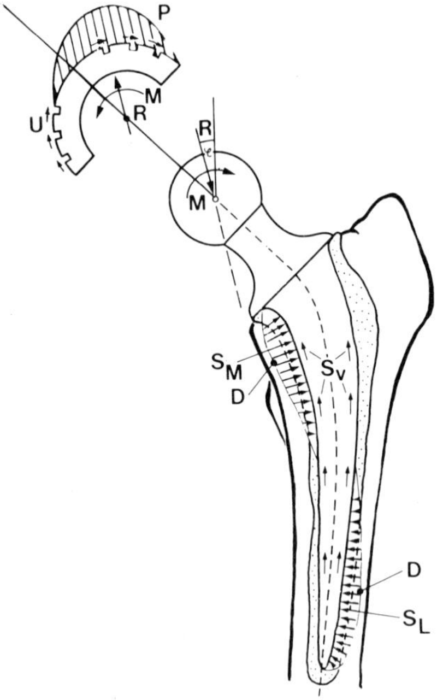

Fig. 12
Compressive stresses and shearing forces at the implant/bone interface.
D,P = pressure,
M = friction torque
R = hip joint force resultant
S_M,S_L = supporting forces
S_V,U = shearing forces

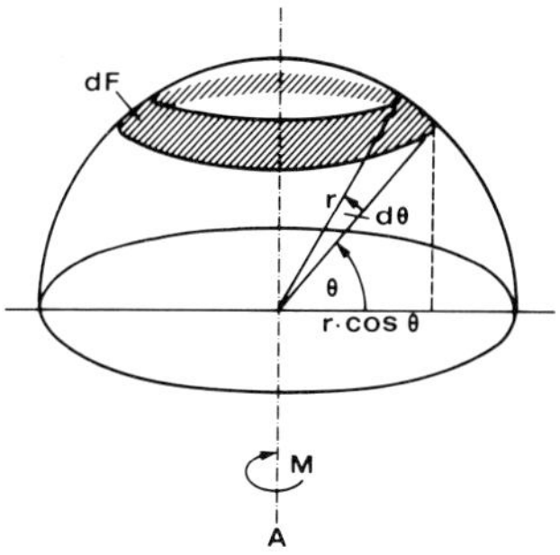

$$M = \tau_c \, 2\pi \, r^3 \int_0^{\frac{\pi}{2}} \cos^2\theta \cdot d\theta$$

$$= \tau_c \, r^3 \, \frac{\pi^2}{2}$$

if $\tau_c = 42 \text{ kgf / cm}^2$

$r = 28 \text{ mm}$

$M = 45{,}4 \text{ kgfm}$

Fig. 13
Calculation of critical torque (M) for critical shearing stress of 42 Kgf · m (τ_c)

bonding of the artificial hip cup. Assuming a hemispherical implant geometry without cement plugs (Fig. 13) we have calculated the friction torque which would be necessary to produce a shearing stress of 42 Kgf/cm^2 in the zone of bonding. For an implant of r = 28 mm this torque would have to be 45 Kgf · m. This is of a different order of magnitude than actual friction torques. On the other hand, experiments by Andersson et al. (1) have shown loosening torques for acetabular components of artificial hip joints cemented into cadaveric pelvis of 9-19 Kgf · m. Considering the conditions under which our test specimens were produced, and those under which acetabula were anchored to pelvis in the experiment, these figures are quite compatible with our values for standard test specimens.

In order to get an idea of the influence of cement plugs in the fixation of artificial acetabula we have assumed the case of an acetabular component fixed to the bone with

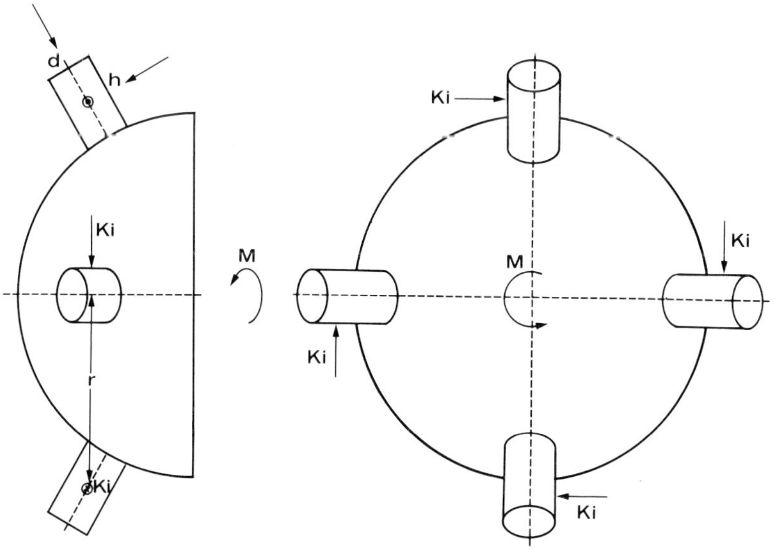

Fig. 14 Assumed implant geometry for calculation of critical torques, critical stresses in plugs (M = torque, Ki = supporting forces, r = distance between centre of plug and axis of rotation)

cement plugs only (Fig. 14). Assuming a torque applied in a fashion similar to that of Andersson (1), Jäger et al. (5) and Chen et al. (3), we found a critical torque of 4.5 Kgf · m (plugs with 10 mm diameter and height of 10 mm and a distance from the axis of 30 mm) due to bending stresses at the bases of the plugs. This torque, in the clinical case, adds to the strength of the bond achieved by the penetration of cement into cancellous bone on the remaining surfaces of the implant.

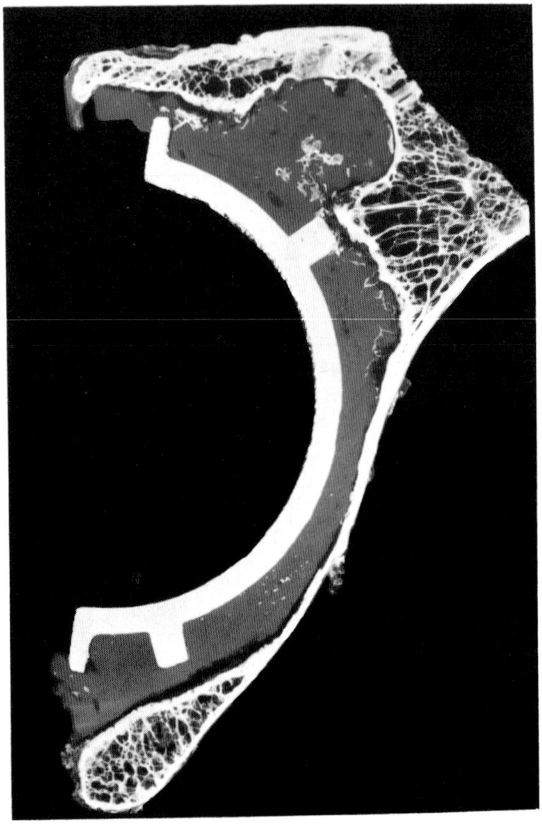

Fig. 15
Radiograph of 2 mm section through acetabulum with McKee replacement, 21 months after implantation. Radiolucent area between cement and bone represents connective tissue. Cement with superficial inclusions of necrotic trabeculae

CONCLUSIONS

From our static and preliminary dynamic tests we may conclude that immediate post-operative weight bearing is justified from a mechanical point of view. This is an indisputable advantage of implant fixation with acrylic cement and will continue to be so in the future.

From morphological studies we know that the bone cement bond does not remain a two-phase transitional zone for very long. This pseudo-continuity will be interrupted, and this interruption is not an abrupt change but a gradual one. However, it changes the mechanics of load transmission profoundly. Stresses are set free i.e. normal and shearing forces which call for the formation of tissue able to negotiate shearing and tensile forces across a discontinuity of bone. This is fibrous connective tissue which, consequently, we shall have to study as to its behaviour under different mechanical conditions. Mechanical conditions do change, not only within a tiny element of the interface, but also overall: Bonding by some kind of a two-phase transitional zone between bone and cement is replaced by an interference fit (mediated by a viscoelastic material) (Fig. 15). Here, overall implant configuration, surface geometry and implant orientation, relative to the skeleton, are even more important. They determine load transmission at the interface, bone remodeling and hence the service life of implant fixation.

On the other side of the interface, acrylic cement is subject to short- and long-term changes which affect its mechanical properties and biological compatibility. Saturation with body water and degradation (8) may be changed in modified bone cements. As long as they are organic polymers, however, changes can only be quantitative ones.

REFERENCES

1. Andersson, G.B.J., Freeman, M.A.R., Swanson, S.A.V.: Loosening of the cemented acetabular cup in total hip replacement. Journal of Bone and Joint Surgery 54-B, 590 (1972)
2. Charnley, J.: Acrylic cement in orthopaedic surgery. Edinburgh: E. & S. Livingstone 1970
3. Chen, S.C., Lowe, S.A., Scales, J.T., Ansell, R.H.: An in vitro experiment to determine the efficiency of fixation of the McKee-Farrar acetabular component in relation to torsional force. Acta Orthopaedica Scandinavica 45, 429 (1974)
4. Hardinge, M.C.: Determination of the strength of cancellous bone in the head and neck of the femur. Surgery, Gynecology and Obstetrics 89, 439 (1949)
5. Jäger, M., Küsswetter, W., Rütt, J., Ungethüm, M., Burkhardt, R.: Loosening of the cemented prosthetic cup in total hip replacement by torsional loading. In: F. Hartmann, edit., 7. Wissenschaftliche Konferenz der Gesellschaft Deutscher Naturforscher und Ärzte "Biopolymere und Biomechanik von Bindegewebssystemen", Berlin: Springer 1974
6. Kummer, B.: Die Beanspruchung der Gelenke, dargestellt am Beispiel des menschlichen Hüftgelenkes. Verhandlungen der Deutschen Orthopädischen Gesellschaft 55, 301 (1969)
7. Wilson, J.N., Scales, J.T.: Loosening of total hip replacement with cement fixation. Clinical Orthopaedics and Related Research 72, 145 (1970)
8. Zarek, J.: Lectures on biomechanics. Biomechanics Course, University of Surrey 1971/72

Chapter 4
Trends in Hip and Knee Prostheses Development

DESIGN CRITERIA OF TOTAL HIP REPLACEMENTS FIXED WITH BONE CEMENT

A.H. Huggler and E. Weidmann

The science of strong materials (metallic as well as nonmetallic) has provided data on the mechanical behavior of these materials under various circumstances. These data provide the framework within which the design of a special device for a specific purpose may be carried out.

In total hip replacement, as in a lesser degree in applied engineering, the design is not so much jeopardized by the mechanical requirement but rather by the biological problems and the surgical feasibility. Therefore, most total hip joints are to a greater or lesser degree compromise solutions.

Before discussing design criteria in cemented prostheses, some comments are in order on mechanical and biological requirements, which are strongly interrelated. There is also an interrelationship between design and material.

Because the foreign implant materials must coexist with the living bone, it is obvious that the behavior of the prosthesis (and the cement) must be compatible with that of the surrounding bone. To determine the behavior of the implant under the forces acting on it, it is absolutely necessary to study the nature of the forces and analyse the effect of these forces on the bone as well as the implant (Table 1).

Table 1 Determining elements for materials evaluation and design in total hip prosthesis

Design	Material
	Static properties
Surgical feasibility in relation to biomechanical properties of the hip joint	Ultimate tensile strength Yield point Ductility Hardness
	Dynamic properties
	Fatigue strength Impact strength Corrosion resistance Wear resistance Coefficient of friction
	Biological properties
	Biological compatibility Material sterilizable

MECHANICAL REQUIREMENTS

Evaluation of the behavior of metals and nonmetals (organic polymers, ceramics) has proved to be difficult because of the special environmental conditions (bone, soft tissue, body fluids) in which these materials are used and which cannot be simulated in in-vitro experiments (wear tests).

In some cases, a metal-on-metal combination for total hip replacement has been developed (13), but the most promising development so far is a combination of a metal with a suitable polymer, e.g. HDP (5). The use of ceramics (Al_2O_3) for weight-bearing components is underway (3). These artificial joints and most of their modifications are cemented into the bone with methylmetacrylate (4,6).

STATIC PROPERTIES

The metal must have sufficient strength to prevent breakage. The yield point (Kp/mm^2), which indicates the stress under which the metal commences to deform plastically, and the ultimate tensile strength (Kp/mm^2) are important.

The ultimate tensile strength (Kp/mm^2) is the nominal stress under which the metal breaks. It is the most common physical test carried out.

Ductility is that property of the material which allows it to be extruded or deformed plastically without breakage (Table 2).

DYNAMIC PROPERTIES

IMPACT STRENGTH (mKp/cm^2)

Impact strength is the energy required to break the test specimen. The value obtained is a measure of its toughness. Impact loading, however, does not occur in the human body as in general mechanical engineering. The joints of the lower extremity would damp shock loads.

Table 2 Minimum values of different mechanical requirements for metallic implants

Ultimate tensile strength (σ_{UTS})	$> 90\ Kp/mm^2$
Yield point ($\sigma_{0.2\,\%}$)	$> 60\ Kp/mm^2$
Ductility (δ_5)	$> 50\ \%$
Vickers hardness number (HV)	$> 300\ Kp/mm^2$

FATIGUE STRENGTH (Kp/mm^2)

The test specimen is usually submitted to a reversed stress between set stress limits, from compression to tension, to determine the number of repetitions before failure occurs. In general, fatigue fractures are also a design problem. Implants should be designed with a large safety margin for use as human artificial hip joints.

STRESS CORROSION

Corrosion is conversion of the material into compound forms by the action of natural agencies. Corrosion occurs preferentially in highly stressed areas.

WEAR RESISTANCE

Wear is governed by:

1. Bearing pressure (Kp/cm^2) is related to the sphericity of joint components. In all cases, the ball is slightly less in diameter than the socket, which means, that there is always some clearance (Fig. 1). The cold flow, which is the primary mechanical problem encountered with polymers, is a nonelastic deformation. In such cases, the joint clearance changes and so does its performance. The clearance may even disappear completely so that eventually clamping occurs. Such clamping not only entails additional frictional torque but also additional wear.
2. Mating surfaces. The nature of materials that must slide against each other is of paramount importance. Generally speaking, it is well known in mechanical engineering, that a hard surface that bears against a softer one, offers a good combination, on the condition that the surfaces are well polished. No rule however exists regarding the selection of materials according to their hardness.
3. Sliding velocity (m/sec).
4. Sliding distance (mm).

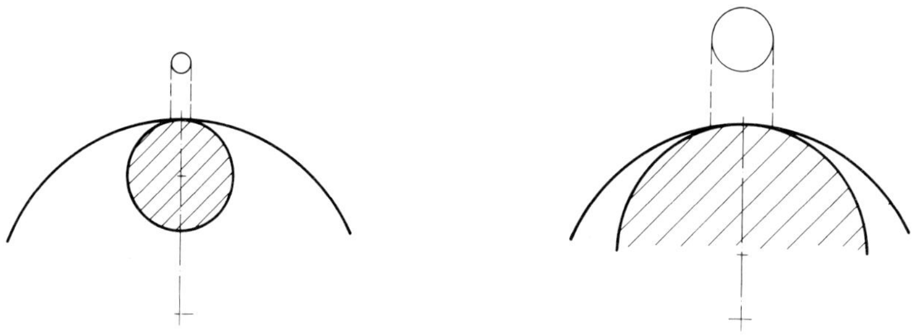

Fig. 1 Contact area between spherical mating surfaces depending on clearance

5. Surface roughness (μm). The rougher the surfaces the more impossible it becomes to separate them by means of a film of lubricant.
6. Lubrication of artificial joints depends on the adhesion of the lubricant (serum with albumines, synovial fluid) to the material of the rubbing surfaces; the layers of lubricant slip over each other instead of the dry surfaces (Fig. 2). The wear problems of organic polymers have been described by Duff-Barclay (8) as follows: "The history of the use of plastic components as part joint replacements has not been a happy one. The wear particles have produced an undesirable biological response (tissue reaction)." So far, only the HDP, under ideal clinical circumstances, has shown a low rate of wear of 0.2 mm/year (5). The wear rate observed in metal-to-metal combinations seems tolerable, but the coefficient of friction is 3 to 4 times higher (14).

BIOLOGICAL REQUIREMENTS

The biocompatibility of materials used in total hip replacement is seldom detectable with tissue culture alone. Experiments in small animals (sheep, rats, rabbits, etc.) also do not seem to be reliable enough.

The elastic properties of the implant under the static and dynamic loads of the hip joint together with those of the recipient cancellous and cortical bone must be carefully considered. The influence of compressive, tensile, and shear stresses, as well as the effect of motion on the behavior of normal bone remodelling (Wolff's law 1887), must be studied before the best way of implantation and especially anchorage to the bone can be discussed (Figs. 3-5).

The material, design, and anchoring of the prostheses involve compromises, which have on the whole proved to be very encouraging and satisfactory within a certain (temporary) framework of reduced daily activities.

Perren et al. (17) demonstrated experimentally that, whenever there is relative motion between an implant and bone, or in the case of fractures between bone fragments, especially in weight-bearing extremities, bone resorption will take place. Neither for cancellous nor for cortical bone is the precise stress, which leads to infraction, microfractures, and secondary instability in relation to the bone, known (Table 3).

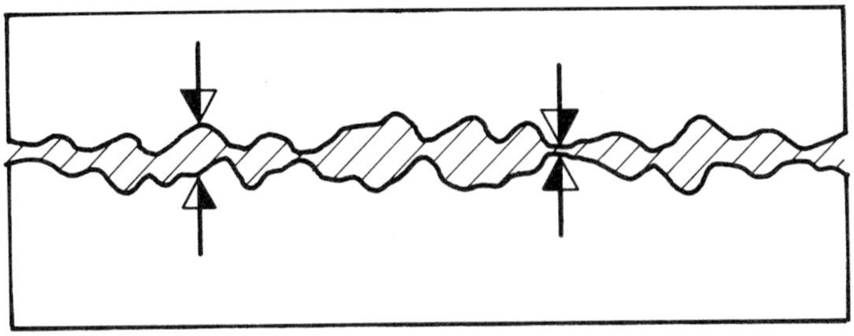

Fig. 2 Separating (lubricating) effect of an adhesive film of fluid at very low rubbing velocities

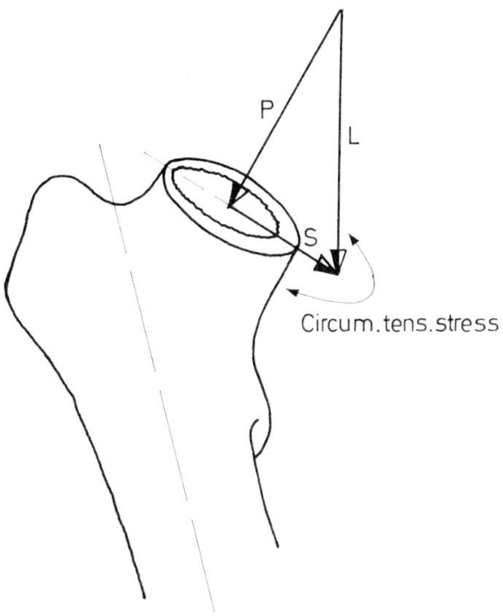

Fig. 3
The vertical load L is resolved into two components, P and S, respectively normal and transverse to the cross-section

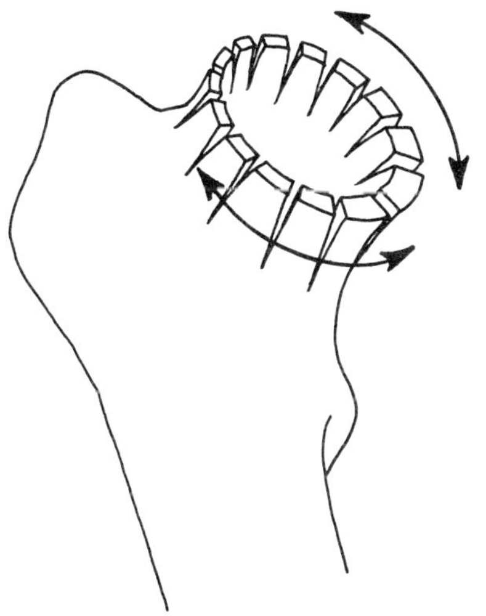

Fig. 4
Circumferential tensile stresses that tend to meridionally split the neck

THE DESIGN

The design concept which finally leads to prototype construction does not necessarily depend on an already existing prosthetic element. The final product, however, is the result of materials evaluation, manufacturing possibilities, performances tests, and clinical trials.

The stress pattern of the hip joint, as it exists in its initial pre-operative state, will certainly undergo a change. The bone remodelling after operation cannot be analysed in clinical (or animal) trials because of the fact, that, even if the complete turn-over of bone takes

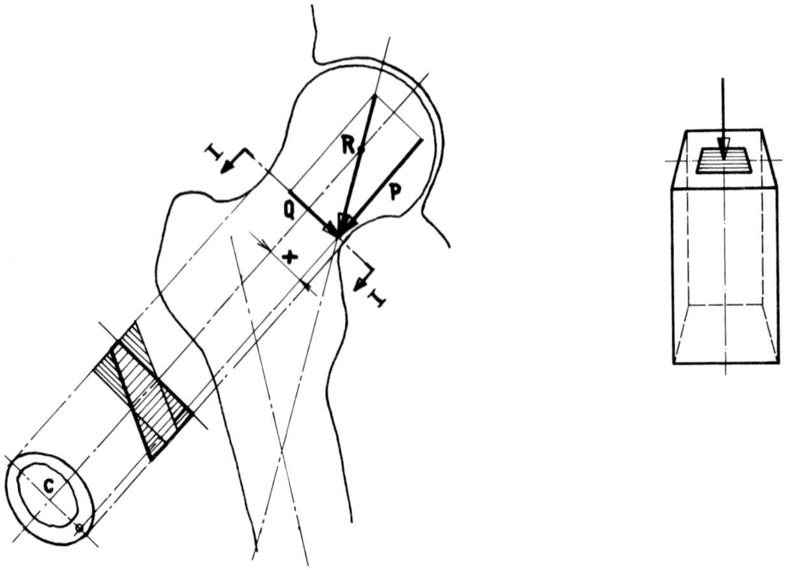

$$\underline{M_b = P \cdot x}$$

Fig. 5 Meridional stresses in the femoral neck resulting from superimposition of bending and pure compressive stresses

Table 3 Mechanical and biological factors which may induce loosening of the implant

Infection "Low grade infection"
Rejection
Microfractures
Lack of stress protection
Osteoporosis
Trauma
Fatigue fracture
Fractures of the bone cement
Biomechanical factors
Defects in the material

about 12 months, more time is needed for long-term changes in bone structure. When the implant must perform the task of weight transmission, not as in osteotomies or internal fixation of fractures, the surrounding bone gets involved in "stress protection" what can be seen with heavy implants which have been used by Jackson Burrows (12) some 25 years ago. It is rather the design than the modulus of elasticity alone which are responsible for this.

1. Head-size. Due to the load P (Fig. 6) and the coefficient of friction μ, the frictional force Q at the bearing surface is given by $P \cdot \mu$. This is the force which must be applied at the contact surface to overcome friction. Because the ball rotates about its center, the torque necessary to overcome friction is given by $R \cdot P \cdot \mu$, and hence a smaller ball requires a lower torque. A smaller ball, however, requires higher specific loading or bearing pressure, but on the other hand, for a given angular movement and angular velocity, the rubbing speed and total surface movement is lower.

   As mentioned earlier, all of these aspects have a considerable influence on wear and the necessity for a compromise again arises. A further point regarding the size of the head is, that for a given neck diameter, the permissible angular movement with a larger head is greater than that with a smaller one.

2. Neck length. The less the femoral neck is resected, the lower are the transversal forces necessary for equilibrium. It must however be pointed out, that the bone in this area may be weaker than at the inferior part of the calcar femorale. These observations have been made without considering the lateral/distal displacement of the trochanter major (5) (Fig. 7). It is well known that a varus position of the prosthetic shaft also increases flexural bending stresses of the implant and the bone (1).

3. Shaft length, material, and shape. In the optimum shaft arrangement, the flexural stiffness of the shaft at its mid-point equals that of the surrounding bone (absolut conformability). Towards its upper end, the flexural rigidity of the shaft should gradually increase, while towards the lower end or tip, the rigidity should gradually decrease. Flexural stiffness is not governed alone by the modulus of elasticity of the material used, but is also affected by the design of the femoral implant. If such con-

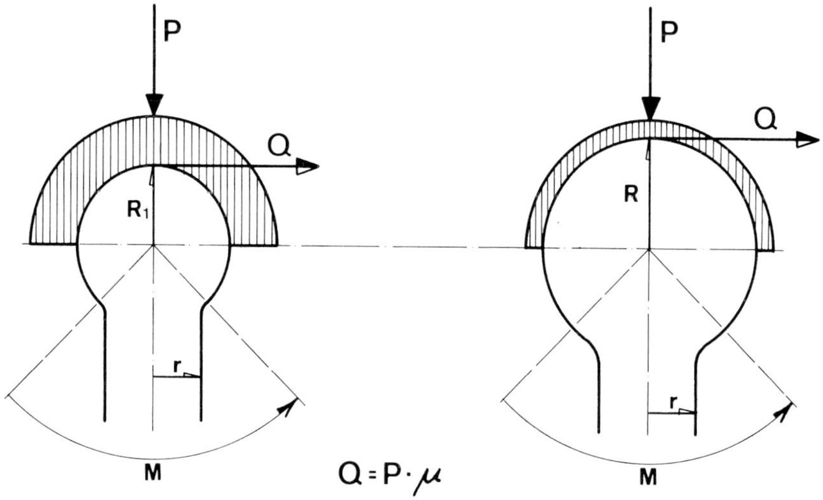

Fig. 6 Comparison of frictional torque and degree of angular freedom between a large and small ball

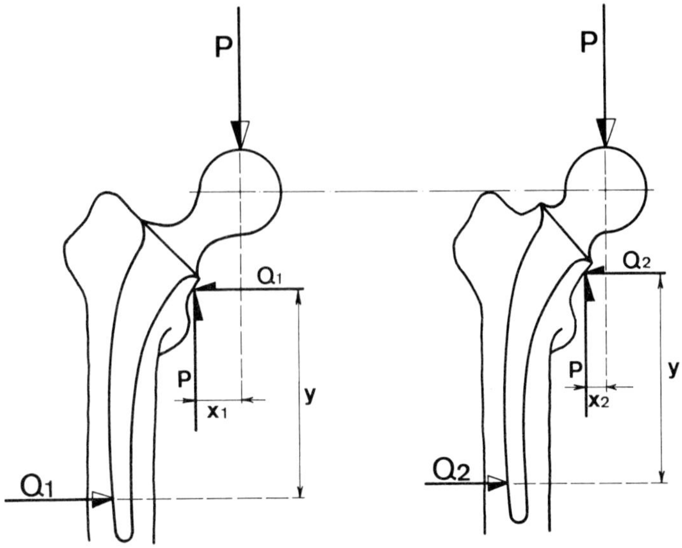

$P \cdot x_1 = Q_1 \cdot y \qquad Q_1 > Q_2 \qquad P \cdot x_2 = Q_2 \cdot y$

Fig. 7 Bending moment resulting from eccentric action of P and restraining moment effected by transversal forces Q

ditions could be met, then a long shaft would certainly enable forces to be transferred to the bone over a large area. If, however, this condition cannot be realised, the implant would tend to transmit the introduced forces either at one proximity or the other (Figs. 8,9). Through such considerations it becomes immediately apparent that, at best, only a compromise could be attained with any design of shaft.

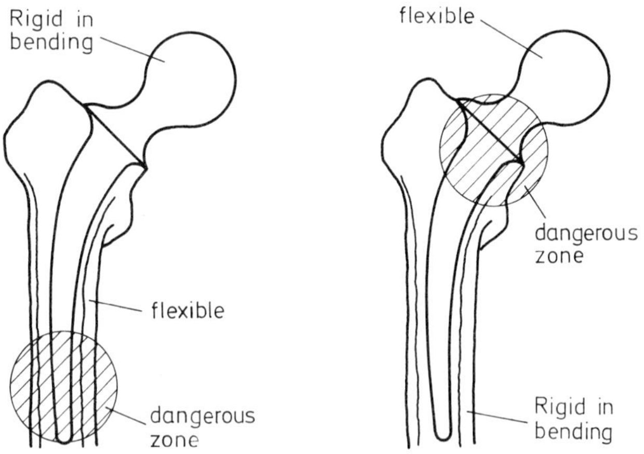

Fig. 8 Areas of stress concentration attributable to abrupt discontinuity of flexural rigidity

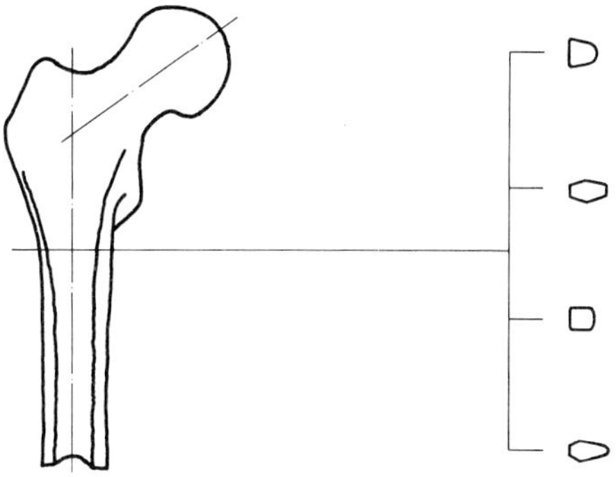

Fig. 9
The four sections of currently used total hip stems in relation to the shape and size of the proximal femur. The cross-sectional shape of the stem and the efficiency of cement filling between the stem and the bone may determine the likelihood of a stem failure (2)

When there is a third medium (e.g. cement), in spite of the original inconformability of the shaft and bone structures, a considerable amount of compatibility can nevertheless be obtained. This, however, necessitates the use of a cement which must exhibit a lower modulus of elasticity than that of the implant and that of the bone. This cement layer then enables distribution of introduced forces over a larger area than would otherwise be the case. The bone structure when stressed must deform. If no overstressing or local stress concentrations are to occur, the bone must be allowed to deform in its natural way. Therefore, only manner for accommodating this is by utilizing an intermediate layer of an elastic substance that, of course, also exhibits the necessary strength characteristics (Fig. 10).

4. Stem taper angle. The transversal force Q (Figs. 11,12) due to the load P and the wedging action of a taper are largely dependant on the angle α as well as the coefficient of friction μ between the implant and the surrounding material. Force Q increases with decreasing angle α and also with a decrease in the coefficient of friction μ. It appears, therefore, desirable either to increase the angle or increase the coefficient of friction.

This means, that if a self-locking shaft is envisaged, the value of μ must necessarily be small and therefore the undesirable transversal force Q could only be reduced by increasing the angle of the shaft α. Since load transmission is by the cement, no big weight-bearing collar is needed as Charnley (4) has pointed out. The mechanically

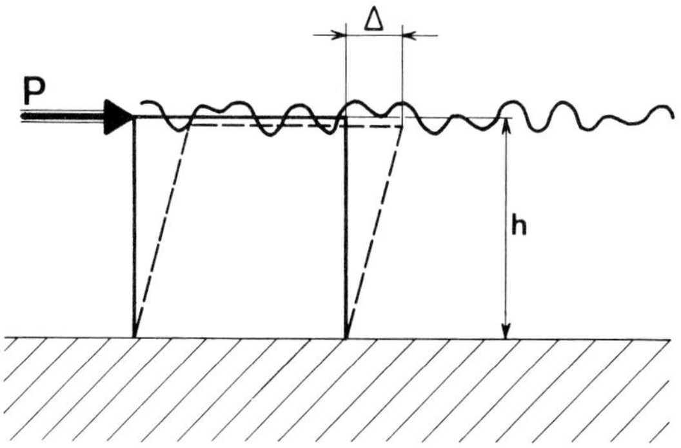

Fig. 10
The compressive and shear components of an obliquely acting force

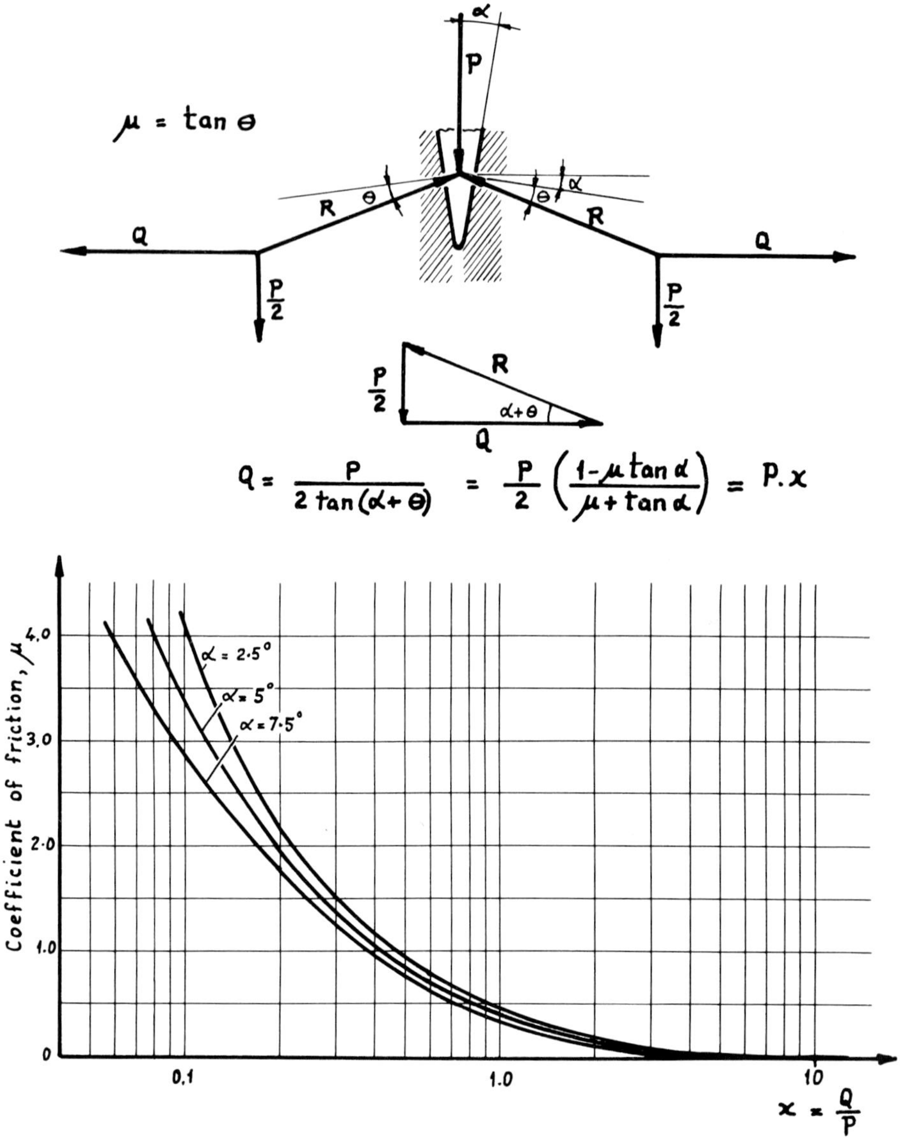

Fig. 11 Forces exerted by a wedge. Not only the angle α of a taper (stem) but also the coefficient of friction μ between the taper and the surrounding material (cement) will influence the wedging action of the force Q (see text)

structured surface of a femoral shaft prostheses (high value of μ) and therefore reduced wedging tendency ensures, furthermore, a better force transmission to the bone cement, which was proved by several repeated extraction tests (20).

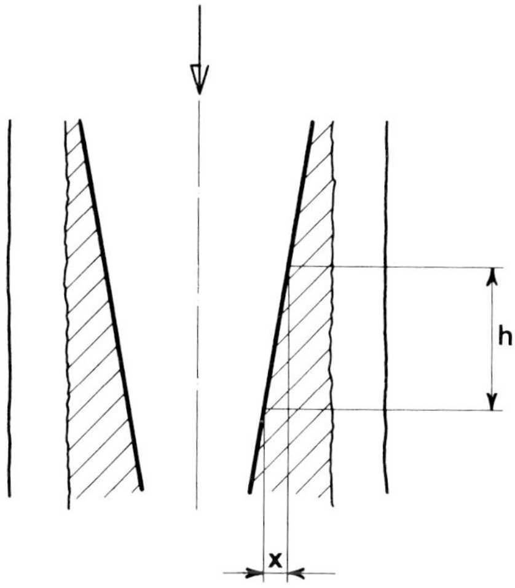

Fig. 12
Splitting action of a wedge

BONE STRENGTH

The dynamic strength of bone is not known, but the static strength has been measured on various occasions (not in vivo). Any attempt to evaluate the dynamic strength of bone in in-vitro experiments must be considered useless for all practical purposes. Only for momentary loading conditions of the bone could the static strength be applied.

The mechanical quality of bone varies in different individuals and with different diseases. Furthermore, some important mechanical features, such as the modulus of elasticity, may not only change at different skeletal locations, but also depends on the direction in which the bone specimen is tested. Finally, it is to be hoped, that experimental and mathematical methods of stress analysis (e.g. finite-element method (19) of Scholten) would provide more understanding of stress conditions in the hip joint.

GENERAL VIEW OF TOTAL HIP JOINTS

All-metal joints exhibit little abrasion and have served well (and are still continuing to do so) over many years, but the HDP-metal combinations outnumber these arthroplasties by far. The trunnion-bearing prosthesis which was used by Scuderi (18) has led to several new concepts in hip replacement (7,10,22,23). There is also a trend to overcome the anchoring problem without the use of cement using Al_2O_3 ceramics (9,15) and the iso-elastic prosthesis made of an organic polymer (14,16).

The problem of stable fixation in bone seems to be, however, basically the same for all biocompatible materials that are in use. On one hand, there is the danger of high stress concentration attributable to the rigidity of the implant (Al_2O_3) and on the other hand, it seems difficult to obtain an isoelastic solution which requires the necessity of individual conformability to the bone. The elastic properties of bone may vary appreciable from case to case.

Cement is still the best compromise for anchoring and load transmission between prosthesis and bone. Additional tension-band wiring should be used to overcome circumferential tensile stresses in the bone and the cement. It must also be emphasized, that it is very difficult to properly handle the cement; there must be a sufficient amount of cement without damaging the natural structures of the joint (acetabulum, femur) and still guarantee a mechanically stable anchorage. The injection of cement into the femur may be advocated only if the consistency of the cement is such that there is no danger of the cement flowing away. Because the acetabular roof (subchondral bone) should be left intact, different sizes of cups will be needed. This also applies for the stem and the neck, so as to fit the prosthesis to the patient rather than the patient to the prosthesis. As Anderson et al. (2) have shown, their special reaming procedure of the acetabulum with circumferential notches is most suitable for stable fixation with cement. However, it should be pointed out, that deep circumferential grooves will certainly adversely affect the stress pattern between the subchondral bone within the acetabulum and the acetabular rim.

In conclusion, it may be said, that although a vast amount of knowledge has been gained in the past regarding behavior of the implant as well as that of the bone, there still remains an enormous amount of investigation required to further define and resolve several unsolved problems that still exist.

REFERENCES

1. Amstutz, H.C.: Complications of total hip replacement. Clinical Orthopaedics and Related Research 72, 123 (1972)
2. Anderson, G.B.J., Freeman, M.A.R., Swanson, S.A.V.: Loosening of the cemented acetabular cup in total hip replacement. Journal of Bone and Joint Surgery 54-B, 590 (1972)
3. Boutin, P.: Arthroplastie totale de la hanche par prothese en alumine fritee. Revue de Chirurgie Orthopedique 58, 229 (1972)
4. Charnley, J.: Anchorage of the femoral head prosthesis to the shaft of the femur. Journal of Bone and Joint Surgery 42-B, 28 (1960)
5. Charnley, J.: Arthroplasty of the hip – A new operation. Lancet, II, 1129 (1963)
6. Charnley, J.: Acrylic cement in orthopaedic surgery, Edinburgh-London: E. and S. Livingstone 1970
7. Christiansen, T.: A new hip prosthesis with trunnion-bearing. Acta Chirurgica Scandinavica 135, 43 (1969)
8. Duff-Barclay, I., Spillman, D.T.: Total human hip joint prostheses – a laboratory study of friction and wear. Symposium on lubric and wear in living and artificial human joints, London (1967)
9. Griss, P., Krempien, B., v.Andrian-Werburg, H.: Urämische Osteopathie als Ursache einer zweiseitigen Hüftendoprothesenlockerung. Zeitschrift für Orthopädie 112, 1157 (1974)

10. Huggler, A.H.: Follow-up study of 122 total hip replacements (1962-1969). In: G. Chapchal, edit., Arthroplasty of the hip, Stuttgart: Georg Thieme Verlag 1973

11. Huggler, A.H., Schreiber, A., Dietschi, C., Jacob, H.: Experimentelle Untersuchungen über das Deformationsverhalten des Hüftazetabulums unter Belastung. Zeitschrift für Orthopädie 112, 44 (1974)

12. Jackson Burrows, H.: Replacement of tumours affecting bone by major internal prostheses. Biomedical Engineering and its Clinical Application in Orthopaedic Surgery. London: The British Council 1971

13. McKee, G.K., Watson-Farrar, J.: Replacement of arthritic hips by the McKee-Farrar prosthesis. Journal of Bone and Joint Surgery 48-B, 245 (1966)

14. Mathys, R.: Stand der Verwendung von Kunststoffen für künstliche Gelenke. Actuelle Traumatologie 3, 253 (1973)

15. Mittelmeier, H.: Zementlose Verankerung von Endoprothesen nach dem Tragrippenprinzip. Zeitschrift für Orthopädie 112, 27 (1974)

16. Morscher, E.: Erste Erfahrungen mit einer zementlosen-isoelastischen Totalprothese der Hüfte. Kongress der Niederländisch-Schweizerischen Gesellschaften für Orthopädie, Lausanne 1974

17. Perren, S.M., Huggler, A.H., Russenberger, M., Allgoewer, M., Mathys, R., Schenk, A., Willenegger, H., Müller, M.E.: The reaction of cortical bone to compression. Acta Orthopaedica Scandinavica Supplement 125, 19 (1969)

18. Scuderi, C.: Personal communication

19. Scholten, R.: Über die Berechnung der mechanischen Beanspruchung in Knochenstrukturen mittels für den Flugzeugbau entwickelter Rechenverfahren. Vortrag vor dem Arbeitskreis Biomechanik an der 22. Jahrestagung der Vereinigung Süddeutscher Orthopäden, Baden-Baden 1974

20. Semlitsch, M.: Implant metals for plates, screws and artificial joints in bone surgery. Engineering in Medicine, 68 (1973)

21. Walker, P.S.: The optimum use of materials in total hip design. In: The Hip. St. Louis: C.V. Mosby Company 1973

22. Weber, B.G.: Die Rotations-Totalendoprothese des Hüftgelenkes. Zeitschrift für Orthopädie 107, 304 (1970)

23. Weber, B.G., Semlitsch, M.: Total hip replacement with rotation-endoprosthesis: problem of woor. In: G. Chapchal, edit., Arthroplasty of the Hip. Stuttgart: Georg Thieme Verlag 1973

PROBLEMATICS OF CURRENT HINGE–TYPE ARTIFICIAL KNEE JOINTS

W. Blauth, W. Skripitz, and G. Bontemps

The hinge-type artificial knee joint consists of a femoral and tibial part, held together on a rigid axis. The joint permits movement in one plane only; consequently a constraint movement around this one axis occurs.

With it, however, we lack the basis for duplicating the extremely complex functioning of the normal knee joint (20,37). Although this target presently seems unattainable and surpasses practical requirements, there appears to be no satisfactory solution in arthroplasty in the form of a single-axis hinge-type prosthesis. Considerable disadvantages are connected with the implantation of this type of prosthesis, so that good results can really only be expected for limited periods. The considerable constructural differences in various models have a distinct effect. Nevertheless, despite serious deficiencies, we cannot presently do without the hinge-type prostheses, and their application is only a question of indication.

The problematics of hinge-type prostheses involve the fundamental advantages and disadvantages of various models. These will be discussed. Thereafter, construction features of single-axis knee joints are compared, with emphasis, on the differences in individual models. This discussion will be limited to the various types of single-axis joints, centered on primary representatives. Multi-axis linked prostheses with rotation components such as models by Herbert (31), Blietz (9), Sheehan (43), Attenborough (4), Deane (15), Trillat (48), and others will not be taken into consideration.

Subsequently, comments are included on the indications of hinge-type prostheses, including some developmental tasks based on a review of current technology. The solution to these tasks could bring about significant improvement in this type of prosthesis.

Finally, a short report is presented on experience with hinge-type prostheses as reported in the literature. However, statistics and clinical observations in individual reports cannot be compared with one another, and operative methods have not been performed under analog conditions. Furthermore, on the whole, extremely short observation periods have been taken as a basis. However, a summary is of interest, especially in view of certain complications in some systems.

The advantages of a hinged joint can be described as follows:

1. In most cases, it is of simple construction and therefore generally allows for technically uncomplicated and less time-consuming implantation techniques than prostheses with sliding surfaces.
2. High-degree axial misalignments can be corrected relatively easily.

3. In the case of severe bone destruction, tumors, and destruction of the ligament system, a stability of the knee, painless mobility, and fast recovery of walking ability can be achieved.

The disadvantages are:

1. Non-elasticity of the motion system resulting from the constraint movement around one axis, abrupt erratic movements, and the lack of rotary movement. The non-elasticity is one of the most important causes for loosening of the prosthesis and complications associated with accidental falls.
2. The extensive bone resections necessary for the installation of many types of knee prostheses, which results in insufficient supporting area of spongious surface and limited potential for correction in case of failure.
3. The application of bone cement is necessary with most models.
4. The considerably more complex design compared with prostheses with gliding surfaces.
5. The danger of infection arising from the quantity of foreign materials or from external injuries and internal pressures.

To examine the differences in the various models and derive conclusions, a classification is suggested of the various models, which could be devided according to principal features. One basic differentiation is between prostheses which are implanted primarily intraosseously, for example, the Letournel and Lagrange (35) or St. Georg (13) models, and prostheses that are located more superficially and therefore are more exposed in the joint area, such as the Walldius (54), Shiers (44), Young (59) or the newer models of GSB- and Guepar-prostheses or our own model (8).

Developers of the St. Georg-type of prosthesis see the main advantage of their construction in the lower degree of danger of infection resulting from the predominantly intraosseous position of the foreign body (13). Present results of treatments seem to agree, although comparable statistics and long-term results are still lacking, and the problem of infection is extremely unpredictable.

Interestingly, the latest St. Georg-model deviates from earlier devices in that two femoral condyle caps have been added, which provide broader distribution of the loads. It seems that, with this alteration of the original concept, an attempt was made to eliminate the disadvantages, as there are the unphysiological intraosseous and intracondylar power transmission, the insufficient support in valgus and varus strain found in narrower models, as well as the danger of sinking in of prosthesis parts.

However, remaining factors are the disadvantages from the extensive intracondylar bone resection. We question, together with Gschwend (26), whether, considering the remaining narrow border area of the condyles, the possible alternative solutions are really easier than with prostheses which require primarily a wider bone resection, e.g. the Walldius joint (Fig. 1). The depth of intracondylar resection is also of concern, because important parts of the main support pylon of the dorsal femoral corticalis are destroyed.

The superficially located hinge-type prostheses show various construction principles, and can only be compared with one another as well as with intraosseous models if divided into two major categories. The first is representative of the technically simple construc-

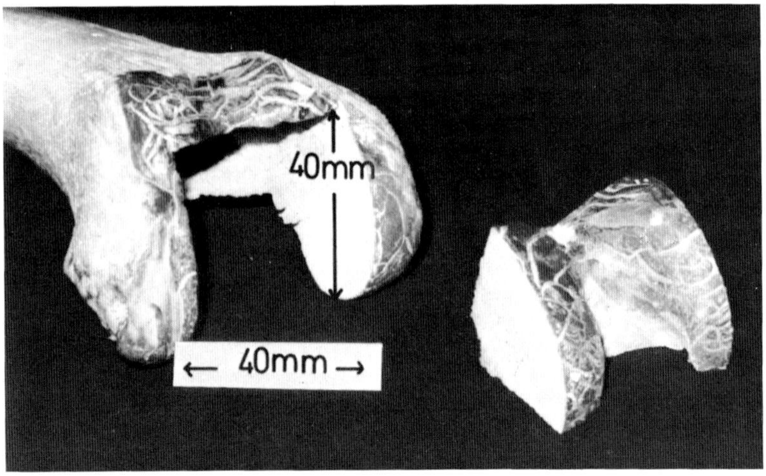

Fig. 1 Example of the extent of intracondylar bone resection when implanting an intraosseous prosthesis, e.g. the St. Georg large model. It is obvious that, in case of failure an arthrodesis is difficult

tions of Walldius (54), Shiers (44), Young (59) and the Guepar group (36). The implantation of these prostheses requires a fairly deep resection across the joint of approximately 2 to 4 cm and therefore is relatively easily managable. The supposition that sacrifice of the natural planes of support is a considerable disadvantage is legitimate, that is, biomechanically as well as with respect to the second line of defense in case of infection and breakage or loosening of the prostheses. The spongious support surfaces favor "sinking in" of the prostheses parts. The danger of loosening and spontaneous fractures augment the progressive bone resorption (Fig. 2).

The GSB prosthesis (25) and our own model (8) are representative of the second category. These require much less resection while preserving the natural femoral condyles. The implantation of these models is therefore slightly more demanding. The advantages lie partly in utilization of the physiological bearing surface. In this respect, it is questionable whether the material in the GSB prosthesis is not used too sparingly or whether our model is built too solidly. To offer a comparison of the bearing surfaces determining the load distribution in different types of prostheses, the values of several well-known models were calculated. It was established that the Shiers and Guepar prostheses have the smallest supporting surfaces, whereas our own model has the largest (Table 1).

In comparing hinged prostheses, the differences of rotational safety and rotational surfaces are prevailing factors. Rotational lips, splints, or plaques have been attached for rotational safety. These are generally embedded in the bone and counteract rotational forces. The surface absorbing these forces is called the rotation surface. The force is the so-called surface moment of inertia, which can be determined approximately by squaring the perpendicular distance from the shaft axis multiplied by the area of the rotation surface (Table 2).

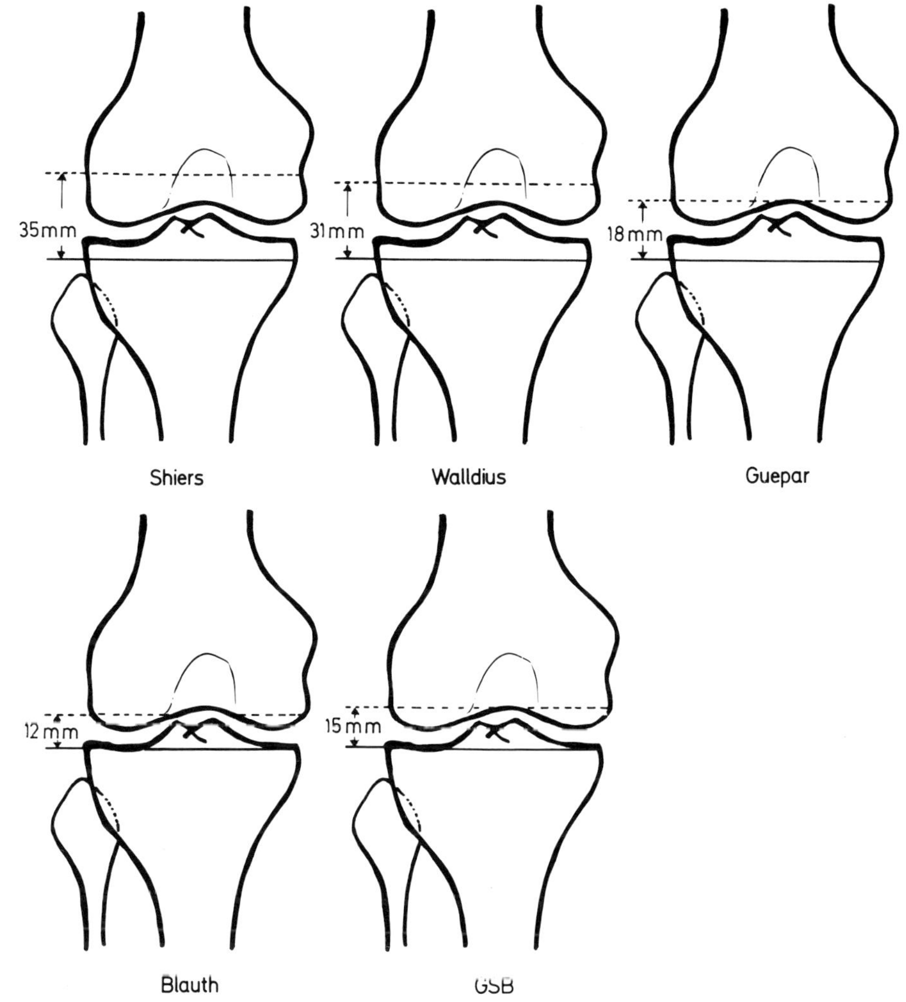

Fig. 2 Extent of resections in different hinge-type prostheses. Shortening of the leg is implied when performing an arthrodesis

Table 1 Prostheses which preserve the femoral condyles have larger supporting surfaces of the bone

	Bearing surface of the bone (cm^2)	
	Femoral part	Tibial part
Shiers	11.0	5.9
Walldius	20.3	18.1
Guepar	13.7	13.2
St. Georg P-model (large)	12.1	14.1
St.Georg M-75 (small)	17.9	14.1
Blauth	31.0	24.5

Table 2 Rotational impediments range from the Shiers prosthesis without rotational safety to the Blauth model with the highest values

	Measurement: Polar moment of inertia (cm^4)	
	Femoral part	Tibial part
Shiers	0	0
Walldius	8.7	6.0
Guepar	12.8	7.2
St. Georg P-model (large)	68.2	7.6
St. Georg M-75 (small)	48.0	7.6
Blauth	130.0	22.5

There are considerable differences in the various prostheses; these range from the Shiers prosthesis without rotational safety to our model with the highest values. However, these values do not consider the effect of bonding with bone cement. When comparing the axes, three aspects must be considered (Fig. 3):

1. The position of the axis with respect to the center of the physiological curve. It is obvious that a rigid axis should be placed in the center of this curve because this more readily allows for normal movement. We have implemented this requirement in our model. Axes positioned centrally between the parts of the prosthesis, e.g. in the Walldius or the Young knee, result in limited flexibility. Cranially positioned axes such as the Shiers knee provide for better mobility, but require much too extensive bone resections. When flexed, dorso-cranial axis positions, as with the Guepar knee, lead to tilting of the femur towards the dorsal on the tibia; the ventral parts of the joint also unfold. This incurs an abnormal tension in the ventral soft tissues, including the extension apparatus. Therefore, the possible flexing range of the prosthesis will

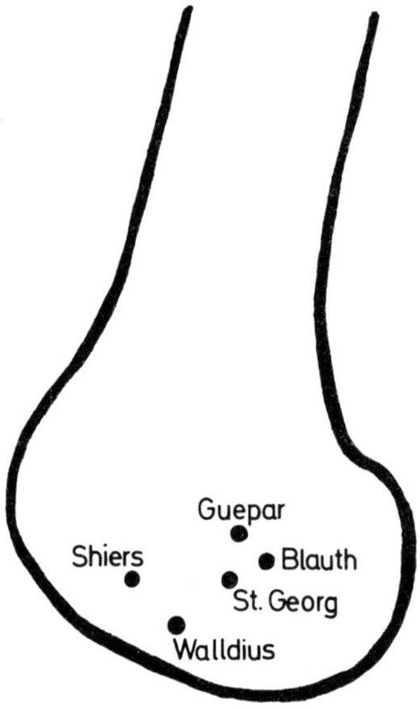

Fig. 3
Projected axis positions of different hinge-type prostheses. The axis of the Blauth prosthesis lies near the center of the physiological curve

never be reached when implanted. It is questionable if, with a migrating axis such as in the GSB prosthesis, the advantages outweigh the disadvantages. With the omission of a rigid connection between the prostheses parts, friction develops between the metal components which can result in metalosis.

2. The axes in most hinge-type prostheses sustain the full load. Therefore, they are subject to considerable stress, depending on position and quality. Wagner (49,50) reports that, when the knee is flexed 45 degrees, loads as high as 500 to 700 Kp act on the axis. Even loads of 800 to 1050 Kp can be experienced when flexing the knee 90 degrees. Accordingly, with a mechanical safety factor of approximately 3, depending on weight, several tons of load could be carried. Therefore, it is of significant advantage that the loads be transferred directly from the femoral condyles to the tibia and that the axis, as the only carrier of the load, is crucially relieved.
3. With regard to the high loads, bearing of the axis must be considered. Metal combinations as in the Guepar, Shiers, McKee, or Walldius knees are inferior to the polyethylene-metal combination working on the low-friction principle. Metal combinations are threatened by metalosis and other damages, which lead to seizing in the axis or to severe irritations caused by foreign bodies (46). For this reason, we had to remove two of a series of 30 Walldius knees to date.

Many of the problems with hinged prostheses are connected with the length, cross-section, and tilting angle of the prostheses stems. Therefore, a comparison of the various models seems appropriate. In principle, the femoral prosthesis stem should have at least 7 ^{o} valgus. Wagner (49,50) demonstrated that otherwise an increased asymmetrical load-bearing of the knee joint would be the consequence. Prostheses stems at right angles show higher bending moments. These are higher in the femur and the tibia than in prostheses with valgus stems. In our opinion, reliable details are not yet available on the ideal size and shape of stems. Overly long stems augment the danger of loosening of the prosthesis. Extremely short stems cause higher deformation in tension and compression of the lower limb. However, further detailed questions, e.g. regarding the optimal cross-sectional form of the stem, are of secondary importance, as long as most hinge-type prostheses are anchored with the aid of bone cement.

There are considerable differences between the various hinge-type prostheses in the sliding bearing of the patella and braking of dynamic forces. In all systems, an unphysiological abrupt braking occurs which, as already mentioned, is an important cause of loosening. Prostheses with metallic stops in both directions, and prostheses that, after implantation, allow only restricted knee flexion (less than 110 ^{o} to 120 ^{o}) are especially unfavorable. Experiments with braking of the dynamic strains in an elastic manner, thereby reducing high deformations in tension and compression, have led to installation of silastic blocks.

According to research on the Guepar prosthesis, silastic blocks reduce dynamic strains by about 25 % (49). It stands to reason, however, that elastic material will become brittle and wear. Therefore, these blocks cannot be a long-term solution; we use them for lack of a better alternative. Additionally, muscles and capsular structures serve for braking. Therefore, the dorsal capsule is generally not resected. We remove only a small amount of bone, which results in a restraint of extension of approximately 10 degrees. In this case, the dorsal structures of the knee joint brake the extension and make hyperextension difficult. The patients must also learn how to catch the abrupt step with their muscles when walking.

Let us consider the influence of various hinge-type prostheses on the patella and patella femoral joint. Almost regularly, arthroplastic measures are required after an implantation, e.g. removal of the osteophytes and shaping destroyed joint surfaces which in themselves or together with synovectomies result in complications such as adhesions of the soft tissues, painful restriction of movement, or irritating effusions. These, however, are not addressed here in the interest of further discussion of the problems with the patella regarding the form and material of the prosthesis parts.

Depending on the flexing range of the lower leg, contact between the patella and the foreign body is encountered in all prostheses, which results in irregularities. Therefore, some models like the Walldius and Guepar or our own prostheses have a femoral patellar plate which receives the shaped patella and which is meant to balance the irregularities. However, even this construction is not fully satisfying, because only a very rough match is possible, and the bone is subject to severe wear. In this respect, the quite frequent complaints of patients about the femoral patellar joint are understandable. It remains to be seen, whether the alternative of prosthetic replacement of the patella is really progress. Removal of the patella, which is obligatory in the Shiers prosthesis, produces an acceptable solution probably only in exceptional cases. In addition to weakening in the quadriceps tendon and the joint being insufficiently covered by tissues on the ventral side, a relatively high percentage of rupture of the patella tendon has been experienced. Arden (2) reported a complication rate of over 20 %.

Comparison of the various prostheses of this type shows that an ideal hinge-type prosthesis is nonexistent and probably cannot exist because, in indicating and planning the operation, we must consider the conditions so that choosing the appropriate prosthesis is possible. To that end, the use of those types of prostheses that demand a broad bone resection during implantation cannot be forced. At present, basic concerns are with the following areas of indication:

1. Severely destroyed painful joints associated with such a high-degree of instability and subluxation of the joint as well as misadjustments of the axis of the limb, that partial prostheses or models without axes are out of the question and arthrodeses are contradicted for reasons of double-sidedness of the process and/or stiffening of the opposite knee or hip joint. In this category also belong joint destructions with therapy-resistant flexion contractions of more than 20 to 30 degrees and misadjustments of the frontal plane, which passively cannot be corrected sufficiently.
2. Knee-joint ankyloses, especially bilateral. Remobilizing one side with the aid of a hinge-type prosthesis can be tried. However, if on the side that is to be operated upon there is a stiffening of the hip joint, this should possibly be eliminated before implantation of the knee prosthesis, because otherwise premature loosening, serious material wear, and stress fractures caused by very unfavorable leverages threaten the success of the knee prosthesis.
3. Hinge-type prostheses are indicated in cases where implantation of partial prosthesis has failed. In these cases, a total hinge-type prosthesis is a second line of defense.
4. Cases of exceptional indications, e.g. treatment of certain tumors proximal to the joint and for which a resection with a bridging of the defects is not advisable because of the age of the patient. In such cases, a special type of prosthesis may be suggested after careful consideration of all factors.

The age of the patient is a very important presupposition for the application of the hinge-type models. Normally, the patient should be over 65 years old. For the rest, all the possibilities of joint make-up must be considered, including the patellectomy, the osteotomies close to the joint, the prostheses with sliding surfaces, and the arthrodeses, before we implant a hinge-type prosthesis. All single-axis knee joints offer compromising solutions, and generally the types which come close to optimal construction, are those that:

1. demand a minimal of bone resection and therefore allow for reversion to other tried methods of treatment,
2. do not forgo the natural joint condyles as load carrying surfaces and therefore provide a broad distribution of the forces,
3. have the axis positioned in the center of the physiological center curve,
4. have an axis that does not carry the full load alone,
5. work according to the low-friction principle,
6. exhibit a sufficient rotational safety and sufficient length of stem and shafts in the valgus position, and
7. allow bending of the lower leg of at least 110 to 120 degrees as well as elastic braking of extension and flexion movements (Figs. 4,5).

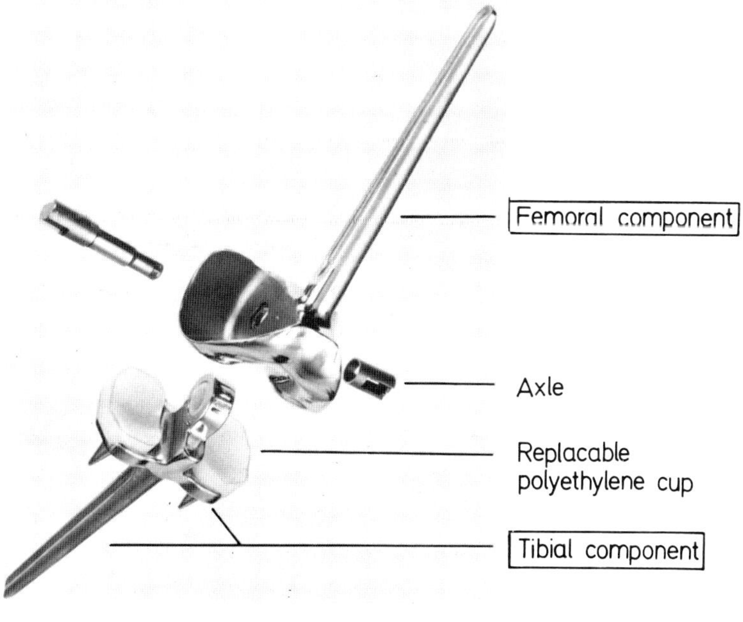

Fig. 4 The Blauth prosthesis before assembly. The articular surface of the femoral part slides over the replaceable polyethylene cups of the tibial component. The load is spread over large areas and the low-friction principle is realized. The axis is unloaded and has polyethylene bearings

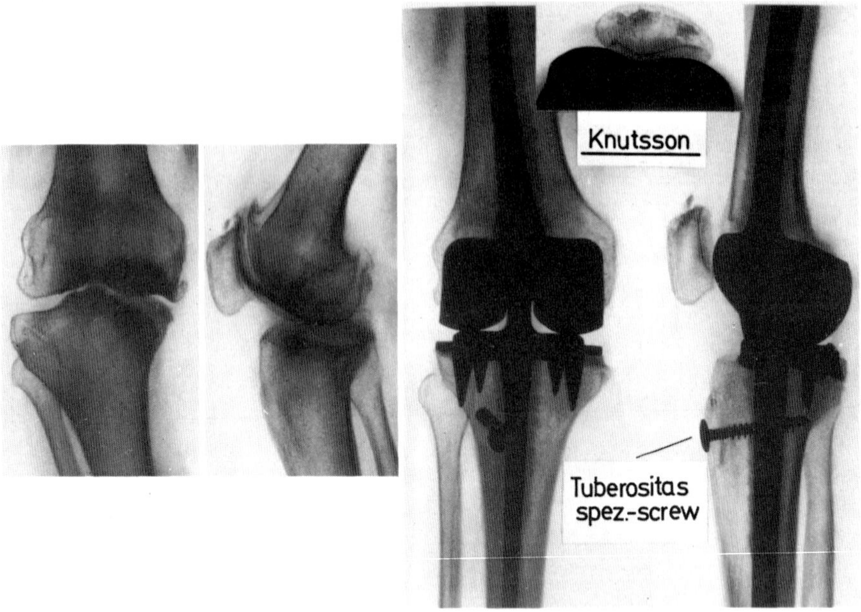

Fig. 5 Implanted Blauth prosthesis. Radiograph of an 82-year old patient with a severe varus gonarthrosis

In the future work should be done on additional improvements in hinge-type prostheses. As short-range goals, the following should be considered:

1. Implantation without cement.
2. Better solutions to the problems of rotation and the patella femoral joint. It should be possible to reach an elastically retarded rotation of the prosthesis parts towards one another, including the extended position, and to diminish high compression on the patella femoral joint.
3. Better braking of dynamic forces in flexion and extension.
4. Progressive development of materials which suggests improvements in hinge-type prostheses.

Further progress in hinge-type prosthesis may be attained by application of new technological systems.

In conclusion, we offer a short summary of published reports, and in doing so, would like to point out the most important complications in various hinge-type prostheses. As mentioned initially, these statistics should only be interpreted very cautiously because they give by no means information on realistic conditions and probably convey a much too optimistic impression. In a great many reports, statements on observation periods and additional details important for the evaluation, are missing. Many reported results (Table 3) are based on very short-term experience, some as little as a few months.

A total of 837 Walldius prostheses are mentioned in the literature, but only 672 include indications of observation periods of more than 6 months. Of this total, 558 were satisfactory, with 94 bad results, 38 severe infections, 4 amputations, 27 loosenings, and 19 bone fractures (1,3,6,7,10,12,14,21,23,24,27,30,33,34,40,55,56,57).

Table 3 Reported results with hinge-type prostheses

	Walldius	Shiers	Guepar	St. Georg	Young
Number	672	309	324	410	143
Satisfactory	558	253	308	389	72
Bad	94	56	16	21	71
Infection	38	36	13	6	20
Amputation	4	3			3
Loosening	27	25	4	2	
Fracture	19	18	1	5	1

Of 552 reported Shiers knee implants, only 309 indicate observation periods of 6 months to 12 years; satisfactory results are reported with 253, bad results with 56 patients. Severe infections occurred in 36 cases. Three patients had limbs amputated, loosening occurred 25 times, and fractures of the prosthesis stem and bone fractures occurred 18 times (2,11,14,16,24,30,33,39,44,45).

Of 470 Guepar knees, 324 show observation periods of 6 months to a maximum of 3 years and report mostly satisfactory results. More precise statements are missing in the remaining 146 cases. The count of patella luxations is strikingly high (12,19,23,24, 29,32,36,38,41,58).

Of 410 St. Georg-prostheses with observation periods from 6 months to 5 years, 389 have shown good results, with 21 bad results. Six infections, 2 loosenings, and 5 fractures are reported; 48 patients had retropatellar complaints (17,18,47).

Of 154 Young prostheses with observation periods of 6 months to 13 years, 72 were satisfactory, 71 had bad results; 20 infections occurred. In 12 cases, the prosthesis had to be removed. In all of the 12 cases, metalosis occurred. In addition, 3 amputations and 17 arthrodeses were necessary (22,23,24,28,59).

All these statistics should make us think in two respects:

1. The superficiality and lack of criteria with which many an author offers his results in so-called "surveys" is disappointing. Such presentations lead nowhere and only obscure the extraordinarily difficult questions that we encounter in knee joint endoprosthetics. What we need are reports on regular test examinations on the same patients from which we can observe developments over long periods. Information on early results should only be stated when the author feels obliged to write such reports. In those cases, emphasis should be on uniform diagnosis as well as assessment guides which allow comparison of the results. If at all possible, the surgeon should not personally conduct these data compilations; he is frequently prejudiced and judges rather optimistically.
2. These statistics show the extent of severe complications which accompany hinge-type prostheses. Furthermore, no mention has been made of drop foot, tendon ruptures, torn tuberositas tibiae, skin necrosis, exchange of prostheses, sinking in of prostheses components, shaft perforations, misalignment, and many more. In this analysis, the

Young and Shiers prostheses were most problematical, followed by the Walldius prosthesis. This may result from the fact that these models have been observed for a longer period. Second generation prostheses, such as the Guepar, St. Georg, Stanmoore (42), or our own model prostheses, permit only preliminary conclusions.

Presently, it appears that the decision to implant a hinge-type prosthesis must be considered with great reservation. In principle, it would be better, if the implantations could be effected in clean-air operating theaters and could be performed only by certain clinics, whose primary effort is directed toward working with these problems. Only if several clinics, working with a certain model, collaborate by operating and documenting according to common rules, can utilizable evidence and a safe basis for further research be established.

REFERENCES

1. v.Andrian-Werburg, H., Jentschura, G.: Total Walldius knee endoprosthesis. Journal of Biomedical Materials Research Symposium 5 (part 2), 289 (1974)
2. Arden, G.P.: Total knee replacement. Clinical Orthopaedics 94, 92 (1973)
3. Armstrong, G.D.: The Walldius total knee prosthesis. Journal of Bone and Joint Surgery 51-B, 778 (1969)
4. Attenborough et al.: Stabilized gliding total knee replacement. In: Ingwersen et al., edit., The knee joint, JCS 324, pp. 234-241, Excerpta Medica (1974)
5. Aubriot, J.H. et al.: La prothese Guepar. Acta Orthopaedica Belgica 39, 257 (1973)
6. Bain, A.M.: Replacement of the knee joint with the Walldius prosthesis using cement fixation. Clinical Orthopaedics 94, 65 (1973)
7. Blauth, W.: Zur Kniegelenk-Totalprothese nach Walldius. Zeitschrift für Orthopädie 109, 417 (1971)
8. Blauth, W.: Bauprinzipien einer neuen Kniegelenktotalprothese. Zeitschrift für Orthopädie 113, 527 (1975)
   and
   Über eine neue Kniegelenk-Totalprothese. Medizinisch-Orthopädische Technik 94, 65 (1974)
9. Blietz, R.: Construction of a simple spherical knee endoprosthesis and clinical trial. In: O.S. Ingwersen, et al., edit., The knee joint, JCS 324, pp. 232-243, Excerpta Medica (1974)
10. Blundell-Jones, G.: Total knee replacement – the Walldius hinge. Clinical Orthopaedics 94, 50 (1973)
11. Brady, T.A., Garber, J.N.: Knee joint replacement using Shiers' knee hinge. Journal of Bone and Joint Surgery 56-A, 1610 (1974)
12. Brussatis, F.: Erfahrungen mit der Scharnierprothese am Kniegelenk. Zeitschrift für Orthopädie 113, 523 (1975)
13. Buchholz, H., Engelbrecht, E.: Die intracondyläre totale Kniegelenkendoprothese "Modell St. Georg". Der Chirurg 44, 373 (1973)
14. Casagrande, P.A., Turner, R.R.: Total knee replacement. Clinical Orthopaedics 89, 150 (1972)
15. Deane, G.: A new concept in knee joint design. In: O.S. Ingwersen, et al., edit., The knee joint, JCS 324, pp. 244-247, Excerpta Medica (1974)

16. Duparc, J. et al.: Arthroplastie du genou par prothese charniere. Revue de Chirurgie Orthopedique 58, 179 (1972)

17. Engelbrecht, E.: Erfahrungen mit den Knie-Endoprothesen "Modell St. Georg". Zentralblatt für Chirurgie 99, 171 (1974)

18. Engelbrecht, E., Tillmann, K.: Vortrag auf dem VIII. European Rheumatology Congress, Helsinki, 1.-7.6.1975

19. Erban, W.K.: Operative Erfahrungen mit der Guepar-Endoprothese. Zeitschrift für Orthopädie 113, 519 (1975)

20. Fick, R.: Handbuch der Anatomie und Mechanik der Gelenke. Jena: G. Fischer 1911, Vol. 3, pp. 521-593

21. Freeman, P.A.: Walldius arthroplasty (a review of 80 cases). Clinical Orthopaedics 94, 85 (1973)

22. Friedebold, G., Radloff, H.: Alloarthroplasties of the knee joint. Reconstruction Surgery and Traumatology 12, 181 (1971)

23. Gandolfi, M., Demartin, F.: Total prosthesis of the knee joint. Off print from Lo Scalpello 1973, pp. 19-44

24. Groeneveld, H.G.: Alloarthroplastik des Kniegelenks. Zeitschrift für Orthopädie 113, 512 (1975)

25. Gschwend, N. et al.: The GSB knee prosthesis. In: O.S. Ingwersen et al., edit., The knee joint, JCS 324, pp. 261-266, Excerpta Medica (1974)

26. Gschwend, N.: Indikation zur Verwendung von Teilprothesen, Schlittenprothesen und Scharnierprothesen am Beispiel des Kniegelenkes. 23. Jahrestagung der Vereinigung Süddeutscher Orthopäden e.V., Baden-Baden, 30.4.-4.5.1975

27. Habermann, E.T. et al.: The knee arthroplasty with the use of the Walldius total knee prosthesis. Clinical Orthopaedics 94, 72 (1973)

28. Hanslik, L.: First experience with the knee joint replacement using the Young hinged prosthesis combined with a modification on the McKeever patella prosthesis. Clinical Orthopaedics 94, 115 (1973)

29. Hanslik, L.: Erfahrungen mit der Kniegelenkendoprothetik und der Alloplastik des patello-femoralen Gleitlagers. Zeitschrift für Orthopädie 113, 516 (1975)

30. Harrison, M. et al.: The hinge total knee arthroplasty. Journal of Bone and Joint Surgery 56-B, 587 (1974)

31. Herbert, J.J., Herbert, A.: A new total knee prosthesis. Clinical Orthopaedics 94, 202 (1973)

32. Insall, J.N. et al.: A comparison of four different total knee replacements. Journal of Bone and Joint Surgery 56-A, 1541 (1974)

33. Jackson, J.B., Elson, R.A.: Evaluation of the Walldius and other prostheses for knee arthroplasty. Clinical Orthopaedics 94, 104 (1973)

34. König, G. et al.: Erfahrungen mit der Kniegelenktotalendoprothese nach Walldius. Zeitschrift für Orthopädie 113, 513 (1975)

35. Lagrange, J., Letournel, E.: Total knee replacement with the "L.L."-type prosthesis. Clinical Orthopaedics 94, 249 (1973)

36. Mazas, F.B. et al.: Guepar total knee prosthesis. Clinical Orthopaedics 94, 211 (1973)

37. Menschik, A.: Mechanik des Kniegelenkes, I. Teil. Zeitschrift für Orthopädie 112, 481 (1974) and
Mechanik des Kniegelenkes, II. Teil, Schlußrotation. Zeitschrift für Orthopädie 113, 388 (1975)

38. Mohing, W.: Erfahrungen mit dem Guepar-Knie. Zeitschrift für Orthopädie 113, 520 (1975)

39. Phillips, R.S.: Shiers' alloplasty of the knee. Clinical Orthopaedics 94, 122 (1973)

40. Phillips, H., Taylor, T.G.: The Walldius hinge arthroplasty. Journal of Bone and Joint Surgery 57-B, 59 (1975)

41. Ritter, H., Overbeck, W.: Unsere Erfahrungen mit der Guepar-Totalendoprothese des Kniegelenks. Archiv für orthopädische und Unfall-Chirurgie 78, 122 (1974)

42. Scales, J.T., Lettin, U.: The evolution of the Stanmoore hinged total knee replacement. In: O.S. Ingwersen, et al., edit., The knee joint, JCS 324, pp. 284-295 Excerpta Medica (1974)

43. Sheehan, J.M.: Arthroplasty of the knee. In: O.S. Ingwersen et al., edit., The knee joint, JCS 324, pp. 296-299, Excerpta Medica (1974)

44. Shiers, L.G.P.: Arthroplasty of the knee. Journal of Bone and Joint Surgery 42-B, 31 (1960)

45. Shiers, L.G.P.: Hinge arthroplasty of the knee. Journal of Bone and Joint Surgery 47-B, 586 (1965)

46. Swanson, S.A.V. et al.: Laboratory tests on total joint replacement prostheses. Journal of Bone and Joint Surgery 55-B, 759 (1973)

47. Tillmann, K. et al.: Zur partiellen und totalen endoprothetischen Versorgung der Kniegelenke. Zeitschrift für Orthopädie 113, 509 (1975)

48. Trillat, A. et al.: La prothese rotatoire du genou. Acta Orthopaedica Belgica 39, 296 (1973)

49. Wagner, J. et al.: A mechanical study of total knee arthroplasty: preliminary report. In: O.S. Ingwersen et al., edit., The knee joint, JCS 324, pp. 58-62, Excerpta Medica (1974)

50. Wagner, J., Bourgois, R.: Biomechanical study of the hinge knee prosthesis. Clinical Orthopaedics 102, 188 (1974)

51. Walldius, B.: Arthroplasty of the knee joint employing an acrylic prosthesis. Acta Orthopaedica Scandinavica 23, 121 (1953)

52. Walldius, B.: Arthroplasty of the knee, using an endoprosthesis. Acta Orthopaedica Scandinavica Supplement 24 (1957)

53. Walldius, B.: Arthroplasty of the knee, 8 years experience. Acta Orthopaedica Scandinavica 30, 137 (1960)

54. Walldius, B.: Arthroplasty of the knee, using an endoprosthesis. SICOT, XI^{ieme} Congres, Mexico 1969, p. 446

55. Walldius, B.: A comparative analysis of different methods for arthroplasty of the knee. Instn. Mech. Engrs. 209, 34 (1974)

56. Wilson, F.C.: Total replacement of the knee in rheumatoid arthritis. Journal of Bone and Joint Surgery 54-A, 1429 (1972)

57. Wilson, F.C.: Total replacement of the knee in rheumatoid arthritis. Clinical Orthopaedics 94, 58 (1973)

58. Witvoit, J. and the Guepar group: Guepar total knee prosthesis. In: O.S. Ingwersen et al., edit., The knee Joint, JCS 324, pp. 305-315, Excerpta Medica (1974)

59. Young, H.H.: Reconstruction of the knee joint with Young-type hinged Vitallium prosthesis. Reconstruction Surgery and Traumatology 12, 176 (1971)

ANCHORING HIP ENDOPROSTHESIS WITHOUT BONE CEMENT

H. Mittelmeier

Despite several important earlier attempts, wider use of replacement hip joints was first initiated by the Judet brothers with their acrylic femoral head prosthesis. The good results initially obtained were, however, only temporary. Prosthesis fracture and surface wear with foreign-body tissue reaction around the abraded particles occurred. It soon became evident that polymethylmethacrylate was inadequate for both mechanical and chemical reasons. Furthermore, the metallic portion of the prosthesis was prone to breakage. Broadly, these problems were associated with implant materials (Fig. 1).

Significantly, in many cases, failure resulted from bone resorption. The canal for the stem of the femoral neck widened, and painful reciprocating movement or fluttering of the prosthesis resulted, especially in transverse implantation. Cases with relatively vertical insertion, in contrast, often became well, thereby emphasizing the importance of biomechanical influence, and demonstrating that the implantation of an endoprosthesis without other means (for instance bone cement) is not unsolvable.

Lacking knowledge of material properties and appreciation of the biomechanical bone reaction, the Judet procedure mostly resulted in a practical failure. Scales in 1967 considered it to be "one of the greatest disasters in surgery," but, if so, it was a major milestone in advancing the technology (Fig. 2).

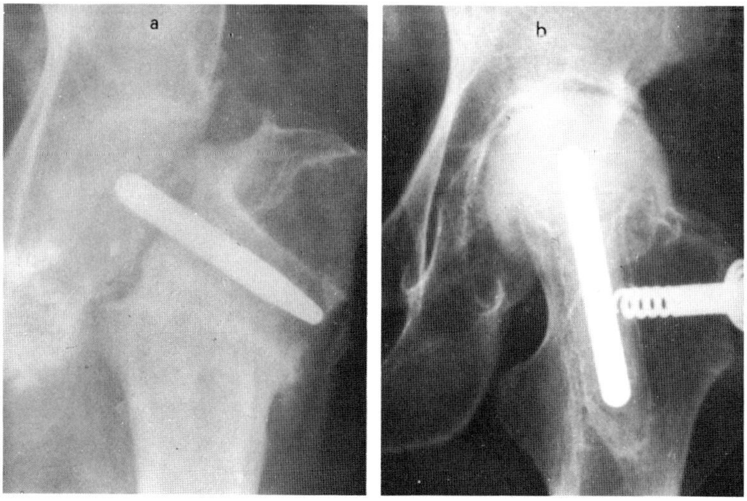

Fig. 1 Early forms of hemialloarthroplasty of the hip joint (type Judet)

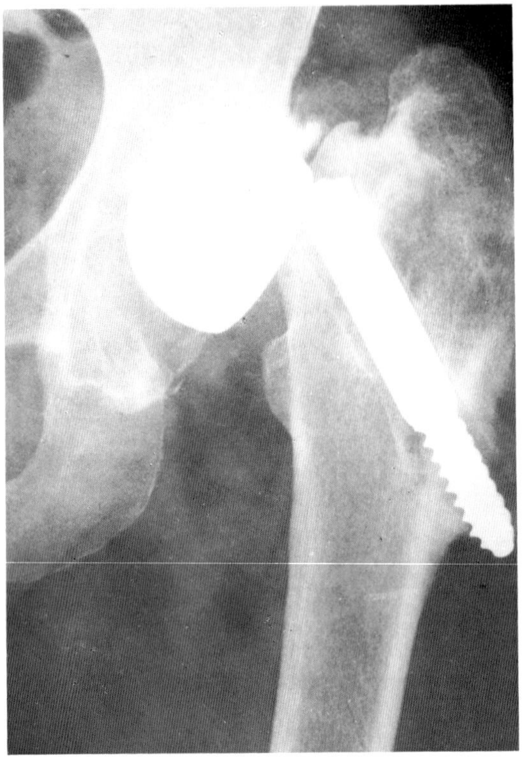

Fig. 2
Failure of a Judet prosthesis due to loosening of the metal stem and fracture of the head

From 1953 through 1956, as Assistant in Pathologic Anatomy, I had the chance to histologically study several hip joints after arthroplasty, and prepared the first comprehensive report on tissue reaction in alloarthroplasty in 1956, that study forming the basis for our further developmental work. We could show that the chemically induced foreign-body reaction occurred only in the capsula where the abraded acrylate powder collected, and that the important bone resorption in the canal of the femoral neck was not produced by this, but for biomechanical reasons (Fig. 3). In contrast, we could see that the body tries to establish a new load bearing layer within the femoral neck, around of the stem of the prosthesis (stimulated by the mechanical influence). Below the surface of connective tissue, a network of a new bone is formed, supported by existing cancellous bone trabeculas, which evidently become stronger by apposition. Later, a transformation into corticalis-like lamellous bone has been observed. In cases with transverse implantation and high shearing forces, a superficial resorption of the new bone by osteoclasts occurred. Obviously, bone adaptation here is overcome by too much stress concentration, thereby resulting in an adaptation inbalance and failure by loosening of the prosthesis.

So we stated the hypothesis that an adaptation balance can be achieved when forces on the prosthesis are distributed below a critical pressure limit (by enlargement of the load-bearing bone layer) and that resorption proceeds when pressure (despite enlargement of the weight-bearing surface) remains over a critical limit. This limit is established by mechanical forces on the prosthesis, by the size of adapted bone surface, and by the biological rules of osteoclastic reaction.

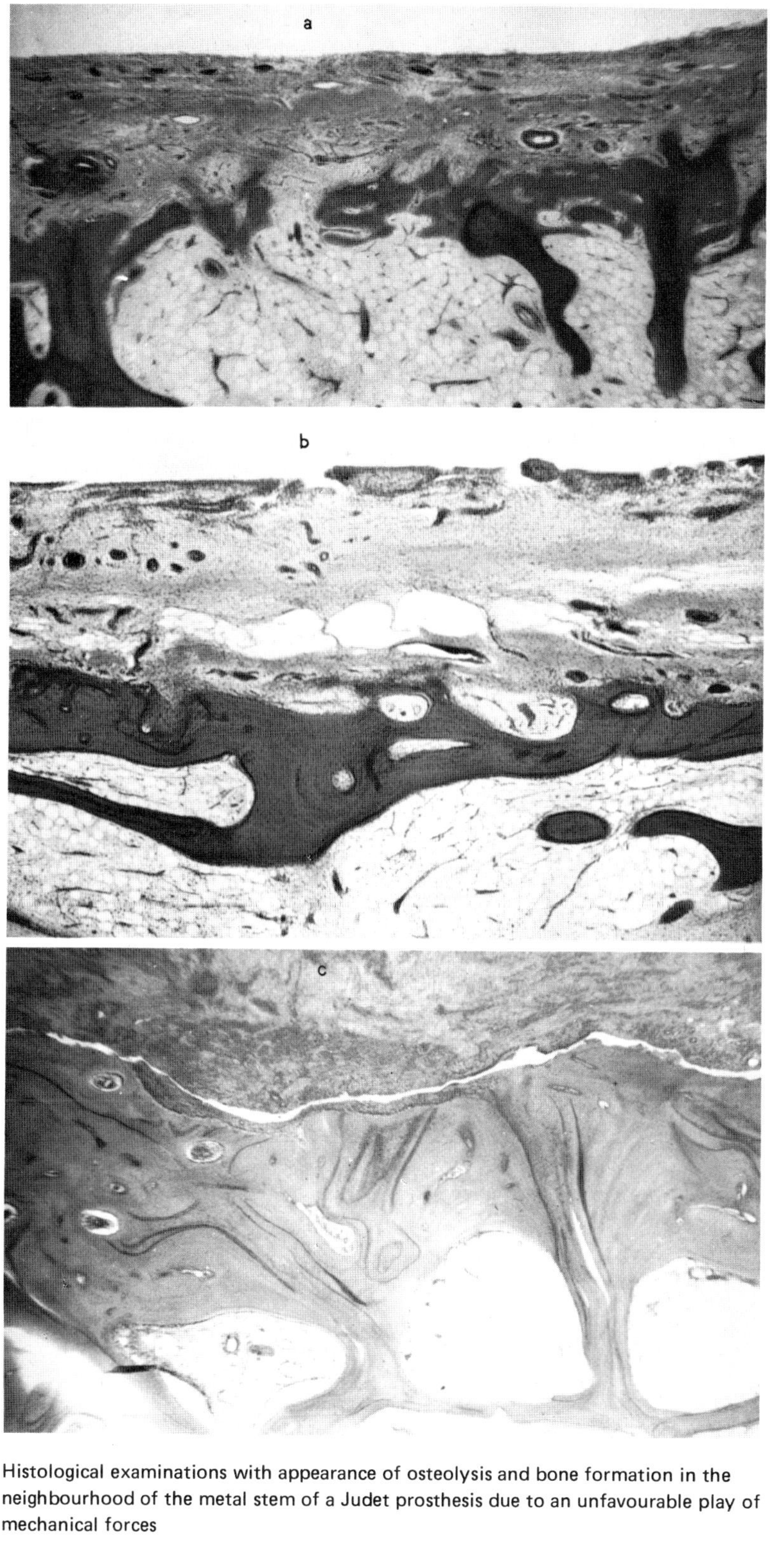

Fig. 3 Histological examinations with appearance of osteolysis and bone formation in the neighbourhood of the metal stem of a Judet prosthesis due to an unfavourable play of mechanical forces

To solve the problem of loosening, the direction of insertion might be improved to achieve a better load distribution within some critical limit. But the real solution to the problem appears to be enlarging the surface of the prosthesis and its bony load-bearing layer, as proposed almost 20 years ago; the main principle of anchorage of endoprosthesis is the reduction of bone pressure by enlargement of the surface.

But this proposal was generally neglected, because the new American endoprostheses of Moore and Thompson were believed to solve the problem by anchoring the stem in the medullary shaft canal of the femur to establish primary contact with the hard corticalis. Early reports over several years showed a permanent success, but according to our recent follow-up studies (60 cases), the success rate approximated 15 %. Despite 85 % of failures, once more there is evidence that implantation without cement may be successful. The failure of most cases resulted from bone resorption in the acetabulum and especially in the femur resulting in a fluttering movement of the prosthesis.

To avoid resorption in the acetabulum and femur, the development of arthroplasty went to the total hip replacement with an additional cup and to implantation using acrylic cement (McKee and Farrar; Charnley). As the metallic combinations showed remarkably high friction and rate of loosening, as well as wear, resulting in metallosis, Charnley used the combination of metal and plastics, which have considerably lower friction.

Anchoring the prosthesis in the bone using cement is not accomplished by the same effect as using a glue. It is based on mechanical contact of cement protrusions in the bone cavities, and long-term stability is the result of indirect enlargement of the surface of the prosthesis by the cement.

The significant advantage of a good immediate fixation of the prosthesis by the bone cement and the excellent tolerance of polyethylene brought this system and its derivations (use of cobalt-chromium alloys instead of stainless steel) to a high success, and its use became world wide.

But polyethylene shows wear after some years and therefore does not appear to be a "lifetime" material, useful even in young patients (Fig. 4). Based on our experience with polyacrylic material in the Judet prosthesis, we were especially sceptical regarding the compatibility and endurance of acrylic cement and predicted resorption of bone surface, fatigue fractures of the cement with loosening of the prosthesis, and the possibility of cancerous metaplasia after a long-term implantation (over 30 years).

The U.S. Food and Drug Administration did not approve the use of acrylic cement for implantation until 3 years ago. Many orthopedic surgeons still restrict the use of cement to patients older than 60 years. Hackenbroch Jr. (Fig. 5) reported about 25 % aseptic loosenings during an observation period of 3 to 6 years. The average securely anchored lifetime of the cemented prosthesis is calculated to be between 5 and 10 years. We therefore state that, until this time has elapsed, we really have no long-term arthroplasty, useful for younger patients, with a good whole-life prognosis. Further efforts to overcome material and loosening problems are evident in the last years in new attempts to develop self-locking prostheses, for instance of the type by Sivash, Ring, and others, and with new materials, for instance titanium, but without convincing success. Judet is presently trying

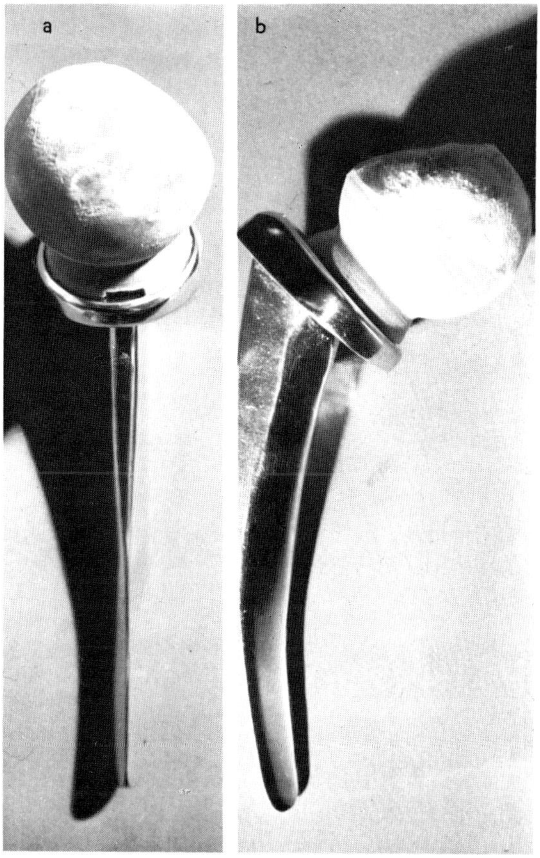

Fig. 4
High degree of wear and resulting change of shape in the polyethylene head of a femur stem prosthesis

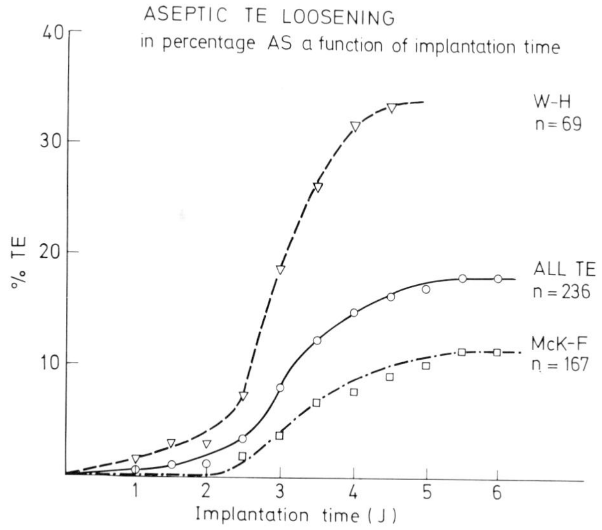

Fig. 5 Latest results of a study on the number of loosening complications in total hip joint replacement over a period of 6 years for various types of prosthesis

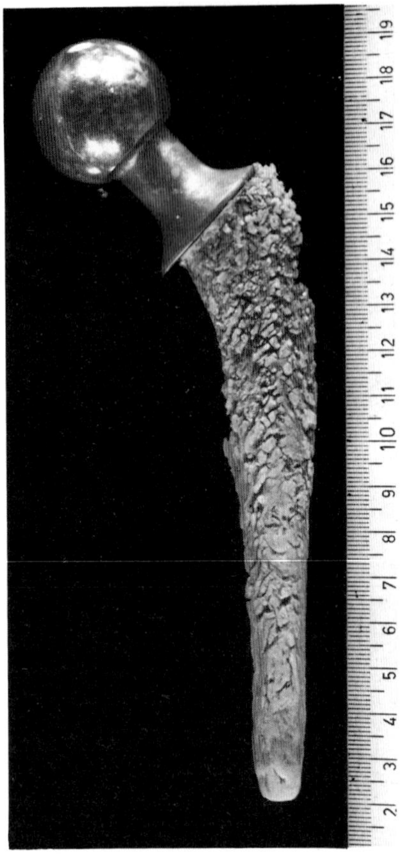

Fig. 6
Possibility of non-cement anchoring of a stem prosthesis due to structuring and thus enlargement of the contact surface area to the bone

a new self-locking prosthesis with a porous metal surface (having the further disadvantage of high friction) (Figs. 6,7).

In 1969, in collaboration with the Osteo-AG Switzerland, development started on our new self-locking prosthesis, based upon the principle of enlargement of the surface. We have named it the "load-bearing-ribs prosthesis" (Fig. 8).

This prosthesis was designed as a total prosthesis. The stem for the femoral head was designed with surrounding ribs (rims) to enlarge its surface and to allow the ingrowth of bone. The head is interchangeable and available in different lengths, fitted to the stem with the self-locking cone. A cup the shape of an obtuse cone with external thread is provided. For the cup, we choose the obtuse conical shape to prevent tilting and to provide good attachement by the cone expanding during installation. The enlarged surface area of the cups is (according to the different sizes) 40 to 50 cm^2 and of the stem 20 to 30 cm^2.

First, we constructed the cup of metal and the ball of polyethylene. We then designed a second type with ceramic cup and ceramic head which we now prefer because the ceramic type has excellent material advantages.

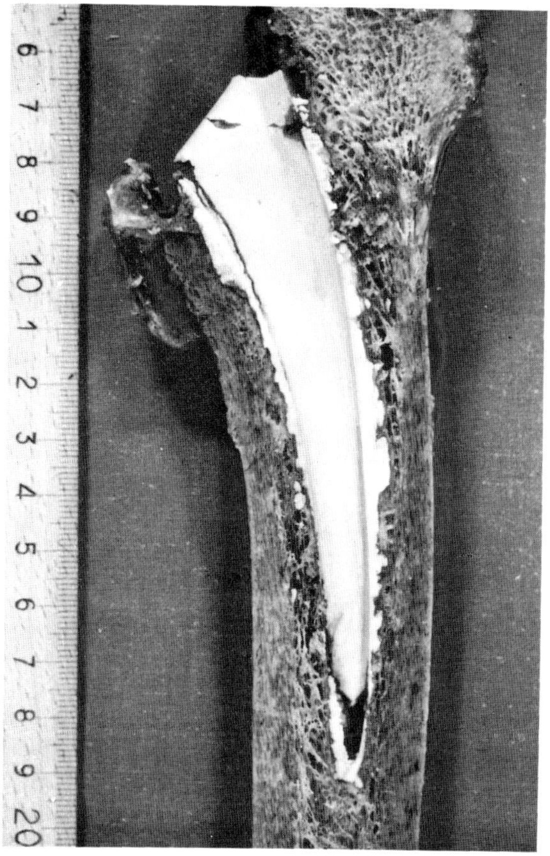

Fig. 7
Possibility of non-cement anchoring of a stem prosthesis due to structuring and thus enlargement of the contact surface area to the bone

Ceramics have been studied as implant material for several years in the U.S., France, Switzerland, and Germany, especially in conjunction with a porous metal to substitute for bone and achieve the ingrowth of bone. It can be proven that a pure aluminium-oxide-ceramic, consisting of 99.5 % Al_2O_3, has no corrosion at all and is better tolerated by the tissue than any other material. The stable oxidation prevents the dissolution of metallic ions and therefore no hydrolysis occurs. But porotic ceramic is not strong enough mechanically and therefore we are trying to use a dense ceramic of high strength, that is useful for both cup and head.

Mechanical investigations of dense ceramic/ceramic showed that friction, in contrast with metal/metal and metal/plastic combinations, decreased to near that of the natural healthy joint (Fig. 9). Wear is less than in other combinations and, after a very short time, approaches zero, while the surface roughness becomes less than 0.1 micron. Thus, ceramic has a self-smoothing effect and, based on results from in vitro accelerated life tests, we can say that it has practically a whole-life endurance capability. Heads and cups were capable of bearing a load higher than one ton (in static and dynamic compression).

Unfortunately, the ceramic has a relative low bending strength (40 Kp/mm^2), only half that of metal, and therefore, to avoid a break, this material is not used for construction

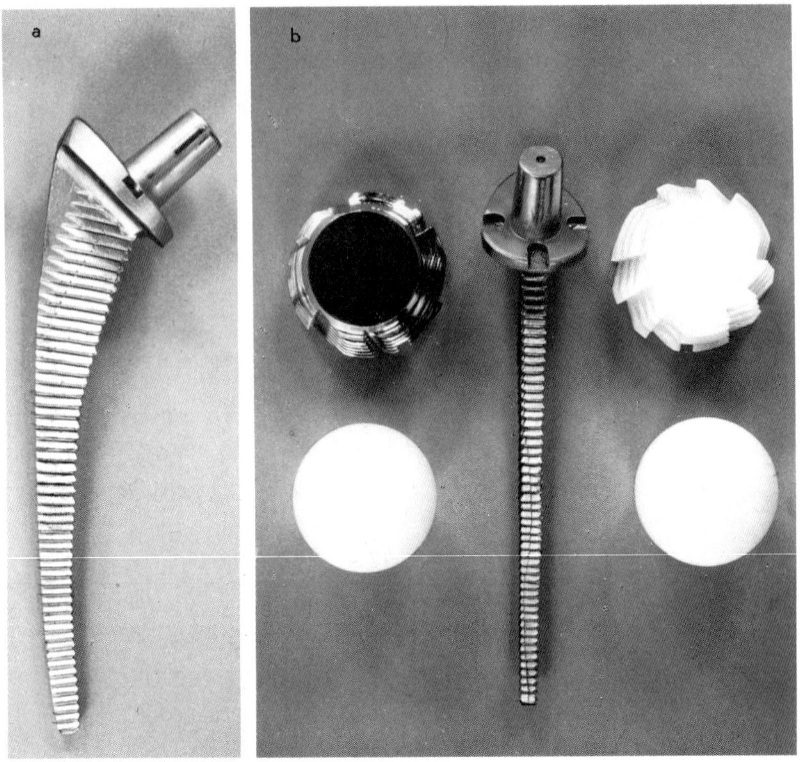

Fig. 8 Further development of non-cement implantation by the application of the "bearing rib" principle for femoral stem and cup anchorage

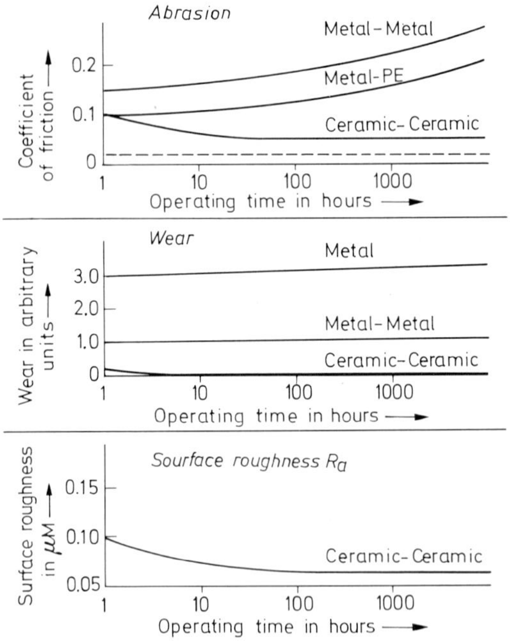

Fig. 9
The nature of articulating surfaces when using different biomaterials for femoral head and cup

of the stem. Instead, proven metal alloys with higher yield strength are used; this is particularly important in striated stems. This produces a compound design. In the future, the stem will be constructed of a new alloy, recently formulated by the Krupp organization in Germany, which is better than the cobalt-chromium alloys (typically Vitallium).

Meanwhile Boutin, in France, in 1971 started the use of ceramics in cemented hip prosthesis. His experience already includes several hundred cases and (as far as we know) he has had no fractures of ceramic cups and heads, but has had some difficulty with anchoring the heads on the stem. These are glued on, and there have been instances of loosening as a result of turning of the ceramic ball, thereby abrading the metal. This is impossible in our type of self-locking conical connection.

In 1971, we first started with animal implantations using dogs (Figs. 10,11). These were performed in collaboration with Harms, Biehl, and Mäusle. The dogs were allowed to

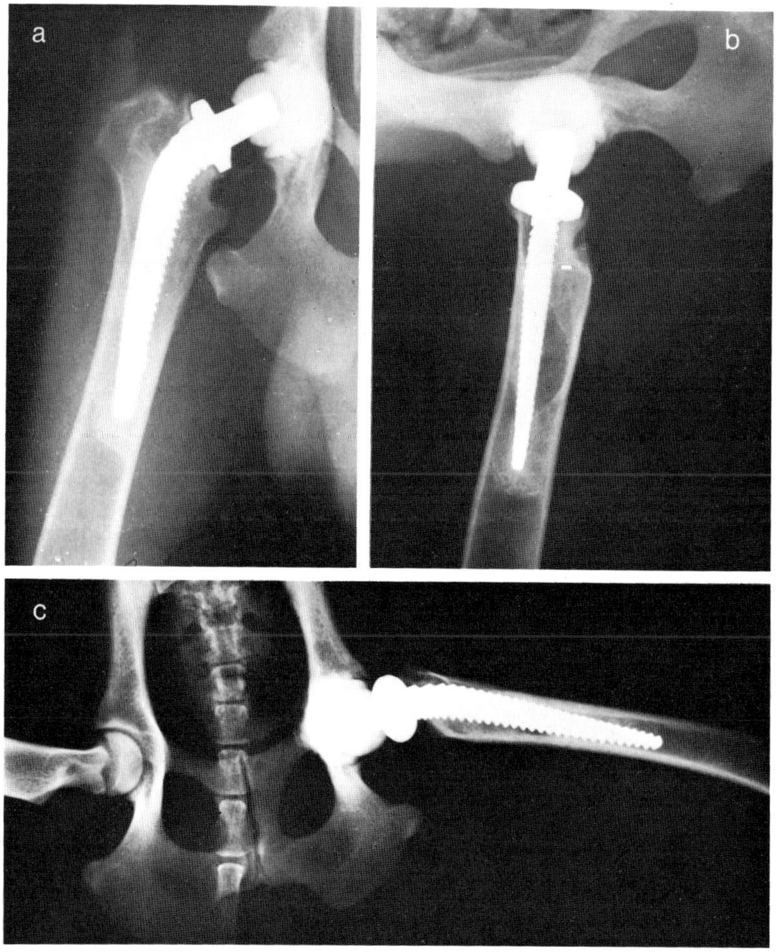

Fig. 10 Radiological follow-up of the behavior of "bearing rib" prostheses in dog experiments

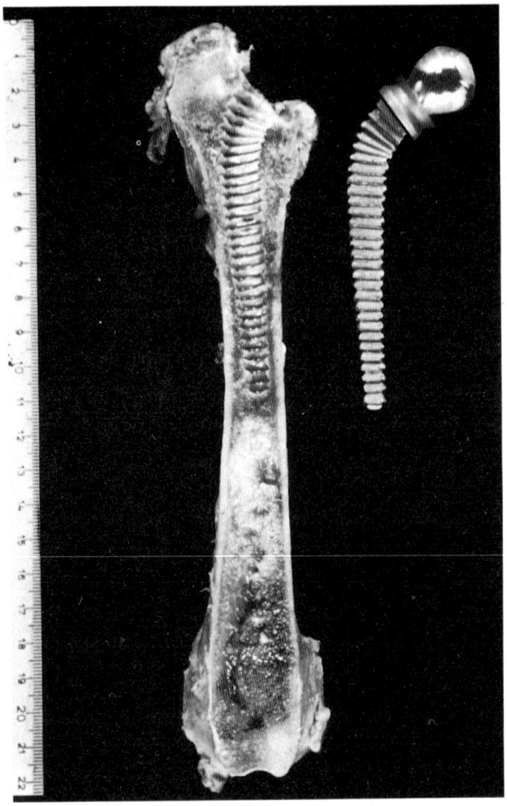

Fig. 11
Preparation of a dog's femur with clearly visible ingrowth of bone structures into the medullary cavity in the direction of the bearing ribs

move freely, and X-rays showed good bone reaction around the stem, building of a new load-bearing layer, with ingrowth of bone into the cavities of the rims.

Histologically, below a thin layer of connective tissue, a callous bone was observed reproducing bony rims in the excavations of the ribbed stem. After one year, a lamellous bone layer without osteoclastic bone resorption was observed. At the top of the stem, was a regular socle (Fig. 12).

For human implants, because of individual anatomical differences, a set of four sizes of cups, equipped with three matching balls (32, 38, and 44 mm in diameter) is needed. Heads of different diameters are available with 2 or 3 different neck lengths in order to provide the necessary muscle tension. In addition, 4 sizes of stems are required which are suitable for all types of balls thereby providing all necessary combinations. This is a significant advantage in comparison to other types of prosthesis with fixed heads.

For older patients with osteoporosis, we have constructed a prosthesis for cement implantation with a hemispherical head and smooth stems, each available in two sizes and to be used with balls 32 and 38 mm in diameter and different neck lengths.

As special instruments, different sizes of conically shaped obtuse reamers are required, as well as conically shaped tapping instruments for preparation of the acetabulum, and cup drivers (with 3 bars fitted into 3 excavations in the rim of the cups). Reamers are

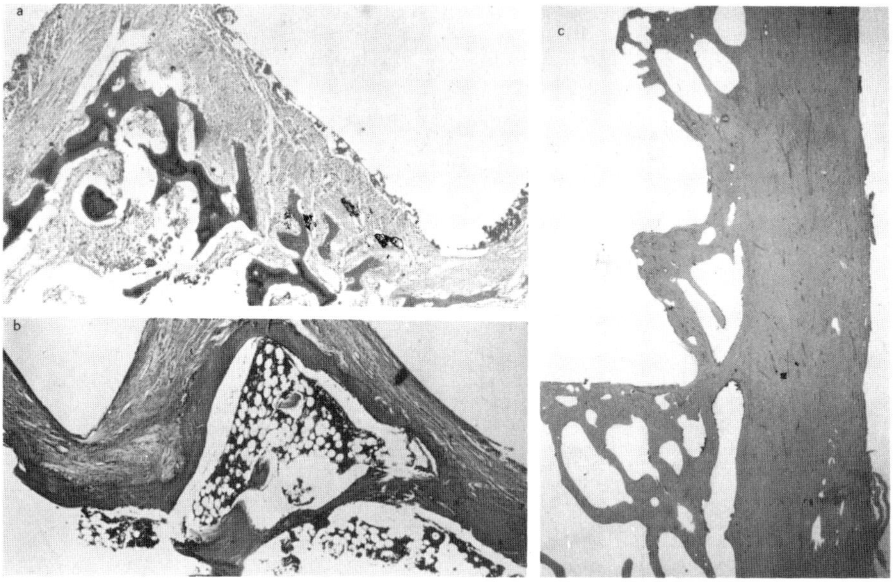

Fig. 12 Histological representation of the newly formed bone structures

required for the femoral cavity, as well as an impactator instrument is required for the stem, and a U-shaped head exchange instrument.

The operative technique is as follows. Normally, the patient is positioned on his posterior, which is a position prefered by the anaesthetist, and gives a better orientation of the position of the pelvis.

Entrance is between the musculus glutaeus medius and musculus tensor fasciae latae (Watson–Jones). To relieve and protect the muscle against hook pressure, we temporarily incide the ventral third of the tendon of the glutaeus medius.

Excision of the ventral capsula is followed by resection of the neck and head (preferable using a saw) and the acetabulum is opened with the aid of several Hohmann elevators. We then remove the resting cartilage and prepare the rough shape of the obtuse cone in the acetabulum using a Lexer chisel and form it exactly with a conical reamer (in 45 ^{o} inclination and 0 ^{o} to 10 ^{o} of anteversion). This is followed by tapping the thread in the acetabulum and driving the cup into position (Fig. 13).

For implantation of the femur part, the leg is brought into uttermost adduction and 90 ^{o} exorotation. Thus, the stump of the neck is directed upwards. The femoral cavity is opened with a chisel (conserving the cancellous bone plug) and reamed so that medial and lateral direct contact with the corticalis is achieved and the proper stem can become inserted with a protrusion of about 1 to 2 cm. Then the cancellous bone plug is brought back into the cavitiy as a support at the top of the stem and finally pushed in by the propulsion instrument, thereby tightly fitted to the bone. It is cramped very tightly into the bone.

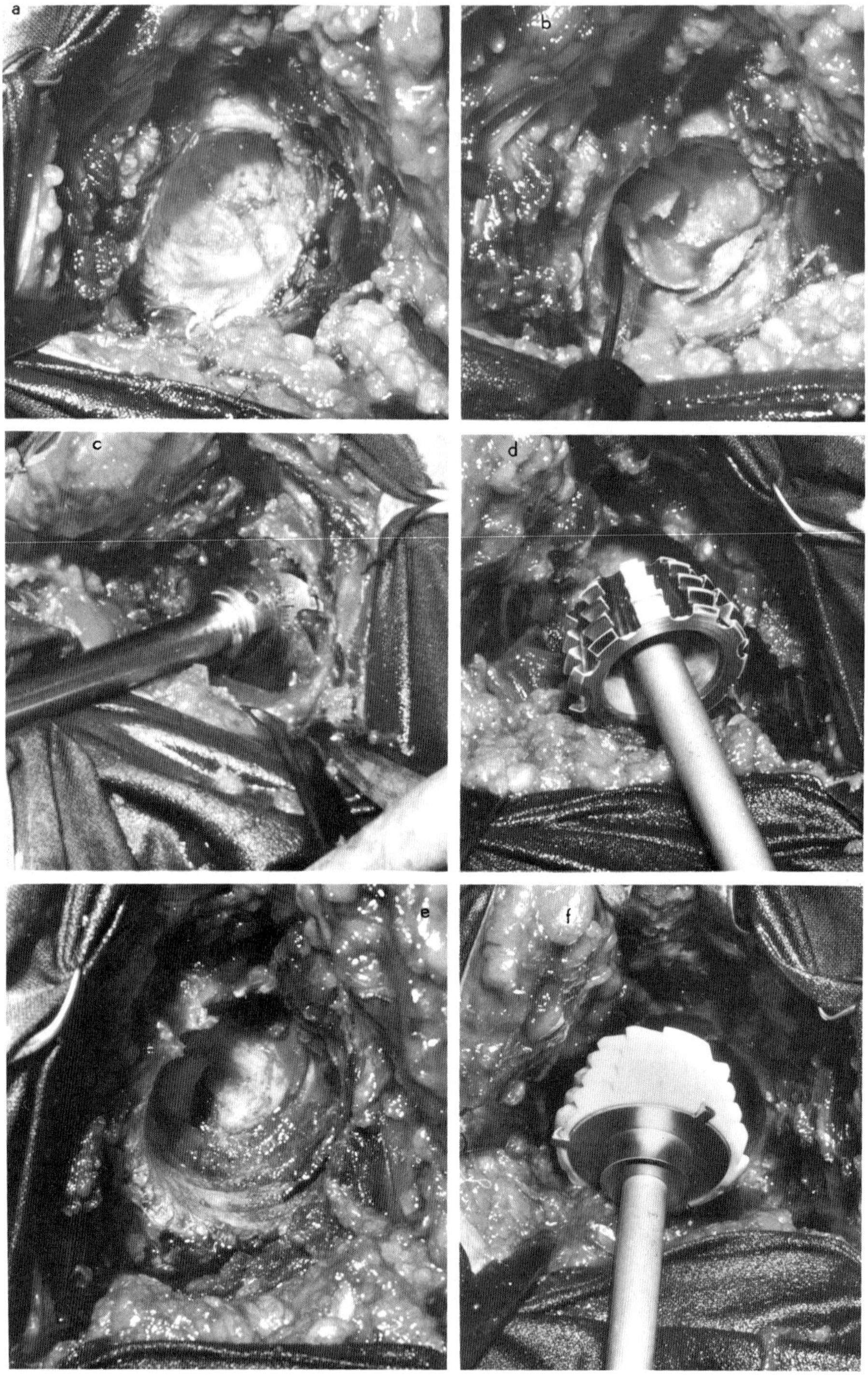

Fig. 13 Stages in the operation for the implantation of a "bearing rib" prosthesis. Preparation of the cup bearing and cement-free cup implantation

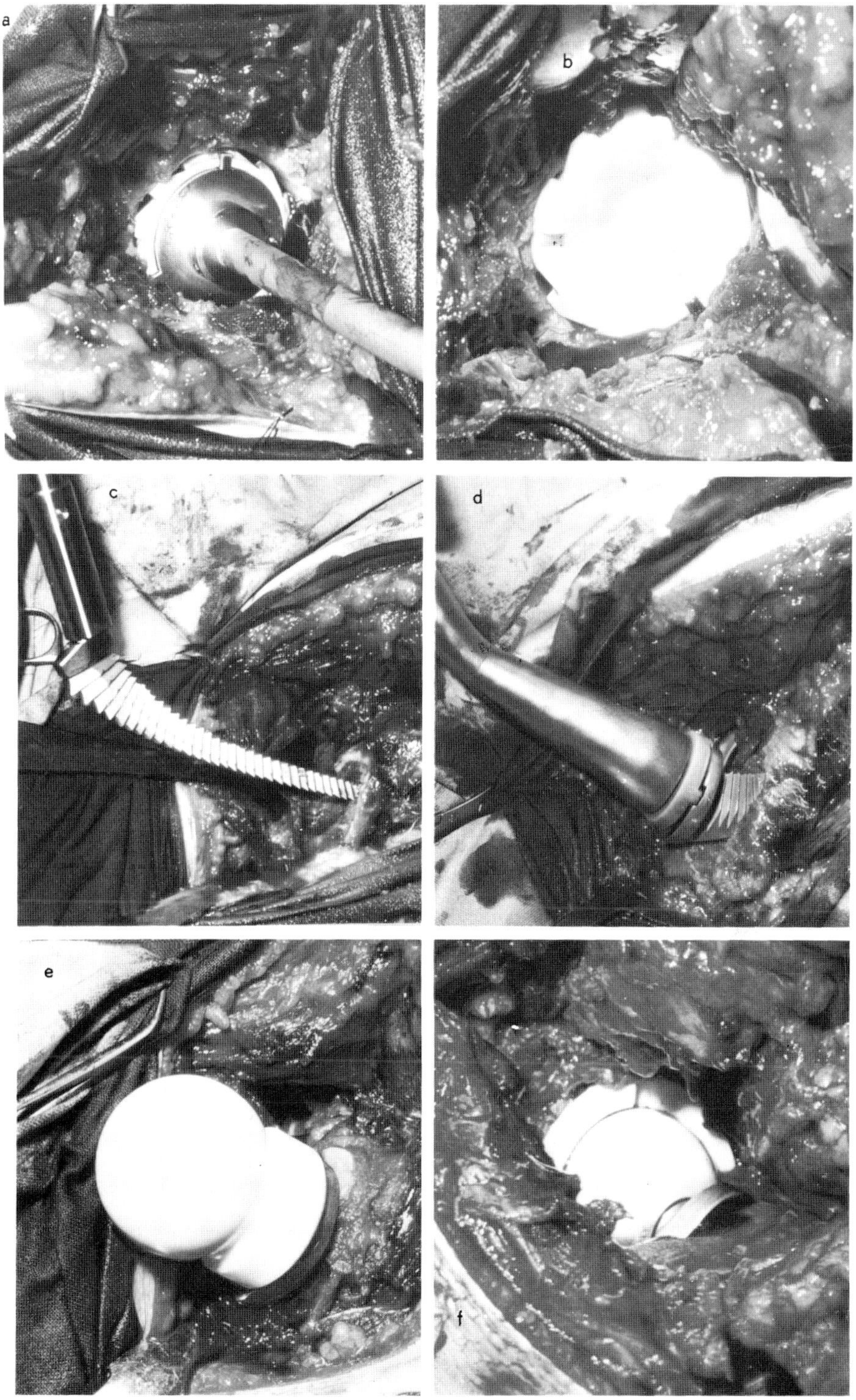

Fig. 14 Following resection of the neck, introduction of the femoral stem prosthesis with bearing ribs, fitting of the ceramic head and repositioning

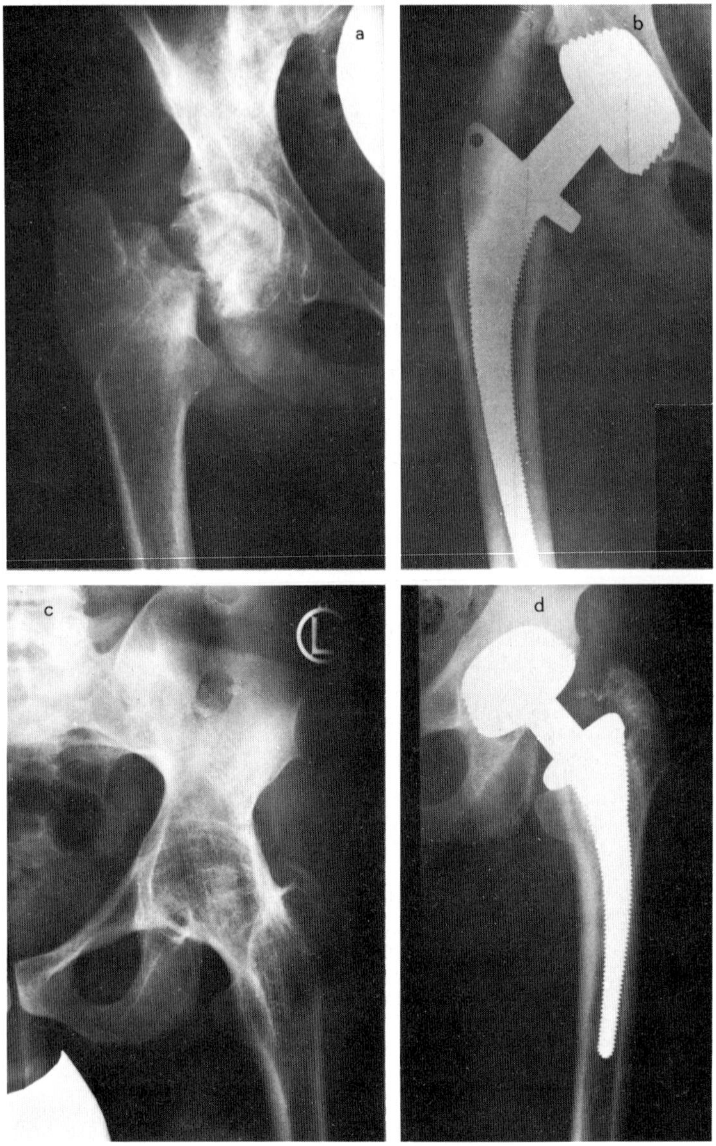

Fig. 15 X-ray images of the non-cemented total hip joint replacement for various indications

Then, the ball is attached to the stem by turning it tightly, and the hip is repositioned by extension and internal rotation of the leg insert, the head being guided by the surgeon's hands (Fig. 14). Sufficient muscle tension is now required. If the head is too long or too short, it may be exchanged by reluxation and removing of the head using the U-shaped instrument, without removing the stem from the femur.

Then follows the application of the drainage, X-ray control and closure of the wound, readapting the ventral third of the gluteus medius tendon, and suturing the fascia lata. In the postoperative treatment, the patient's leg is put into a foam-rubber splint.

Normally, the patient gets up the next day with the aid of a physiotherapist and two crutches. He is allowed to move the hip joint in flexion and extension, but should avoid extreme spreading, adduction, or rotation. He may put the leg on the floor, but without much weight bearing. Hospitalization is normally 2 weeks.

X-ray controls are provided 6 and 12 weeks after the operation. When there is no complication, the patients may increase weight bearing after 6 weeks to about 20 Kg; after 12 weeks they may walk with a simple cane, and after 16 weeks without any support.

Our experience presently is with nearly 100 cases, two thirds of which were implanted without cement, one third (older patients) with bone cement (Fig. 15). Results are generally good. Some difficulties were experienced with early implants when we had only two medium sizes of cups and stems, which were sometimes too large or too small. Now we have overcome these difficulties by the use of additional sizes.

In two cases, we observed an infection, but could control it without removement of the prosthesis. Naturally, because of the short observation time, we cannot give exact prognoses about stability. The cups without bone cement seem all to be stabile. In the stems, we observed some cases which seemed to loosen.

In conclusion, we cannot arrive at a final judgement of the cemented-type prosthesis. For older patients, there will probably be no special problem, except cement problems. But with the self-locking prosthesis, further follow-up of our patients must be carried out. To get more experience, we started recently with 15 other hospitals a wider clinical investigation. Within 1 year we hope to have a better survey. We may have to change some flattering or wobbly stems, but we are sure that we will be able to optimize the stem. Finally, we hope we are making progress toward solving the problems of arthroplasty in younger people; this will indeed be significant progress in orthopedic surgery.

REFERENCES

1. Biehl, G., Harms, J., Mäusle, E.: Tierexperimentelle und histopathologische Untersuchungen über die Anpassungsvorgänge des Knochens nach der Implantation von "Tragrippen-Endoprothesen". Archiv für orthopädische und Unfall-Chirurgie 81, 105 (1975)
2. Boutin, P.: Arthroplastie totale de la hanche par prothese en alumine frittee. Revue de Chirurgie Orthopedique 58, 229 (1972)
3. Charnley, J.: Clinical and laboratory observations on the rate of wear of different plastic materials in the sockets of artificial hip joints. 55th Scientific Meeting "Materials for Use in Medicine and Biology", Cambridge 1974
4. Dörre, E. et al.: Anforderungen an oxidkeramische Werkstoffe als Biomaterial für künstliche Gelenke. Archiv für orthopädische und Unfall-Chirurgie 83, 269 (1975)
5. Esser, M.: Die Hüftgelenksarthrose und ihre operative Behandlung durch plastische Eingriffe. Dissertation Köln 1958
6. Griss, P., Krempien, B., Andrian-Werburg, H. v., Heimke, G., Fleiner, R.: Experimentelle Untersuchung zur Gewebeverträglichkeit oxidkeramischer (Al_2O_3) Abriebteilchen. Archiv für orthopädische und Unfall-Chirurgie 76, 270 (1973)

7. Hench, L.L.: Histo-chemical responses at a biomaterials interface. Clemson University 5th Ann. Biomat. Symposium April 1973

8. Hench, L.L., Paschall, H.A.: Direct chemical bond of bioactive glass-ceramic materials in bone and muscle. Journal of Biomedical Materials Research Symposium 4, 25 (1973)

9. Hulbert, S.F., Klawitter, J.J.: History of ceramic orthopedic implants. Material Research Bulletin 7, 1239 (1972)

10. Hulbert, S.F., Young, F.A., Mathews, R.S., Klawitter, J.J., Talbert, C.D., Stelling, F.H.: Potential of ceramic materials as permanently implantable skeletal prosthesis. Journal of Biomedical Materials Research 4, 433 (1970)

11. Judet, R., Judet, J.: Technique and results with the acrylic femoral head prosthesis. Journal of Bone and Joint Surgery 94-B, 173 (1952)

12. Judet, J.: Entwicklung und gegenwärtiger Stand der Orthopädie in Frankreich. Zeitschrift für Orthopädie 113 (1975)

13. Leonhäuser, I.: Nachuntersuchungsergebnisse der partiellen Hüft-Alloarthroplastik. Dissertation Saarbrücken 1975

14. Mittelmeier, H., Singer, L.: Anatomische und histologische Untersuchungen von Arthroplastikgelenken mit Plexiglas-Endoprothesen. Archiv für orthopädische und Unfall-Chirurgie 48, 519 (1956)

15. Mittelmeier, H.: Zementlose Verankerung von Endoprothesen nach dem Tragrippenprinzip. Zeitschrift für Orthopädie 112, 27 (1974)

16. Mittelmeier, H.: Selbsthaftende Keramik-Metall-Verbund-Endoprothesen. Medizinisch-Orthopädische Technik 6, 152 (1975)

17. Moore, A.T.: The self locking metal hip prosthesis. Journal of Bone and Joint Surgery 39-A, 811 (1957)

18. Pauwels, F.: Grundsätzliches über Indikation und Technik der Hüftgelenksplastik. Archiv für Klinische Chirurgie 276, 322 (1953)

19. Rettig, H.: Die Hüftarthroplastik mit Spezialendoprothesen. Zeitschrift für Orthopädie 290 (1952)

20. Ring, P.A.: Complete replacement arthroplasty of the hip by the ring prosthesis. Journal of Bone and Joint Surgery 50-B, 720 (1968)

21. Scales, J.T., Zarek, J.M.: Biomechanical problems of the original Judet prosthesis. British Medical Journal 1, 1007 (1954)

22. Sivash, K.M.: The development of a total prosthesis for the hip joint from a partial joint replacement. Wiederherstellungschirurgie und Traumatologie 11, 53 (1969)

23. Scheier, H., Sandel, J.: Abrieb an der Kunststoffpfanne bei Metall-Kunststoffendoprothesen. Kongreß der Niederländisch-Schweizerischen Ges.f.Orthop. Lausanne, Mai 1974

24. Schoch, J.: Die Arthroplastik der Hüfte mit der Judet-Endoprothese. Ann. Univ. Sarav. Med. 1963

25. Thompson, F.R.: Experience with a intramedullary hip prosthesis. Tex. St. J. Med. 49, 749 (1953)

26. Ungethüm, M., Refior, H.J.: Ist Aluminiumoxidkeramik als Gleitlagerwerkstoff für Totalendoprothesen geeignet? Archiv für orthopädische und Unfall-Chirurgie 79, 97 (1974)

27. Willert, H.G., Puls, P.: Die Reaktion des Knochens auf Knochenzement bei der Allo-Arthroplastik der Hüfte. Archiv für orthopädische und Unfall-Chirurgie 72, 33 (1972)

ISO–ELASTIC ENDOPROSTHESIS – A NEW CONCEPT IN ARTIFICIAL JOINT REPLACEMENT

E. Morscher, R. Mathys, and H.R. Henche

Bone surgery shows that the "stress protection" of too rigid implants leads to bone resorption and even structural changes of cortical bone to cancellous bone. This phenomenon always appears when the implant discharges too much of the weight bearing function of the bone (Figs. 1,2).

For temporary fixation of bone fractures, correctly dimensioned metallic implants are certainly indicated. With a stable fixation, primary bone healing can be achieved in a short time, but the implant should be removed as soon as possible after bony union. We shall always find unfavourable conditions in the long term, when too rigid implants are used, e.g. metallic hip joint prostheses permanently fixed with bone cement. It is conceivable, that because of the unphysiological weight bearing of the bone, after an implantation of a hip joint prosthesis, bone resorption or even structural changes of the bone will take place, similar to what we find in too rigid implants in bone-surgery.

Fig. 3 shows doubtful stable conditions after bone resorption leading to loosening and destruction of the cement-bed and later to fatigue fracture of the stem of the prosthesis. The enormous difference in elasticity between bone and the cement-supported metal implant is an important factor in this process. The application of bone-cement for the fixation of prostheses is still associated with a number of unsolved problems such as toxicity and uniform structural strength.

In designing a new type of endoprosthesis, our aims were the following:
- cementless fixation of the implant, and
- deformation behaviour under load similar to that of bone.

For the development of prostheses showing an "iso-elastic" behaviour with the bone, a number of facts had first to be studied. Problems such as deformation and elastic behaviour of bone, strength and bio-compatibility of plastic materials had to be solved.

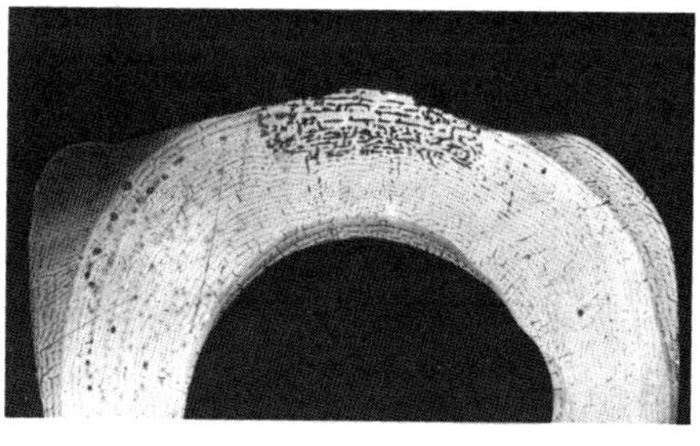

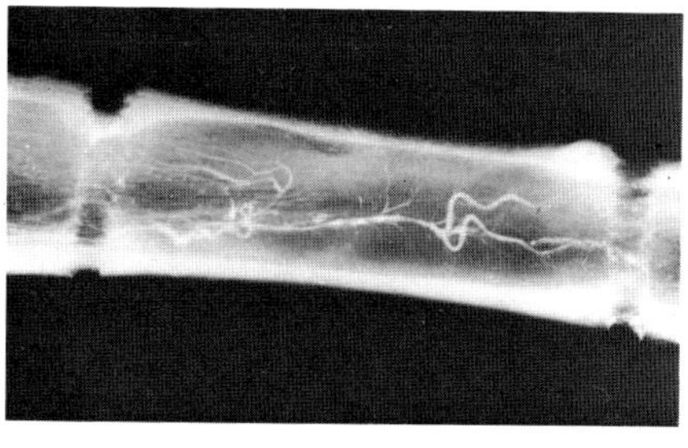

Figs. 1,2 Bone resorption under rigid bone plate

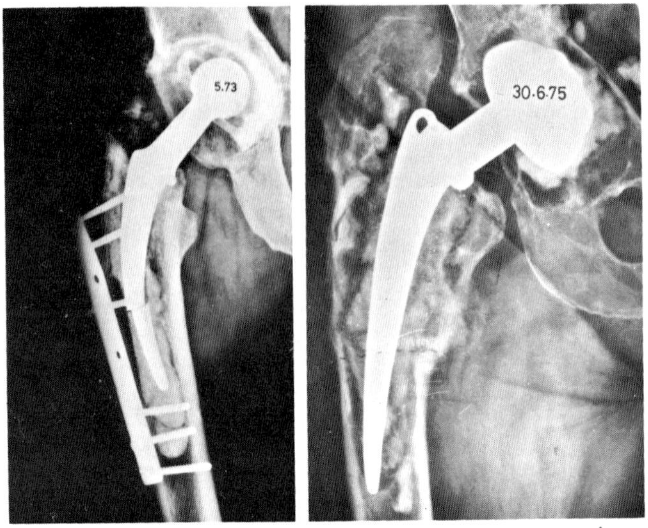

Fig. 3 Doubtful stable conditions after bone resorption

Mechanical and biomechanical tests were carried out at the research department of Rob. Mathys, Manufacture of Instruments. Biocompatibility and incorporation studies were made at different research institutes.

IMPLANT MATERIALS

MECHANICAL PROPERTIES

The tests to establish the suitability of plastics for its use as highly stressed implant materials for long-term implantation were also applied to high-density polyethylene (RCH 1000) and polyester (Hostadur).

Fig. 4 shows the compressibility of various plastics. The acetal-copolymer (POM/POM+R) shows a similar behaviour to that of the rigid polyester (PETP). The fact that high-density polyethylene creeps under load precludes this material from being used for highly stressed components.

Fig. 5, shows various, characteristic mechanical properties of plastics so far found suitable as implant materials. The acetal-copolymer (POM), the material we use for the highly stressed components, shows very good properties with a high fatigue strength.

Fig. 6 shows the structure of the acetal-copolymer. This copolymer has, in addition to the homopolymer, carbon-carbon links statistically distributed along the molecule. These carbon-carbon links increase the thermo- and chemical stability. Hostaform C is a partially crystalline thermoplastic material and reaches a crystallinity of 70-75 % with optimal manufacturing processes. The melting point of the crystalline sections is 164 ^{o}C. There-

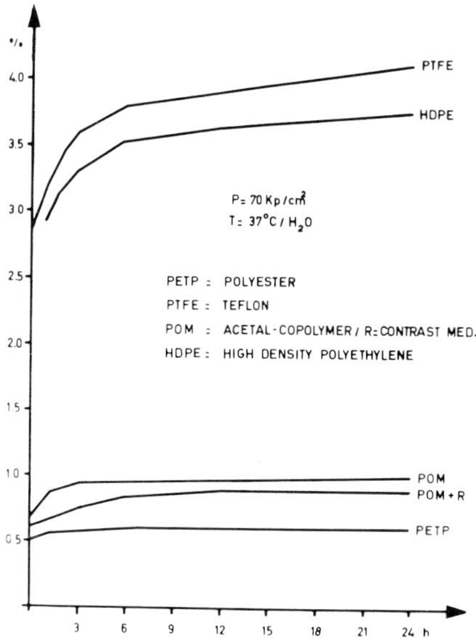

Fig. 4 Compressibility of plastics

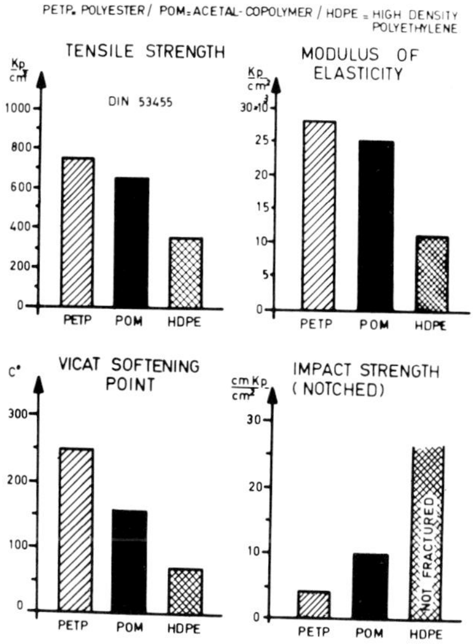

Fig. 5 Mechanical properties of plastics

Fig. 6
Structure of acetal-copolymer

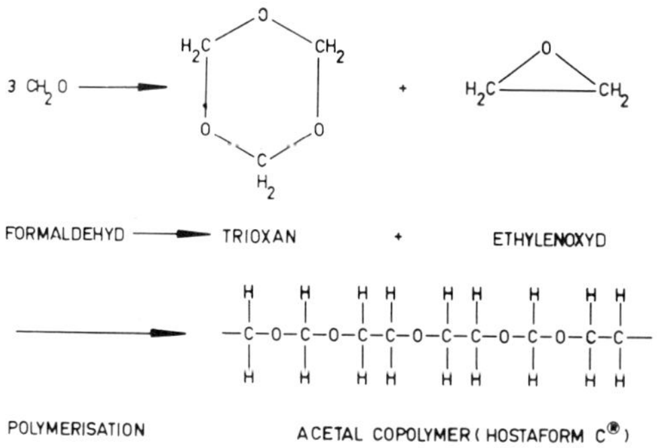

fore, sterilization by autoclave at 140 °C is possible. Even after 10 autoclave sterilizations, no changes could be found in the plastic. This allows easier handling in the operating theatre, as X-ray contrast medium, 3 % by wt. of chemically pure barium-sulfate, is added to the plastic (Hostaform CR, POM + R).

High-density polyethylene as material for acetabular prostheses shows, in combination with steel and Cr/Co/Mo-alloys, most suitable coefficients of friction (Table 1). The

Table 1 Dynamic coefficient of friction, μ.
$p = 2.5 - 22.5$ Kp/cm^2
$v = 10$ m/min

Test specimen	Shaft	μ
polyethylene HDPE	steel	0.15 – 0.20
acetal-copolymer POM	steel	0.15 – 0.20
polyester PETP	steel	0.15
acetal-copolymer POM	polyester PETP	0.05 – 0.10
polyester PETP	acetal-copolymer POM	0.05 – 0.08

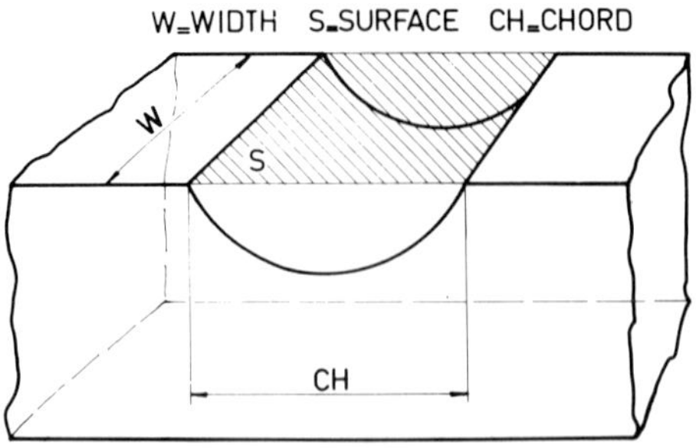

Fig. 7 Wear test

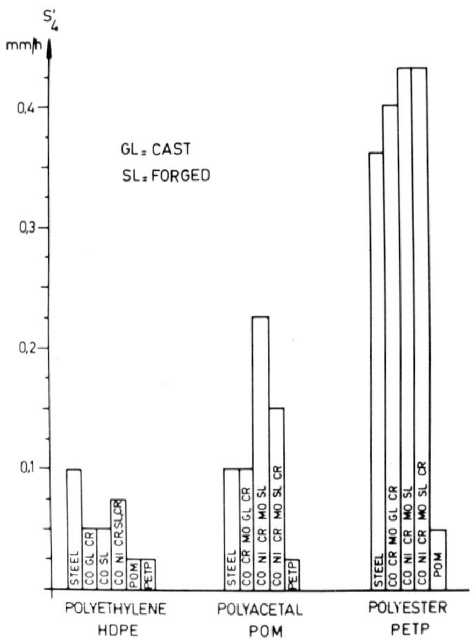

Fig. 8 Wear rate

wear tests were carried out in the following manner: the plastic test specimen was pressed (10 Kp) against a shaft (diam. 10 mm), rotating backwards and forwards ($\pm$ 40 ^{o}). During the test period, the specimen was fully immersed in a physiological salt solution at 37 ^{o}C. The amount of wear was checked by measuring the length of chord S (Fig. 7).

Fig. 8 shows the wear rates (after 4 hours of test) of different material combinations. Polyethylene combined with metals gives the most satisfactory results. Even better resistance to wear is shown by combinations of two plastic materials, e.g. HDPE-POM or PETP.

One-year results with total hip replacements in sheep, showed this fact to be realistic. Further experiments on dogs will have to be carried out to confirm this experience.

BIO–COMPATIBILITY

The bio-compatibility tests were carried out at the Swiss Research Institute at Davos. The results of subcutaneously implanted plastic threads proved to be statistically inadequate. Therefore, a test specimen has been designed to eliminate movements between the implant and the tissue (Fig. 9). These specimen to be tested were also implanted subcutaneously.

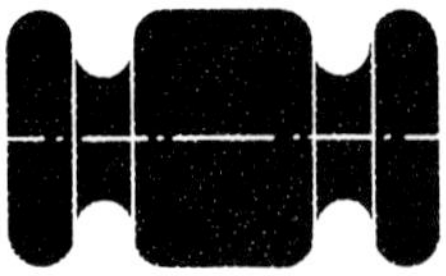

Fig. 9 Test specimen for bio-compatibility tests

The tests included the following materials: polyethylene (HDPE), polyester (PETP), acetal-copolymer (POM) and stainless steel (AISI 316 L of AO-quality).

Fig. 10 shows the histological preparations of the interfaces of the test specimen and the tissue. Stainless steel proves to be a very well tolerated implant material. All the various plastics induced a minor reaction of the surrounding tissue.

After an experience of 6 years with shoulder prostheses and of 3 years with finger joint replacements, we believe the bio-compatibility of the acetal-copolymer (Hostaform C) to be proved. Special consideration must be given to the wear particles.

ISO–ELASTICITY

An implant can only be incorporated by bone if all movements at the interfaces are absolutely eliminated. For components to be implanted without cement, this means a very precise operative preparation of the "bone-bed", and a stable primary fixation of the implant to the bone is necessary. If this can be achieved, the stem of the prosthesis is forced to follow the elastic deformation of the bone and an integral system is formed.

For an implant manufactured of plastic material it is possible, on account of its elasticity, to follow the deformation of the bone on the compression and the tension side. Any movements at the interface implant/bone are therefore eliminated and the stability required to enable the bone to grow into the indentations of the surface of the implant is achieved. If this is the case, one can refer to an iso-elastic behaviour of the implant with the bone.

The experiments to confirm this iso-elastic behaviour, have been carried out with a transparent plastic tube with the dimensions of a medium sized long bone (Fig. 11a). The rods representing the implant (Figs. 11b,c) fit precisely into the tube representing the bone. The marking lines on the tube and the rods are placed at exactly the same distance apart.

In the bending device (Fig. 12), the tube with a rod inserted can be bent, and any movement at the interface can be observed by inspecting the aligned markings.

When bending the tube with the inserted rods of different elasticity, no shifting of the markings could be observed (Fig. 13). Therefore, the linear changes of the two components, on the tension and compression side, are exactly the same.

These experiments show that elastic components of prostheses, well fitted into the medullary cavity, co-act iso-elastically with the bone, if the implant is more flexible, but also if the implant is more rigid.

The only difference we observe when inserting rods with different elasticity into the tube, is the deflection at the loading point. Fig. 14 shows the deflections (mm) under

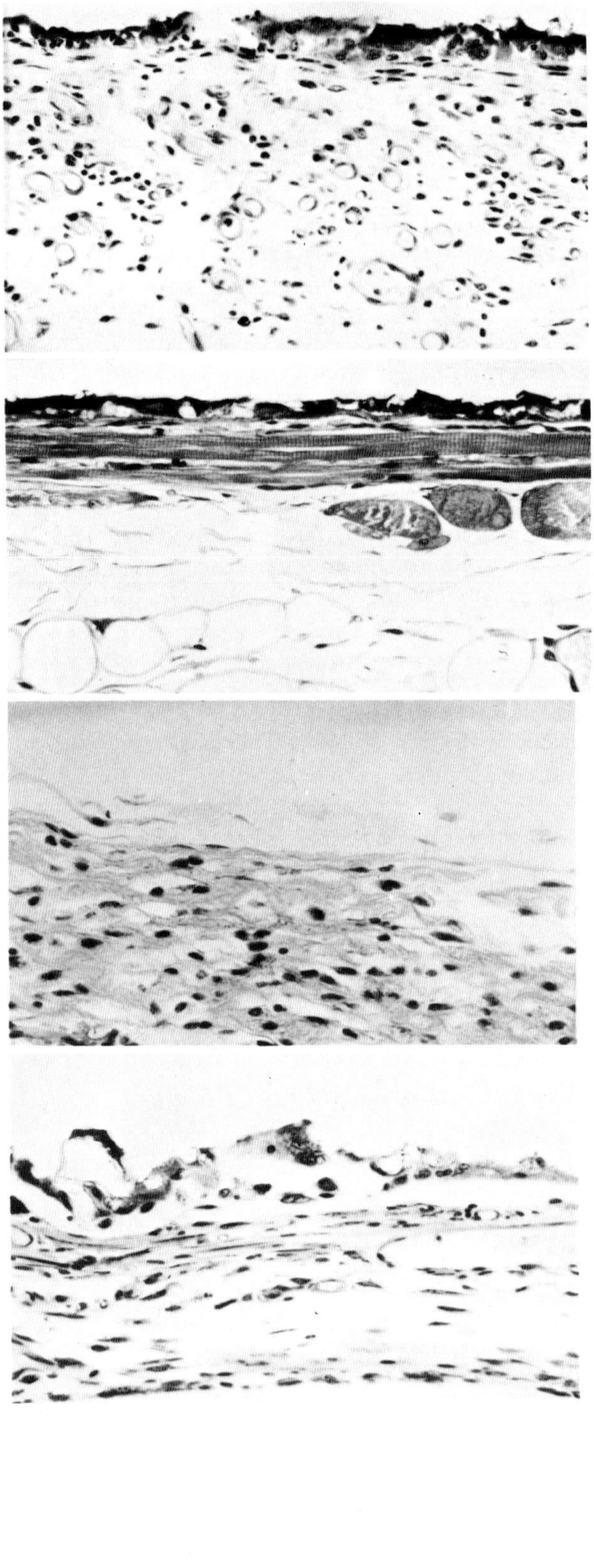

a. PETP

b. POM

c. AISI 316 L

d. HDPE

Fig. 10
Histological preparation of the interfaces of the test specimen and tissue (after 3 weeks)

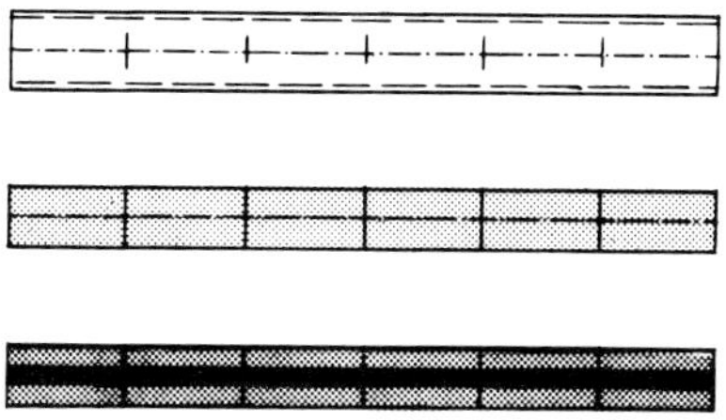

Fig. 11
Test specimens in bending tests
a. Tube representing the long bone,
b. Rod representing medullary stem of prosthesis, with lower modulus of elasticity than that of the tube,
c. Rod with higher modulus of elasticity than that of the tube

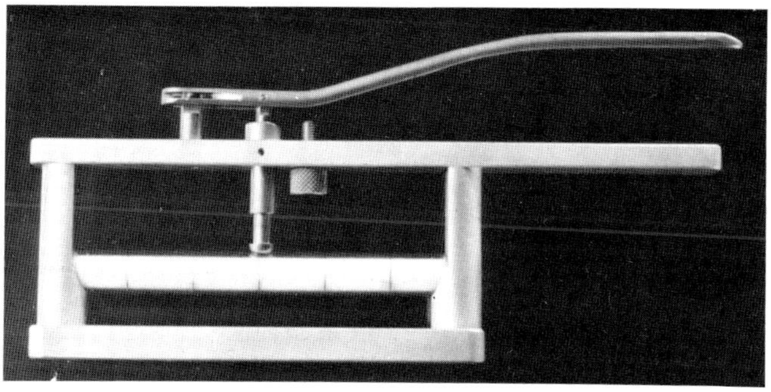

Fig. 12
Bending device

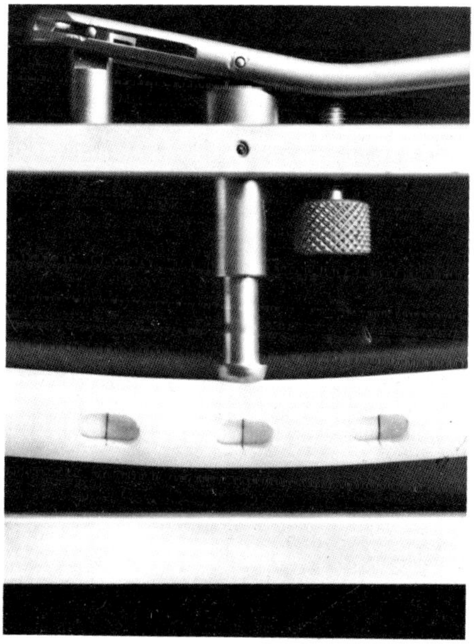

Fig. 13
Bending of a test specimen

a load of 10 Kp. No shifting can be seen at the interface of the tube and the rod reinforced with a metal wire.

One can see that there is a difference in elasticity between the bone and the bone plus implant. This difference depends on the amont of bone removed when locating the prosthesis (Fig. 15).

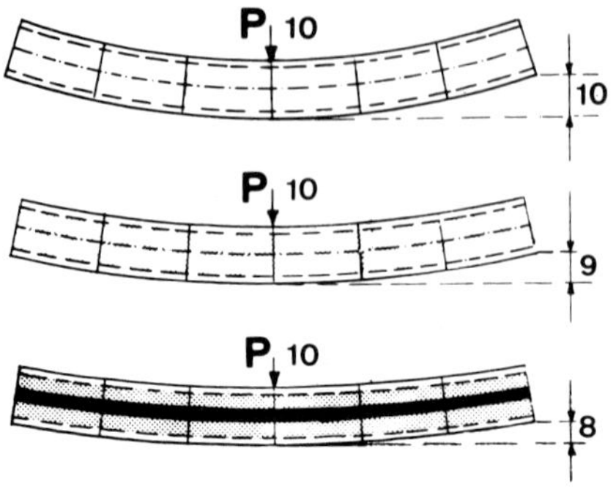

Fig. 14 Deflection of the test specimens

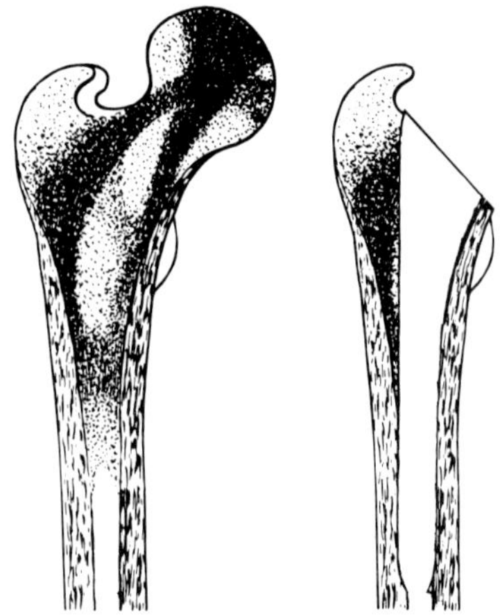

Fig. 15 Increase of elasticity in the proximal femur when preparing the bed for the implant

THE DEFORMATION OF THE PROXIMAL FEMUR

Fig. 16 represents the results of the deformation studies of the proximal femur. Narrow hatched, the deformation of the bone. The load required to cause a neck-fracture depends on the size and the age of the bone and ranges from 300 Kp to 700 Kp. The maximum deformation at fracture ranges from 1.6 mm to 2.0 mm. Wide hatched, the large field of load-deformation behaviour that can be covered by variously reinforced elastic implants.

The implantation of a metal prosthesis with cement fixation reduces the deformation to 0.12-0.26 mm within the normal range of loading (300 Kp - 500 Kp). This means a substantial loss of elasticity of the proximal femur.

Photo-elastic studies provided us with further information about the stress distribution in the proximal femur after implantation of a prosthesis (Fig. 17). In Fig. 17a we can see the unfavourable stress distribution in the bone model after "implantation" of a metal prosthesis fixed with cement. The stress is concentrated around the tip of stem. Along the stem, the stress-protecting action of the rigid implant can be noticed. Fig. 17b shows a virtually ideal stress distribution in the bone model, after "implantation" of an iso-elastic prosthesis. A stress concentration around the tip cannot be seen. For the bone, this means:

- maintenance of vitality, and
- elimination of a possible fatigue fracture in the distal part of the stem.

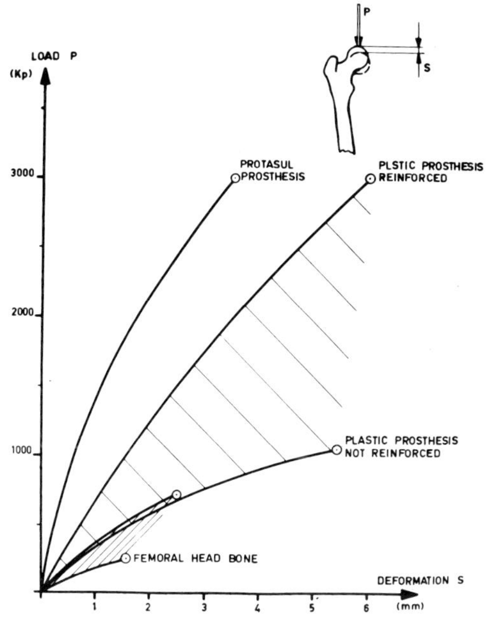

Fig. 16
Deformation studies of proximal femur

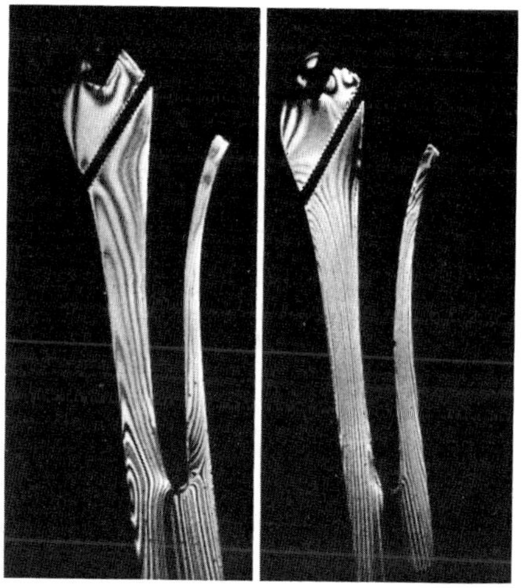

Fig. 17
Photo-elastic experiments
a. Rigid metal implant fixed with cement,
b. Iso-elastic implant incorporated

ANIMAL EXPERIMENTS

The second step in animal experiments, to prove the concept of the iso-elastic prosthesis, was carried out in sheep at the Medizinische Hochschule Hannover.

On the components used for these experiments (Fig. 18) it must be said that the design of the acetabular cup was optimal, but the femoral component was dimensioned too small. Therefore, primary stable fixation of the stems could not be achieved in the widely

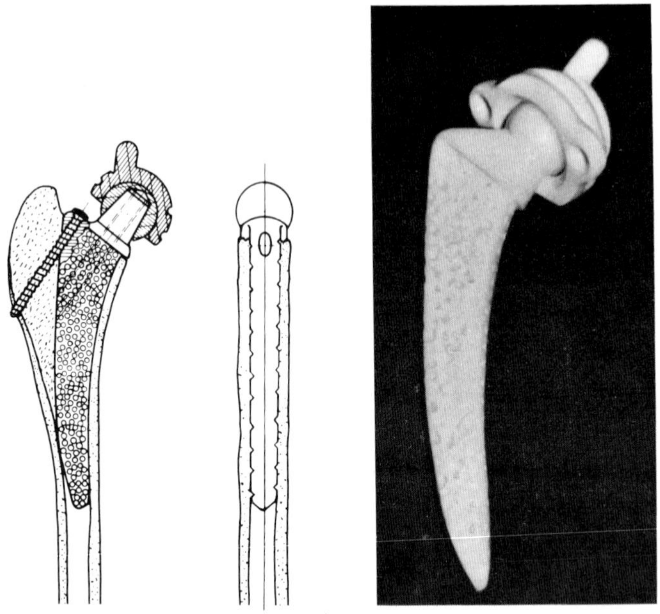

Fig. 18   Components for total hip replacement for animal experiments

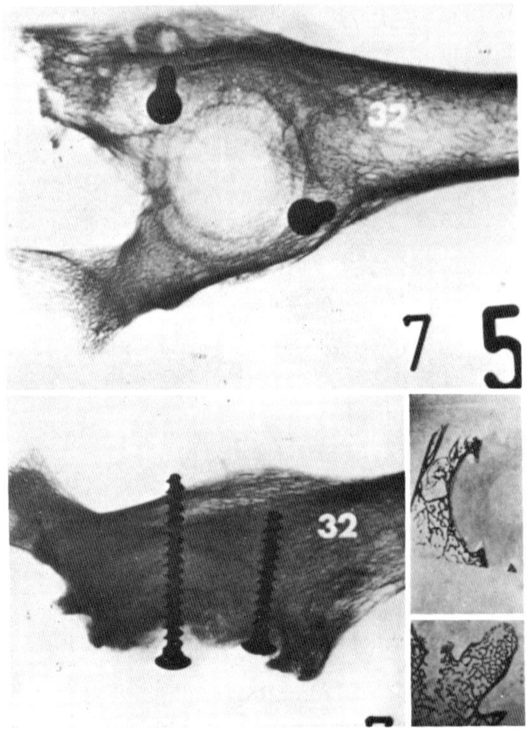

Fig. 19a
Experiments with sheep:
Acetabular cup

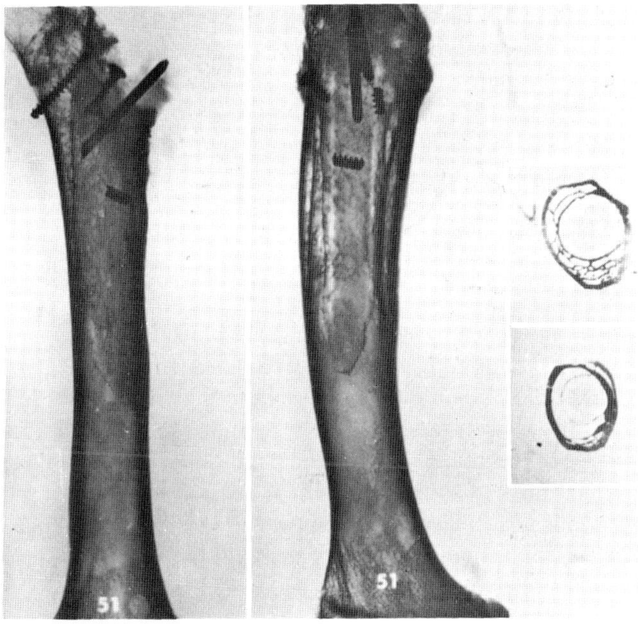

Fig. 19b
Experiments with sheep: Femoral component

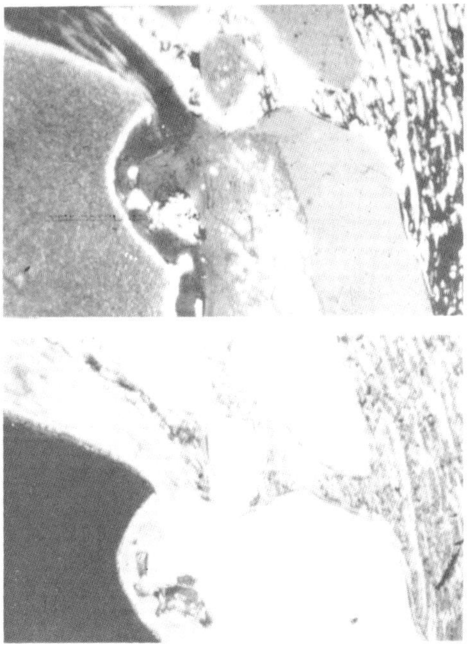

Fig. 19c
Experiments with sheep: Implant/tissue interface

diverging medullary cavity of the sheep. Figs. 19a-c show the results of the sheep experiments. Fig. 19a shows a healed-in acetabular cup, 32 weeks postoperatively. The X-ray shows good anchorage of the cup and the screws. Fig. 19b shows the stabilization of a femoral component, 51 weeks after insufficient fixation at implantation. After the component had moved distally, a bony sleeve supported and stabilized the implant. We can also see the formation of cancellous bone as a structural support of the sleeve. In Fig. 13c stabilizing bone trabeculae in an indentation of the stem and a fine layer of connective tissue at the interface can be seen.

ACETABULAR PROSTHESES

When developing the acetabular cup we aimed for a design to be fixed without cement. A possible solution to this problem can be seen in Fig. 20. The cup is fixed with two screws. Two pins on the outer surface of the implants are intended to give additional stability against rotation (Fig. 21). Because of the required form-stability and a simple process of manufacturing, the cup has been made of acetal-copolymer (POM+R). The difficult manufacturing process of the sheet-metal head of the femoral prosthesis led to inadequate congruency of the two articular surfaces. The result was excessive wear of the acetabular component. Therefore, we returned to the established cement-fixed high-density polyethylene cup.

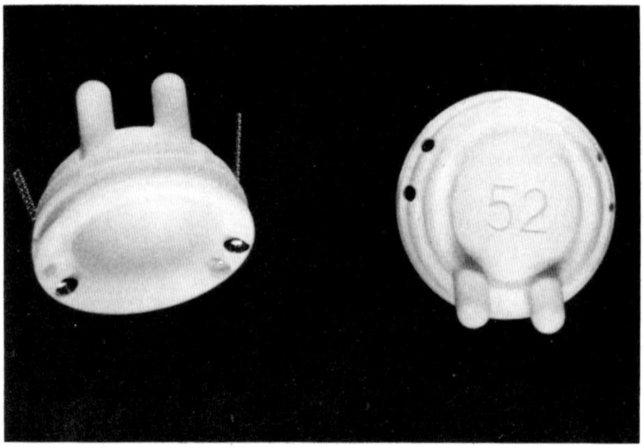

Fig. 20
Acetabular component

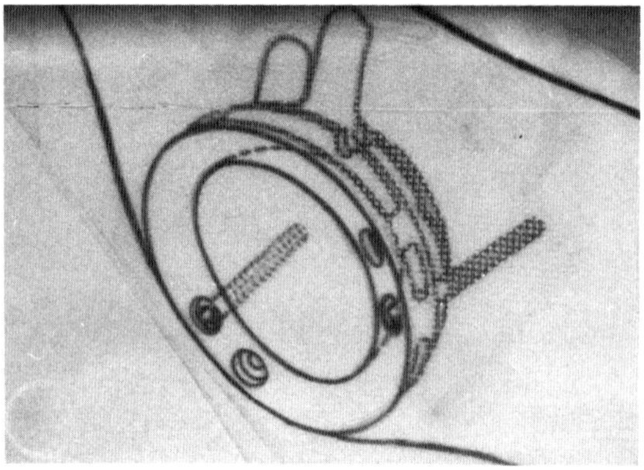

Fig. 21
Implantation of acetabular cup

Latest designs again aim at a cementless fixation of the acetabular component. Fig. 22 shows a HDPE cup with a conical thread on the outer surface. After the cutting of a thread in the acetabulum with a suitable instrument, the cup is twisted into position and finally fixed with two screws.

FEMORAL PROSTHESIS

Because of the very high intermittent forces in the hip joint, difficult problems had to be solved when designing an elastic prosthesis to be fixed without cement. The X-ray (Fig. 23) shows very well the tension and compression trabeculae in the femoral neck. This bone structure represents the basis for the design of our femoral component.

Fig. 24 shows the virtually physiological design of the prosthesis. A lag-screw on the tension side transmits the traction forces to the lateral cortex. The well supported collar of the component takes the compressive forces on the medial side. The third element of fixation is the stem of the prosthesis extending into the diaphysis. As mentioned before, precise seating of the prosthesis is absolutely necessary to achieve primary stability.

The femoral prosthesis is also manufactured of acetal-copolymer (Fig. 25). To achieve the required structural strength in the neck portion, the component is reinforced by a thick metallic wire. To increase the elasticity of the stem, the reinforcement is tapered towards its tip. This allows the stem of the prosthesis to follow the deformation of the bone. The articular surface of the component is formed by a metal cover welded to the reinforcing wire. The reinforcement used at the beginning (Fig. 25a), proved to be too elastic in the neck. This meant instability in the head of the component, and fatigue fractures of the weld between wire and cover occurred. This experience led to the concept with the conical neck and the interchangeable heads (Fig. 25b). This design always permits the application of the most suitable head-materials, e.g. metals or ceramics. In addition to this change, the cross section of the reinforcement in the area of the neck has been enlarged and, because of insufficient rotational stability, the lateral shape of the stem has been changed too (Fig. 25b, below).

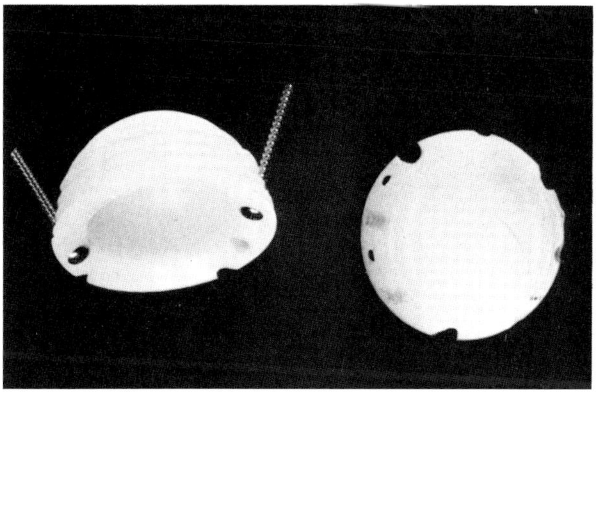

Fig. 22
HDPE cup with conical thread

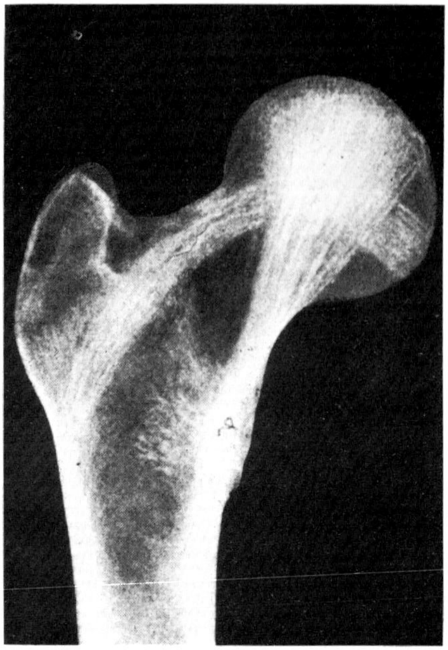

Fig. 23
Tension and compression trabeculae in femoral neck

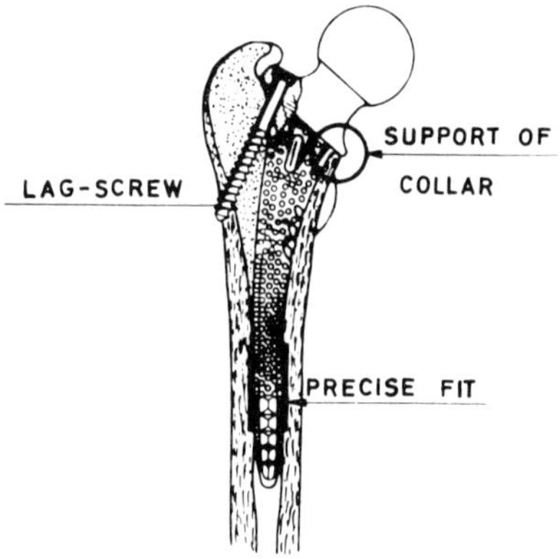

Fig. 24 Design of a physiological prosthesis

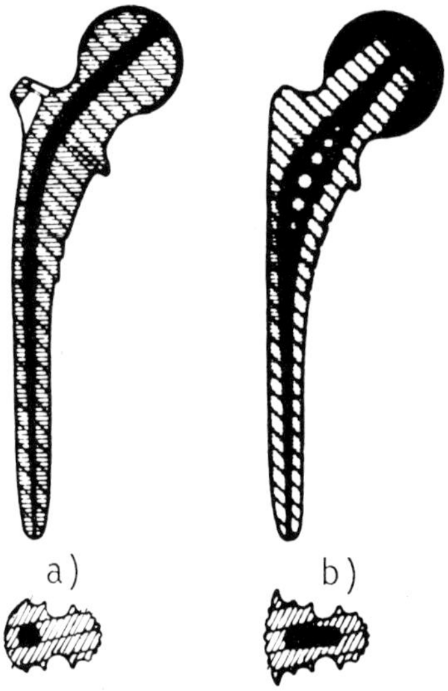

Fig. 25 Femoral prosthesis
a. Old model
b. Latest model

CLINICAL EXPERIENCE

Between March, 1975 and October, 1975, 73 iso-elastic prostheses were inserted in 68 patients in the Orthopedic Department of the University of Basle. Four different types were employed. Up to the beginning of 1974, the clinical results could be regarded as good or very good. In 1974, and particularly in 1975, there were set-backs. Our original optimism was considerably damped by the poor clinical results. We were forced to replace 18 of the prostheses by conventional models. Analysis of the failures showed the following:

- Six cup fractures were the result of a technical error in the manufacture of the material. The latter caused increased wear and loosening of the prosthesis because of marked friction in the artificial joint.
- Loosening of the shaft was certainly due to lack of rotation stability and probably also to the considerable elasticity of the neck. The clinical complaints of the patients, in whom loosening of the shaft was confirmed operatively, were typical. They reported cramp-like pains in the muscles of the thigh. When examining the range of rotation, severe pain was reported in extreme outward and inward rotation. 11 cases were reoperated on the basis of these severe complaints, revealing a loosening of the shaft. Intraoperatively a layer of connective tissue was found to have formed between the bone and the plastic material. In the region of the medial supporting surface, osteolysis and secondarily rotation of the prosthesis into the varus position had taken place as a result of the loosening. This phenomenon is also observed in conventionally cemented prostheses (Fig. 26).
- Marked calcification should also be sought as a further reason for the rejection of a prosthesis. It has been observed that this calcification occurred primarily in the patients operated in 1973. We think that this is due to the very intensive preparation of the femoral shaft. The resulting bone dust is most probably the cause of the cal-

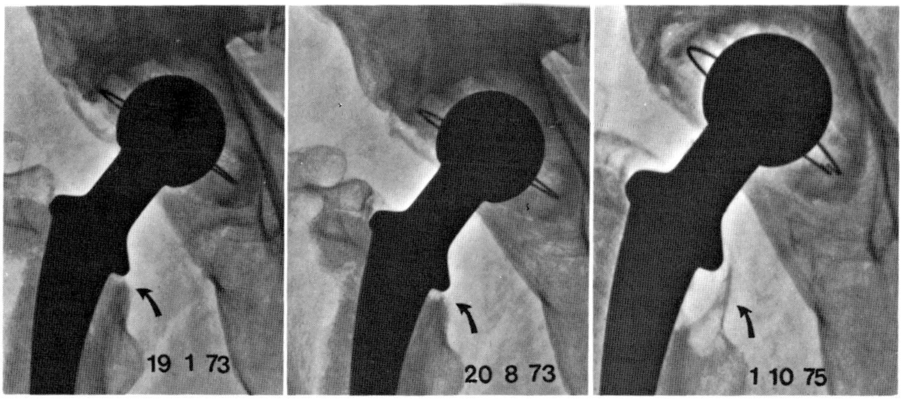

Fig. 26 Osteolysis at the medial support, secondary rotation of the prosthesis into the varus position and therefore loosening can be found with prostheses conventionally cemented into place

cification. We have since then altered our operative technique so that calcification is, as in conventional prostheses, an exception.

It appears to us at the present time that a further 5 to 6 total prostheses will have to be replaced in addition to the 18 which have been reported. These patients are already complaining of severe muscle cramps in the thigh and some of them of resting pain lasting up to an hour after weight bearing.

These patients with poor results can be compared with two further groups. One includes some 35 patients who also have slight to moderate pain in the thigh related to weight bearing. The discomfort is not permanent, however, and can vanish for several weeks. Unfortunately, only 12 patients can be included in the last group. In these patients, the result is good to excellent (Fig. 27). Surprisingly, they are mainly patients with rheumatoid arthritis or Bechterew's disease. It also appears that the increased physiotherapy in the first weeks and months disturbs the incorporation of the prosthesis, and the excess activity of the patients in the first weeks can lead to an earlier loosening. These 12 patients with good results up to a period of two years after implantation, give us some

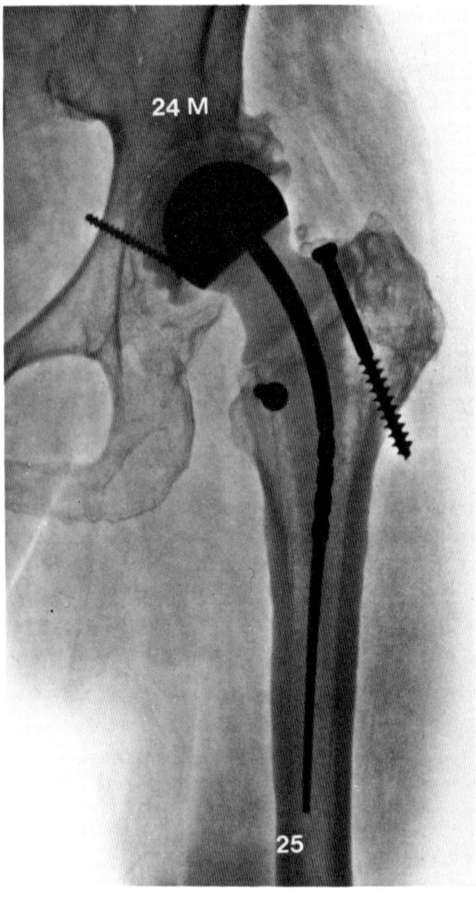

Fig. 27
2-year control of an iso-elastic total prosthesis which shows a very good result

encouragement to proceed, even though with caution. They confirm that the principal of the new prosthesis cannot be wrong.

I would now like to mention our last operated case, in which we implanted the latest 75b model. The 41-year old woman suffered from severe necrosis of the left femoral head. The iso-elastic prosthesis of the new type was implanted in September. The conventional cup of polyethylene was cemented in place in order to avoid any unknown factor. We did this although we are convinced that the problem does not lie in the fixation in the acetabulum but rather in the fixation of the stem. The shaft prosthesis carries a massive metallic head which can be set on it. The artificial femoral neck is secured by a reinforced metallic stem. The lateral stem fixation screw was only slightly altered (Fig. 28).

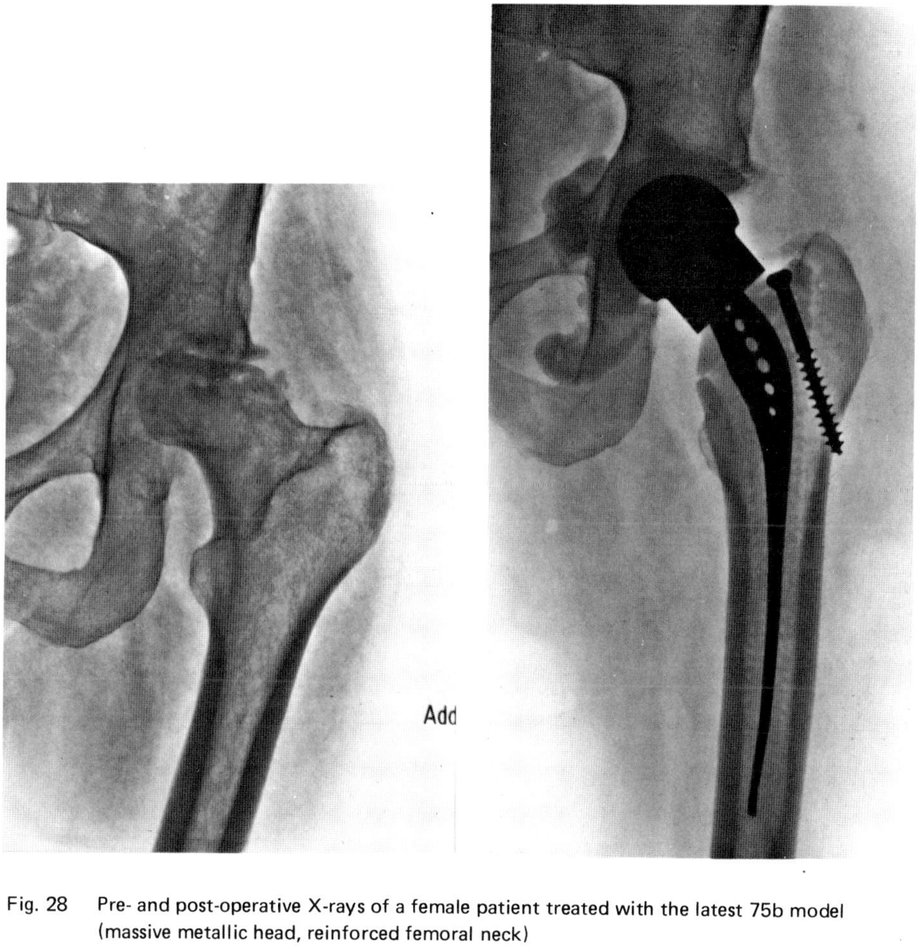

Fig. 28 Pre- and post-operative X-rays of a female patient treated with the latest 75b model (massive metallic head, reinforced femoral neck)

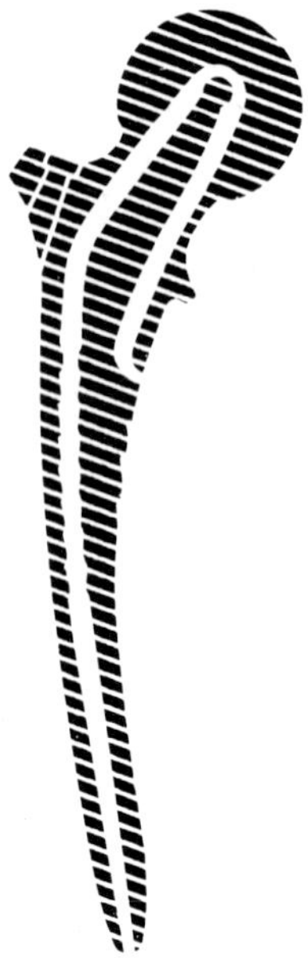

Fig. 29
New design of hip joint prosthesis

FUTURE PROSPECTS

We see a possibility of completing the concept of this prosthesis in the combination of two plastics as bearing surfaces. Table 1 and Fig. 8 show the extremely favorable conditions of two articulating plastic materials with respect to wear and friction.

Our idea of the femoral prosthesis might be as shown in Fig. 29. The plastic component would again be reinforced by wire. The material of the articulating surface would be the same as for the stem (POM). This hip joint prosthesis is still in the process of being developed. The shape of the components and their surface structures (recesses) are not yet optimal. The instruments needed to achieve optimal primary stability of the implants, have also to be improved.

After a too optimistic beginning, evoked by good short-time results, we are now in a second phase of careful reconstruction.

REFERENCES

1. Debrunner, H.U., Eulenberger, J.: Der Einbau von Fremdkörpern aus Kunststoff in Spongiosa. Aktuelle Traumatologie 4, 277 (1974)
2. Mathys, R.: Stand der Verwendung von Kunststoffen für künstliche Gelenke. Aktuelle Traumatologie 3, 253 (1973)

3. Mathys, R. sen., Mathys, R. jun.: Die Grenzflächen Metall–Metall, Metall–Kunststoff, Kunststoff–Kunststoff. 7. Wissenschaftliche Konferenz Deutscher Naturforscher und Ärzte, Biopolymere und Biomechanik von Bindegeweben, Berlin, Heidelberg, New York: Springer Verlag 1974

4. Morscher, E., Mathys, R.: La prothese totale de hanche iso-elastique fixee sans ciment. Premiers resultats cliniques. Societe Belge de Chirurgie Orthopedique et de Traumatologie, Bruxelles, Mai 1974

5. Morscher, E., Mathys, R.: Erste Erfahrungen mit einer zementlosen isoelastischen Totalprothese der Hüfte. Zeitschrift für Orthopädie und ihre Grenzgebiete 113, Heft 4 (1975)

6. Müller, W.: Möglichkeiten des plastischen Ersatzes bei tumorbedingten Resektionen großer Gelenke. Therapeutische Umschau 29, Heft 11 (1972)

7. Bedeschi, P., Luppino, T.: Endoprotesi articolari del polso e della mano. LIX Congresso Della Societa' Italiana di Ortopedia e Traumatologia, Cagliari 30 settembre – 3 ottobre 1974. Modena: Poligrafico Artioli

TISSUE INGROWTH AND MECHANICAL LOCKING FOR ANCHORAGE OF PROSTHESES IN LOCOMOTOR SYSTEM

J.J. Klawitter, A.M. Weinstein, S.F. Hulbert,and B.W. Sauer

Orthopaedic prosthetic devices currently used are fastened to the skeletal system by one of three methods:

1. mechanical fixation using screws, nails, etc.,
2. impaction of the prosthesis into bone,
3. use of an acrylic bone cement polymerization in situ as a filler at the bone/prosthesis interface.

Due to many reasons, these methods leave much to be desired.

Impaction or fixation by the use of screws, etc., has shown to result in unnatural stress concentrations within the bone. These stress centers are relaxed by either biological or physical processes (1). When the stress concentrations are greater than physiologically acceptable, bone resorption will occur and if the stress concentration exceeds the strength of the implant material, mechanical failure will result. Both reactions to stress concentrations will ultimately loosen the implant, and the attachment strength is reduced or entirely lost.

The use of an acrylic bone cement such as methylmethacrylate has its disadvantages (34). Nevertheless, this material is extensively used to cement many prostheses to bone in order to secure attachment and distribute stress concentrations caused by a load-bearing prosthesis. Some of the disadvantages of the acrylic bone cement are:

1. polymerization of the cement in situ is exothermic and bone pyronecrosis results,
2. the monomer has been reported to have toxic properties,
3. eventual loss of stability over the long term,
4. variable properties.

Klawitter and Weinstein (2) have reviewed the problems of obtaining prosthetic fixation and conclude that the problems are further complicated by the fact that mechanically ideal methods of attachment must often be compromised out of biological necessity. Additionally, it was stated that the requirements of maintaining blood supply, as well as tendon and ligament attachments, often force compromises in the method of skeletal fixation which may be mechanically less desirable but biologically necessary.

Trying to alleviate the enigma of prosthetic fixation, researchers have explored new methods of anchoring a prosthesis to living bone. Two potential solutions to this problem have arisen:

1. possible development of primary chemical bonds between the implant and bone matrix,

2. the use of porous materials fabricated to accept bone tissue ingrowth as a means of stabilizing prosthetics to skeletal bone.

The possible development of primary chemical bonds between the bone matrix and synthetic materials has been demonstrated (3-8). A number of studies have been conducted on Ca, P, Na, and SiO_2 containing glasses and glass-ceramic implants. These materials show stable interfacial osteogenesis when correct combinations of implant surface chemistry and implant sites are met. These primary chemical bonds have been reported to result in interfacial bond strengths of approximately 3/4 the strength of the host bone. Use of chemical bonds with the bone matrix must be considered clinically applicable for orthopaedic implants in the future.

A more foreseeable development to possibly alleviate the bone implant attachment problem is the application of porous materials to allow for bone ingrowth. Ingrowth attachment requires a controlled physiological interaction between the implant and the adjacent living tissue. A knowledge of the physiological functions and structure of bone tissue has resulted in the proper design of porous materials able to accept bone ingrowth.

A porous material provides a scaffolding into which bone may invade to anchor it to the skeletal system. This large surface area of ingrowth provides a distribution of local stresses so that the possibility of pressure necrosis of the bone tissue is minimized. Since large mechanical stresses or loads could be applied to the prosthesis in orthopaedic reconstructive surgery, high strength materials are a necessity.

Porous metallics (9-17, 33, 34), porous polymers (18-20) and porous ceramics (21-32) are being investigated for possible application for skeletal attachment, reconstruction, and support. These materials represent a broad spectrum of engineering properties.

The primary physiological considerations for porous structures such as inertness in the body environment, proper surface pore size, and appropriate pore size interconnection have been established. Concerning proper pore size and pore size interconnection, Klawitter et al. (21) have determined that "mineralized" bone ingrowth is restricted if pore interconnections are less than about 100 microns in diameter. Furthermore, it was determined that osteonal bone ingrowth occurred with pore sizes and interconnections of 250 microns or greater.

RATE OF BONE INGROWTH

The initial attempts to determine the rate at which bone grows into a porous structure were undertaken by Klawitter (21) and Hulbert (25).

In these first studies of ingrowth, calcium-aluminate pellets 6.35 mm in diameter were produced having different pore structures, and were implanted in canine femurs up to 22 weeks duration. Special evaluation techniques were developed by Klawitter (21) to substantiate ingrowth of bone into the ceramic material. The depth of bone growth into three pore structures of calcium-aluminate pellets are shown in Table 1. The results give one an indication of the rate at which bone proliferates into specific porous structures.

Bowman (23) examined bone growth into porous pellets of titania (TiO_2), porcelain, and calcium-aluminate. The porous calcium-aluminate was the same as that used by Klawitter and had a pore size range of 150–200 microns. All specimens were implanted in canine femora for 6 and 12 weeks. A summary of Bowman's measurements of pore size and relative depth of bone ingrowth is shown in Table 2.

Greer (26) reported that complete filling of interfacial porosity of porous calcium-alumino-silicate implants required 8 to 16 weeks. Bagwell (20), working with porous polyethylene, reported that bone ingrowth occurs in pores less than 69 microns, and that the rate of bone ingrowth increased with increasing size up to 100 microns. Above 100 microns, no further increase in rate of bone ingrowth was observed. A summary of this work is presented in Table 3. The present pore volume filled with bone is shown as a function of mean pore diameter and implant duration.

Table 1 Maximum depth of mineralized bone ingrowth into calcium aluminate

Pore size	Depth in microns	
Microns	11 weeks	22 weeks
75–100	50	50
100–150	200	500
150–200	600	1500

Table 2 Depth of bone ingrowth into porcelain, titania, calcium aluminate

	Avg. pore size		Depth ingrowth (microns)	
Material	Microns	Porosity (%)	6 weeks	12 weeks
Calcium-aluminate	265	51.4	400	900
Porcelain	478	46.2	1100	1800
Titania	295	57.6	1150	1750

Table 3 Bone growth into porous polyethylene

Mean pore diameter (microns)	% Pore volume ingrowth 4 weeks	8 weeks	16 weeks
39	0	0	0
65	21	0	78
115	51	54	100
163	47	56	100
179	47	59	100

BONE/POROUS MATERIAL INTERFACE MECHANICS

Galante (10) reported on a study of bone growth into porous titanium fiber pellets, produced by sintering short fibers. Rabbits and dogs were used as experimental animals in this research. Depth of bone ingrowth was measured for both species, but bone/implant interfacial shear strengths were only calculated for the dogs. A summary of the depth of ingrowth as reported by Galante is shown in Table 4, and shear strength measurements are reported in Table 5. Intimate contact between bone and metallic titanium fibers was evident in all fiber composite implants. Galante reported bone ingrowth in all the two week implants and showed deep penetration from 3 weeks on. The shear strength was reported to increase up to the second week and then remain relatively constant thereafter. Different shear strength values calculated for individual time periods were evaluated with a "T" test and were found to be not significant after the second week.

Nilles and Coletti (15) measured the mechanical strength of the bone/porous material interface of metals, ceramics, polymers, and carbon. Implants were placed transverse to the long axis of the long bones of dogs. The shear strengths were measured by pushing the implanted cylinders out of the bone. It was concluded that porous metals displayed the greatest interfacial shear strength, with values ranging from 1/3 to 2/3 those of cor-

Table 4 Maximum depth of bone ingrowth into titanium fiber pellets

Implantation time	Animal	Depth (microns)
10 days	rabbit	300
2 weeks	rabbit	300
2 weeks	dog	350
3 weeks	rabbit	1500
3 weeks	dog	900
6 weeks	rabbit	2680 *
6 weeks	dog	2200
12 weeks	rabbit	2680 *
12 weeks	dog	3125 *

* radius of pellet

Table 5 Interfacial shear strengths at different time intervals

Duration of implant	No. of implants	Average shear strength (Kg/cm^2)
24 hours	4	2.55
1 week	4	5.84
2 weeks	4	18.72
3 weeks	9	23.76
6 weeks	4	21.56
12 weeks	4	17.82

tical bone. Also reported was a reduction of elastic mismatch of the metal and bone in the ingrowth region or area of bone/metal composite.

Welsh, Pilliar, and McNab (12) reported pushout tests for cerosium and a porous ceramic. These materials had relatively small surface pores (18 to 23 microns). The results for the pushout testing of the cerosium and ceramic embedded in bone is shown in Table 6. The authors suggested that the lower values obtained for the ceramic was the result of the fracture of the ceramic spicules before the fracture of the bone spicules. This fracture of the ceramic implant before bone demonstrates the need for proper choice of implant material.

In 1974, Klawitter (29) and associates reported the interfacial shear strengths between intramedullary canine bone and porous structures of an alumina ceramic, a cobalt-chromium alloy, and a high density polyethylene. The (HDPE) implants were cylindrical in shape and were placed in the proximal end of the canine femur. Mechanical tests on the HDPE were performed using a pull-out technique, and a push-out technique was applied for the mechanical tests of the ceramic and cobalt-chromium alloy. Table 7 presents their data. Klawitter reported that the shear strength increased with increasing time and that strengths measured for the ceramic and cobalt-chromium were much higher than those found for the HDPE. This, it was noted, could be the result of the different specimen configurations tested, as well as the different methods of testing, but was primarily a reflection of the vastly different mechanical properties of the porous materials.

Karagianes (31) implanted a porous titanium alloy void metal composite (VMC) and a porous ceramic material, alumina porcelain, into fresh and healed sockets of miniature swine incisor and premolar teeth. The VMC was fabricated to allow for approximately 55 % porosity and pore diameters of 275 and 450 microns. The alumina porcelain, composed of 95 % Al_2O_3 and 5 % nepheline syenite which was volatilized to form pore diameter ranges from 200 to 400 microns.

Three animals (two fresh and one healed socket approach) were sacrificed at 111, 147 and 246 days respectively. No evidence of adverse tissue reactions was observed. Extensive bone ingrowth was seen in the VMC and alumina porcelain implants. Maximum interfacial shear strengths of 98, 169 and 165 Kp/cm^2 were measured on VMC implants pressed from the surrounding bone by pure shear loading. Of the three ceramic implants tested, shear strengths of 148, 117 and 198 Kp/cm^2 were calculated. Complete filling of the porosity of the VMC was observed. The ceramic implants were not completely

Table 6 Bone/porous material interfacial shear strength (Kp/cm^2) for ceramic and cerosium

Time (months)	0	1.5	3	4	6
Ceramic	.35	1.9	7.6	7.0	6.8
	.56	2.2	9.1	8.0	9.1
	.56	2.5	10.6	8.4	10.1
Cerosium	.42	3.0	26.0	28.8	29.2
	.56	3.7	28.2	31.5	31.5
	.56	4.1	29.2	31.5	32.4

Table 7 Interfacial shear strengths

Material	Mean pore size	Implant duration (weeks)	Number of specimens	Type of bone adjacent to implant	Interfacial shear stress (Kp/cm^2)
HDPE	206 microns	2	1	cortical cancellous	3.0
		4	1	cortical cancellous	6.9
		8	1	cortical cancellous	9.5
		16	1	cortical cancellous	8.4 *
Cobalt-chromium	180 microns	4	2	cancellous	71.7
		4	2	cortical	35.9
		8	2	cancellous	84.7
		8	2	cortical	40.7
Alumina	350 microns	8	4	cancellous	31.2
		8	6	cortical	46.7

* bone fractured before implant was pulled out

filled, but this impedance of bone ingrowth was apparently caused by the small diameter of the interconnecting porosity.

Wheeler (33) designed and fabricated VMC intramedullary (I.M.) pins with pore size of 275 and 460 microns to be implanted in the femoral medullary canals of 18 adult African pygmy goats. The implants were designed to be placed in sites permitting apposition of the endosteum of the cancellous and cortical bone similar to the shaft of a femoral head prosthesis. Two I.M. VMC test pins were surgically implanted in the proximal femora of each goat.

Post-sacrifice VMC/bone interfacial shear strength tests were performed on I.M. pins having ingrowth from cortical and cancellous bone at 1-1/2 and 4 months post-implantation. The shear tests were performed by a conventional procedure in which the porous VMC plug is pushed from its implantation site while measuring the push-out force and the displacement to failure. The shear tests showed an increase in strength with implant time for 275 microns pore size VMC in cortical bone. Table 8 shows the results of the static shear tests for 1-1/2 and 4 months VMC implants.

Wheeler further reports that a layer of new bone formed between the VMC and the older, mature compact bone. This new bone formed from the reamed intramedullary cavity surface or resulted from natural growth of young bone as the goat ages during implant periods. Plotting the I.M. pin push-out force as a function of the percent coverage of pin surface by ingrowth would be expected to show increasing push-out force with increasing ingrowth area coverage. Wheeler noted that there was no apparent correlation between push-out force and area coverage, indicating that the shear strength is strongly

Table 8 Static shear tests of one and one-half and four month VMC implants

Implant time (mo.)	Bone type	Pore size (μm)	% Area covered by bone ingrowth	Interface strength (Kp/cm^2)	Interface displacement (mm)
1 1/2	cortical	275	18	56.5	.46
1 1/2	cortical	460	0	7.7	.23
4	cancellous	460	56	19.7	.25
4	cortical	275	17	67.4	.25
4	cancellous	275	8	19.0	.36

related to the structure and properties of bone. Histological results corroborated the mechanical results in most cases. There appeared to be little difference in depth of hard tissue ingrowth between the 275 and 460 microns pore size material. Bone trabeculae in the cancellous region had a tendency to penetrate through the specimens while cortical bone was found mainly in the surface pores. One would not expect cortical bone to entirely fill the medullary cavity, and the deep invasion of cancellous bone into the pores of the VMC suggests that attempts were being made by body osseous tissues to follow a normal pattern of bone geometry. Wheeler concluded that:

1. Interface strength increased with implant time.
2. Cortical bone appeared to be stronger with the 460 microns pore size as compared to the 275 microns pore size. (This trend was evident for all specimens implanted longer than 1-1/2 months).
3. The comparison of interface strength with area of pin surface coverage by bone ingrowth showed no direct correlation between strength and coverage. This inferred that interface strength is dependent upon such morphologic factors as composition and arrangement of bone collagen and the extent of mineralization of the new bone.
4. Cancellous bone was seen to penetrate the VMC deeply while cortical bone was found mainly in the surface pores.
5. A 50 % dense material seemed to be optimum for interface strength while a 30 % dense material was optimum for bone ingrowth. VMC density should be in the range of 30 to 50 % for best attachment to bone. The values of 30 and 50 % density appeared to be dependent on pore structure.

In this review of data presented by many investigators it has been established that:

1. Bone growth could occur into pores less than 69 microns.
2. Ingrowth rate increases with increasing pore size up to 100 microns.
3. When ingrowth did occur, the porous material/bone composite demonstrated a reduction in the elastic mismatch between the bone and implant material.
4. The maximum shear strength between porous material and bone is achieved in about 8 weeks.
5. Complete filling of interfacial porosity takes about 8-16 weeks.

IMPLANT PERFORMANCE

DESIGN CONSIDERATIONS

When viewing attachment of orthopaedic implant devices by tissue ingrowth, a number of characteristics associated with implant performance can be identified and related to specific structural parameters. The characteristics are shown in Table 9. The interrelationships between the attachment characteristic and the structural parameter have been optimized for items 1 and 3 in Table 9. Table 10 lists the mechanical properties of a number of materials which have been shown to be of interest as porous biomaterials. The percent porosity of the porous materials listed in Table 10 corresponds to porosities concomitant with tissue ingrowth. In general the strength of porous materials decreases monotonously with increasing porosity as, typified by the behavior of porous high density polyethylene as shown in Fig. 1. The experimental points shown in Fig. 1 between 30 and 60 % porosity again represent the porosity range of interest for tissue ingrowth attachment. The materials shown in Table 10 and Fig. 1 present a broad spectrum of engineering properties, to the designer, ranging from soft, low strength, compliant porous HDPE to the hard, high strength, noncompliant, brittle, porous aluminum oxide. However, the interrelationship for items 4 and 5 have not been clearly defined. Characteristics 4 and 5 are directly associated with the mechanical function of an implant device utili-

Table 9 Prosthesis attachment by tissue ingrowth

Attachment characteristic	Structural parameter
1. Rate of bone ingrowth	Pore size
2. Strength of porous material	Volume fraction pores
3. Depth of tissue viability	Interconnection pore size
4. Attachment strength	Volume fraction pores at surface
5. Bone/porous material interface deformation	Pore size, pore morphology and pore volume

Table 10 Porous material engineering properties

Material	Porosity (%)	Y.T.S.* U.T.S. (psi)	U.C.S. (psi)	Flexural strength (psi)	Elastic modulus (psi)
Co-Cr-Mo	0	75000*	–	–	30×10^6
Co-Cr-Mo	44	10500	–	43500	4×10^6
Ti	0	80000*	–	–	16×10^6
Ti	40	7000	–	–	6×10^5
Al_2O_3	0	30000	400000	50000	50×10^6
Al_2O_3	50	–	15000	5-6000	9×10^6
PMMA	0	10000	15000	16000	3.5×10^5
PMMA	32	1200	2750	1800	5.5×10^4

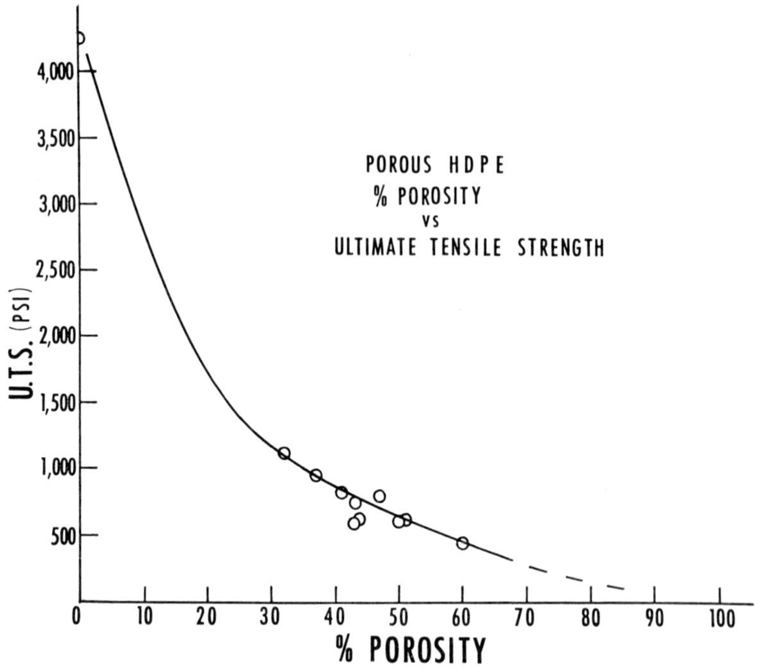

Fig. 1 Ultimate tensile strength vs. percent porosity for high density polyethylene

zing attachment by ingrowth and therefore are of prime importance. Optimization of these characteristics is essential to provide the basis for establishing sound criteria for prostheses design. Item 4, being primarily dependent on a single variable, lends itself to direct experimental determination. However, item 5 is dependent on three variables and optimization of this characteristic does not lend itself to an experimental determination. It should be possible, however, using appropriate analytical techniques, such as finite element stress analysis, to optimize the bone interface deformation characteristics. In order to achieve this goal it is essential that the model generated be tested and confirmed in the light of actual experimental data. Heretofore, the use of finite element techniques has been restricted to establishing stress distributions in implants and surrounding structures based on variations in gross implant geometry and material properties (35-38).

CLINICAL APPLICATIONS

Limited clinical applications involving porous materials to obtain ingrowth attachment to bone have been reported. These, for the most part, do not involve the high load areas associated with the lower extremities with the majority of application being associated with facial reconstruction and oral surgery. One research group has reported on the clinical trial of porous coated metallic orthopaedic implants. In this study the application of several cobalt-chromium alloy implant devices having a porous coating designed to accept bone ingrowth has been reported (39). Total shoulders have been implanted in patients with no loosening observed.

We have performed limited clinical trials using cobalt-chromium alloy implants having a porous HDPE coating. To date one total elbow and two femoral prostheses (one distal and one proximal) have been implanted in humans, as shown in Fig. 2. Initial fixation was achieved by impaction in the medullary canal in all cases. The results after 6 months in situ indicate the potential of ingrowth attachment for high load bearing implant devices.

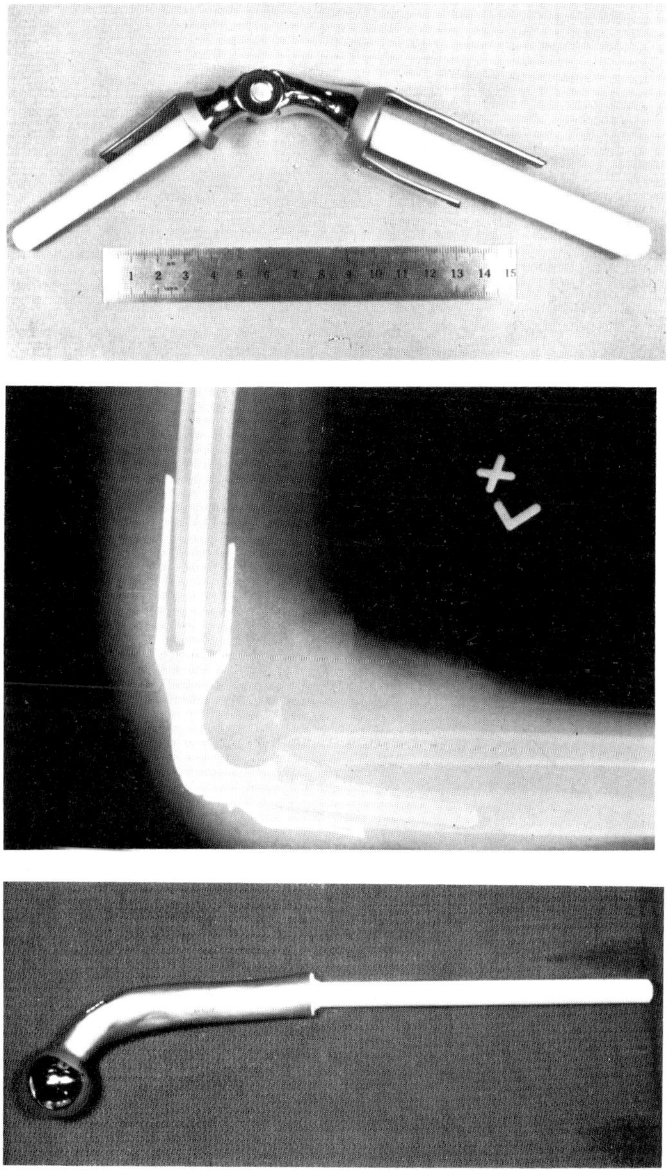

a

b

c

Fig. 2 Elbow and femoral prostheses having a porous coating designed for attachment by bone tissue ingrowth

CONCLUSION

In summary the concept of prosthetic attachment by tissue growth into porous materials has been demonstrated experimentally and limited clinical trials have begun. Time is now required to confirm the efficacy of ingrowth attachment for improved prosthetic function. Exhaustive studies remain to be carried out before broad clinical application; however, such continued work is well justified by the results obtained to date by numerous investigators.

REFERENCES

1. Charnley, J.: Journal of Bone and Joint Surgery, 47 b, 354 (1965)
2. Klawitter, J.J., Weinstein, A.M.: The status of porous material to obtain direct skeletal attachment of tissue ingrowth. To be published in Acta Orthopaedica Belgica (1975)
3. Hench, L.L., Splinter, R.J., Allen, W.C., Greenlee, T.K.: Journal of Biomedical Materials Research, Symposium 2, 117 (1972)
4. Hench, L.L., Greenlee, T.K., Allen, W.C.: An investigation of bonding mechanisms at interfaces of a prosthetic material. Reports Nos. 1, 2, and 3, August, 1970, 1971, and 1972, U. S. Army Med. R. and D., Contract No. DADA-17-70-C-0001
5. Greenlee, T.K., Beckham, C.A., Crebo, A.R., Malmorg, J.C.: Journal of Biomedical Materials Research 6, 235 (1972)
6. Hench, L.L., Paschall, H.A.: Histo-chemical responses at a biomaterials interface. To be published in Journal of Biomedical Materials Research, Symposium (Prostheses and Tissue: The Interface Problem), Clemson University 1973
7. Hench, L.L., Paschall, H.A.: Direct chemical bond of bioactive glass-ceramic materials to bone and muscle. Journal of Biomedical Materials Research 7 (1973)
8. Beckman, C.A., Greenlee, T.K., Crebo, A.R.: Journal of Calcified Tissue Research 8, 2 (1971)
9. Peterson, C.D., Miles, J.S., Solomons, C., Predecki, P.K., Stephen, J.S.: Journal of Bone and Joint Surgery 51-A, 805 (1969)
10. Galante, J., Rostoker, W., Lueck, R., Ray, R.D.: Journal of Bone and Joint Surgery 53-A, 101 (1971)
11. Hirschhorn, J.S., McBeat, A.A., Dustoore, M.R.: Journal of Biomedical Materials Research 6, 49 (1971)
12. Welsh, R.P., Pilliar, R.M., MacNab, I.: Journal of Bone and Joint Surgery 53-A, 963 (1971)
13. Hirschhorn, J., Reynolds, J.: Powder metallurgy fabrication of cobalt-base alloy surgical implants. In: E. Korostoff, edit., Research in Dental and Medical Materials, New York: Plenum Press 1960
14. Karagianes, M.T.: Biomaterials, Medical Devices and Artificial Organs 1, 171 (1973)
15. Nilles, J.L., Colletti, J.M.: Journal of Biomedical Materials Research 7, 231 (1973)
16. Hahn, H., Polich, W.: Journal of Biomedical Materials Research 4, 571 (1970)
17. Galante, J., Shafer, S.J., Meltzer, W., Ray, R.D.: Journal of Bone and Joint Surgery 52-A, 835 (1971)

18. Taylor, D.F., Smith, F.B.: Journal of Biomedical Materials Research 6, 467 (1972)

19. Struthers, A.M., Plastic Reconstructive Surgery 15, 274 (1955)

20. Bagwell, J., Klawitter, J., Sauer, B., Weinstein, A.: A study of bone growth into porous polyethylene. Sixth Annual Biomaterials Symposium, Clemson University, Clemson, S.C., U.S.A., April 20-24, 1974

21. Klawitter, J.J., Hulbert, S.F.: Journal of Biomedical Materials Research 5, 161 (1971)

22. Hentrich, R.L., Graves, G.A., Stein, H.G., Bojpai, P.K.: Journal of Biomedical Materials Research 5, 25 (1971)

23. Bowman, L.: Characterization of tissue growth into pellets, partial sections of porous ceramics implanted in bone. M.S. Thesis, Clemson University 1971

24. Predicki, P., Auslander, B.A., Stephen, J.E., Monney, Stanitski, C.: Journal of Biomedical Materials Research 6, 347 (1972)

25. Hulbert, S.F., Young, F.A., Mathews, R.S., Klawitter, J.J., Talbert, C.D., Stelling, F.H.: Journal of Biomedical Materials Research 4, 443 (1970)

26. Greer, W.: A quantitative determination of the rate of bone growth into a porous ceramic material. M.S. Thesis, Clemson University, Clemson, S. C., 1973

27. Smith, L.: Archives of Surgery 87, 653 (1963)

28. Jameson, L.H.: An evaluation of a porous high alumina ceramic as an artificial tooth root material. M.S. Thesis, Clemson University, Clemson, S. C., 1974

29. Klawitter, J.J., Sauer, B.W., Weinstein, A.M., Hulbert, S.F.: Characterization of tissue growth into porous biomaterials. Technical Report No. 7, ONR Contract No. N00014-71-A-0339-0001 (Project No. NR 032-529) 1974

30. Karagianes, M.T., Westerman, R., E., Rasmussen, J.J., Lodnell, A.A.: D.D.S., Submitted to Journal of Dental Research

31. Karagianes, M.T., Westerman, R.E., Rasmussen, J.J., Marshall, R.P.: Journal of Biomedical Materials Research Symposium 5, 391 (1974)

32. Lyng, S., Sudmann, E., Hulbert, S.F., Sauer, B.W.: Acta Orthopaedica Scandinavica 44, 694 (1973)

33. Wheeler, K.R., Karagianes, M.T.: Porous metals for orthopedic/prosthetic application. Final Report to the National Institute of Arthritis, Metabolism, and Digestive Diseases on Grant AM 15092, Battelle Pacific Northwest Laboratories, Richland, Washington, 1974

34. Black, J., Nunamaker, D.N., Tronzo, R.G.: Prosthetic implant stabilization: A comparative study of cementation and biological ingrowth fixation in the total hip joint replacement. Submitted to Clinical Orthopaedics and Related Research

35. Andriacchi, T.P., Galante, J.O., Rostoker, W., Hampton, S.: An analytical study of stresses in a femoral stem of a total hip prosthesis. 21st Annual Meeting of Orthopaedic Research Society 1975

36. Forte, M.R.: Structural analysis consideration in the design of the total hip prosthesis. 21st Annual Meeting of Orthopaedic Research Society 1975

37. Bartel, D.L., Ulsoy, G.A.: The effects of stem length and stem material on stresses in bone-prosthesis systems. 21st Annual Meeting of Orthopaedic Research Society 1975

38. Swenson, L.W., Hayes, W.C., Schurman, D.J.: Finite element stress analysis of normal and prosthetic knee joints. 21st Annual Meeting of Orthopaedic Research Society 1975

39. Pilliar, R.M., Cameron, H.U., MacNab, I.: Porous surface layered prosthetic devices. Biomedical Engineering 4, 1 (1975)

EXPERIMENTAL INVESTIGATIONS OF DENSE ALUMINA CERAMIC FOR HIP AND KNEE JOINT REPLACEMENTS

D. Geduldig, R. Lade, P. Prüssner, H.-G. Willert, L. Zichner, and E. Doerre

Before using dense alumina ceramics clinically as materials for artificial joint construction, animal studies are necessary to examine the tissue compatibility and performance of these materials in the physiologic environment.

Experimental studies of dense alumina ceramics have shown their potential as well as their limitations for use as prosthetic material. The ultimate goal of the following studies has been to develop prosthesis designs for animal implantation which satisfy the mechanical properties of these materials and extend this knowledge for the development of human prostheses. Using a model implant system, the bone segmental defect replacement prosthesis for sheep and dogs, the tissue compatibility and ingrowth kinetics were studied. The results of these initial studies led to the development of dense alumina hip and knee joint prostheses suitable for implantation without bone cement.

The results of this research indicate that ceramic does have considerable potential as a bearing surface for joint prostheses. However, the unique mechanical properties of ceramic materials must be kept in mind when designing prostheses for clinical use.

Recently, the dense aluminum oxide ceramic has become the focal point of interest as an implant material. Based on its high chemical resistance and its advantageous tribologic behaviour, the use of this material seemed appropriate, in particular as a bearing surface for artificial joints. The following three criteria must be fulfilled:

- high purity
- high density
- fine standard of grain

The results of tribologic investigations have shown a polishing effect on the ceramic-to-ceramic joint surfaces. Therefore the friction diminishes continuously and the normally extremely low wear proceeds to zero (Fig. 1).

Using the conventional metal to polyethylene bearing surfaces, we normally see a fraying on the surfaces, which increases the friction and leads to an increase of the wear rate, especially in the polyethylene component.

A disadvantage of the ceramic materials is their inherent brittleness which we believe limits their range of application. Dense alumina ceramic is therefore unsuitable for use as plates, bent plates, nails, long screws and long stem prostheses.

In order to take advantage of the excellent wear characteristics of dense alumina ceramics, new prosthesis designs must be utilized, in which the ceramic is stressed primarily by compression and not by bending or tension.

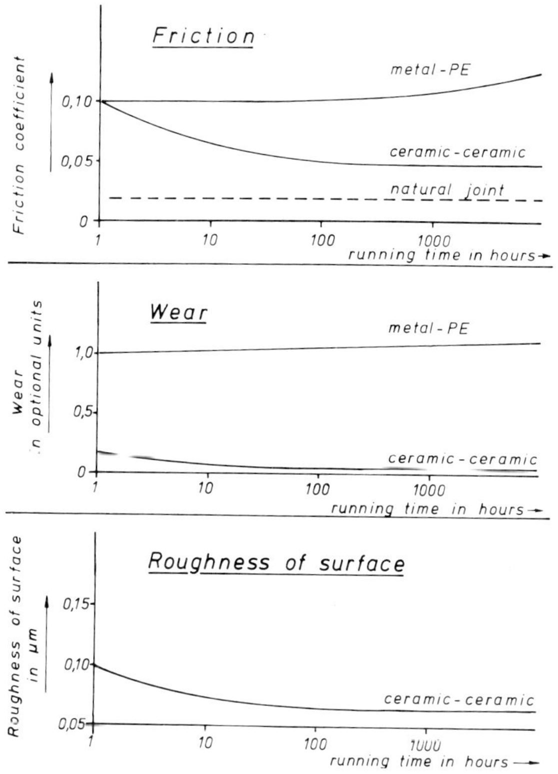

Fig. 1
Long-term behaviour of matching metal-polyethylene and ceramic-ceramic for friction, wear and surface roughness

The first clinical application of dense alumina ceramics "Biolox" was in a total hip prosthesis, normally stressed by friction and wear, in which the head was replaced by a ceramic ball (which articulated in a ceramic cup). A taper joint was used to fix the ceramic ball to the metallic stem. This type of joint provides increasing strength of fixation with increasing load (Fig. 2).

The ultimate goal of these long tests is to develop prostheses made entirely of ceramic and to fix them solidly to the bone without bone cement.

In the orthopaedic department of the university of Frankfurt/Main we have studied the bone/ceramic interface for three years using a bone segmental replacement in the canine

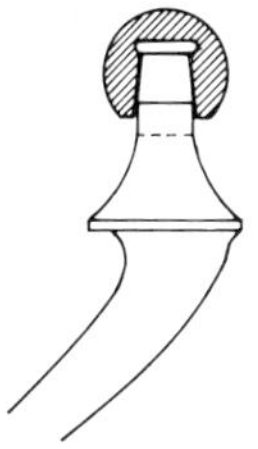

Fig. 2
Taper joint for fixing the femoral head to the stem

and ovine femur as a model system. The implants consist of a threaded intramedullary rod which is held in place by a threaded washer, which also serves as a spacer (Fig. 3). A specially formed plate is used to provide stability of the implant system for 12 weeks (Fig. 3 A). After this time the bone plate is removed and the implant subjected to full weight bearing (Fig. 3 B).

The newly-formed bone is not resorbed but develops further to lamellar bone. The implant is separated from the bone only by a thin connective tissue membrane (Figs. 4-6).

On the basis of the results of the bone segmental replacement studies, we designed two prostheses – a hip and a knee – which take into account the special properties of the dense ceramic (Figs. 7-8).

The hip joint prosthesis consists of a ball-shaped cap which is pinned to the femoral head following appropriate milling. The inner surface of the cap is cuboidal in form with rounded edges to avoid the notch effect. In addition there are rill-like grooves on the inner wall which serve as anchorage for the newly formed bone. The branches of the medial and lateral circumflex femoral arteries which are not damaged with the chisel, supply the medial part of the femoral neck.

Earlier pilot studies using a longer ball shaped cup which covered more of the femoral neck resulted in aseptic necrosis of the femoral head and neck which led to loosening and dislocation of the prosthesis. This failure was not observed with the design we are using now. To get a relative state of rest and stress prevention, we do a temporary

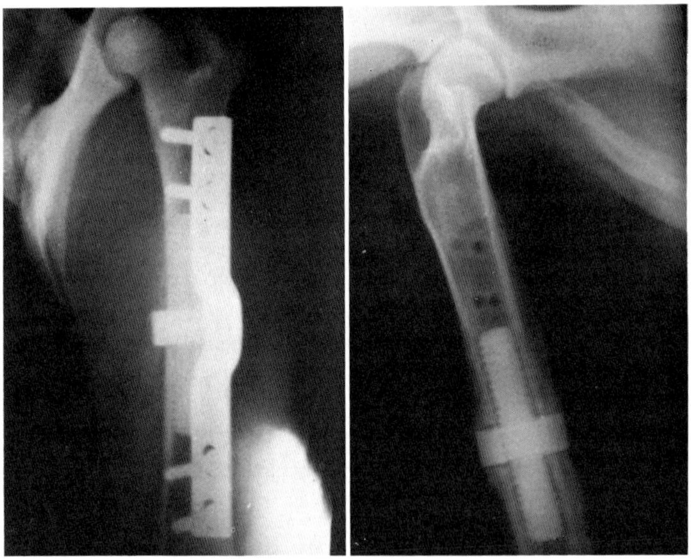

Fig. 3 X-ray after cement-free implantation of a dense ceramic spacer in a foxhound.

A. left: with fixation by a bent metal plate for 12 weeks

B. right: after removal of the plate and full stress of the bone/implant anchorage

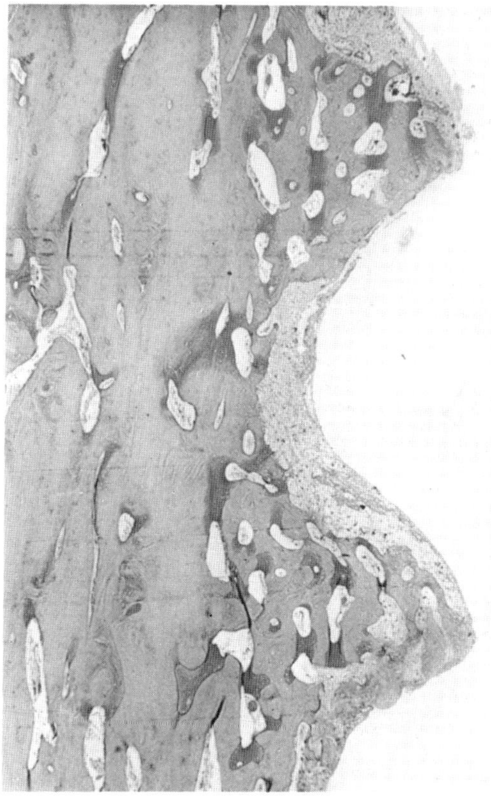

Fig. 4
Histological thin sections 12 weeks after surgery. In the threads of the bar, the fibrous bone is well developed and closely approximates the ceramic material (x 4)

limited arthrodesis of the knee with two spongiosa screws in maximal bending for 12 weeks (Fig. 9). In our future implantations we shall use external fixation effected by a double three point fixation (sacral bone, ilium and femur) of the hip to achieve absolute immobility.

The hip socket is also put in without cement after preparing the acetabulum with an appropriately shaped punch. The outline of the socket, which is in part angular and in part corrugated in form, is adapted to the anatomical proportions of the experimental animals. Rotational stability is guaranteed by the angular form of the acetabulum. The outer walls also have grooves to ensure firm fixation. The articulating surfaces are polished to a high-gloss with an average roughness of 0.07 microns.

Recent histologic results (Figs. 10-14) after an observation time of 16 weeks, of which the hip was fixed for 12 weeks with an arthrodesis of the knee, show a tissue response identical to that seen around the segmental defect implant. In the region of the femoral cap (Fig. 10) we find, adjacent to the ceramic implant, a connective tissue zone which consists of relatively dense packed collagen fibers parallel to the implant surface. Sporadically there is osteoid tissue. At the endosteal surface we find active signs of bone remodelling with new formation of woven bone and with bone resorption at the same

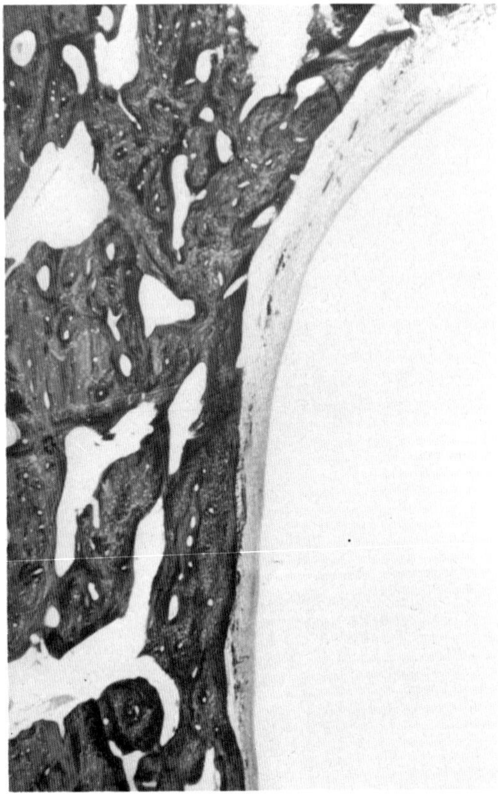

Fig. 5
Histological thin sections 24 weeks after implantation. At the top of the bar there is a thin dense connective tissue membrane (x 4)

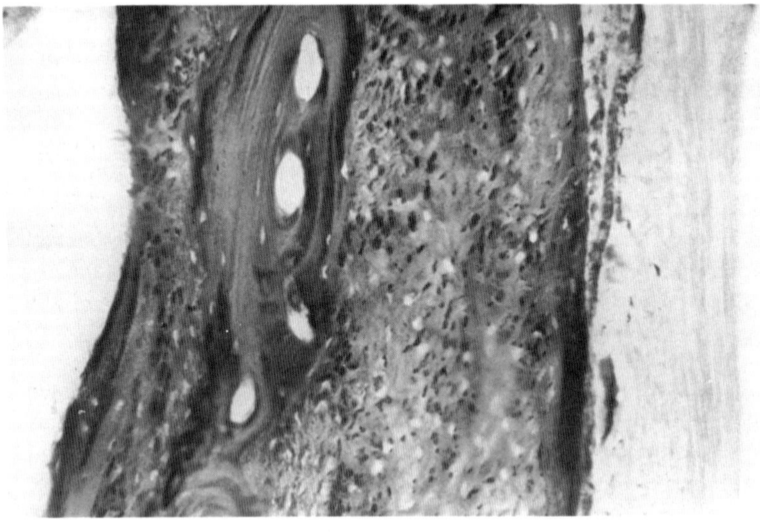

Fig. 6 Detail: lamellar remodelling of the fibrous bone (x 10)

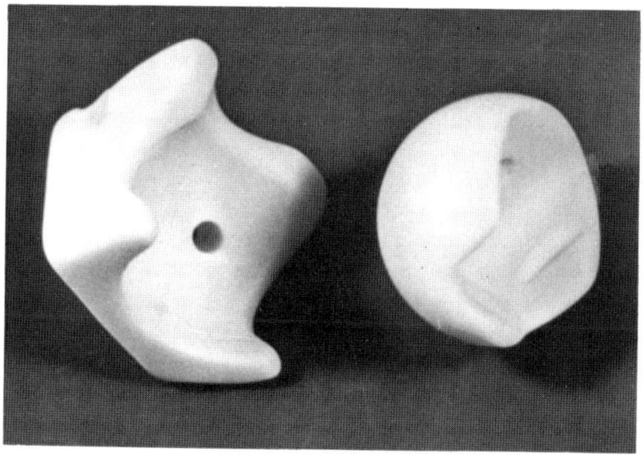

Fig. 7
View of the hip joint. Both components, the socket and the cap are made of dense alumina ceramic for cement-free implantation in animal studies (sheep and foxhound)

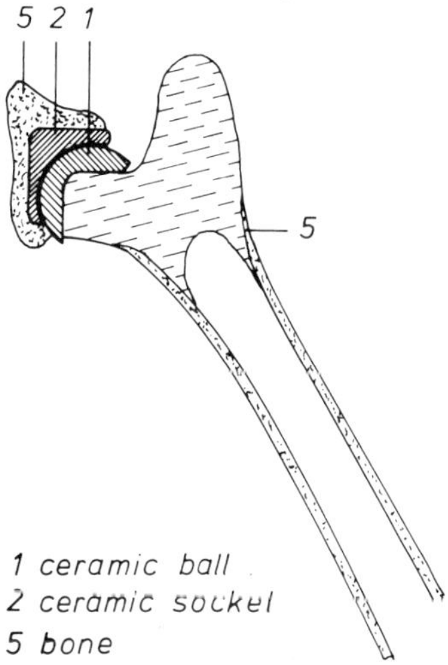

Fig. 8
Schematic representation of a hip prosthesis of dense alumina ceramic for cement-free implantation in animal studies (sheep and dogs)

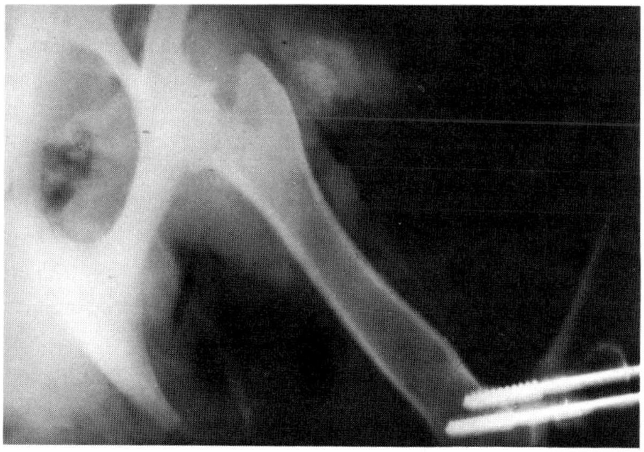

Fig. 9 Radiograph 12 weeks after implantation of a hip prosthesis of dense alumina ceramic with temporary arthrodesis of the knee by 2 spongiosa screws for 12 weeks (sheep)

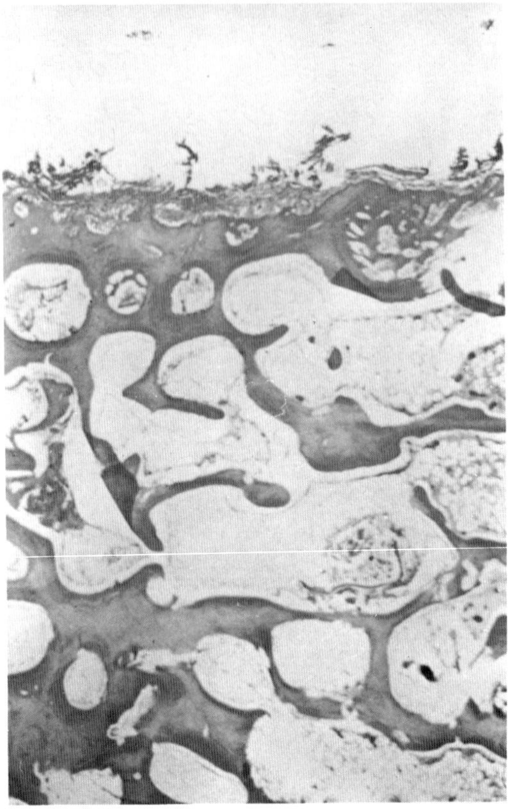

Fig. 10
Histological thin section of the femoral neck, which supported the ceramic cap for 16 weeks, 4 of which were completely weight bearing: the border to the implant consists of a connective tissue membrane followed by woven bone with anchors to the spongy neck bone (x 2.5)

time. This occurs even in the peripheral areas. The result is a largely longitudinally directed lattice of spongy bone. The same is seen around the acetabular component (Figs. 11-12). Interspaced with the remnants of the original acetabular structures, compact and cancellous bone and articular cartilage, we see a lattice-like structure of newly formed woven bone. In places this new bone formation extends virtually to the acetabular component. The zone of demarcation consists of variably thick connective tissue with closely spaced collagen fibers. The anchorage holes of the socket implant are also filled with connective tissue. An alignment of the fibers is not seen. In addition, calcified tissue was not present.

In comparision to the hip the problems of knee replacement are more difficult in experimental animals. Because of the special anatomical proportions, for example the additional ligamental apparatus and the small spongiosa zones in the femoral and tibial condyles, the space which can be resected is limited. To obtain an acceptable dimension of the knee prosthesis a design in the form of a sledge prosthesis was developed (Figs. 15-16). A resection of the cruciate ligaments is necessary for implantation. The height of the femoral and tibial component is determined by the level of resection and also by the outline of the implant area. For anchorage, a grooved rectangular plug was chosen which during the standing phase is loaded mainly by compression. To diminish the notch effect and to simplify fabrication, the connection between the

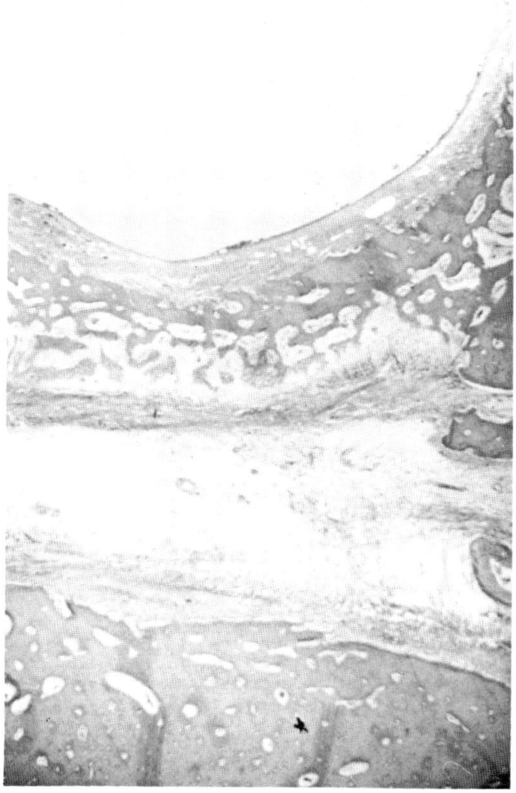

Fig. 11
Histological thin section of the acetabulum showing the tissue layers surrounding the implant: fibrous connective membrane, woven bone lattice and residual cartilage (x 2.5)

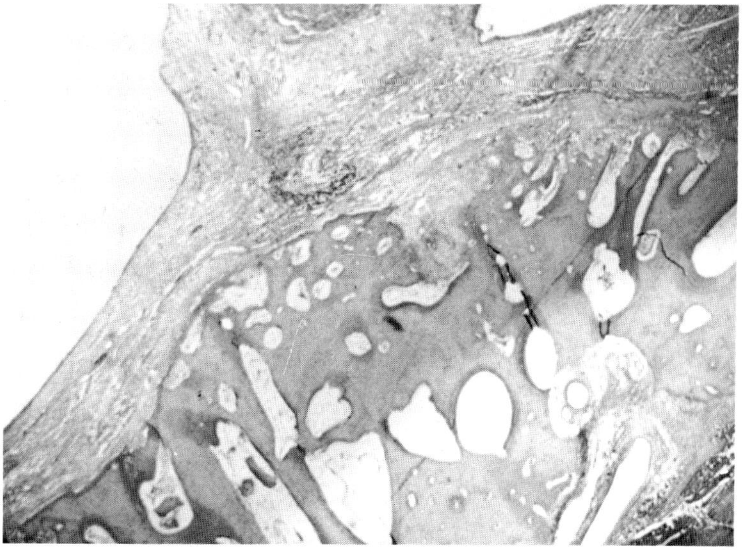

Fig. 12 Histological thin section of the connective tissue, which fills the holes in the ceramic socket. There is no alignment of the collagen fibers (x 4)

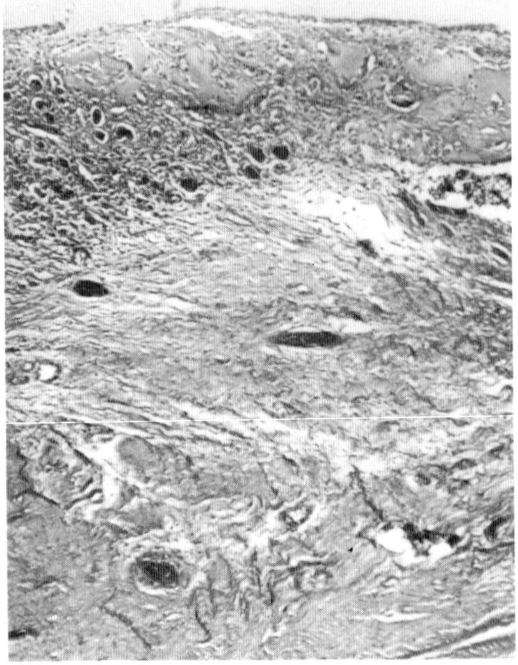

Fig. 13
Detail of the junction membrane/ woven bone (x 10)

anchor and the base plate was formed with the greatest radius equivalent to that of the grooves. Using this technique, the differences in thickness of the walls are reduced. This leads to a shear strength of 650 Kp. The joint surface of the femoral condyle has the form of a complex curve with a continuously changing radius. This form is approximated with the natural form of the knee joint. The implantation of the knee prosthesis is also carried out without using bone cement. The implant bed is prepared by accurately punching out the anchor holes so as to achieve a press fit with the anchor plugs. Postoperatively the resting phase is guaranteed by external fixation. In addition, a measured initial stress can be applied to the ceramic knee joint during the healing period (Figs. 17-19).

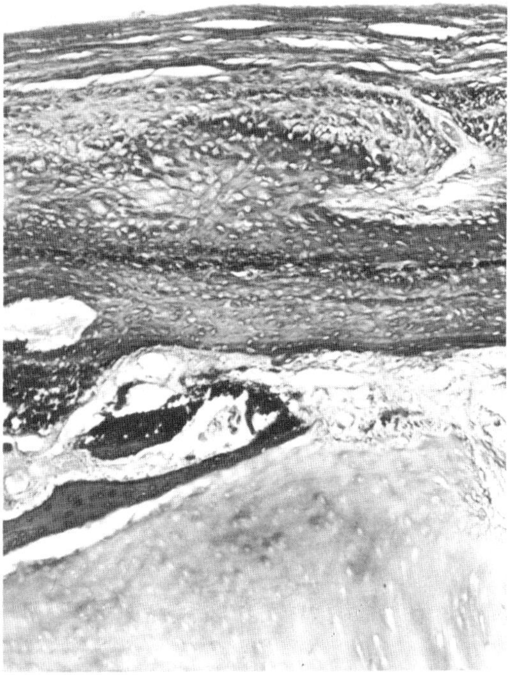

Fig. 14
Detail of the junction membrane/
woven bone (x 10)

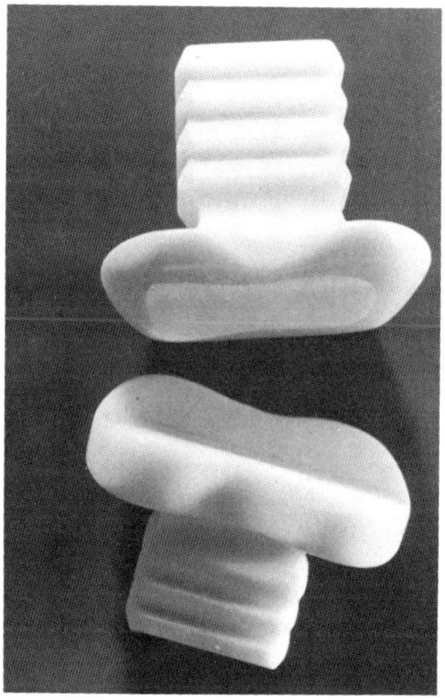

Fig. 15 View of the knee joint. Both components, the femoral and tibial part are of dense alumina

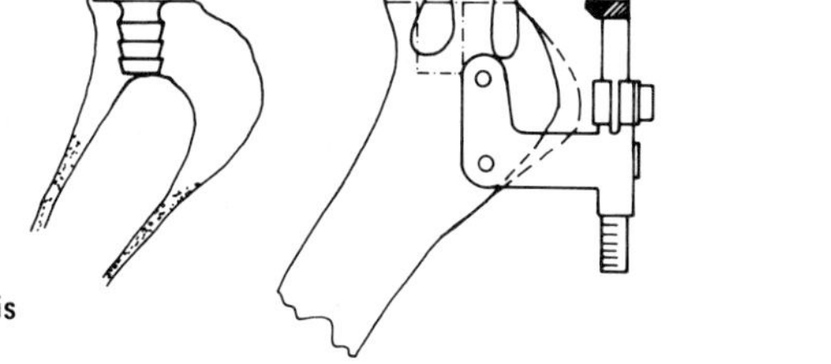

Fig. 16 Schematic representation of the knee prosthesis of dense alumina ceramic for cement-free implantation. The guide instrument is shown in situ

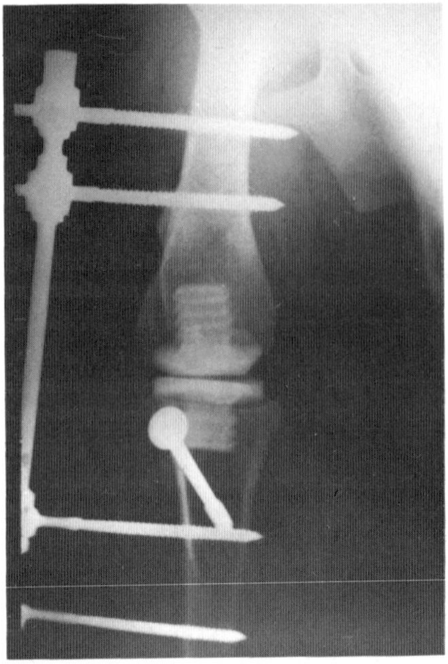

Fig. 17
Radiograph 12 weeks after implantation of a knee prosthesis of dense alumina ceramic without use of bone cement. Temporary fixation with external fixator for 12 weeks, ap-view

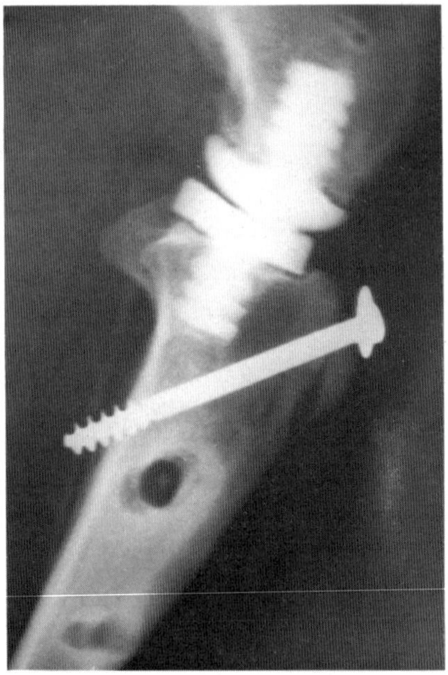

Fig. 18
4 weeks after removal of the external fixator in lateral view of the same sheep

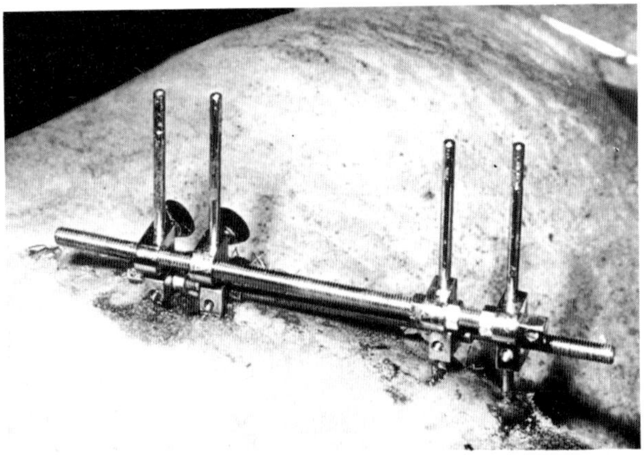

Fig. 19 View of the external fixator for temporary arthrodesis of the knee after cement-free implantation of a hip prosthesis of dense alumina ceramic

REFERENCES

1. Dörre, E., Beutler, H., Geduldig, D.: Anforderungen an oxidkeramische Werkstoffe als Biomaterial für künstliche Gelenke. Archiv für orthopädische und Unfall-Chirurgie (1975)
2. Geduldig, D., Happel, M., Lade, R., Prüssner, P., Willert, H.-G., Zichner, L., Dörre, E.: Animal studies on bone ingrowth kinetics of ceramic material under dynamic stress. International Biomaterials Symposium, University of South Carolina, Clemson, 1975
3. Geduldig, D., Happel, M., Lade, R., Prüssner, P., Willert, H.-G., Zichner, L., Dörre, E.: Welche Aussicht hat die Biokeramik als Implantatmaterial in der Orthopädie? 23. Jahrestagung der Süddeutschen Orthopäden e.V., Baden-Baden 1974
4. Geduldig, D., Happel, M., Lade, R., Prüssner, P., Willert, H.-G., Zichner, L., Dörre, E.: Tierexperimente zur Anwachskinetik von keramischen Werkstoffen unter Entlastung und dynamischer Belastung. Societe Internationale de Chirurgie Orthopedique et Traumatologie, 13. World-Congress, Copenhagen 1975
5. Geduldig, D., Happel, M., Lade, R., Prüssner, P., Willert, H.-G., Zichner, L.: Neuester Stand der tierexperimentellen Untersuchungen mit Gelenkendoprothesen aus dichter Al_2O_3-Keramik. 62. Tagung der Deutschen Gesellschaft für Orthopädie und Traumatologie, Tübingen 1975

CERAMIC HIP JOINT REPLACEMENT – EXPERIMENTAL RESULTS AND EARLY CLINICAL EXPERIENCE

P. Griss, G. Heimke, B. Krempien, and G. Jentschura

Alumina oxide ceramic was proposed by several investigators as a candidate biomaterial for joint replacement based upon morphologic studies with small implants in bone and soft tissue of different animals (1,4-9,15,17,21). In addition, tribologic studies showed this material to have excellent gliding properties with only minimal wear rates (2,12-14,22).

Summing up the biocompatibility studies in small animals it can be stated that this material is highly biostable and biocompatible, permitting the surrounding tissue virtually undisturbed differentiation. Depending mainly on implant site and load condition of the implant, the interface is a highly vascularised soft tissue with synovial cell linings, fibrocartilage or mature bone in close contact with the implant surface. This last observation promised direct fixation of alumina in bone, avoiding the use of cement and thus recommending its application in human joint replacement (2,6-10,15).

EXPERIMENTAL RESULTS WITH ALL–CERAMIC HIP JOINT REPLACEMENT

Since 1972 several series of sheep experiments (45 animals, post-operative survival max. 16 months) have been performed in order to develop and test different designs and implantation techniques for direct fixation of ceramic hip joints to bone, avoiding the use of cement substance. The results that have been published subsequently (6-11,18) allow the following statements to be made.

The response of the bioenvironment to directly implanted and immediately loaded ceramic prostheses must be divided into two categories:

1. the interface reaction
2. the reaction of the supporting bone around the implant.

Both reactions are dependent on a number of factors affecting the type of tissue response along the implant surface as well as the amount of bone remodelling within the supporting structures around the alumina hip prosthesis. We have to consider design-dependent influences, biomechanical interrelationships and technical facts such as the rigidity of the primary implant fit and biological implications caused by the introduction of an implant into the well vascularised bone and soft tissue composite. Most of the reactions now to be described can basically also be observed with other materials such as chrome-cobalt alloy or polyethylene RCH 1000. The already described superior biostability and biocompatibility of alumina, however, still seems to give better results with respect to close bone/implant contact and hence mechanical interlocking of the bone/alumina composite. Adverse effects caused by toxic metal ion release and polymerization, or degradation or wear products of polymeric implants can be avoided. This allows a better interpretation of tissue reactions around loaded implants.

Alumina hip prostheses which did not fit exactly into the bone bed primarily, thus permitting relative movements along the interface, became loose within a short time. The interface was composed of a highly vascularised thick fibrous tissue layer, the underlying bone showed osteoclastic resorptive seams and sporadic new fiber cartilage and woven bone formation. These findings are in agreement with those of Geduldig et al. (3) using alumina screws pushed into the medullary canal without exact bone bed preparation allowing a rigid primary fit. This type of reaction can be called a "pseudarthrotic interface reaction".

Alumina cup designs such as the square cup (Fig. 1a) and the screw cup, (Fig. 1b) exactly fitted to the bone by special techniques (6,10) gave better results. Along the bottom and within the screw windings and also within macroscopic grooves along the outer surface of the square cup, well organized bone was found. This gave good stability to the cup by mechanical interlocking of bone and alumina (Fig. 1a,b). Within the range of routine hard tissue histologic technique, areas of up to 5 mm length were found where the supporting healthy bone was obviously in close contact with the implant surface (Fig. 2a,b). Yet there might still have been a thin cellular layer between, attached to the alumina on removal of the implant before histologic preparation (7).

The restoration, or in part permanence, of bone implant contact was mainly observed along those implant areas, where pressure transmission could be expected (Fig. 2a,b). Other areas along the implant surface showed a fibrocartilage or fibrous tissue interface still present even after 13 months of implantation, area F in Fig. 1b. This indicates biomechanic rules to be responsible in interface differentiation along alumina surfaces under load conditions. In other words, any hip implant design which is not loaded exclusively by pressure stresses will show areas of a fibrous interface "non union". This was most obvious along the intra-medullary interface of the femoral design (Fig. 3a). Bone support developed only beneath the neck and around the tip of the prosthesis while the smooth stem was surrounded by a thick layer of soft tissue which did not permit a bone – alumina interlocking. As a result all stems became loose within 3-6 months.

From these observations it can be concluded that any stem design should possess profiles allowing pressure stress transmission in order to distribute the load more evenly along the endosteum of the femoral tube. Taking into consideration proposals of McBride (19) and Mittelmeier (20) we proposed a stem design made of alumina having big and individually shaped steps according to local stress patterns and inverse steps along the lateral surface to convert shearing stresses into compressive stresses onto the lateral structures of the femur. This design is still under test in sheep (Fig. 3b).

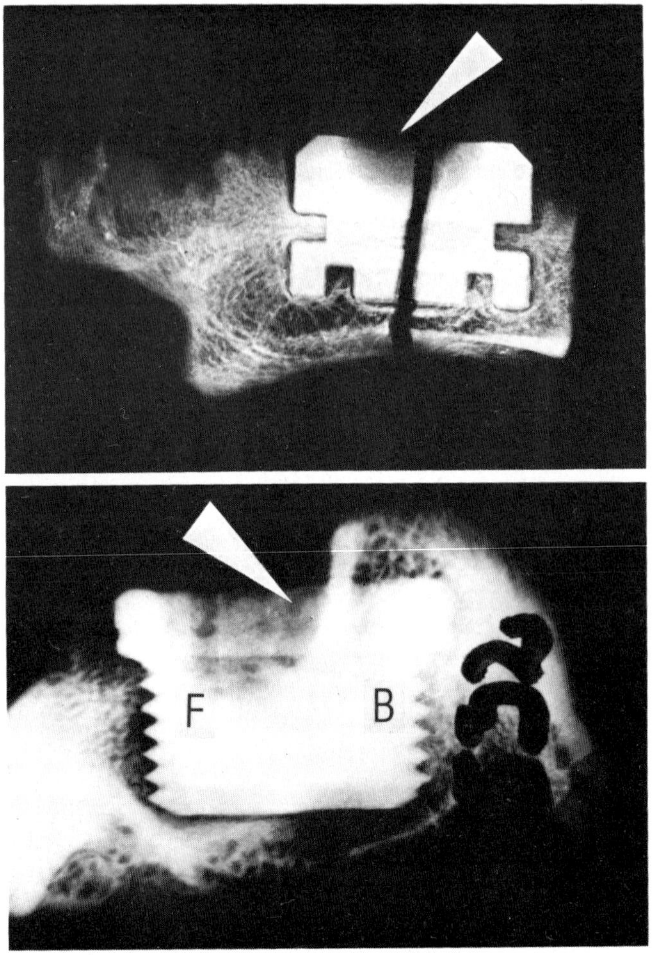

Fig. 1
a. X-ray of square-shaped cup 6 months after surgery in a sheep. Arrow indicates main direction of load transmission. Mechanical interlocking of the socket by bone ingrowth into microprofiles, trabecular reorientation at left.
b. X-ray of a screw cup 13 months after surgery in a sheep. Area B represents main load transmitting zone, the bone is in close contact with the thread of screw. Area F represents a zone of fibrous tissue "non union"

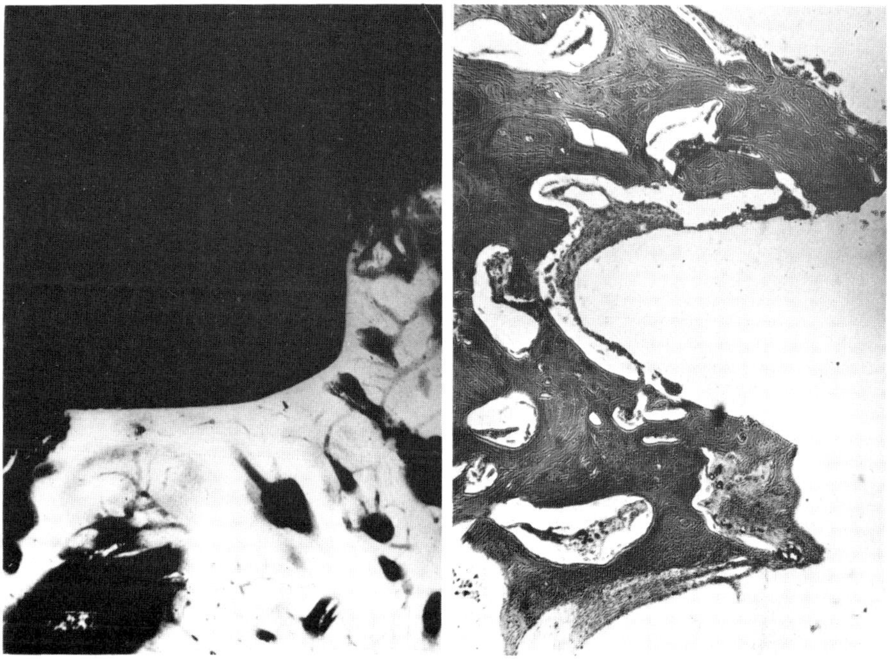

Fig. 2 a. Microradiogram from pelvic bone in close contact with a square-shaped cup surface 3 months after surgery in a sheep.
b. Decalcified thin section of bone in direct contact with alumina screw profiles 3 months after insertion of a screw socket. Arrows show areas of lamellar bone directly transmitting load from the cup to the bone interface, x 40 (ref. Goldner)

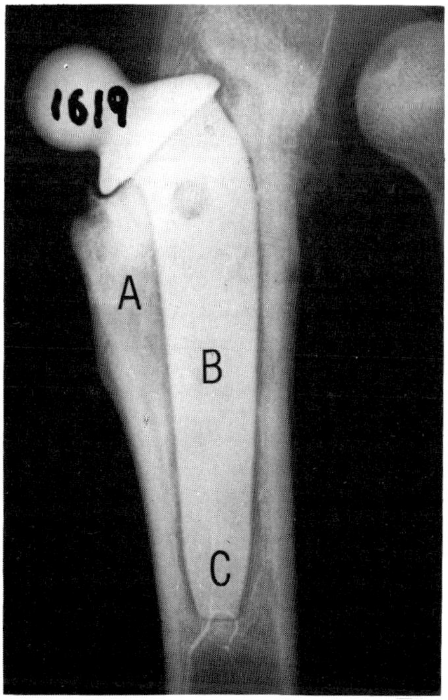

Fig. 3a
X-ray from an alumina stem implant in a sheep 3 months after surgery. Load transmitting areas A and C with considerable new bone formation; area B smooth stem surface with thick fibrous tissue interface. Stem was loose on sacrifice of the animal

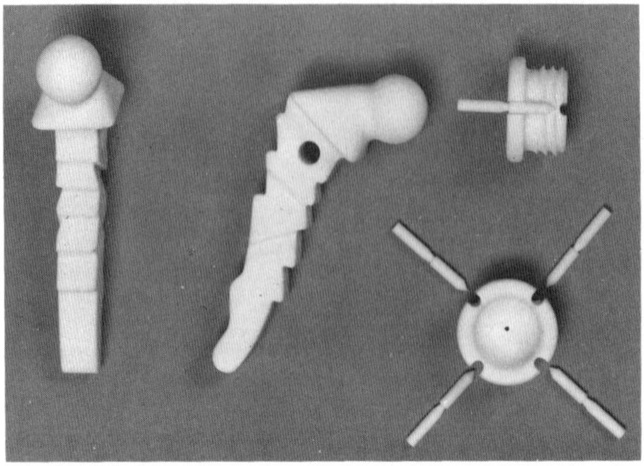

Fig. 3b
New stem design for better load transmission along the whole stem area. Further explanation see text

EARLY CLINICAL EXPERIENCE WITH TWO ALUMINA–METAL COMPOSITE PROSTHESES

Both the square and the screw cup were chosen for human implantation. In combination with a still cemented modified Weber or Charnley stem, both cups are used mainly in selected cases of unilateral hip disease (Fig. 4). The ceramic balls are attached to the stem by means of a self-locking cone. The screw cup is indicated in patients between the age of 40 and 60 years, the square cup is used in individuals older than 60, together with only a small amount of cement along the side walls to allow early ambulation.

Both prostheses can be implanted by an anterolateral or posterior approach. A set of new instruments including a front-, rim- and screw cutter and a square shaped chisel, facilitate accurate preparation of the bone bed and assure a rigid primary fit with extended initial bone implant contact.

The Lindenhof prosthesis has, to date, been used in 15 cases, including those with degenerative coxarthrosis, idiopathic or Cortisone-mediated femoral head necrosis, hip dysplasia and posttraumatic coxarthrosis. Postoperative observation time ranges up to 13 months. Full weight bearing on the operated leg is allowed 8 to 12 weeks after surgery in order to facilitate the experimentally observed remodelling of the interface under exclusion of unphysiologically high local stresses (7,8). In all cases up to now no resorptive border has appeared along the ceramic cups on X-ray control. On the contrary, bone grows into the profiles showing by the time progressive sclerosis along the load-bearing areas (Fig. 5a,b). All patients have regained a full range of motion and can walk and work without a cane.

The small screw cup, 45 mm, can be inserted fully into the original acetabulum in most cases. Even the rim can be countersunk completely under the level of the acetabular rim

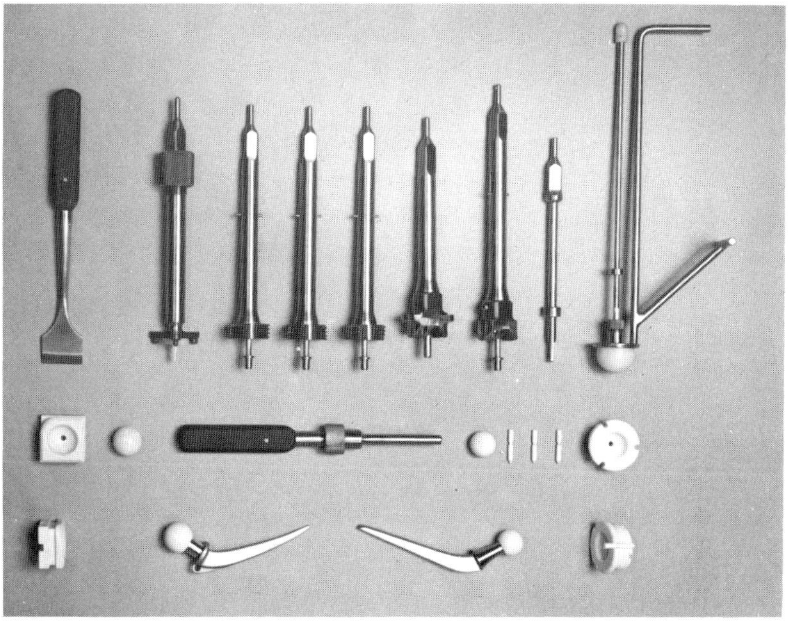

Fig. 4 Instruments and alumina-metal composite prostheses for human application.
Bottom right: screw socket type Lindenhof with three pins to block the screw thread,
Bottom left: square socket type Friedrichsfeld

offering additional surface for load transmission (Fig. 6a,b). As was pointed out by Huggler et al. (16) after biomechanical studies of the acetabular stress distribution this rim seems to be very essential.

The square-shaped cup has been employed in 5 patients up to now. It can be used in any case of acetabular destruction and with special advantage in protrusio acetabuli or acetabular dysplasia. In the latter condition a shaped femoral head segment can be screwed along the straight lateral wall of the cup to reconstruct a complete bony bed (Fig. 7a,b).

During surgery the acetabulum is prepared with the smallest front cutter of the Lindenhof prosthesis (screw cup), whose diameter is 4 mm smaller than the largest diameter of the Friedrichsfeld cup (square cup). This results in a cylindrical hole with a plain bottom. A square shaped chisel is now used to remove four slices of bone from the wall of this hole exactly corresponding to the edges of the cup. The cup can now be pushed into place, the correct position being given by the plain bottom. Cancellous bone from the femoral neck stump or a very small amount of cement can now be pressed along the four side walls of the cup to fill the small spaces left by the cylindrical cutting tool. The cup is well secured against tilting and rotational forces by virtue of its shape and by this implantation technique. The patient can walk with full weight bearing soon after surgery.

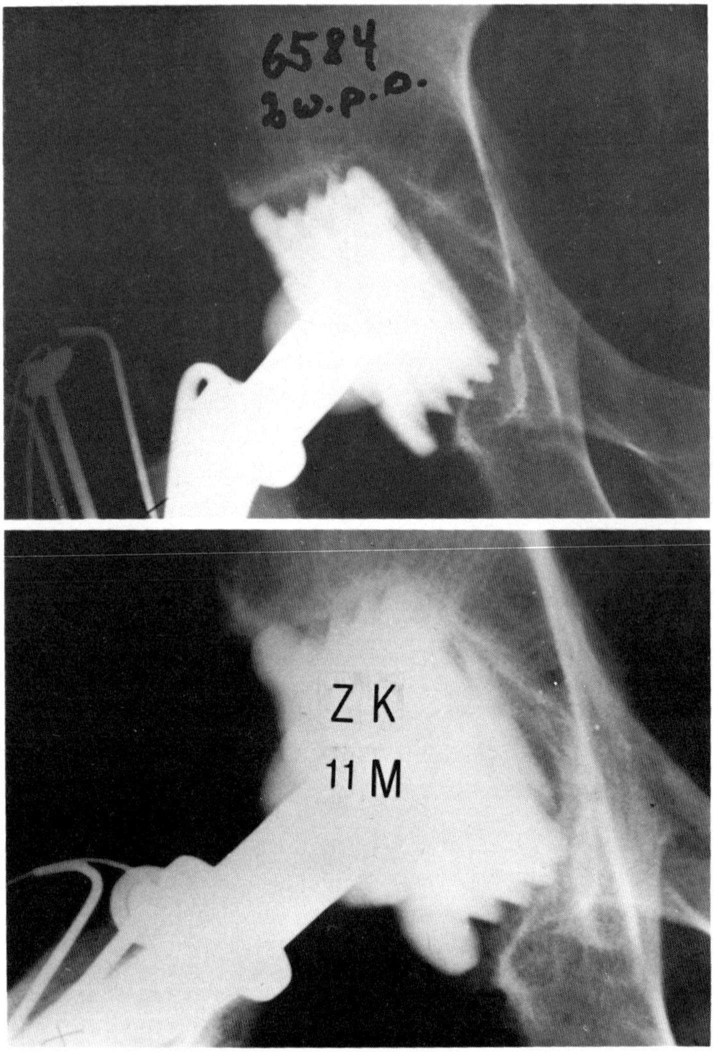

Fig. 5 a. X-ray of right hip 2 weeks after implantation of a screw socket because of idiopathic femoral head necrosis. Poor interlocking because of technical difficulties during surgery. No bone within the screw thread and along the bottom.

b. X-ray of the same hip 11 months after surgery. Full integration of the socket into the pelvic bone. Weight bearing allowed 3 months after surgery

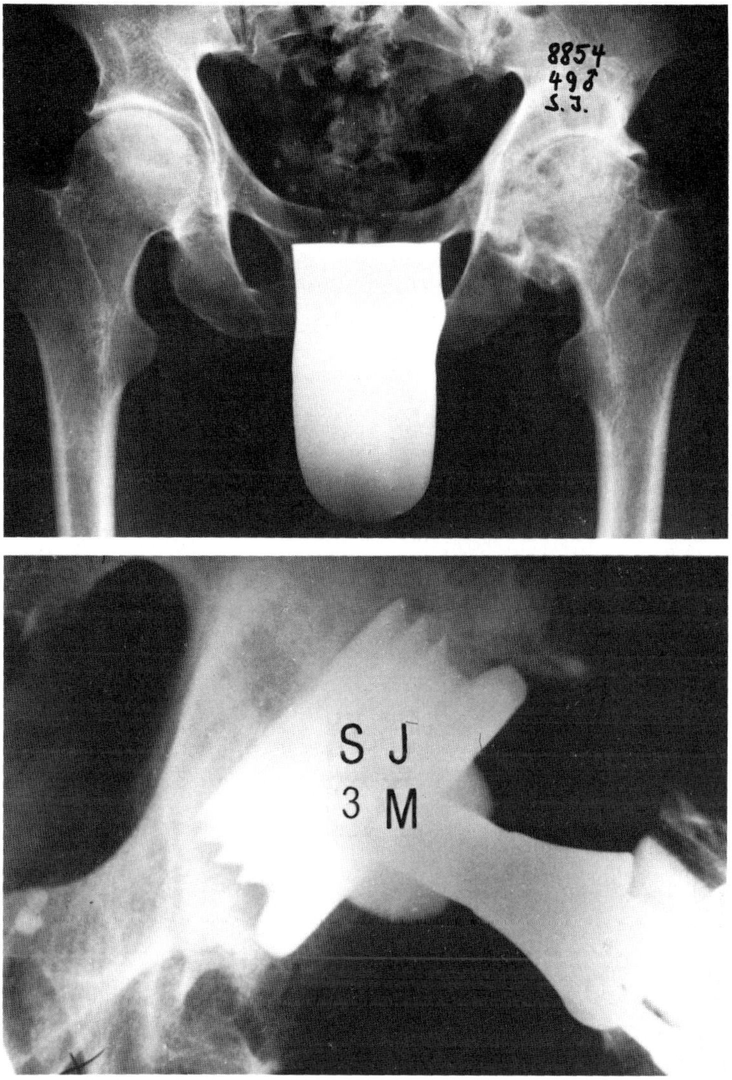

Fig. 6 a. preoperative X-ray of a 49-year-old male with unilateral coxarthrosis.
b. left hip 3 months after insertion of a small Lindenhof socket and 2 months after full weight bearing. Perfect integration of the cup without a visible soft tissue interface

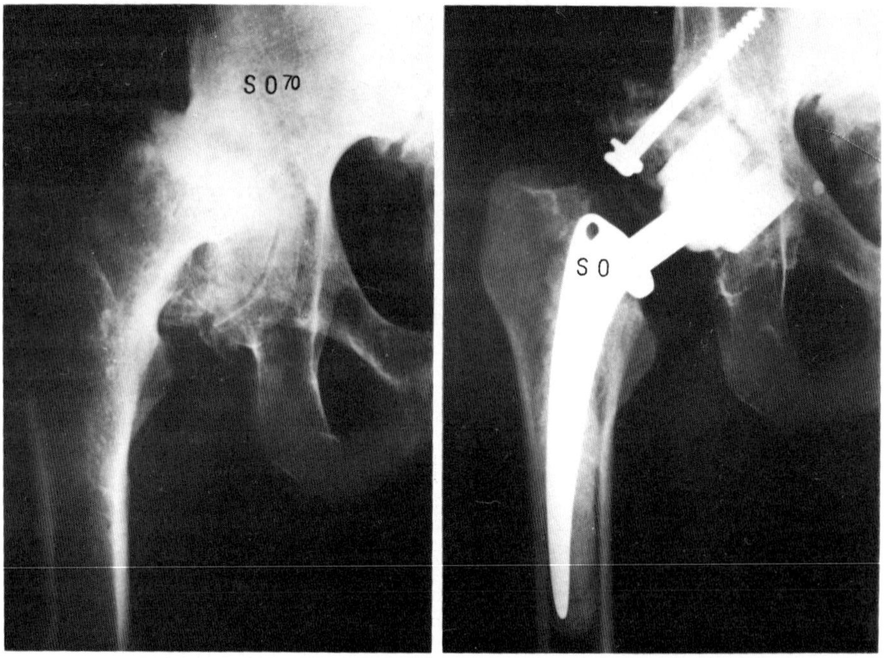

Fig. 7 a. Preoperative X-ray of the hight hip of a 70-year-old male. Coxarthrosis following slipped capital femoral epiphysis in adolescence with a shallow acetabulum.
b. Postoperative X-ray of the same hip after insertion of a Friedrichsfeld socket together with a segmental femoral head reimplantation to restore bone continuity around the cup

CONCLUSIONS

Both prostheses are experimentally proven designs that hold out hope for a permanent bone/alumina interlocking when correct positioning is achieved and a correct implantation technique is used. A primary rigid fit of the implant in the bone is essential for success. A cement-free stem design is still experimental. Therefore, neither prosthesis is implanted in individuals under the age of 40 years. The experience in humans is to date very preliminary but positive. A careful selection of patients and only unilateral hip replacement is recommended until a large number of cases and late information about this procedure is available.

REFERENCES

1. Boutin, P.: Presse Med. 79, 639 (1971)
2. Boutin, P.: Revue de Chirurgie Orthopedique 58, 229 (1972)
3. Geduldig, D., Happel, M.W., Lade, R., Prüssner, P., Zichner, L., Willert, H.G.: Medizinisch-Orthopädische Technik, in press

4. Griss, P., v. Andrian-Werburg, H., Krempien, B., Heimke, G.: Journal of Biomedical Materials Research Symposium 5, 39 (1973)

5. Griss, P., Krempien, B., v. Andrian-Werburg, H., Heimke, G., Fleiner, R.: Archiv für orthopädische und Unfall-Chirurgie 76, 270 (1973)

6. Griss, P., Krempien, B., v. Andrian-Werburg, H., Heimke, G., Fleiner, R., Diehm, T.: Journal of Biomedical Materials Research Symposium 5, 39 (1974)

7. Griss, P., v. Andrian-Werburg, H., Heimke, G., Krempien, B., Reipa, S., Hartung, H.J., Lauterbach, H.J.: Zeitschrift für Orthopädie 113, 756 (1975)

8. Griss, P., Heimke, G., Krempien, B., Silber, R., Haehner, K., Merkle, B.: Medizinisch-Orthopädische Technik, in press

9. Griss, P., Heimke, G., v. Andrian-Werburg, H., Krempien, B., Reipa, S., Lauterbach, H.J., Hartung, H.J.: Journal of Biomedical Materials Research Symposium 6, 177 (1975)

10. Griss, P., Heimke, G., v. Andrian-Werburg, H.: Archiv für orthopädische und Unfall-Chirurgie 81, 259 (1975)

11. Griss, P., Heimke, G., Krempien, B.: Zeitschrift für Orthopädie, in press

12. Heimke, G., Beisler, W., v. Andrian-Werburg, H., Griss, P., Krempien, B.: Berichte der Deutschen Keramischen Gesellschaft 50, 4 (1973)

13. Heimke, G., Griss, P., v. Andrian-Werburg, H., Krempien, B.: Archiv für orthopädische und Unfall-Chirurgie 78, 216 (1974)

14. Heimke, G., Griss, P., Krempien, B.: Acta Medicotechnica 23, 243 (1975)

15. Hentrich, R.L., Graves, G.A., Stein, H.G., Baipai, P.K.: Journal of Biomedical Materials Research 5, 25 (1971)

16. Huggler, A.H., Schreiber, A., Dietschi, C., Jacob, H.: Zeitschrift für Orthopädie 112, 44 (1974)

17. Hulbert, S.F., Morrison, S.J., Klawitter, J.J.: Journal of Biomedical Materials Research 6, 347 (1972)

18. Krempien, B., Griss, P., Heimke, G., v. Andrian-Werburg, H., Harung, H.J., Reipa, S., Lauterbach, H.J.: Acta Orthopedica Belgica 40, 624 (1974)

19. McBride, E.D.: Journal of Bone and Joint Surgery 34-A, 989 (1952)

20. Mittelmeier, H.: Zeitschrift für Orthopädie 112, 27 (1974)

21. Predecki, P., Stephan, J.E., Auslaender, B.A., Mooney, V.L., Kirkland, K.: Journal of Biomedical Materials Research 6, 375 (1972)

22. Ungethüm, M., Refior, H.J.: Archiv für orthopädische und Unfall-Chirurgie 79, 97 (1974)

IMPROVED UHMW POLYETHYLENE LOW FRICTION HIP ENDOPROSTHESIS USING AL_2O_3 CERAMIC INSTEAD OF METAL FOR THE ARTICULATING BALL

M. Semlitsch

The principle of "low friction arthroplasty", devised and introduced in 1963 by Charnley (1) and shortly afterwards by Mueller (2), is generally preferred nowadays with total hip endoprostheses. With the polyethylene/metal combination used for the joint socket and the articulating ball, the moment of friction is initially very low. However, owing the wear phenomena on the polyethylene socket (3,4,5,6) – and to a minor extent on the metallic ball as well (7) – a limited service life of the polyethylene socket is to be reckoned with.

A tribological study conducted at Sulzer over several years has been concerned with the following points:

- Continued application of the polyethylene socket (proven in over ten years' clinical experience).
- Reduction of the wear rate on the polyethylene socket.
- Elimination of the release of metallic wear particles from the articulating ball into the adjacent tissues.
- Maintaining the low moment of friction between the polyethylene socket and the articulating ball for a longer period of time than presently possible.

It appears that in the highly-polished Al_2O_3 ceramic BIOLOX (8), which is characterized by minimal grain size and maximal strength, we have found an ideally suited implant material for the ball articulating with the polyethylene socket (9). The extremely good behaviour of the polyethylene/ceramic combination with a low moment of friction and a very small wear rate can be explained by the material properties of this ceramic, which are much better for this purpose than those of the currently employed implant metals such as FeCrNiMo stainless steel AISI-316L and CoCrMo cast alloy (Table 1).

Following the animal experiments with total hip endoprostheses using the optimized new material combination, which are now being conducted at the Orthopaedic University Clinic in Frankfurt/Main (10,11), Müller- and Weber-type total hip joint replacement prostheses with this combination are soon to be implanted in patients at a number of clinics in Switzerland and Germany. Without having to effect any basic changes in the present design and implantation principles, the functional life of these hip endoprostheses based on the following material concept will, in all probability, be considerably prolonged:

1. Joint socket of UHMW polyethylene RCH-1000 with good elasticity in the acetabulum.
2. Joint ball of Al_2O_3 ceramic with optimal properties as a sliding partner for the polyethylene.

Table 1 Ceramic/polyethylene-pairing for articulating parts of hip joints

Properties	Metal FeCrNiMo AISI-316	Metal CoCrMo HS-21	Ceramic Al_2O_3 BIOLOX
Biocompatibility	++	++	+++
Biostability	+	++	+++
Corrosion resistance	+	++	+++
Compression strength	++	++	+++
Impact strength	++	++	++
Fatigue strength	++	++	++
Hardness	+	++	+++
Scratch resistance	+	++	+++
Polish of surface	+	++	+++
Wetability with fluids	+	+	+++
Sterilization	+++	+++	+++
Tribology against Polyethylene UHMWPE	++	++	+++

+++ very good ++ good + satisfactory

3. Anchorage stem of CoNiCrMoTi wrought alloy PROTASUL-10 with extremely high fatigue strength, toughness, corrosion resistance and biocompatibility (12,13,14,15).

A step-by-step further development of each joint endoprosthesis type will minimize the risk both for the patient and the surgeon, because researchers and designers in the area of endoprosthetics can safely build upon their experience gained over many years.

REFERENCES

1. Charnley, J.: Total hip replacement by low-friction arthroplasty. Clinical Orthopaedics. 72, 7 (1970)
2. Müller, M.E.: Total hip prostheses. Clinical Orthopaedics 72, 46 (1970)
3. Charnley, J.: The long-term results of low-friction arthroplasty of the hip performed as a primary intervention. Journal of Bone and Joint Surgery 54-B, 61 (1972)
4. Willert, H.G., Semlitsch, M.: Kunststoffe als Implantatwerkstoffe. 62. DGOT-Tagung, Tübingen 1975
5. Scheier, H.: Der Abrieb bei der Totalprothese. Kongress der Niederländisch-Schweizerischen Gesellschaften für Orthopädie, Lausanne 1974
6. Charnley, J.: Ten years experience with low-friction arthroplasty. 13. SICOT Congress, Copenhagen 1975
7. Charnley, J.: Clinical and laboratory observations on the rate of wear of different plastic materials in the sockets of artificial hip joints. Conference of the Biological Engineering Society, "Materials for use in medicine and biology", Cambridge/GB 1974

8. Doerre, E.: Al_2O_3-Keramik als Implantatwerkstoff. 62. DGOT-Tagung, Tübingen 1975

9. Semlitsch, M., Willert, H.G., Doerre, E.: Neue Werkstoffpaarung Al_2O_3-Keramik/ Polyäthylen zur Verminderung des Polyäthylenabriebs bei Gelenkpfannen von Hüftprothesen. 62. DGOT-Tagung, Tübingen 1975, Medizinisch-Orthopädische Technik 95 (1975)

10. Willert, H.G., Geduldig, D., Happel, M.W., Lade, R., Preussner, P., Zichner, L.: Tierexperimentelle Testung von keramischen Knochenersatzwerkstoffen. Dokumentation zur wissenschaftlichen Ausstellung der 62. DGOT-Tagung, Tübingen 1975

11. Geduldig, G.: Neuester Stand der tierexperimentellen Untersuchungen mit Gelenkendoprothesen aus Al_2O_3-Keramik. 62. DGOT-Tagung, Tübingen 1975

12. Swiss SNV-Working Group 129 for Surgical Implants: CoNiCrMoTi-Wrought Alloy (No. 056.5 09) VSM/SNV Normen-Bulletin, 23, 172 (1974)

13. ISO/TC-150/SC-1/WG-1: Swiss Proposal No. 30 on Biocompatibility of CoNiCrMoTi-Whrought Alloy. SNV-Switzerland (1975)

14. ISO/TC-150/SC-1/WG-1: Draft Proposal for CoNiCrMoTi-Wrought Alloy (No. 31) ISO/TC-150 Symposium, Copenhagen (1975)

15. Escales, F., Galante, J., Rostocker, W., Coogan, P.S.: MP-35N a corrosion resistant, high-strength alloy for orthopaedic surgical implants, bio-assay results. Journal of Biomedical Materials Research 9, 303 (1975)

EXPERIENCE WITH BIOCERAMIC ENDOPROSTHESES OF THE HIP JOINT

M. Salzer, H. Locke, H. Plenk jr., G. Punzet, N. Stärk, and K. Zweymüller

As far as we know, the earliest mention of alumina as a material for endoprostheses was made in 1933 in a German patent (1) by Rock. In 1971 to 1972 Hulbert and his co-workers reported positive results of animal tests on porous alumina implants (2,3,4). The reaction of bone tissue to porous ceramics was also tested by Rhinelander and co-workers (5). In 1972 Predecki published results on experimental work on the kinetics of bone growth into cylindrical channels of titanium and alumina (6). In Germany, Heide and Hofmann reported the application of ceramics in medicine in 1972 (7). In 1973 Heimke et al. published results on testing implants of high-purity dense alumina (8). All this scientific work was concerned with "in vitro testing" of materials and with animal tests. In 1972 a publication was produced by Boutin reporting on human implantations of total hip joint endoprostheses (9). He described implants consisting of a metal stem on one side and of alumina ceramic ball and socket on the other. The ball of this implant is fixed to the stem. In a first stage, socket and stem were implanted in a conventional manner using bone cement. In 1975 he published a report on his further work doing implantation of the socket without bone cement (10).

In 1973 Engelhardt and Zeibig reported on implantation of bioceramic humerus prostheses in human patients (11); this was followed by publications of Salzer and his co-workers (12,13), who did a number of implantations in human patients suffering from bone cancer. Bioceramic endoprostheses for several parts of the skeleton were implanted.

All this work demonstrates that alumina may be a material which can be used in endoprosthesis designs for human patients.

PROPERTIES OF ALUMINA CERAMICS

There are two known modifications of pure aluminium oxide (Al_2O_3). The crystal structure of α-alumina is cubic. Heated to temperatures of about 1000 ^{o}C it is transformed to an hexagonal crystalline structure called α-alumina. This modification is a very stable material. As a single crystal α-aluminum oxide is known to be precious stone. In the polycrystalline state it is used as ceramic material with advanced electrical and mechanical properties. Its main mechanical properties are listed in Table 1. The characteristic data of alumina depend on the purity of the material, its medium grain size, its porosity and on the surface quality of the samples. The data listed are the properties of pure dense α-alumina (Al_2O_3 content 99.7 %; density 3.90 g/cm^3). Samples are polished to a CLA-value of 0.15 μm. The medium grain size of the material is about 5 μm (Fig. 1).

Table 1 Mechanical properties of alumina ceramics

Al_2O_3 content	99.7 %
medium grain size	< 5 μm
bulk density	> 3.90 g/cm^3
Vickers hardness	2300 N/mm^2
pressure strength	4000 N/mm^2
bending strength	500 N/mm^2
tensile strength	300 N/mm^2
Young's modulus	$3.8 \cdot 10^5$ N/mm^2

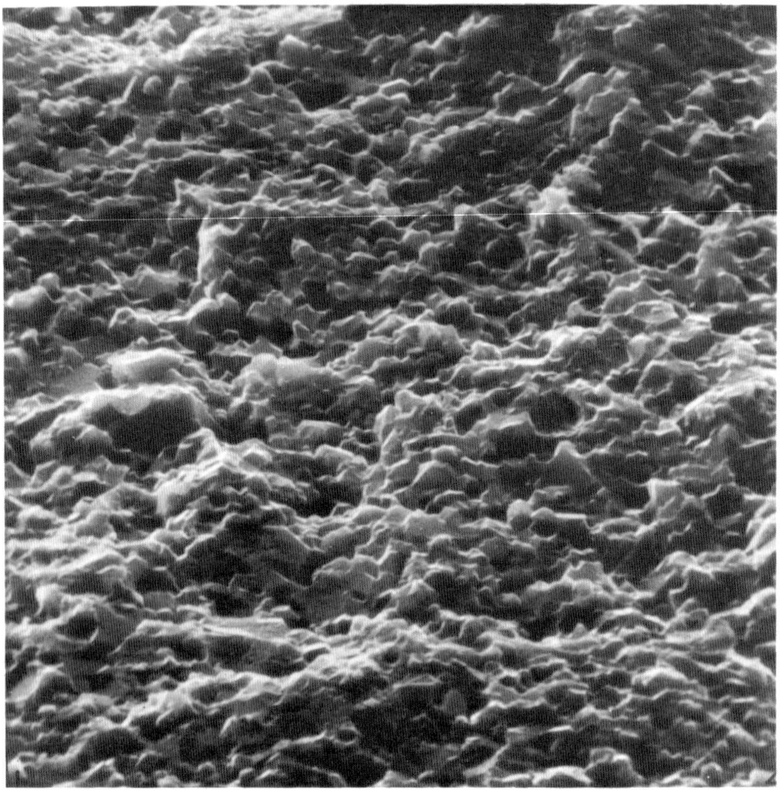

Fig. 1 SEM-picture of pure dense alumina. The medium grain size of the material (Al_2O_3-content 99.7 %) is about 5 μm

Young's modulus and compressive strength are very high, tensile and bending strength are considerably lower. When designing technical components of alumina one has to take account of the difference in bending and compressive strength and the fact that alumina is a brittle material; this means that loaded samples after having suffered elastic deformation (Hooke's range) lack any of the plasticity known from metals. Therefore ceramic material will break immediately when the load exceeds Hookian range.

Another advantage of pure dense alumina ceramics is low abrasion and friction of polished surface. So it is a very useful material for designing joints which have to work under severe conditions (load, body fluid) over a long period of time.

DESIGN OF BIOCERAMIC ENDOPROSTHESES

As is known from the results of animal tests, alumina is to a large degree biocompatible. In order to utilize the biocompatibility of the material, implantations have to be done without bone cement. It is expected that a durable fixation of the implant is obtained by bone growth into the indentations of the surface of the implant. The basic requirement for bone tissue ingrowth is a stable fixation of the implant to bone during the initial period after implantation. To obtain a stable fixation of the implant to bone the "conical sleeve technique" is applied. The exterior of the long bone is shaped conically by means of a special milling cutter. The length of the cone is about 1.5 x the diameter of the cross-section of the bone. In this way damage to the bone can be minimized. A bioceramic sleeve fitted to the bone results in a press fit (Fig. 2). By doing this, the technique of the implantation is made relatively simple and gives a good primary fixation.

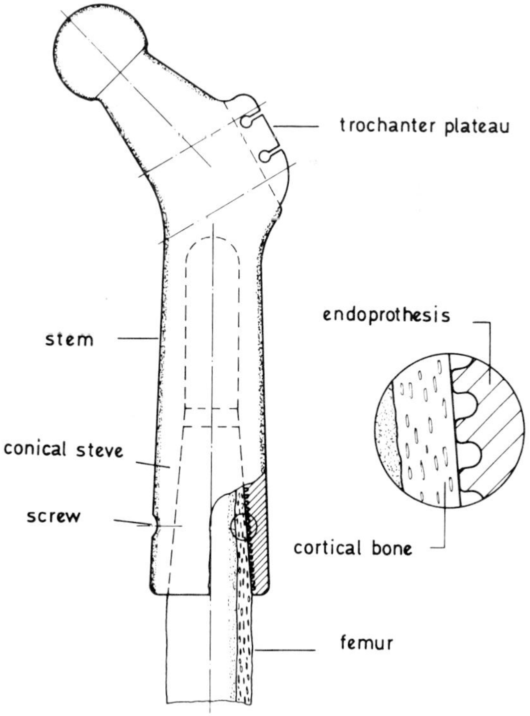

Fig. 2
Hip joint endoprosthesis for bridging defects. The implant consists of the conical sleeve, the stem and the ball. At the inner surface of the sleeve there are indentations

Another advantage of this design is that the bending moment of the sleeve is higher than that of the average stem which is often used for fixing an implant intramedullarily. Therefore the sleeve is able to withstand bending-loads better than a stem. Furthermore, the sleeve, due to the small length of fixation, will stiffen the bone to a lower degree than fixation of the endoprosthesis by a stem. By shaping the exterior of the long bone to a cone, the periosteal blood supply is damaged. Therefore the remaining cortical bone has to be nourished from the intramedullary vessels. It was questionable whether this intramedullary blood supply would be adequate.

Initially, we have designed a hip joint endoprosthesis for bridging defects of the proximal part of the femur of human patients. The implant consists of the conical sleeve, the stem and the ball. The trochanter major can be attached to the trochanter plateau. The securing of the implant against rotation is effected by a metal screw. There are indentations, like grooves, at the inner surface of the bioceramic sleeve (Fig. 2). To test this endoprosthesis in animal experiments the design was modified in size.

Following the principle of the fixation of the implants by means of conical sleeves we designed the so-called "femur cap endoprosthesis". It is intended to be implanted in patients suffering from osteoarthritis. When implanting this endoprosthesis, only one part of the femoral head has to be replaced. After milling the femoral head conically, the cap is fitted to the spongy bone cone. Additionally, a supporting plate can be implanted for better distributing external load (Figs. 3,4). It is provided to permit implantation of this type of endoprosthesis in human patients in the future. At the moment we are testing this cap endoprosthesis by implantation in corpses, animal and in vitro experiments.

In combination with both the femur long shaft endoprosthesis and the cap endoprosthesis a ceramic socket implant is used. In this way a total ceramic hip joint can be achieved which has low friction and wear resistance in accordance with the mechanical properties of alumina. The socket consists of a spherical cup and three pins for the anchorage of the socket into the pelvic bone (Figs. 5,6). Loading the hip joint physiologically the resultant force is always directed between two pins. In this way any rotational movement of the socket can be avoided.

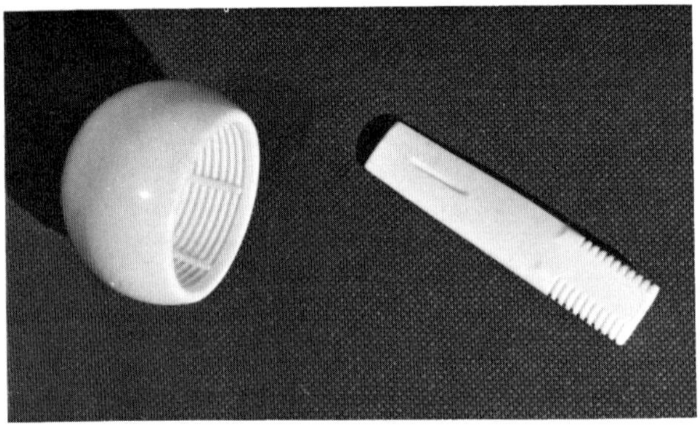

Fig. 3
Femur cap endoprosthesis to be implanted in patients suffering from osteoarthritis

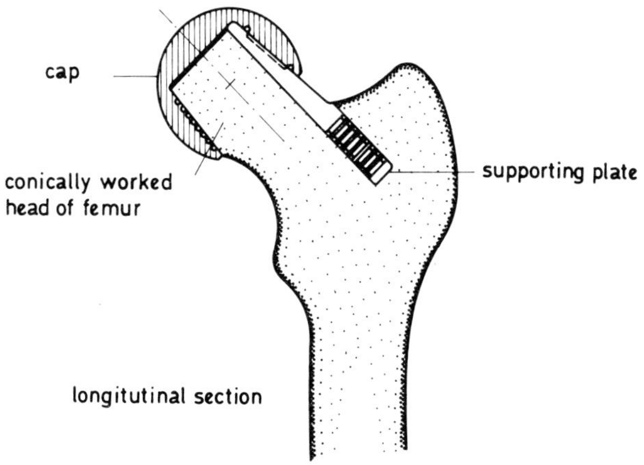

Fig. 4
Femur cap endoprosthesis. The cap is fitted to a spongy bone cone. In addition a supporting plate may be used

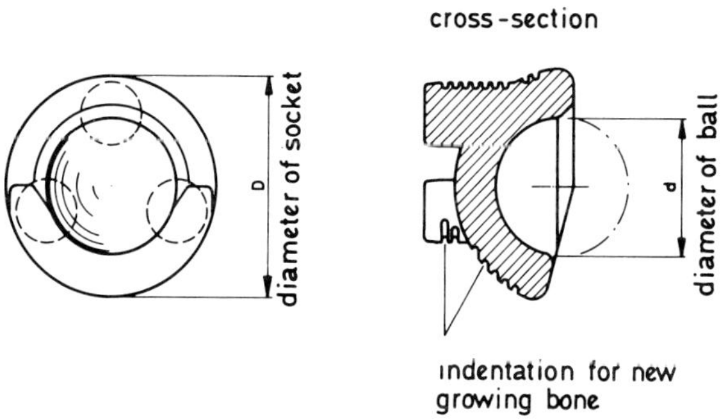

Fig. 5
Schematic drawing of socket design

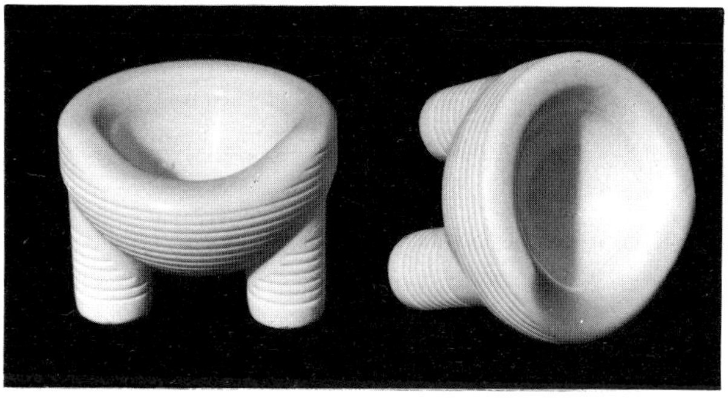

Fig. 6
Bioceramic sockets consisting of a spherical cap and three pins. When loading the hip joint physiologically the resultant force is always directed between two pins

TEST RESULTS

The following experiments were done to test the design of the endoprosthesis. We now have available results of both mechanical in vitro experiments and histological examinations of femur long shaft endoprostheses implanted in animals as well as in man.

Evaluated was the breaking load of the composite of fresh human bone and implant. Because of the range in strength of human bones, pairs of bones were used in the experiments. One femur of each pair was loaded to breaking point. After combining the second femur and the endoprosthesis, this composite was broken too. The axis of the femoral shaft was adjusted to the vertical at an angle of about 6 ^{o} in the valgus position and loaded vertically (Fig. 7). Results showed that the ultimate load of the composites of bone and implant was 100 % to 200 % of the ultimate load of the bones. It must be noted, however, that natural femora are broken in the neck area, whereas the composites broke below the implant.

Animal tests were done in dogs. On the one hand the primary fixation of the implants was to be examined. The other questions were whether intramedullary blood supply of the bone would be sufficient to avoid necrosis, and whether a durable fixation of the endoprosthesis to the bone could be achieved by bone tissue growth into the indentations of the bioceramic implant.

To implant this endoprosthesis the trochanter was first cut. After removing the femoral head from the acetabulum, resection of the femoral shaft was performed. Then the exterior of the long bone was shaped using a conical milling cutter. In a second stage of the implantation the acetabulum has to be shaped by exact milling and drilling to obtain an

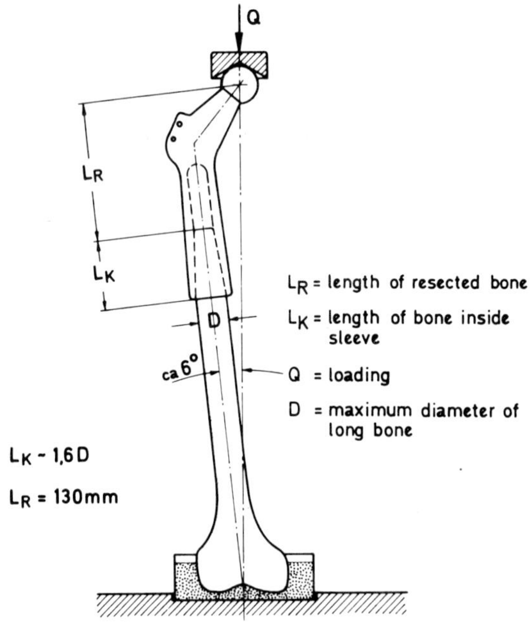

Fig. 7
Mechanical tests of the long shaft endoprosthesis. The axis of the femoral shaft was adjusted to the vertical at an angle of about 6 ^{o} in the valgus position

exact press-fit of the socket. Now the long shaft endoprosthesis is fitted to the conically shaped femur and the trochanter is fixed to the plateau. The operation can be finished conventionally (14,15).

To date 15 implantations of the femur endoprosthesis in dogs have been done. Apart from a number of difficulties at the beginning good results are now obtained. Histological evaluation is available over a period of 6 months after implantation. Two animals are still alive for testing the fixation by a sleeve over a longer period of time.

A special technique of preparing samples for histological examination was developed. After sacrificing the animal, bone and ceramic implant are excised together with surrounding tissues and embedded in methyl methacrylate. Using a diamond saw the specimens are cut into sections of about 0.1 to 0.2 mm thick. Applied to special slides the sections are then ground to a thickness of about 50 μm. In all cases the sections included the undecalcified bone together with the ceramic implants.

In order to evaluate bone formation histologically, the animals were labeled several days before being sacrificed with tetracycline. Recently in some cases an additional labeling was effected with alizarin-complexon and calcein. In this way different stages of bone reaction can be made visible. At a second stage of our work the time dependence of bone formation and remodelling will be evaluated.

Fig. 8 shows a longitudinal section of the distal part of the sleeve 3 months after implantation. The resection plane of the femoral shaft is indicated by the dotted line. Inside the

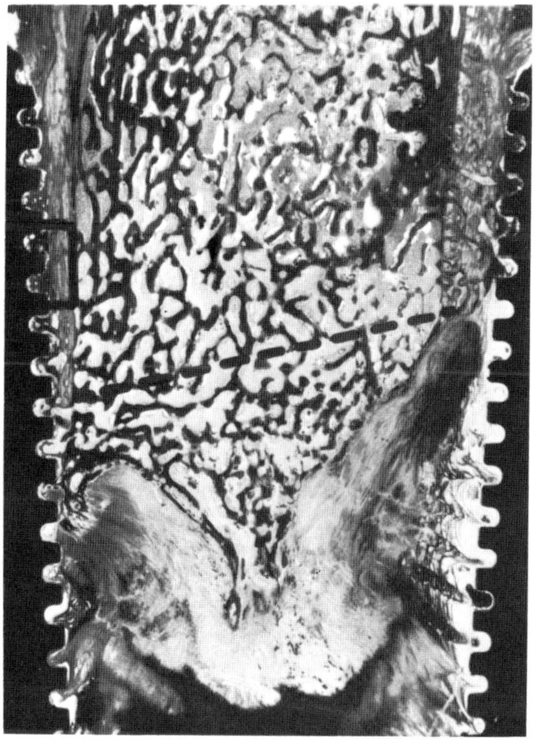

Fig. 8
Histological evaluation of animal tests: Longitudinal ground section of the distal part of the sleeve 3 months after implantation (magnification ca. x 3)

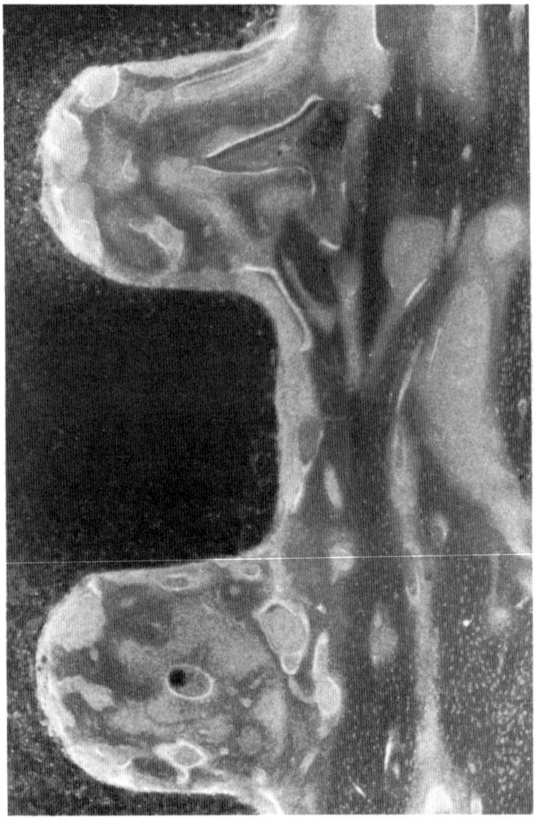

Fig. 9
Histological evaluation of animal tests: Bony ingrowth into the indentations of the bioceramic implant 3 months after implantation (UV-light, magnification ca. x 30)

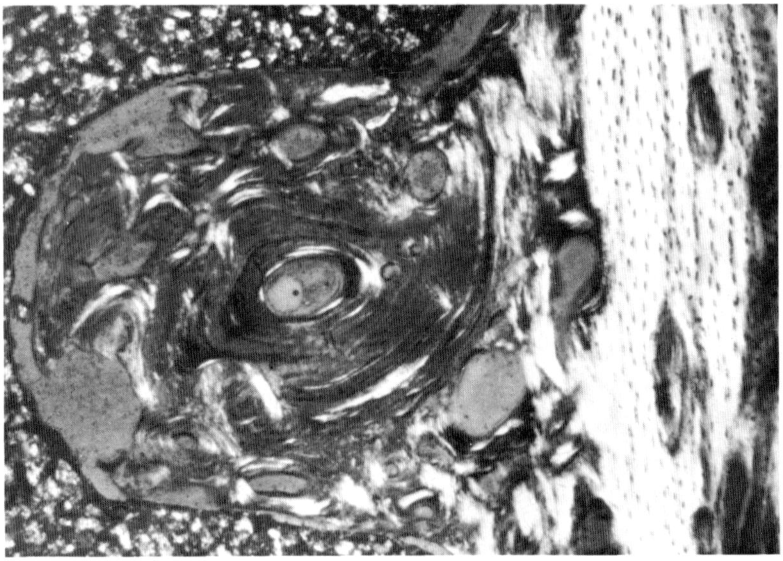

Fig. 10 Histological evaluation of animal tests:
Lamellar structure of newly formed bone 3 months after implantation (polarized light, magnification ca. x 60)

bone and also above the resection plane, newly formed spongy bone can be seen. The contact zone between the cortex and the ceramics (rectangular area indicated) is shown in Fig. 9 at a higher magnification. Within the grooves of the sleeve, newly formed bone can be seen showing yellowish fluorescence at sites of bone formation. The newly formed bone has a lamellar structure (Fig. 10).

In the case of sockets, we have similar results of bone growth into the indentations of the bioceramic implant. In Fig. 11 it can be seen that the grooves on the surface of the pin are also filled with bone tissue 5 months after implantation. Finally Fig. 12 demonstrates bone growth into the surface of the trochanter plateau 3 months after implantation.

On the basis of these results, it can be concluded that new bone formation occurs into the indentations of the bioceramic implant. Bone tissue finally has a lamellar structure. Therefore a durable fixation of the implant can be achieved. These active processes of bone formation point to viable bone within the sleeve. These results are presently limited to an observation period of 5 to 6 months after implantation.

Further research will be done in the future using polyfluorochrome sequential labeling to examine the time dependence of bone reaction. This study will include the evaluation of tissue response after longer periods of time.

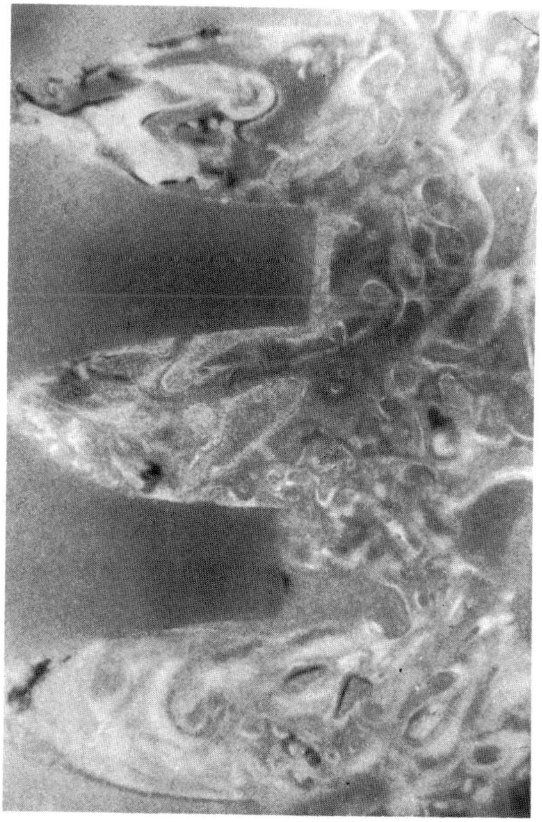

Fig. 11
Histological evaluation of animal tests: Indentations in the pins of the socket; filled with new woven bone tissue 5 months after implantation (U.V. light, magnification ca. x 30)

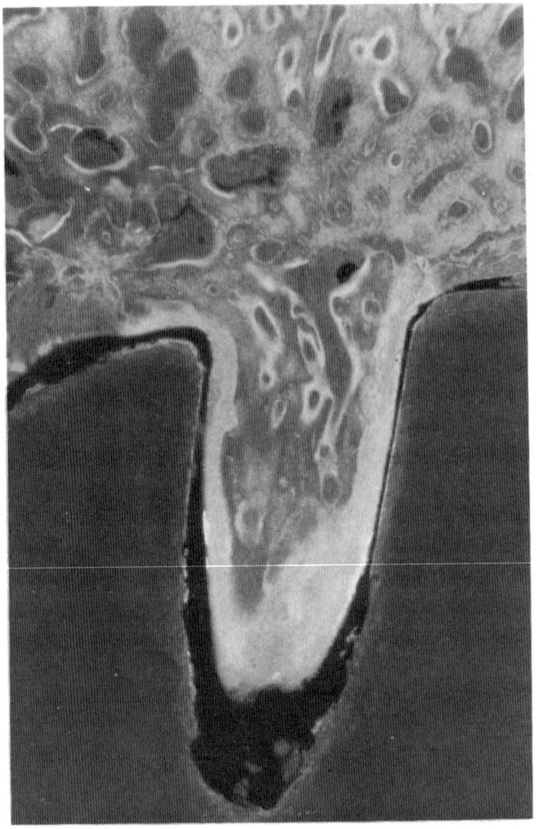

Fig. 12
Histological evaluation of animal tests: Bony ingrowth into an indentation of the trochanter plateau; femur endoprosthesis 3 months after implantation (U.V. light, magnification ca. x 20)

HUMAN IMPLANTATIONS

On the basis of the good results obtained both with mechanical experiments and in animal tests, implantations of bioceramic endoprostheses were performed in humans. In order to collect experience with bioceramic implants in man, the first implantations were performed in patients with bone metastases. In these cases the opportunity is given, due to the short life expectancy, to recover the endoprosthesis and the surrounding tissues for morphological studies.

To date 8 patients have been treated with the long shaft endoprosthesis described. At the time of the operation the patients were between 36 and 72 years old. Amongst them was only one case of chondrosarcoma, the others showed metastases of carcinomas, most of them generalized. The surgical intervention was very well tolerated by all patients also by these whose general condition was bad due to generalized metastases. Two patients died of generalized carcinosis after 2 and a half and 3 and a half months, respectively. The endoprostheses of these two patients were recovered post mortem. The other patients are still alive, the operation dating back 4-5 months (Table 2).

Table 2 Human implantations

Patient	Indication	Remarks	
S.F., male, 72	meta (hypernephroma)	2.5 m. p.o.	+
Z.R., female, 48	meta (hypernephroma)	15 m. p.o.	alive
S.H., female, 61	meta (synovialoma)	3.5 m. p.o.	+
A.K., female, 65	meta (hypernephroma)	8 m. p.o.	alive
W.M., female, 62	myeloma	7 m. p.o.	alive
J.R., male, 61	meta (hypernephroma)	7 m. p.o.	alive
E.A., male, 36	meta (thyreoid cancer)	6 m. p.o.	alive
B.S., female, 54	chondrosarcoma	5 m. p.o.	alive

In an analysis of the results obtained so far, 3 connections between ceramic material and bone have proved of special interest. The conical sleeve connection to the shaft of the femur, the seat of the remaining trochanter on the prosthesis and the connection between the ceramic socket and the pelvic spongy bone.

At the junction of the conical sleeve to the femur, a good primary fitting was always achieved, leaving a cone of 4-5 cm. The final fixation of the endoprosthesis, though, is of decisive importance for the success of the implantation.

In 2 of 8 patients signs of loosening were observed after approximately 3 months, manifested in bone resorption of the conical femur stump, shown by X-ray examination. After breakage of the screw which protects against rotation an impression of the bone into the conical sleeve occurred (Fig. 13). In the first case, this event caused no clinical symptoms, so that a conservative therapy was sufficient.

The second case was one of metastases secondary to hypernephroma; a metallic long stem prosthesis was implanted and fixed with bone cement. A local recurrence of the tumor occurred. For this reason the prosthesis had to be removed and the large bone

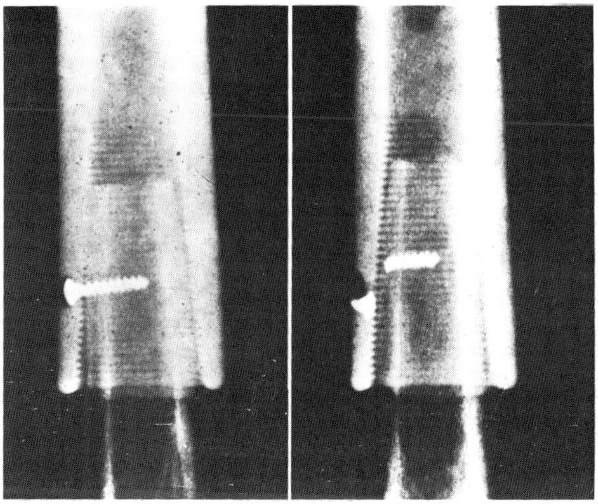

Fig. 13
B.S., 63 years old. Chondrosarcoma right prox.femur.
a. Junction of conical sleeve to femur 2 months after implantation. Incipient resorption of conic femur stump.
b. 3 weeks later, breakage of screw, impression of bone cone into conical sleeve

defect was bridged by a ceramic long shaft endoprosthesis. After some weeks signs of loosening were manifested clinically as well as in the X-ray. Therefore the conical bone stump was resected and the ceramic endoprosthesis was reimplanted. The histological examination revealed the cause of loosening in this case to be a nutritional distrubance of the conically shaped bone due to the intramedullary bone cement of the metallic endoprosthesis.

In two other cases histological examination was performed post mortem. Two and a half months and three and a half months after implantation no or only little formation of new bone towards the grooves of the ceramic implant was observed (Fig. 14). This lack of bone-forming capacity may be due to the tumor cachexia. However, both patients showed clinically stable implants.

The X-rays and the clinical results of the other 4 patients have to be judged favorably 4-15 months after implantation (Fig. 15). The patients are able to put their full weight on the extremity and have retained only a moderate limp due to tumor surgery.

Summarizing the problems of joining the conical sleeve to the femur shaft it must clearly be said that there are still a number of hazards which can lead to clinical failure. Only after identifying them exactly and eliminating their causes can this type of endoprosthesis be recommended on a larger scale.

There are major problems with regard to the seat of the prosthesis on the trochanter which are not only present in ceramic but also in the metallic tumor-endoprostheses. A permanent fixation can be achieved only in rare cases.

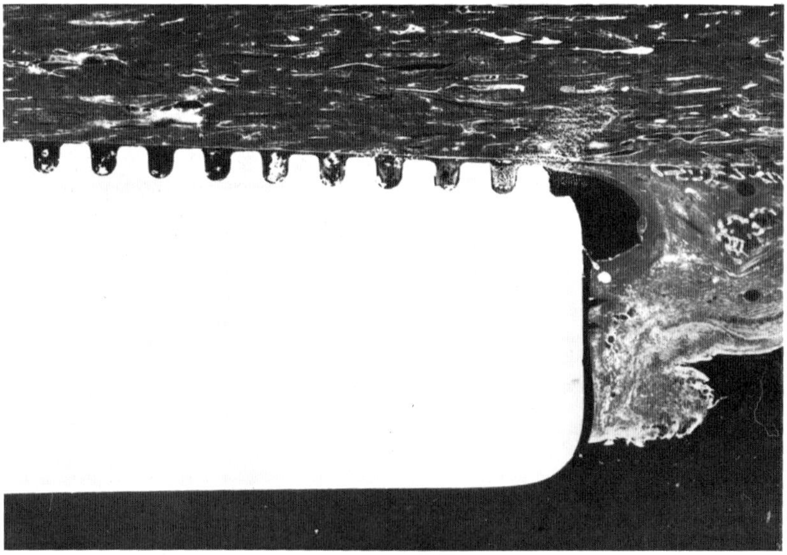

Fig. 14 St.F., 72 years old. Metastases secondary to hypernephroma. Good contact of conical sleeve to femoral cortex, no new bone formation towards the grooves of the ceramic. Periosteal bone distal to cone

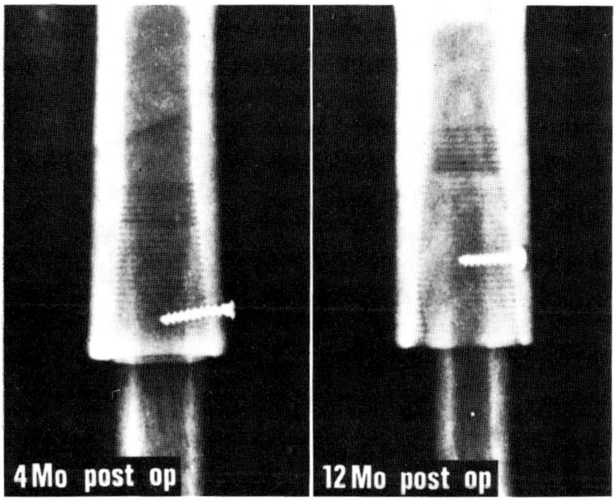

Fig. 15
Good fitting of conical sleeve to femoral stump.
a. A.K., 65 years old. Metastases secondary to hypernephroma, 4 months after operation
b. Z.R., 48 years old. Metastases secondary to hypernephroma, 12 months after operation

The most important experience was made with regard to the socket, since this part of the endoprostheses can also be used for patients suffering from osteoarthritis (Fig. 16). In the first three implantations the sockets were additionally fixed by cortical screws in the pelvic bone. However in these first operations the preparation of the bed in the bone was so exact that an additional fixation did not seem to be necessary. Therefore, the last 5 sockets were implanted without additional screws. The first two sockets had an intermediate layer of polyethylene which was omitted later on. X-rays of all the sockets showed good fitting and no signs of protrusion (Fig. 16), at up to 15 months of observation. In the patient operated first, a thin seam around the socket appeared in the X-ray

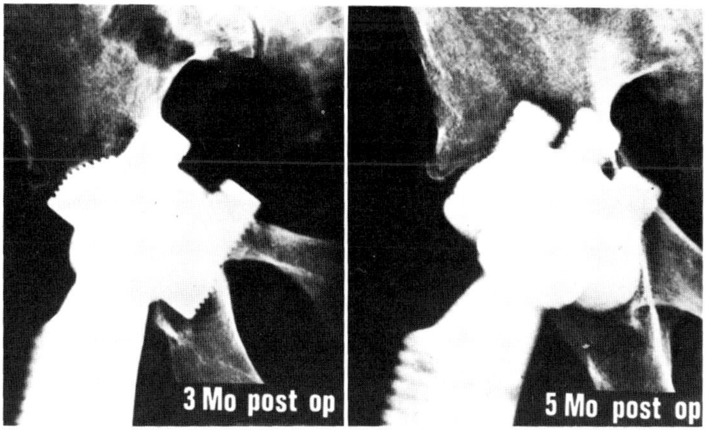

Fig. 16 a. W.M., 62 years old. Myloma, good position of socket, 3 months after operation
b. E.A., 36 years old. Metastases secondary to thyreoid cancer, good position of socket 5 months after operation

soon after surgery (Fig. 17a) and has remained unchanged up to the present. Therefore we do not believe that a loosening has taken place. This view is also supported by the fact that a distinct sclerotic zone has formed around the pedicles (Fig. 17b).

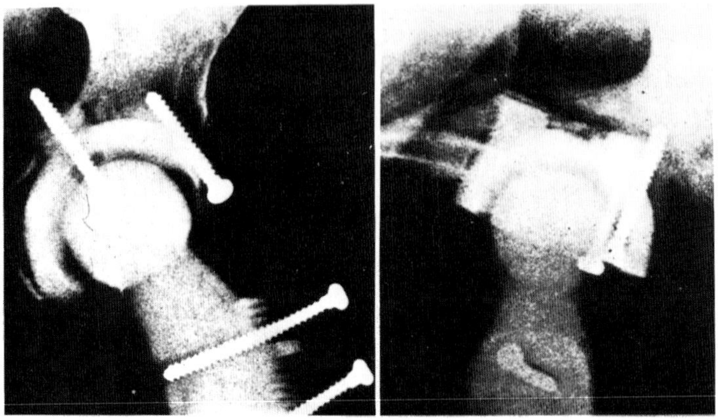

Fig. 17 Z.R., 48 years old. Metastases secondary to hypernephroma, 12 months after operation.
a. thin seam at the medial part of the socket
b. axial X-ray: sclerotic zone around the pedicles

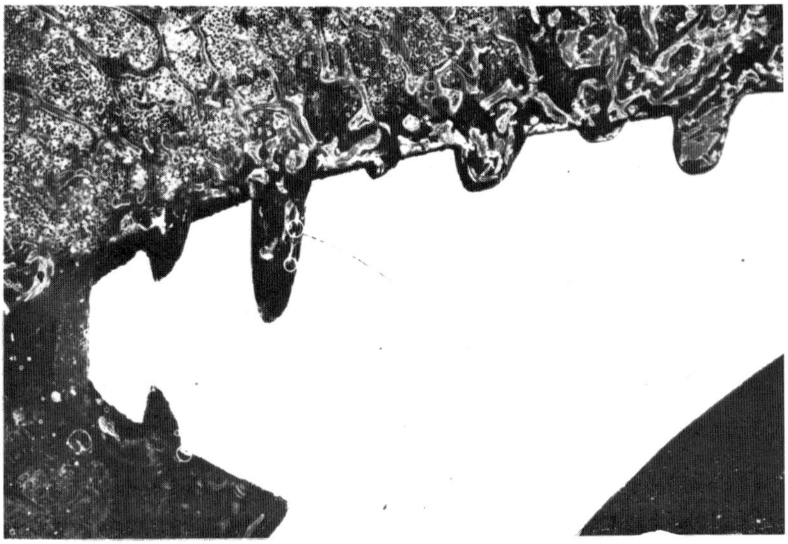

Fig. 18 Sch.H., 61 years old. Synovioma, good new bone formation towards the grooves of the socket 3 1/2 months after operation

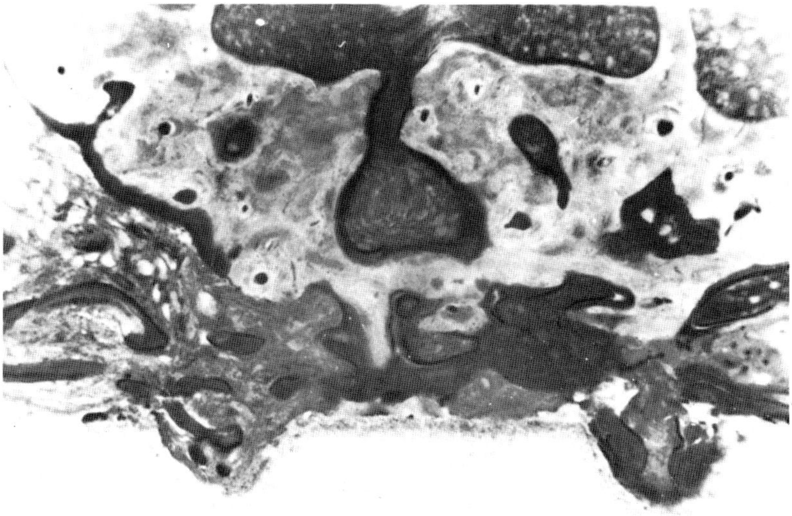

Fig. 19 St.F., 72 years old. Metastases secondary to hypernephroma, new bone in the grooves of the socket 2 1/2 months after operation

Histological examination of the two sockets obtained after 2 1/2 and 3 1/2 months, respectively showed formation of new bone tissue into the grooves of the surface of the endoprosthesis (Figs. 18,19). This new bone formation can be well compared with similar observations in animals.

CONCLUSIONS

It can be concluded from these results that bioceramic endoprostheses can be implanted in human patients suffering from bone tumor. The anchoring of implants to the long bones can be effected by the conical sleeve. The bioceramic socket can be recommended for implantation also in patients suffering from osteoarthritis. For this indication a cap-like femoral part – implanted also without bone cement – was developed. Animal and mechanical experiments with these implants are encouraging.

REFERENCES

1. Rock, M.: DRP Nr. 583 581

2. Hulbert, S.F., et al.: Technical Report No. 1, Office of Naal Research Contract No. N 00014-71-0339-0001. "Characterisation of tissue ingrowth into porous bioceramics". Division of Interdisciplinary Studies, College of Engineering, Clemson University, Clemson S.C., 29631 (Sept. 1971)

3. Hulbert, S.F., et al.: Technical Report No. 2, (Mai 1972)

4. Hulbert, S.F., Morrison, S.J., Klawitter, J.J.: Compatibility of porous ceramics with soft tissue, application to tracheal prostheses. Journal of Biomedical Materials Research Symposium 2, 269 (1972)

5. Rhinelander, F.W., et al.: Microvascular and histogenic responses to implantation of a porous ceramic into bone. Journal of Biomedical Materials Research 6, 81 (1971)

6. Predecki, P., et al.: Kinetics of bone growth into cylindrical channels in aluminium oxide and titanium. Journal of Biomedical Materials Research 6, 375 (1972)

7. Heide, H., Hofmann, U.: Keramische Werkstoffe in der Humanmedizin. Berichte der Deutschen Keramischen Gesellschaft 49, 185 (1972)

8. Heimke, G., et al.: Untersuchungen an Implantaten aus Al_2O_3-Keramik. Berichte der Deutschen Keramischen Gesellschaft 50, 4 (1973)

9. Boutin, P.: Arthroplastic totale de la hanche par prothese en alumine frittee. Revue de Chirurgie Orthopedique et reparation de l' appareil moteur 58, 229 (1972)

10. Boutin, P.: Direct attachment of ceramic joints. 6th Annual International Biomaterials Symposion Clemson S.C., USA (1974)

11. Engelhardt, A., Zeibig, A.: Development of non-metallic implants under consideration of Wolff's law and human implantation experiences. 5th Annual International Biomaterials Symposion Clemson S.C., USA (1973)

12. Salzer, M., et al.: Biokeramische Endoprothesen. Medizinisch-Orthopädische Technik 95, 40 (1975)

13. Salzer, M., et al.: Further experimental and clinical experiences on endoprostheses made of alumina. 7th Annual International Biomaterials Symposion Clemson S.C., USA (1975)

14. Eisenmenger, E., et al.: Knochen- und Gelenkprothetik mit Al_2O_3-Keramik beim Hund: Konstruktionsprinzipien und biologische Aspekte. Proceedings of the XI. Congress of the European Society of Veterinary Surgery, Kopenhagen (Mai 1975)

15. Punzet, G., et al.: Knochen- und Gelenkprothetik mit Al_2O_3-Keramik beim Hund: Implantationstechnik und Erfahrungen. Proceedings of the XI. Congress of the European Society of Veterinary Surgery, Kopenhagen (Mai 1975)

TRENDS IN THE DEVELOPMENT OF PERMANENT CERAMIC IMPLANTS

A. Engelhardt, H. Grell, D. Komitowski, H. Scharbach, W. Heipertz, M. Sencar, D. Kooke, J. Zeitz, and P. Bunz

Permanent implants are being used with increasing regularity to replace defective parts of the human skeleton. By this increasing number of implantations, especially in the hip region, the advantages and limits of endoprosthetics are disclosed. The primary objective of our investigations is to increase the biocompatibility of a skeletal replacement part. The term "biocompatibility" expresses the degree of adaptive interaction between the implant and biological tissue (Fig. 1). Therefore, it is not sufficient either to change only a few constructive details, use improved materials, or apply different surgical procedures or therapies. All conceivable parameters must be considered. Corrosion and metallosis, different E-moduli, alteration of plastics in the sense of water absorption, aging, volume variations, exothermic heat reaction, and liberation of monomers represent negative factors of today's endoprosthetics. The same is true concerning the neglecting of biomechanical laws.

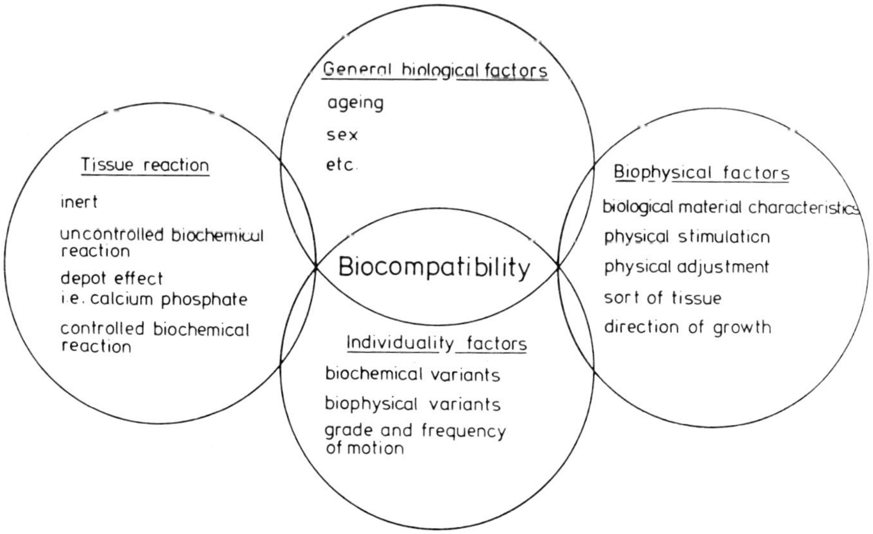

Fig. 1 Factors influencing the design of endoprostheses for skeletal parts

CONCEPT OF DEVELOPMENT

The long-term influence on a permanent implant has a large number of parameters. These can vary among each other in different ways. At present, it is not possible to give a comprehensive presentation of all possible parameters. However, the known parameters can be combined and applied for a classified program (Fig. 2). As tissue remodelling in the musculo-skeletal system cannot be duplicated, therefore, according to our experience, a biologically inert implant must be used. In this case, design limitations must eventually be accepted because of material properties.

PROSTHESES MADE OF ALUMINIUM OXIDE–CERAMIC

Ceramics are produced in a wide range of variations using different basic materials. Since publication of the investigations by Hulbert et al. as well as Hench et al., the high degree of bioinertness with respect to the differentiated possibilities of their application are well known. Considering the results of Hulbert et al. (8,9), we believed that it was possible to comply with the following conditions when using Al_2O_3 (Table 1). In the first phase, high-density ceramic implants were developed and clinically applied for bridging resection defects in tumor patients. Thus, partial functional restorations were reached. In addition, new clinical tests in humans were initiated. They were performed under unfavorable conditions, attributable to the post operative tumor treatment.

Because of the inertness of the material, implants were manufactured for bridging humerus, radius, proximal femur defects, and a vertebral body (Figs. 3,4). Initially, the design was based on individual X-rays of the patient. For inserting the implant, special instruments had to be developed.

This first stage of development and examination of implants led to the following results. By conical adaptation and using intramedullary screws, Al_2O_3 can be used to anchor implants without bone cement (Fig. 5). By primary fixation and following the secondary processes of adhesion and ingrowth, an endoprosthesis free from corrosion can be implanted. However, a special surgical technique must be considered. The material is hard and wear resistant (Table 2), but on the other hand, it presents considerable disadvantages. As a consequence of its brittleness, solid ceramic parts must be manufactured. The manufacturing of the gliding surface requires expensive procedures. Small parts, screw threads, short radii, porous surfaces with corresponding deminuation of the cross-section cannot be supplied. Trying to avoid these disadvantages by accepting metal parts (Fig. 6) we are confronted with wear problems and consequent defects of the interacting ceramic and metal surfaces, starting during the operation. The lower hardness of the metal produces wear particles, surface defects with an increased corrosion rate, metallosis, and possibly premature fractures of the implant.

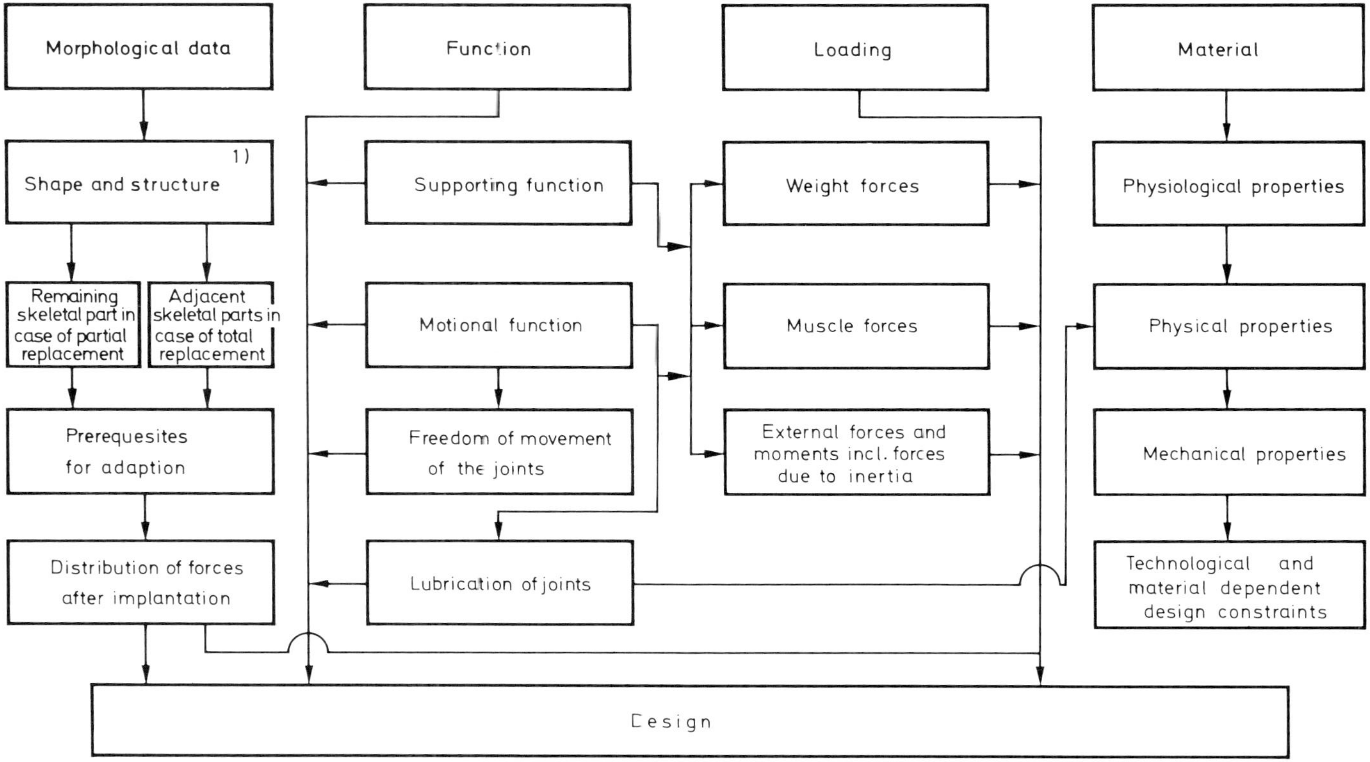

1) = Operative possibilities, surgical technique

Fig. 2 Interaction of known parameters

Table 1 Al_2O_3 implant design conditions

1. Elimination of bone cement (mechanical anchoring) = primary fixation
2. Early mobilization of the patient
3. Physiological transmission of forces
4. Lifelong stability of the implant-tissue interface
5. Secondary fixation by ingrowth of bone
6. No toxicity
7. No corrosion
8. No wear
9. Long-term stability of the implant, i.e. under alternating-load

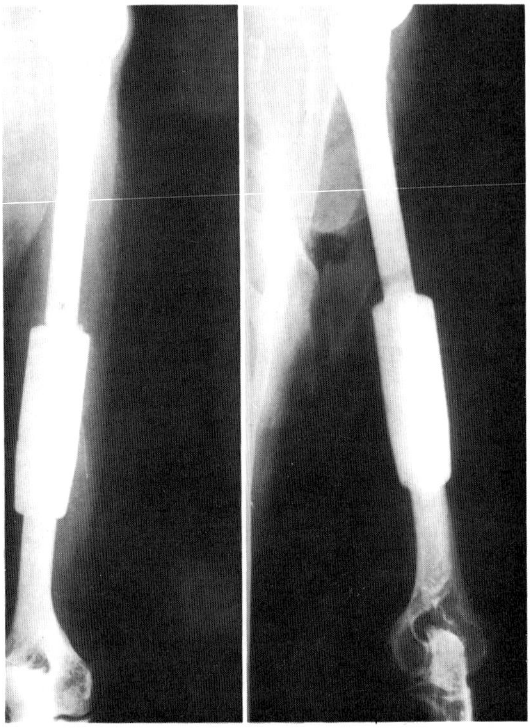

Fig. 3
Al_2O_3 modular endoprosthesis with sleeve and screw (X-ray)

Five years ago, Boutin developed a ceramic prosthesis with a metal shaft. Later, other groups in Homburg/Saar and Mannheim have followed this concept. They report on partial or entirely cementless implantations. However, the use of a metallic stem limits the Al_2O_3 material. Comparative load tests performed by the Vienna-Rosenthal bio-engineering group on femura of cadavers cannot be quoted as proof.

The soft tissue layers showed by many investigators who used metal, combined metal/ Al_2O_3 or solid Al_2O_3 implants in the lower extremities are additional arguments. Under certain circumstances, for instance under alternating loads, unphysiological transmission of forces on small load bearing surfaces, shear-stresses occur because of the implant design and/or the higher E-modulus in comparison to bone. The relative motions, dependent on

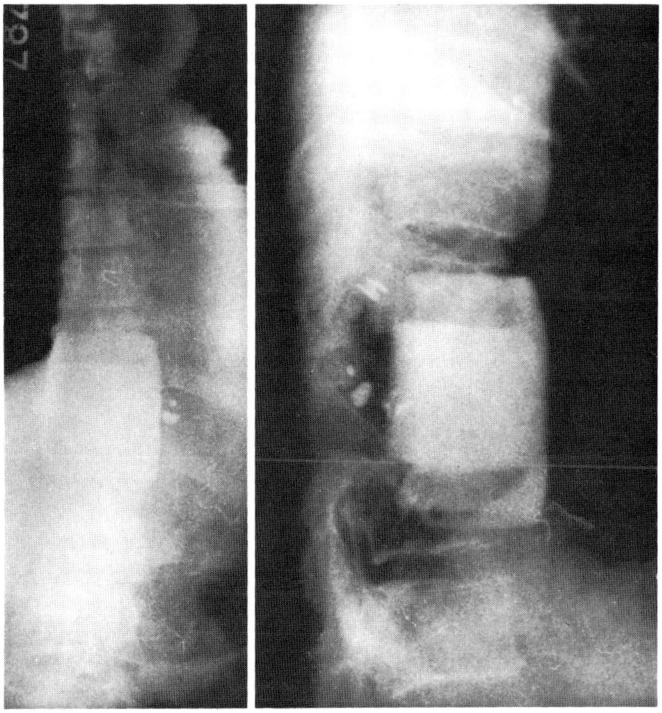

Fig. 4
Vertebra-body in-situ
(X-ray)

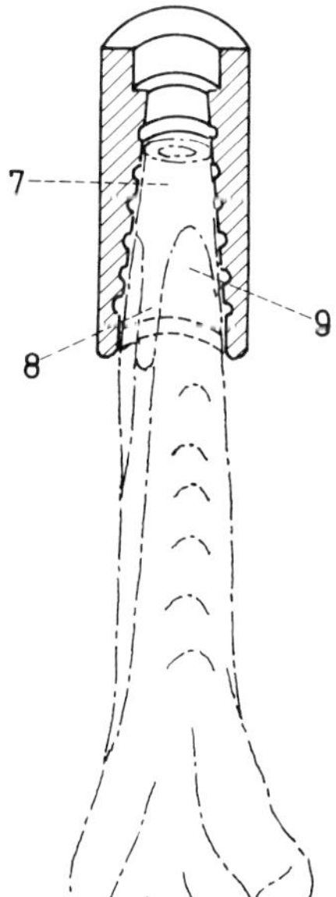

Fig. 5
Conical anchoring

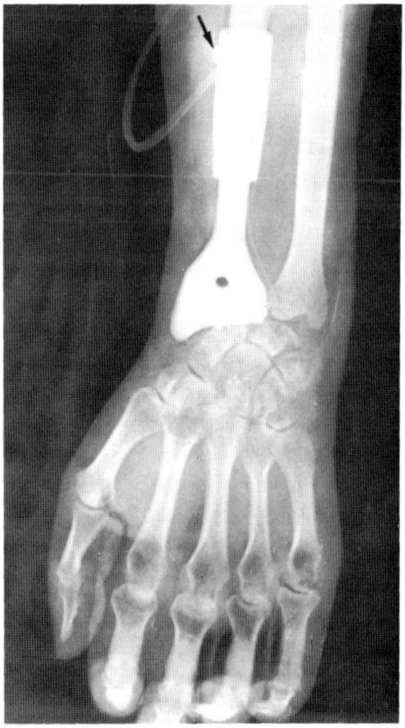

Fig. 6 Implant fixation with metal screw
(arrow indicates metal screw)

Table 2 Physical properties of Rosenthal-Stemag bioceramics

Material	Stemalox A19
Content of Al_2O_3 (%)	99.7
Color	white
Specific gravity (g/cm^3)	3.9
Water absorption (%)	0
Tensile strength (psi)	38 500
Compressive strength (psi)	> 420 000
Flexural strength (psi)	57 000
Volume resistivity ($\Omega \cdot$ cm)	$> 10^{14}$
Chemical resistance:	Resists acid and alkali

design and material, lead to tissue reactions similar to the pseudarthrosis mechanism, which in turn, is a basis for the increasing symptomatic of implant loosening. These findings forced us to search for new materials.

PLASTIC MATERIALS

We considered temporarily an endoprosthesis made from isoelastic plastics, these materials do not comply with our requirements, as the problems of aging, water absorption, etc. could not be solved. The only material within this group that we used was bone cement for assembling the Al_2O_3 modular prosthesis parts. In this case, no negative reactions were observed, because there was no contact between methylmethacrylate and living tissue.

CERAMIC–METAL COMPOUND PROSTHESIS

The present development shows that bioinert biodegradable ceramics can be produced with surface macro- and micro-structures, and with different Young's moduli. The combination of metal and differentiated ceramic coatings in various layers opened new constructive possibilities, without the need to abandon ceramics. This led to an implantable system with high biocompatibility and individual isoelastic characteristics. A comparison with the conventional hip endoprosthesis permits a simple presentation of the principle.

PRINCIPLE OF CONSTRUCTION

Gait analyses show that, dependent on the gait sequence, angular and value variations of the phase dependent maximum of the resulting force occur. The privileged direction of the resultant is from medio-cranial to lateral-caudal. On a conventional hip endoprosthesis, reduced to the point A on the resection plane (collum femoris), the force component $F_R \cdot \cos\alpha$ acts vertically and in the direction of the resection plane, the component $F_R \cdot \sin\alpha$. The acting couple of forces $F_R \cdot a$, after the parallel shift of F_R, is demonstrated (Fig. 7) by the plane of the parallelogram. A practically constant surface pressure p results from the component $F_R \cdot \cos\alpha$ acting vertically on the bone section plane. From $F_R \cdot \sin\alpha$ and the couple of forces $F_R \cdot a$ result the surface pressures q and r, vertically acting on the inner surface of the bone. These calculations show an essential difference to the physiological stress conditions (Figs. 8,9). In our opinion, the findings of Wolff (16), Roux (14), Pauwels (13), and Kummer (10), and others explain the reason for necrotic processes in the medial region of the femur-neck, the basis of the major trochanter, as well as in the area at the end of the stem. After a partial loss of the support caused by the disappearing of bone, loosenings, increased relative motions, and formation of connective tissue result. Furthermore, fractures of the cement coating might occur. Differential stresses and relative motions impede a direct connection between implant and bone, the so-called secondary fixation. According to Münzenberger (11) or Judet, a

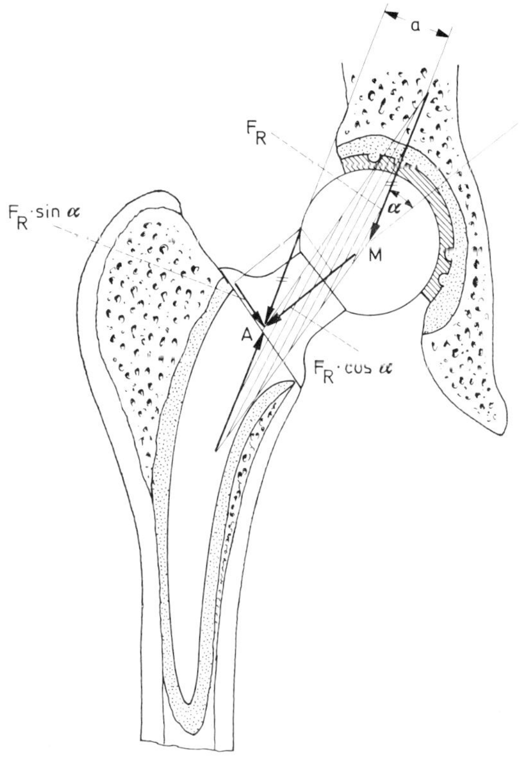

Fig. 7
Load transmission in conventional prosthesis

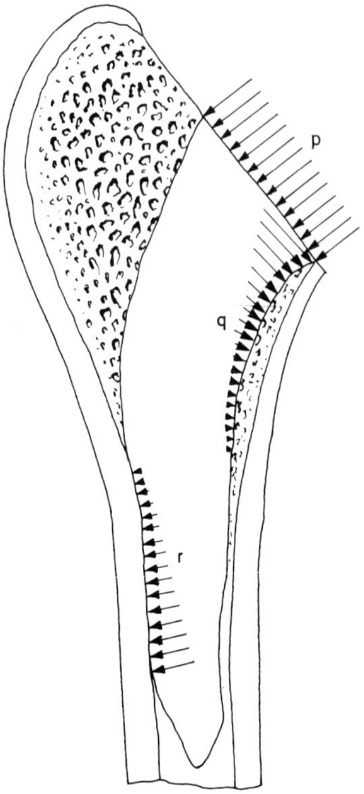

Fig. 8
Unphysiological stress conditions in conventional prosthesis

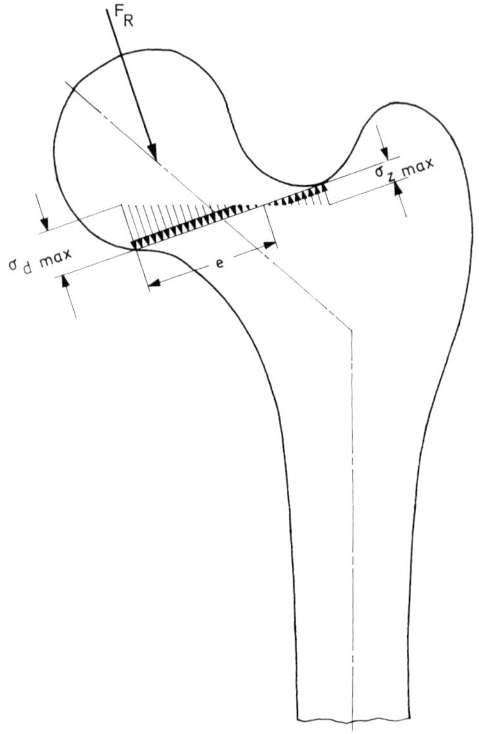

Fig. 9
Physiological stress conditions in femur

connection between bone, cement, and metal might be possible. Ceramic materials have an advantage over bone cement and metals because of their inertness, which might eventually be increased by biodegradable layers. Although the different corrosion processes dependent on the material and surface shape are eliminated, solid ceramic prostheses have a disadvantage, in contrast to those with metal shafts, because of the higher Young's modulus and lack of plasticity.

Unphysiological stress conditions can be avoided by interposing a joint. Thus, the remaining bone can be used for implant support because the remodelling process is stimulated through the simulation of physiological stress conditions. The small forces appearing in the region of the intramedullary thread surface are directly transmitted to the cortical bone. Bone formations for secondary fixation cannot be sheared; because relative motions are reduced to a half diameter of an osteon at maximum (Fig. 10).

MATERIAL

To maintain the advantages of ceramic contact with the bony tissue, a special ceramic coating for alloys has been developed under the name of "Osteoceram". According to the principles and techniques of enameling, the layered coating provides a high degree of adhesion to the metal and permits exactly determinable compound stresses. At the same time, and absolutely liquid and gas-tight coating of any chosen thickness is possible. The range in variation of glass, ceramics, and their combination allows compliance with varied demands on the same implant (Fig. 11). The qualities which can be obtained are universal and extreme chemical stability, biological compatibility, high electrical resistance, a high degree of hardness, and good behaviour in wear and gliding. Degradable inorganic substances, as for instance calcium phosphate, can be added into the layer in any desired concentration. The quality of the surface can be chosen arbitrarily, and ranges from anti-adhesive polish to micro-rough and macro-rough structures with good surface conditions for ingrowth. Porous layers with cross connections to avoid interruption of intercellular liquid circulation present good conditions for ingrowth (Table 3).

Table 3 Material data

	Steel	Osteoceram G	Osteoceram N
Adhesive strenght (Kp/mm^2)		> 10	> 10
Tensile strength (Kp/mm^2)	56-70	8	12
Compound tensile strength (Kp/mm^2)		30	40
Modulus of elasticity (Kp/mm^2)	18500	8000	16000
Volume resistivity ($\Omega \cdot$ cm)	0.004	10^{13}	10^{13}
Specific gravity (g/cm^3)	8.13	2.5	2.5
Layer thickness (mm)		0.5 – 2	
Color		white	
Water absorption (%)		0	
Chemical resistance		Resists all acids (except HF), alkalines, water and organic media	

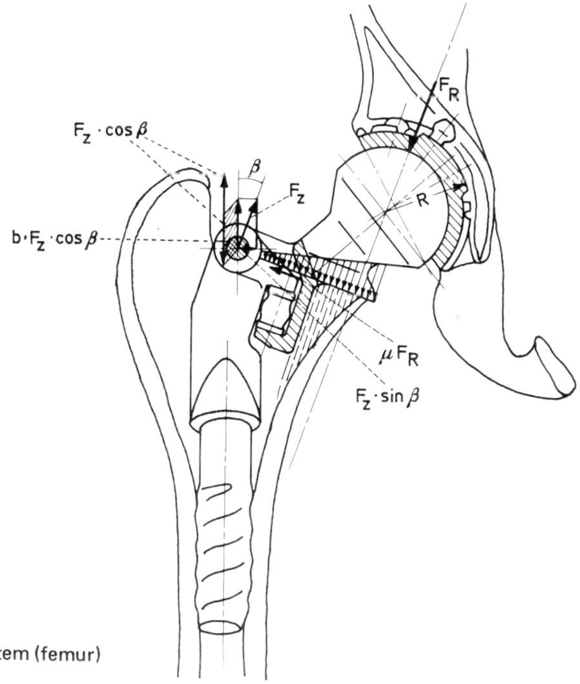

Fig. 10 Forces in new implant system (femur)

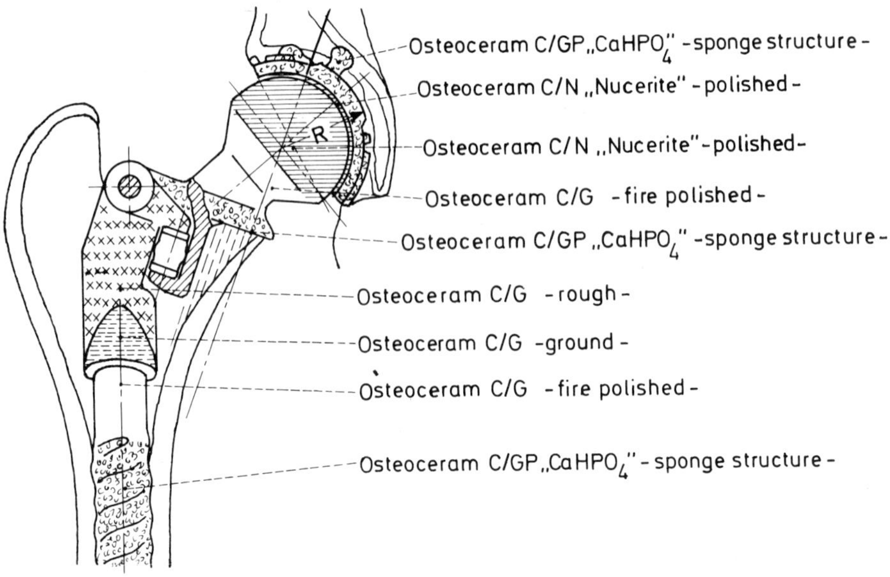

Fig. 11 Osteoceram materials for hip joint implant

The Osteoceram compound can be combined with self-supporting materials such as Al_2O_3 and carbon, without the loss of its chemical and biological advantages.

ADJUSTMENT TO THE SKELETON MORPHOLOGY

A good adjustment of the implant to the surrounding skeleton is required if bone cement, moldable during insertion, is eliminated. The adaptation is ensured by gathering specific data easily taken from X-rays, and by a surgical procedure supported by instruments adjusted to this new system.

X–RAY METHOD

With a coordinate map grid on the table plane, vertical to the traverse axis of the focus, two shots in the same position of the skeleton are taken. The first X-ray is taken with a vertical beam (a.p. position), the second after swinging the focus by a defined angle of 25 ° (Fig. 12). Through the differential movement of certain significant points, the three-dimensional position of these points can be calculated with the aid of trigonometric functions. This method allows a more exact determination of femoral data, as for example, the CCD-angle, AT-angle or the position of the principal plane.

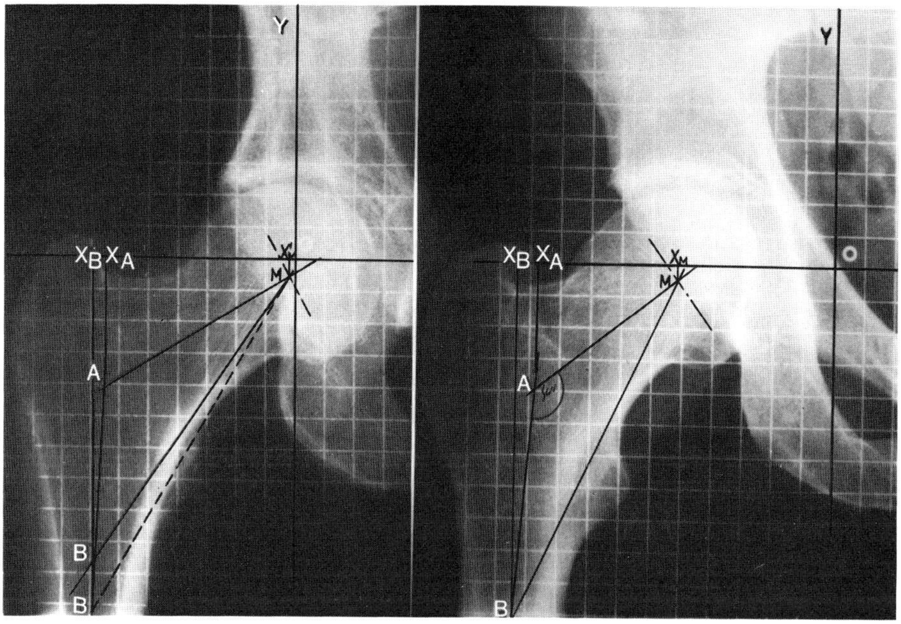

Fig. 12 X-ray for determining three-dimensional femur data

To verify this, we have started X-ray examinations on 13 femora of cadavers. With a especially developed device, ten shots of each femur were taken in exactly defined positions. By these pre-tests, the errors resulting from rotation and/or pathologic skeletal deviations could be estimated. In addition, measurements were made on 75 X-rays taken in the clinic. These disclosed aberrations, for instance, of angles measuring 20 degrees and more. By determining the CCD-angle, the method will be explained. For the calculation, three points on the femur are defined on the two X-rays (Fig. 13):

(1) M = Center of head

(2) A = True point of intersection of the collum and shaft axes of the femur (Backmann)

(3) B = Irreal point of intersection of the resultant of the osteon direction with the axis of the femur shaft, coming from M

Through the fluctuation X of these points (Figs. 12,13) and with the aid of the trigonometric function $\tan\alpha = \frac{x}{n}$, the differing altitudes of these points can be calculated. With the distances measured in the a.p. X-ray l_1 = MA, l_2 = AB, l_3 = MB and the calculated altitudes, the true distances can be obtained:

$$l_1'^2 = l_1^2 + (h_M - h_A)^2$$

$$l_2'^2 = l_2^2 + (h_A - h_B)^2$$

$$l_3'^2 = l_3^2 + (h_M - h_B)^2$$

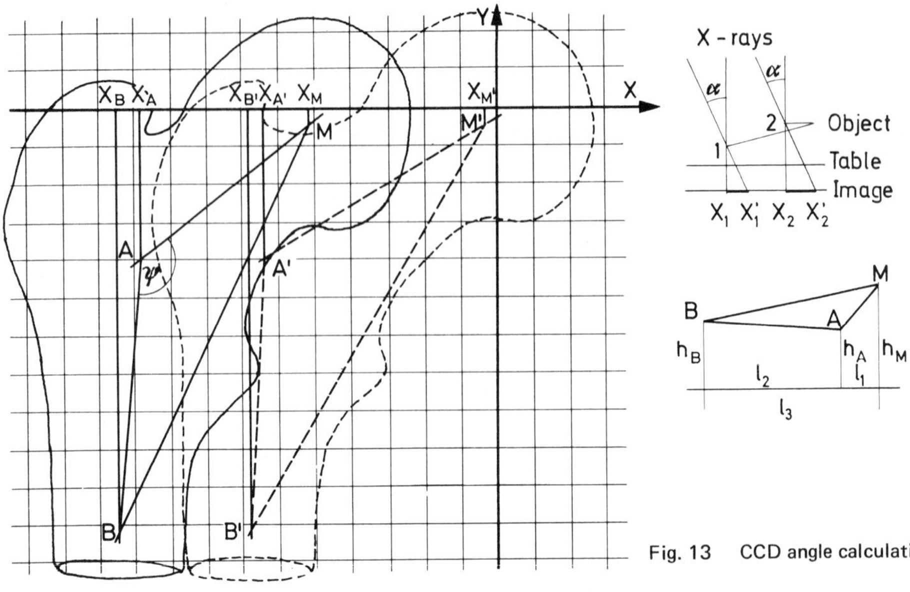

Fig. 13 CCD angle calculation

The true distances contain the true CCD-angle, which can be calculated with the cosine equation:

$$\cos(\mathrm{CCD}) = \frac{l_3'^2 + l_2'^2 + l_1'^2}{2\,(l_2' \cdot l_1')}$$

With this simple method, a method which, in contrast to stereometry, can be conducted in every clinic, objective and exact data are obtainable from the X-rays.

TEST METHOD

Examination of the construction, material, and surgical procedure was accomplished in six stages, with corresponding tests which can only partially be presented because these tests are not yet terminated.

ANIMAL TESTS

Respective technical pre-tests, under defined conditions, are followed by examination of the reaction of unloaded implants. These are implanted in the major trochanter of rabbits (Fig. 14). Extracted and summarized histological results show that, in the early phase (Fig. 15) after insertion of the implant, as a result of the mechanical treatment of bone, necrotic and resulting resorptive processes in the interface region occur. Accumulations of osteoclasts in a typical way are not detected. According to the situation and the kind of implantation, a coat of connective tissue is forming with spindle-shaped fibroblasts.

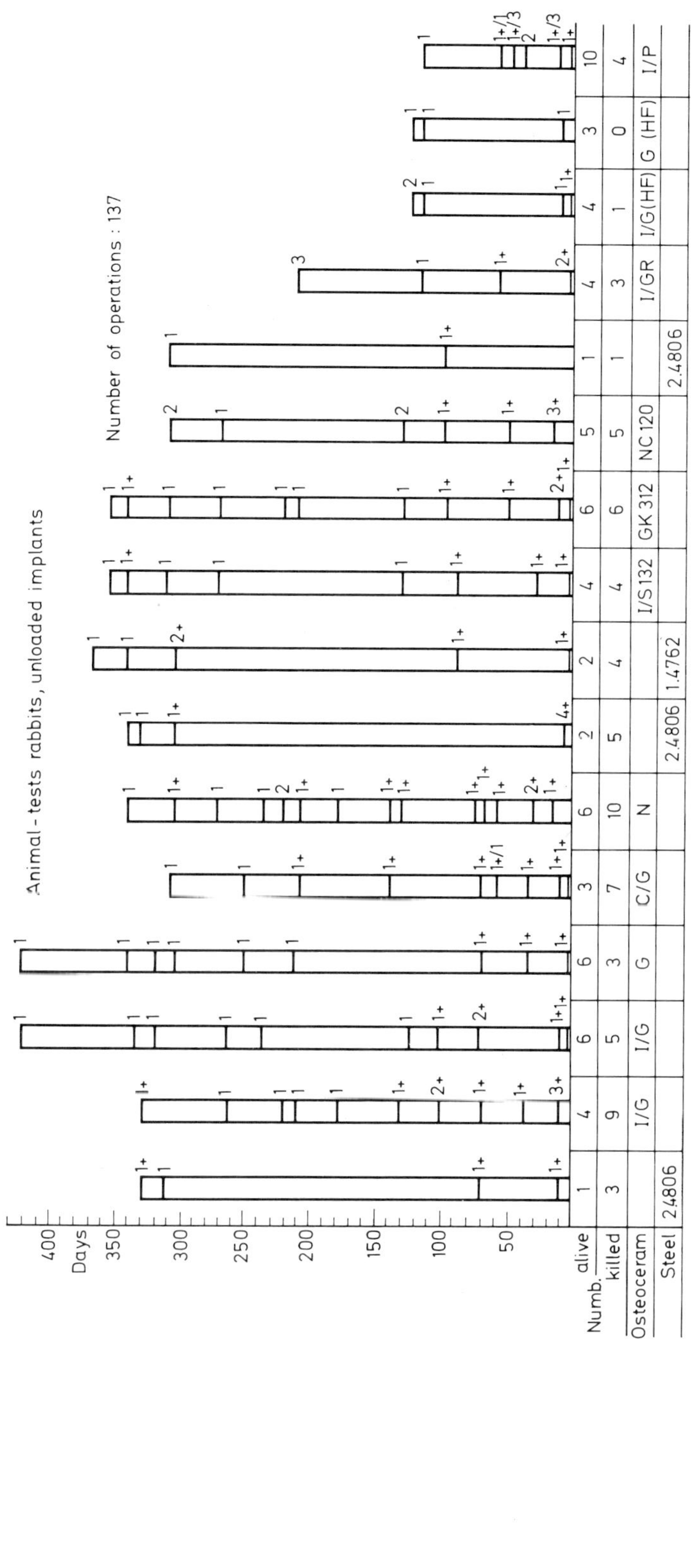

Fig. 14 Tissue compatibility of Osteoceram

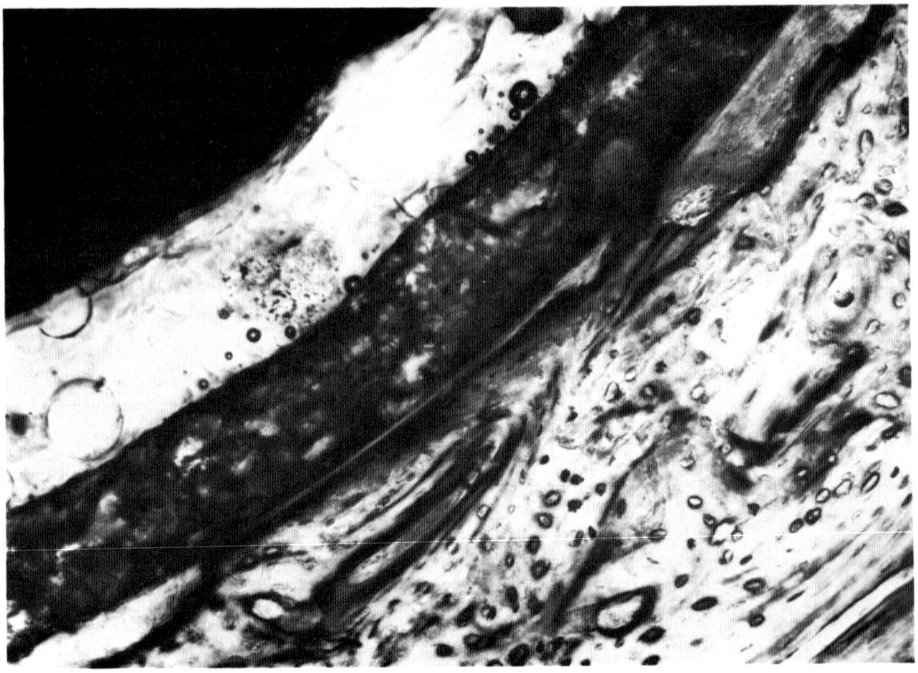

Fig. 15 Phase 1 – Unloaded implant in a femur of rabbit shortly after implantation. Ceramic layer in section and residual bone (about x 50)

The second phase (Fig. 16) is characterized by a clear increase of coarse-grained connective tissue. At some points in the adjacent area of the so-called unloaded implant, concentrations of collagenous fibre structures with a few basophil osteoblasts can be observed, marking a premature osteogenesis, the formation of osteoid. In the resorptive process, still noticeable now, typical osteoclasts take part.

The last phase (Fig. 17) shows an increasing differentiation and development from fibroblasts to osteoblasts. An appositive osteogenesis in the interface area in contact with the bone becomes visible. The marking with Tetracycline shows a clearly increased content of minerals in the new bone with the remaining bone being unchanged.

Extraction tests with considerable power proved a stable fixation of the implant with the skeletal part, which only slightly increases after another four weeks.

A miniature implant is examined in tests on dogs. As a result of the physiological load transmission we expect data interpreting the direction of osteons. Results from animal tests, however, are more limited than usually expected.

TECHNICAL TESTS

Taking into account different mathematical methods, the reaction of the implant is simulated.

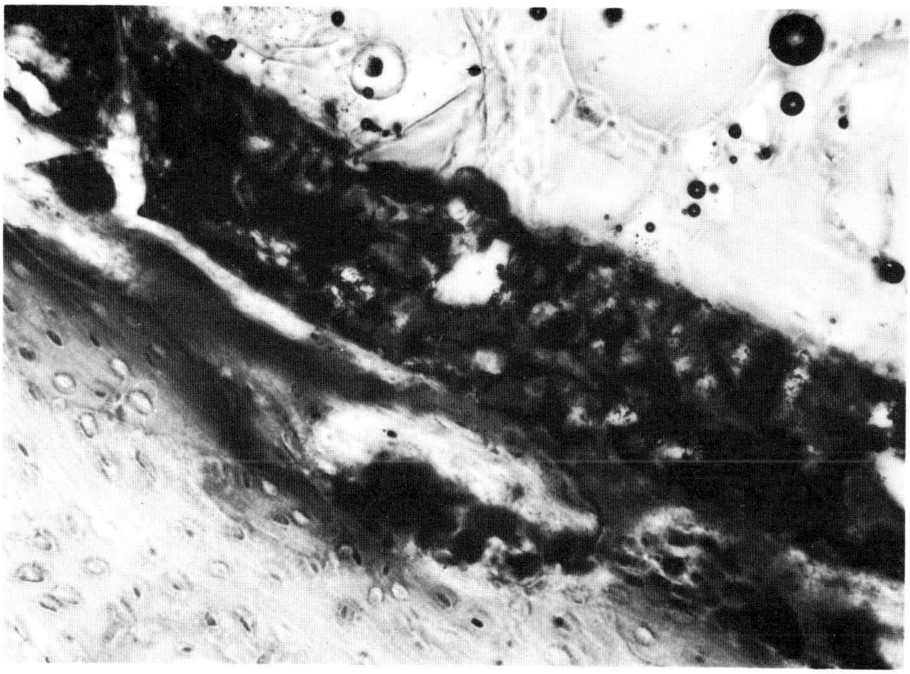

Fig. 16 Phase 2 – Formation of osteoblasts (about x 70)

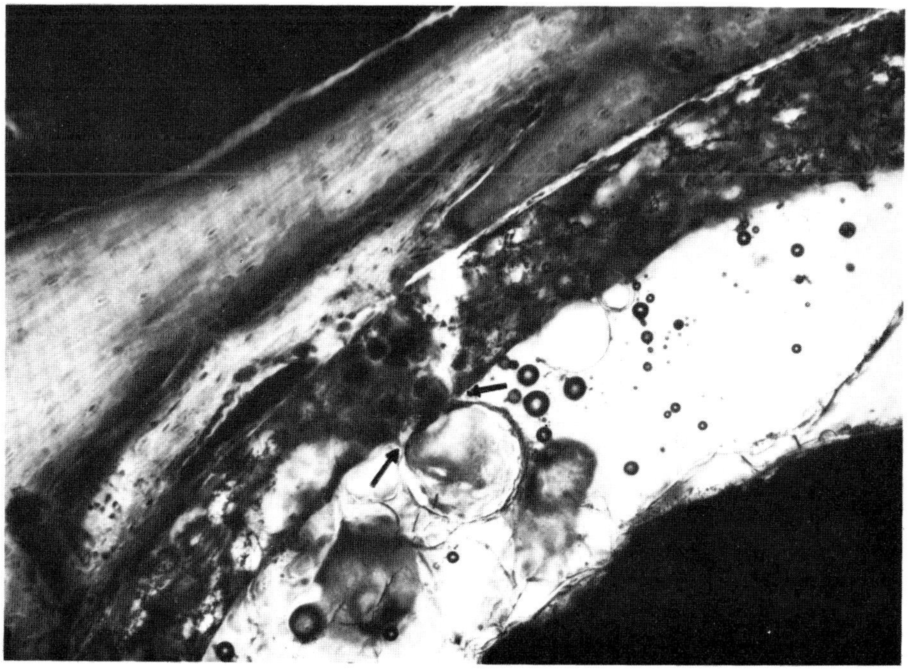

Fig. 17 Phase 3 – Ingrowth of ossifying soft tissue into preformed pores (about x 70)

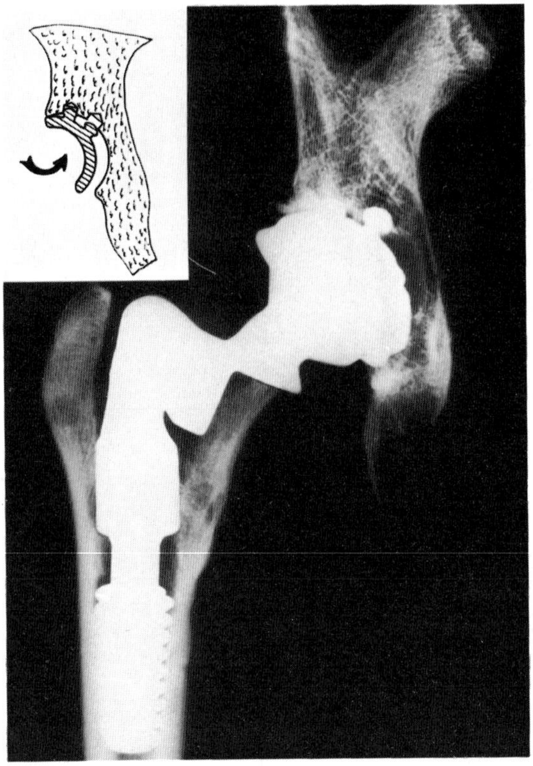

Fig. 18
New implant in the skeleton (X-ray)

These mathematical results are verified by static and dynamic tests, including skeleton elements. Measurements are taken using strain gages. Immediately after resection, the bone is coated to prevent liquid loss. Depending on the projected measuring process, strain gages must be attached immediately.

COMBINED TESTS ON CADAVERS

Examinations are performed to test the material and construction, and to improve the instruments and surgical procedure. The method of implantation and the result is again controlled in laboratory examinations. Extraction tests at the anchor still show a stable fixation up to a load of 690 Kp.

CLINICAL EXAMINATION

The clinical examination was conducted in the same way as with aluminium-oxide endoprostheses, but using a simplified implant system. Present implantations bridging two humerus resections show good results.

DESCRIPTION OF IMPLANT

The implant consists of the femur part already described in the system explanation above. The anchoring screw is connected with the head and neck by the interposed joint. The socket is provided on the reverse side with three plugs, the upper two having an eccentric protrusion; the lower protrusion is centrically located. The plugs are placed so that the resultant force passes through the triangular plane. The lower edge of the socket is cut out like the incissura acetabuli, and the ventral edge is adapted to the m. iliopsoas (Fig. 18).

SURGICAL PROCEDURE

After the femur axis has been determined, a round section of the corticalis in the area of the basis of the femur-neck is cut out. The marrow cavity is milled. When the screw threads are cut, the anchoring piece is placed. An instrument is attached to it, which, after removal of the femur head, mills planely the resection plane in the femur-neck area adjusted to the axis of the anchoring screw, so that a vertical transmission of forces can take place. After the head and neck parts are attached, the femur implantation is completed. Before the socket is inserted, the cartilage must be removed, without damage to the bone, as far as possible. Three holes for anchoring are drilled using a jig. Both upper holes are located excentrically to the axis of the anchoring plug. The protrusions of the anchoring plugs are pressed into the drilled holes with a rotary movement, thereby anchoring the plugs in the socket, without bone cement, resistant to both rotation and pressure.

REFERENCES

1. Backman, S.: The proximal end of the femur. Acta radiol. (Stockh.) Suppl. 146 (1957)
2. Cotta, H., Schulitz, K.P.: Der totale Hüftgelenkersatz, Stuttgart: Thieme Verlag 1973
3. Engelhardt, A.: Experiences with the development and use of human implants made of Al_2O_3. Acta Orthopaedica Belgica 40, 699 (1974)
4. Engelhardt, A.: Experiences with Al_2O_3 implantations in humans to bridge resection defects. Journal of Biomedical Materials Research Symposium 6, 227 (1975)
5. Engelhardt, A.: Individual stress calculation by the method of finite elements as basis for orthopaedic operations on the skeleton. Proceedings of the 12th Congress of the International Society of Orthopedic Surgery and Traumatology, Tel Aviv 1972
6. Engelhardt, A.: Can high density Al_2O_3 ceramic meet the requirements of modern implants? Proceedings 5th Annual International Biomaterials Symposium, Clemson 1974
7. Griss, P.: Experimental analysis of ceramic tissue interactions. A morphologic study on dense aluminia oxide ceramic in various animals. Proceedings 6th Annual International Biomaterials Symposium, Clemson 1974

8. Hulbert, S.F., Matthews, J.R., Klawitter, J.J., Sauer, B.W., Leonard, R.B.: Effect of stress on tissue ingrowth into porous aluminum oxide. Journal of Biomedical Materials Research Symposium 5, 85 (1974)

9. Hulbert, S.F., Young A., Matthews, R.S., Klawitter, J.J., Talbert, O.D. Stelling, F.H.: Journal of Biomedical Materials Research 4, 433 (1970)

10. Kummer, B.: Die Beanspruchung des menschlichen Hüftgelenks. Zeitschrift für Anatomie und Entwicklungsgeschichte 127, 277 (1968)

11. Münzenberger, K.J., Dennert, R.: Zur Bindung von Methylmetacrylat an Knochen. 62. Tagung der Deutschen Gesellschaft für Orthopädie und Traumatologie, Tübingen 1975

12. Paul, J.P.: Bioengineering studies of the forces transmitted by joints-engineering analysis. Biomechanics and Related Bio-Engineering Topics, Oxford: Pergamon

13. Pauwels, F.: Gesammelte Abhandlungen zur funktionellen Anatomie des Bewegungsapparates, Berlin: Springer Verlag 1965

14. Roux, W.: Das Gesetz der Transformation der Knochen. Berliner Klinische Wochenschrift (1893)

15. Rydell, N.W.: Intravital measurements of forces acting on the hip joint. Studies on the anatomy and function of bone and joints, Berlin-Heidelberg-New York: Springer Verlag 1966

16. Wolff, J.: Gesetz der Transformation der Knochen, Berlin: Hirschwald 1892

REQUIREMENTS OF OPERATIONAL TESTS AND TEST RESULTS IN TOTAL HIP AND KNEE ARTHROPLASTY

M. Ungethüm

The total replacement of hip and knee influenced by disease or trauma has gained increasing importance in orthopaedic surgery. During the last decade progress has been made in the further development of the artificial joint, and the quickly growing literature reports many encouraging successes, new techniques and models. Yet the variety of designs and materials of the types of prosthesis now in use, and the clinical problems in their application show the necessity of further research.

The most important basis for a treatment result satisfying long-term is the lasting and trouble-free function of the endoprosthesis parts.

In view of the stresses arising in a hip or knee replacement, the material for a sliding surface in such an implant should have the following properties: high wear resistance under conditions of sliding friction in order to ensure a sufficiently long life; low coefficient of friction to minimize the moving forces required; sufficiently high compressive strength to avoid cold flow and pitting; a modulus of elasticity which is substantially as low as that of bones so that shocks can be effectively absorbed and low stresses are involved in a transmission of socket deformation.

In order to obtain some knowledge about these mechanical data, model tests and experiments in testing machines and simulators are necessary. In these experiments a fatigue test of material and design of the different joint combinations must be effected under simulated physiological conditions. For the development and design of these testing machines we must have some knowledge about the forces and movements correlated to hip and knee.

Literature reports on a number of details, the most important results of which will be reviewed in the following.

FORCE AND MOVEMENT ANALYSIS IN THE HUMAN HIP AND KNEE JOINT

For an approximative and simplified mathematical model of the forces and movements correlated to the hip, the use of an orthogonal system of coordinates which has its origin in the femoral head, is essential. In this system the forces and movements can be split up into the following components:

- anterior-posterior force, F_x,
- vertical force, F_y,
- lateral force, F_z,
- rotation in the frontal plane about the x-axis: abduction-adduction,
- rotation in the transverse plane about the y-axis: internal-external rotation,
- rotation in the sagittal plane about the z-axis: flexion-extension.

Moreover, there exist further minor linear movements in the three axis directions, as a kind of self-alignment of the joint.

The resulting force on the femoral head, which is due to the body weight and muscle forces, runs from a medial high point to a lateral low point and manifests an angle of 16 ^{o} (25). There are different analyses regarding the amount of compression force and the load pattern with respect to the hip in normal gait. 1935 Pauwels (25) calculated the pattern and amount of the load on the femoral head during the standing phase in a physiological gait process. With a test person body weight of approximately 60 Kp, a maximal force of 260 Kp (that is to say 4.5 times body weight) can be measured at the femoral head. The characteristic double-peak-pattern of the load was also confirmed by Rydell (27) and Paul (24) in a series of experimental tests. Both diagrams show that the load rises to a peak when the body weight is transmitted on the standing leg and that it falls to zero as soon as the standing leg is lifted from the ground. The minimum between the two peaks during the time of the standing leg period is caused by the effect of dynamic forces (positive and negative acceleration).

All authors (24,25,27) agree that the duration of a walking cycle, that is to say, the sum of the period of a standing and a swing phase, is approximately 1-1.2 seconds in normal gait. Each femoral head is hit by 1-2.5 million impacts (standing phase) a year. The speed with which the joint surfaces glide on each other is some 5 cm/sec. According to Duff-Barcley and Spillman (10), who presented a graphical series of comprehensive studies regarding movement phases when walking, the range of rotation in normal gait is 45 ^{o} flexion-extension, 12 ^{o} abduction-adduction and 14 ^{o} internal-external rotation.

With respect to the knee joint there are much more complicated conditions according to anatomy and mechanics. While the load in the main direction shows a similar picture to the double-peak pattern at the hip, rotations occur predominantly in the sagittal plane. During the standing phase the flexion lies within a range of 20 ^{o}. Abduction and adduction are largely prevented and the rotation about the long axis is ca. 9 ^{o} in normal gait.

While surgeons performing alloarthroplasties dream of a possible durability and function of the implants of 50-60 years, engineering does not make such high demands on bearings.

For testing tribological properties, special testing methods are therefore necessary; for these tests we can, in part, return to model apparatuses which have already been applied in technology. In detail the following methods apply (Fig. 1).

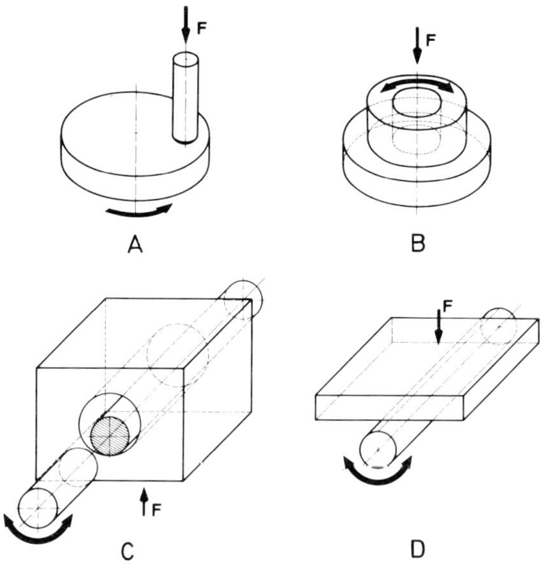

Fig. 1
Schematic presentation of different wear and friction testing machines
A. pin-on-disc
B. ring-on-disc
C. journal-and-bush
D. block-on-journal

MODEL APPARATUS FOR TRIBOLOGICAL TESTS

A simple and comparatively reliable testing apparatus is the pin-on-disc machine. In it a pin, operating in liquid, rubs against the surface of a rotating disc. The wear volume is calculated from the wear track profile, which is observed and enlarged by means of the Talysurf. In Fig. 2 the pin-on-disc machine developed and used in our hospital is shown. Via a strain-gauge chamber, the horizontal frictional force can be measured directly. In accordance with a proposal by the British Standards Institution the conditions for testing are:

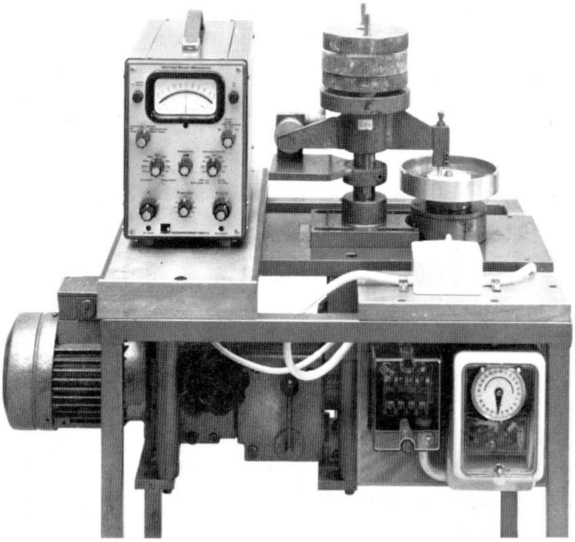

Fig. 2
Pin-on-disc machine

- diameter of pin not less than 6 mm; end face of pin 20 mm spherical radius; surface finish: metal – better than 0.03 μm CLA, plastics – better than 1.0 μm CLA; mean diameter of wear track 25 mm; load 100 N; mean rubbing velocity 0.05 m/sec; lubricant bovine serum; duration 48 hours.

Various disadvantages of the pin-on-disc machine mean that the results achieved can be applied only with restrictions to the facts of the artificial joint. The continuous movement effects a different surface temperature and a different lubrication pattern than an oscillating movement. The pin-on-disc method was also inadequate for testing ceramic materials. Under test conditions microcracks and spalling of particles appeared in the wear track of test discs. In contrast, experiments with the simulator showed excellent wear behaviour when using complete total hip replacements of the same material.

A better possibility of calculating friction and wear behaviour of new materials for total joint replacements is offered by the "journal and bush" machine, which is used by Scales (30) in the Institute of Orthopaedics in London. A journal oscillates horizontally in a screening rig, measuring the friction torque using a strain gauge arm (to determine the stick-slip effects).

Another possibility of the oscillating rig is the machine employed by Mathys (20). In this machine a thermoplastic block is pressed against an oscillating journal with constant force. For the special testing of ceramic materials in the biomechanical laboratory of our hospital we use the principle of the ring on disc. In this principle the flat surfaces of a ring and disc rub in an oscillating movement against each other. Both test specimens consist of the same material. Before the beginning and after the end of the test the macro- and micromorphologies of the gliding surfaces were examined with the help of an electronic stylus.

In all these test machines, friction and wear results depend exclusively on the material data and the lubricating mechanism. Thus differences in quality which are due in particular to the material, can easily be proved. For the tribological behaviour of a prosthesis, however, other factors such as head diameter, accuracy of form, surface roughness, clearance between head and cup etc. are responsible.

For an investigation of these influences depending on design and processing, the joint simulator seems to be ideal, as it is an optimal testing method for completely artificial knee or hip joints.

JOINT SIMULATORS

A number of hip-joint simulators have been described in the literature. Some of these simulators show one or several shortcomings with regard to an optimal imitation of the actual physiological conditions. These simplifications represent definite compromises resulting from the technical efficacy and costs in the development of such simulators with consideration to all parameters obtaining in physiological movement and loading.

In 1965 the literature reported on the first hip simulator invented by Scales et al. (30). In the following years numerous further simulator modifications were developed. The following names must be mentioned: Bousquet and Grammont (3); Boutin (4); Buchholz and Strickle; Dowson et al. (8); Hoffmann-Daimler (18); Miller (22); Thomas and Uhr (38); Shikita and Oonishi (34); Swanson, Freeman and Heath (36); Walker and Gold (47); Weightman et al. (50).

In an optimal imitation of the movement and load conditions of the human hip joint, the following requirements must be met by a hip simulator on the basis of the present state of the art:

1. Rotating movements in frontal, transverse and sagittal plane (abduction/adduction, internal/external rotation, flexion/extension).
2. Stepless variability in the range of the movements (stride).
3. Compression forces in form of the characteristic double peak cycle.
4. Maximum and minimum values of the double peak cycle stepless variable (values depending upon body weight and walking speed).
5. Stepless variability of cycle speed (walking speed).
6. Possibility of testing commercially available prostheses without special preparation.
7. Presence of a temperature controlled lubricant.
8. Filtering off of wear particles for analysis.
9. Possibility of determining frictional moment, deformity, compressive loading, damping, and temperature of the sliding surface of the tested prosthesis.

With the aid of the following example, the function of a hip joint simulator will be explained in detail.

The complete set-up consists of four main parts, the hydraulic converter including power supply, the kinetic testing jig, the electronic control device and the measuring unit (Fig. 3).

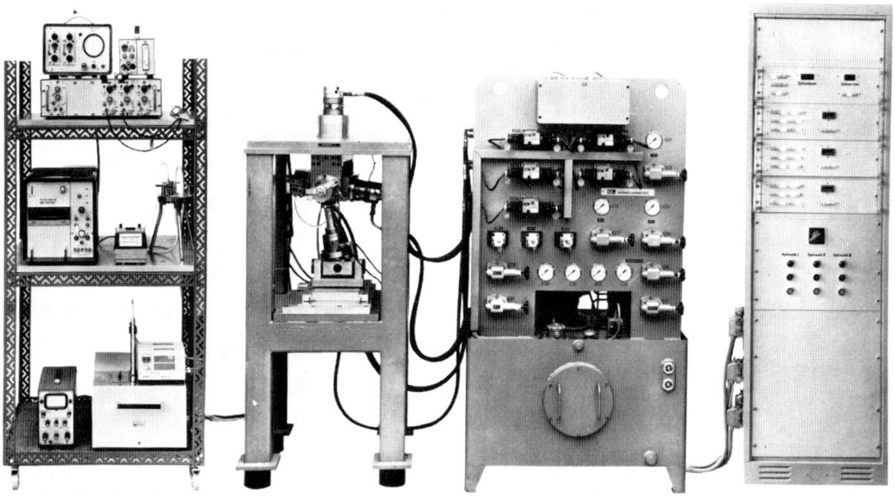

Fig. 3 Hip joint simulator type München

The prosthesis is fixed as in the human body with special holding devices (Fig. 4). While a vertical force acts on the prosthesis in the form of a characteristic double peak cycle, the simulated acetabulum moves against the head of the prosthesis. Swivel movements in all three planes are possible. The range of the movements and subsequently the stride, as well as maximal and minimal values for force can be regulated steplessly. Movements and load are produced by a special hydraulic system. The articulating surfaces are covered with a rubber collar, through which a pseudo-synovial fluid elevated to body temperature is pumped.

A filter built into this circulating system filters off wear particles. Thus, this simulator permits optimal imitation for normal walking, fast running, jumping, climbing stairs etc., for any selected body weight. We believe we have solved the problem of centering the head and cup by using a universal joint underneath the prosthesis for continuous self-alignment and a special embedded anchoring construction. Via a piezoelectric registration of force and moment, the vertical compression loading and the frictional moment between head and cup can be registered. Additionally, the simulator contains gauges for the registration of elastic deformation, damping, and surface temperature of the test prosthesis. All data are registered with a 12-channel UV-recorder.

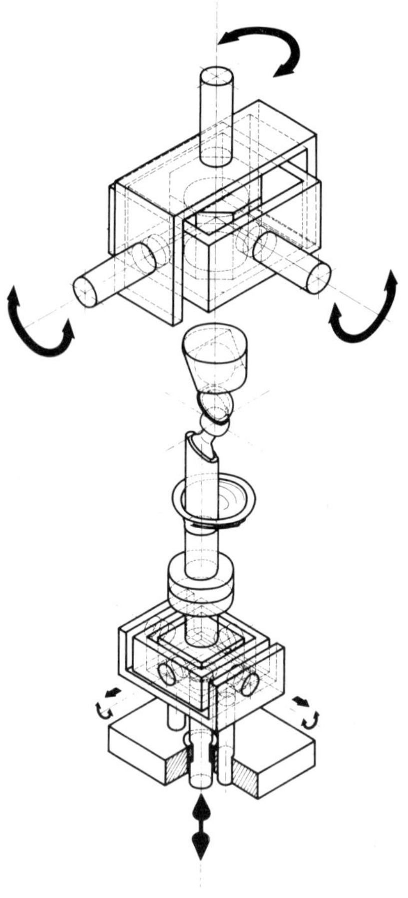

Fig. 4
Schematic presentation of the hip joint simulator type München

There is, without doubt, a need for an effective testing device. Yet we are well aware of the fact that artificial joints will not necessarily show the identical tribological behaviour under in vivo conditions as registered with a simulator, since experimental conditions can only be approximated to those of a living organism.

In addition, there are certain limitations in the interpretation of simulator testings. We can calculate the wear rate for certain test conditions, but we do not know how much each individual patient will stress his prosthesis; this means that the degree of activity of the patient will always remain an unmeasurable, unknown quantity. Also the problem of "material aging" with respect to simultaneous alteration of its mechanical properties, particularly with thermoplastic materials, cannot be solved by simulator testing. On the other hand, testing in a joint simulator is still the best way of testing new implants, comparing known prostheses of different designs, and of obtaining quantitative estimates for predicting the long-time behaviour of the articulating surfaces.

In order to specify the rate of wear of the prostheses in simulator experiments, the test specimens must be removed at regular intervals to be submitted to exact measuring. To do this, special measuring methods are necessary. Weightman et al. (50,51) have developed a special wear gauge instrument: "Based on an electromechanical gauge, the instrument compares radial depth measurement, before and after periods in the joint simulator, at twelve points of ten latitudes within the cup".

Dumbleton, on the contrary uses an essentially simplified system. He places the mounted acetabular cup on a precision surface plate and measures the thickness of the cup along the axis of load application.

Numerous new developments of prostheses with increasingly low wear rates caused us to design our own instrument (Fig. 5). The base for the complete set-up is an air-sup-

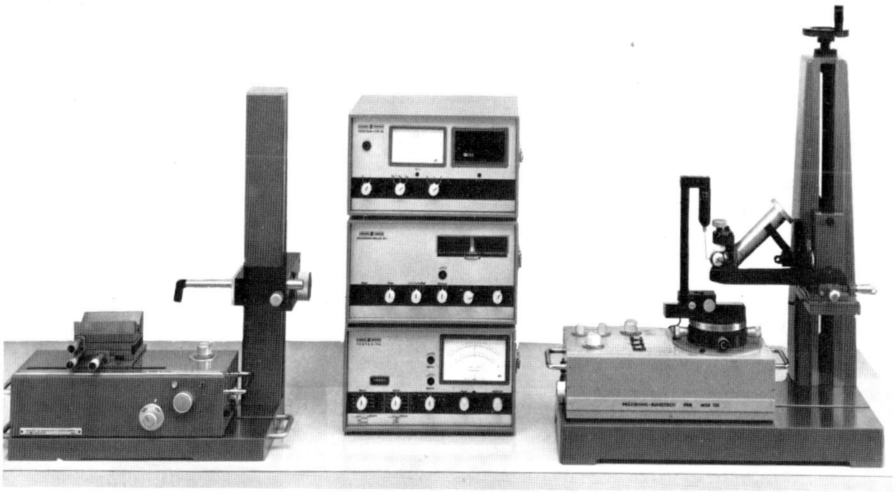

Fig. 5 Measuring unit for determination of roundness and surface roughness of joint components

ported precision round table. Head and cup are measured for roundness (magnification up to x 10,000) and surface (magnification up to x 100,000) by a stylus in 36 meridians. The results are recorded in polar and/or linear diagrams. For all surfaces that are not curved the instrument is equipped with an air-supported measuring carriage. With this apparatus it is possible to detect the smallest differences in quality due to processing techniques or changes due to wear in the micro- and macromorphologies of prosthesis gliding surfaces.

None of the measuring methods known to date, however, can differentiate between mechanical wear and distortion components (cold flow) of polymers. This would be possible by accurately weighing the test specimens before and after the experiment, since the resulting lost of weight corresponds to the wear volume. The unfavourable relationship between mass lost and total mass, however, does not permit the establishment of minor wear rates by measuring.

As pointed out before, we have even more unfavourable mechanical and anatomic conditions in the knee joint. In the development of a simulator to test a total knee replacement we must, therefore, deal with various simplifications, so that the simulation of movement and load can only correspond approximately to the physiological conditions. The implantation of an artificial knee joint can create totally different geometric conditions and thus different load conditions, e.g. a change in the position of the rotation axes and consequently a change in the length of the moment arms. Moreover, different valgus angles can effect moments about the joint axis running from anterior to posterior, which cause an essential additional load of the side bearing surfaces of the replacement.

The physiological load of the knee is formed primarily by the vectorial addition of two components. The first component is made up of those forces to support and accelerate the body mass. The second component develops from the muscular effects (flexor and extensor) on the knee joint.

There are not very many reports on knee joint simulators in the literature. In particular the work of Thull (39,40), Shaw and Murray (33), Swanson, Freeman and Heath (36) must be mentioned. In Thull's simulation machine (Fig. 6) the dynamic load of the knee joint is effected by means of a system of chains and levers by two compressed air cylinders, imitating flexor and extensor forces. The levers and attachment angles anatomically effective for the single force components were taken from the literature. Flexor and extensor levers as well as compression force are variable according to different gait patterns. With the omission of the swinging phase, the test joints are exposed to the load of the standing phase, which is repeated periodically. The conditions of testing are:

– standard load in the direction of the axis of the tibia:	300 Kp
– number of load changes:	10^6
– range of angle of flexion:	0–20 ^{o}
– frequency of load changing:	0.5 Hz
– electrolyte:	phys. NaCl, 35 ^{o}C

The Shaw and Murray simulator (Fig. 7), however, needs only one controlling force component related to the quadriceps muscle group which again is transmitted by means of a chain. The second component – comparable to the external forces – is loaded by

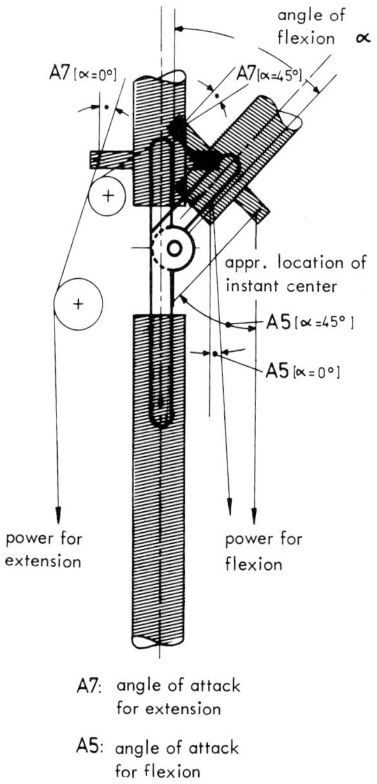

Fig. 6
Knee joint simulator after Thull

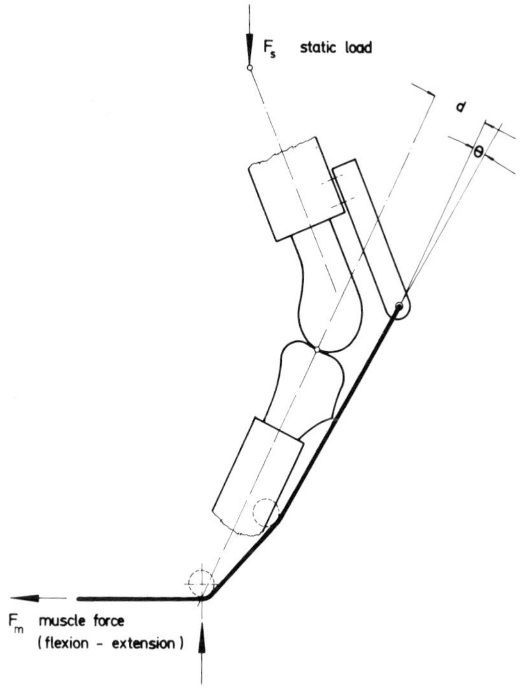

Fig. 7
Knee joint simulator after Shaw and Murray

a set of lead weights. In contrast to the Thull-simulator the swinging phase is also taken into consideration through the unloading of the test joint in a wider range of flexion (0–60 °). Different gait patterns and special joint loads can be simulated by means of a variation of the flexion angles and the force patterns of the cycle.

Swanson, Freeman and Heath use a simulator in which artificial knees as well as hip joints can be tested under chemical, thermal and mechanical conditions and also report on their respective results.

Beside the above-mentioned measuring test for a quantitative determination of wear rates, the scanning electron microscope has proved to be an essential help for the micro-morphological testing of prosthesis components. In particular after testing artificial joints in the simulator, valuable details about the wear mechanisms (adhesion, abrasion, fatigue) involved in the process can be given with regard to the gliding surface of the prosthesis using a scanning electron microscope. Together with the test of prosthesis wear products with regard to their shape, size and surface quality, an analysis of their chemical composition can be carried out at the same time by means of the energy and wavelength despersive material analysis. But the limit for their identification lies within an order of magnitude of 2-3 μm for particle diameters.

TEST RESULTS AND CURRENT STATE OF TRIBOLOGY WITH RESPECT TO ARTIFICIAL HIP JOINTS

At the present time the following materials are used most often for the bearing components in total hip replacement: while some models are still being made from AISI 316 L stainless steel just as they were twenty years ago, most metal parts are today made from a cast CoCrMo-alloy. High-density polyethylene (HDPE) is the only plastic material which has proved satisfactory so far in hip replacements from technical and clinical points of view. High density aluminium oxide ceramic is a promising new development. We shall refer to this material later.

While biology creates optimal gliding and wear conditions in a healthy human joint by special lubricating mechanisms, in an artificial joint we can find tribophysical wear mechanisms which can be divided into adhesion, abrasion and fatigue. Fatigue wear occurs mainly from thermoplastic parts of the prosthesis. Abrasive wear is suffered by both thermoplastic and metal sliding elements. Adhesive wear seems insignificant over long periods of time as it occurs mainly during the initial period.

Because a hip replacement is to be used under varying loads and for movements which are not always uniform, it is difficult to make definitive statements on the actual thickness of the liquid film. A condition of boundary lubrication is certainly typical of artificial hip joints.

In this condition we can find both solid contact as well as surface layer contact due to the molecular film between the surfaces.

In biological joints, more favourable lubrication patterns are to be found. On the basis of classical hydrodynamics in the case of surface roughness of the cartilage of $R \simeq 0.02-0.2\ \mu m$, film thicknesses of $0.01-0.02\ \mu m$ can be determined. These figures, however, cannot explain the actual coefficient of friction of 0.005–0.02. Film thicknesses between 10 and 20 μm according to the elasto-hydrodynamic calculation might rather make possible a correlation with the lower friction torques in biological joints.

On the properties of joint capsule fluid after an alloplastic replacement we know comparatively little. Yet, we can assume in most cases that the rheological characteristics resemble those of the synovial fluid. This fluid has a "non-newtonian" behavior because it has pseudoplastic properties caused by the existence of hyaluronic acid. This means that with the shear rate increasing, the viscosity decreases in a non-linear curve.

Opinions differ with respect to the determination of the pressures to be expected between the head and socket of total hip replacements. These pressures cannot be determined satisfactorily by a calculation of the mean pressure, because the maximum pressure in the zone of contact may be a multiple of the mean pressure. The equation of Hertz is only applicable, however, in the case of low pressures and a relatively large difference between the radii of the ball and the socket.

In Fig. 8 one can see the varying results of four calculating methods in the example of a hip prosthesis now in use. In the case of high load it appears to be more advisable to assume a distribution of the stress in accordance with a sine function, as proposed by Erhardt and Strickle (13). Experimental test results of the real bearing surface, however, show considerable differences with regard to the analytical process (Fig. 9).

From this you can see how difficult it often is for the designer and developer to make quantitative predictions about the wear rates of the gliding components. Only in relation with large-scale processes for calculation of structures under static and dynamic load, can more exact data be worked out. In most cases, however, only an experimental test leads to definite results.

Friction in an artificial hip joint is the resistance of the sliding surfaces to movement, flexion and extension producing the highest torque. In the case of adequate clearance between ball and socket the contact area is near the pole, so that a relatively low friction torque results. However, if the ball is a tight fit in the socket, the bearing area is located near the equator and this effects an increase of friction torque. Walker and Bullough (46) are of the opinion that if the contact between the ball and socket occurs within a solid angle of about 45 degrees from the pole, the frictional torque will be minimized for a given joint.

Wilson and Scales (52) and many other authors have found that the static and dynamic friction is much smaller between surfaces of plastic materials and metal than between metal and metal (Fig. 10). In addition, the friction torque increases in proportion with the size of the head.

Swanson et al. (36) used a hip simulator as well as the Stanton pendulum for the determination of the friction moment. They discovered that the frictional moments in cobalt-

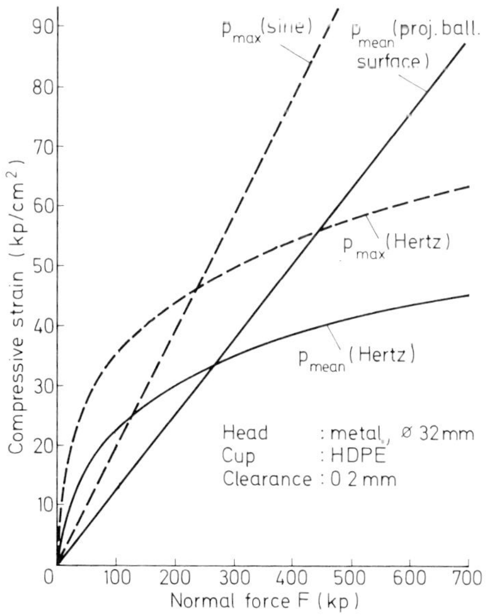

Fig. 8
Specific compression stress in a HDPE cup calculated by different methods

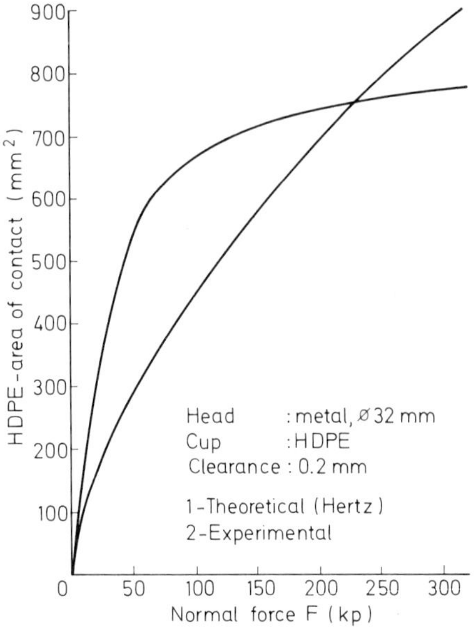

Fig. 9
Differences between the calculated and experimental determination of the real bearing surface in dependence on compression force (material of cup: HDPE)

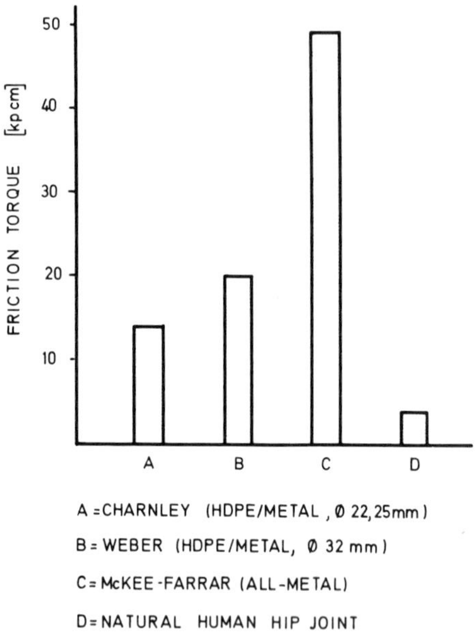

Fig. 10
Frictional moments in total hip replacements

chromium-molybdenum hip prostheses were higher than in stainless steel polyethylene hip prostheses by a factor of at least 2 to 1.

In simulator tests, Walker and Gold (47,48) have measured, in the McKee-Farrar total hip joint, a friction torque which is as much as ten times higher than in the Charnley hip joint. The disadvantage of a high friction torque in all metal joints is that it means a higher stress on the anchoring.

Ruckelshausen (28) has shown statistically that this is the reason why metal-to-metal prostheses become loose in a much higher percentage of cases (5.8 %) than Charnley type metal-to-plastics prostheses and their modifications (0.95 %).

Simon et al. (35) studied the "stiction-friction" (static friction) of McKee-Farrar and Charnley hips in the joint simulator. In their tests they found that the static friction under physiological conditions differed little from dynamic friction in both types of prostheses. Frictional values in joint replacements are, moreover, at least forty times higher than in normal joints. Thus they also came to the conclusion that frictional moments produced in artificial joints may be high enough to cause clinical loosening. In all metal prostheses, the comparatively high friction is influenced by the following factors:

1. position of load transmitting surface (near the pole or equator),
2. irregular geometry of load transmitting surface of head and cup,

3. surface finish,
4. head diameter, and
5. amount of clearance between head and cup.

As regards the irregular geometry, we have checked the sphericity of total hip replacements in our hospital and have found that the roundness values of the articulating surfaces of replacements of the same type, but from different manufacturers, varied greatly and often exceeded the specified tolerances used in precision mechanical engineering (Fig. 11). Some remarks are necessary with regard to the problem "finish of the prosthetic bearing surfaces". We tested the sliding surfaces of a great variety of different types of prostheses by scanning electron microscope technique and Talysurf-profile diagrams. Although when inspected with the naked eye, all metallic surfaces presented an appearance similar to that of a mirror, essential differences in quality could be seen under magnification. When testing metallic bearing surfaces we were able to recognize pits, inclusions and scores. Fig. 12 shows an extract of these results for the surface roughness of two hip joints of different producers. On the whole the rates for CLA lay between 0.04 µm and 0.5 µm. In the case of the thermoplastic gliding components irregularities were much higher. On the other hand we must take the following facts into consideration: as long as there are no final and definitive data for optimal surface roughness, no statement can be made as to whether a "super microfinish" has a favourable or unfavourable effect on friction and wear.

Therefore we require that the deviation from roundness should be less than 5 µm and the mean of the roughness of the surface should be less than 0.025 µm. Good roughness values in the metal parts are required also in metal-to-plastics bearing surfaces in sliding contact, because the rate of wear of thermoplastic materials typically increases with the depth of roughness of the metal part in sliding contact therewith.

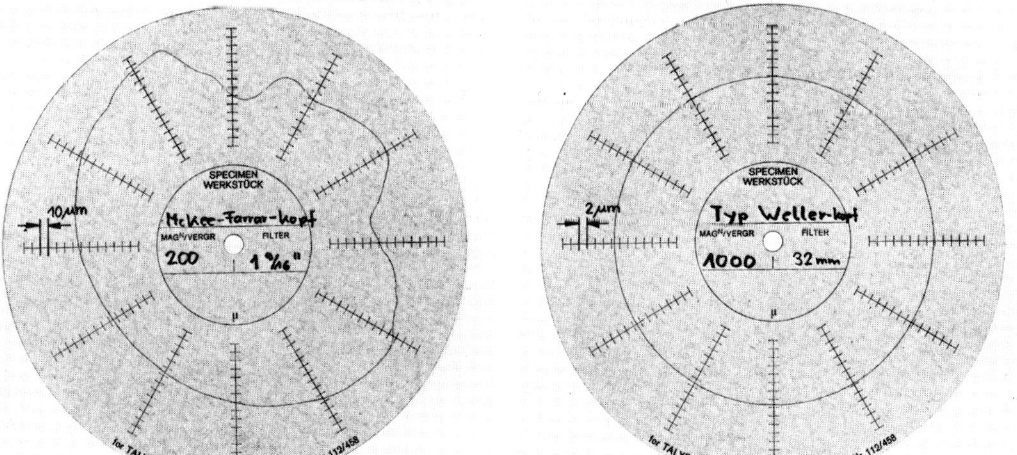

Fig. 11 Varying roundness qualities in two prosthesis heads
left: magnification x 200
right: magnification x 1000

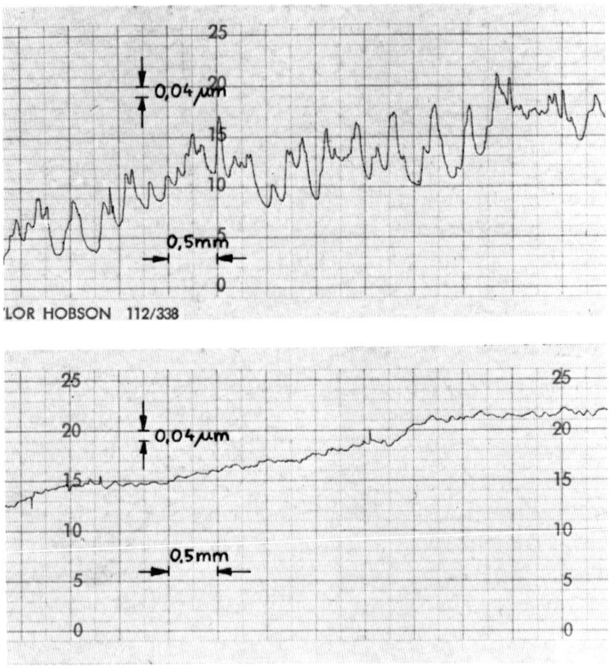

Fig. 12 Extract from measuring results on surface roughness of gliding surfaces. Roughness diagrams of two identical types of prosthesis made by different manufacturers

Scales and Lowe (30) state that the more perfect the finish of a bearing has to be, the higher the cost of the components will become and thus there must be a compromise between what is theoretically desirable and what is economically possible and clinically satisfactory. We feel that the highest possible technical standard has to be achieved in order to avoid catastrophic failures caused by seizures under load and a subsequent loosening of the artificial joint.

To minimize the friction torque between the sliding parts, the radius of the parts of the joint must be minimized, too. On the other hand, the rate of wear increases almost linearly with pressure, so that the pressure in the stressed zone should be minimized, and it is desirable to increase the diameter of the femur head.

To ensure an optimum supply of liquid into the stresses zone, a sufficiently large clearance between the articulating surfaces is required. While the St. Georg type total hip replacement is made with a clearance of 1.5 millimeters, designers of artificial joints believe that a clearance of 0.2 millimeters is sufficient. It may be desirable to provide the parts subjected to sliding friction with a surface which is similar in texture to orange peel and has microscopic pits for holding lubricant and for receiving any abraded particles.

The wear on total hip prostheses is dependent upon:

1. the material of the parts between which sliding takes place and their mechanical and tribological qualities,

2. the diameter of the head (influence of surface compression and contact surface sliding distance),
3. the amount of clearance between head and cup,
4. the activity of the patient, and
5. the body weight of the patient.

A comparative investigation of the wear of artificial joints of the Charnley and Müller types has been carried out by Weightman and his co-workers (50) in the hip joint simulator. In the replacement of these two types, parts of HDPE and metal slide on each other, the heads being 22 and 32 millimeters in diameter respectively. The authors have observed that after 1.8 million load-motion cycles, corresponding to a use of about one year by a human being, the Charnley replacement exhibited removal of the socket wall due to wear of about twice the depth and with about the same abraded volume as the Müller replacement. When Charnley (5,6) inspected removed teflon sockets of his replacements, he found a maximum wear of somewhat more than 5 millimeters after five years of use. Other artificial hip joints did not show any wear after seven years. Because he found no, or little, wear in replacements used by heavy patients, and vice versa, he believes that the "degree of activity" is more significant for the rate of wear than the weight of the patient. On the other hand, it is emphasized that a low friction coefficient need not necessarily result in a low rate of wear and vice versa.

All metal hip joint replacements have a very long life as far as wear is concerned. While in Müller and Charnley total hip joints, a wear of up to 1 millimeter was measured after five years, it has been reported in the literature that a McKee-Farrar all-metal hip joint which was reoperated after three years did not exhibit any measurable wear and that wear to a depth of 1/100 millimeter was observed after a 1000-hour test in the simulator.

Freeman, Swanson and Heath (14) found abraded metal particles of a size up to some μm in diameter in simulator-tested prostheses of the same type.

Fig. 13 shows the transmission electron microscope micrograph of a new McKee-Farrar socket surface. The fine grooves have been produced in the last manufacturing operation. In contrast to this, Fig. 14 is an incident-light microphotograph showing zones of severe wear in a reoperated replacement of the same type. These zones are shown on a still larger scale in Fig. 15 in a transmission electron microscope micrograph. The range of scratch marks lies between 1 and 2.5 μm. Compared with Fig. 13, where the roughness consists only of fine grooves, one can see that Fig. 15 shows scratches and deep grooves which are due to wear debris and bone cement particles. The width and direction of these scratch marks vary significantly and are often superimposed. An influence which should not be underestimated is the presence of a carbide phase between the grain boundaries in the CoCrMo-alloy in the wear process shown here. These carbides are approximately four times harder than the original basic material and therefore can have an abrasive effect.

Thermoplastic materials show a completely different wear pattern. Depth measurements of grooves on reoperated rotating polyester heads revealed, in the area covered by the spherical cup, similar figures as with the metal cup. The initial traces had been smoothed and a highly polished plastic surface resulted.

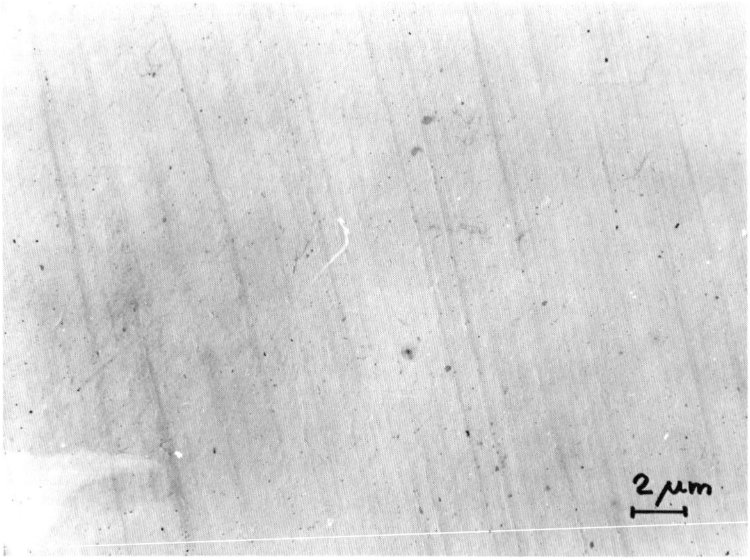

Fig. 13 Transmission electron microscope micrograph (replica) of a new McKee-Farrar socket surface

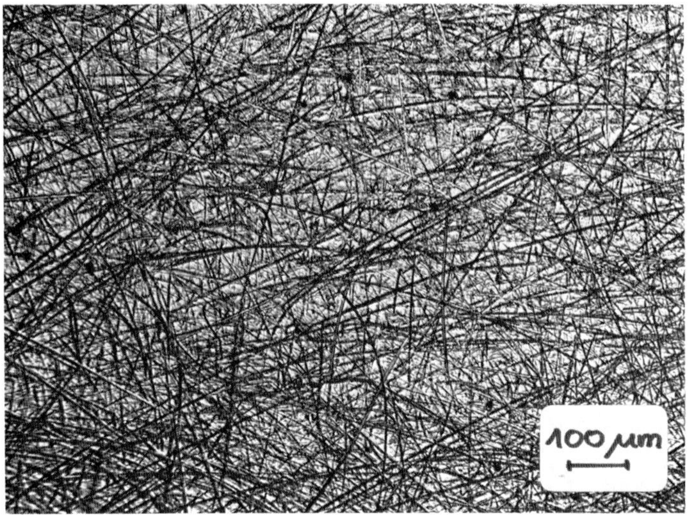

Fig. 14 Incident-light microphotograph of a contact zone showing very heavy scratch marks in a McKee-Farrar socket which was reoperated after three years of use

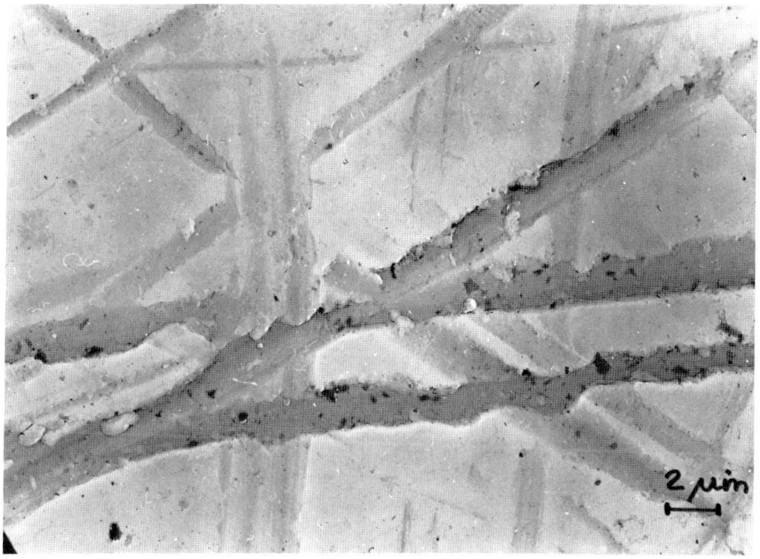

Fig. 15 Transmission electron microscope micrograph (replica) of the scratch marks of Fig. 14

In the wear zone of simulator-tested polyethylene cups of the type Müller, Weightman and his co-workers (50,51) found a combination of abrasive and brittle fracture wear. Rabinowicz (26) has offered an explanation for this: during sliding, a characteristic series of cracks is observed in the wear track. Subsequently, large wear particles tend to be produced as a result of surface breakup.

TEST RESULTS OF ARTIFICIAL KNEE JOINTS

At this point a brief word about the presently used total knee prostheses may be permitted. We have to differentiate between hinge and non-hinge joints. The latter depend, as a prerequisite, on completely efficient ligaments. Additionally, the relatively large bearing surfaces provide more advantageous mechanical conditions than do hinge joints.

Much less information about friction and wear tests of artificial knee joints can be found in the literature. The first report was by Walldius in 1957 (49). The knee prosthesis he used at that time was made of acrylic resin and consisted of a femoral and a tibial part, joined together by a stainless steel rod to form a hinged joint. With the aid of an essentially simplified testing machine, two questions were to be solved:

a. would acrylic surfaces slide against each other and against metal, and
b. would the frictional heat be a potential source of damage within the prosthesis.

Lacking appropriate materials for a rubber collar intended to contain physiological saline, Walldius carried out his tests under "unlubricated conditions". With a maximal load on the tibial parts of between 90 and 140 Kp he came, at the end of the experiment after 242,520 load cycles, to the following result: the diameter of the central rod was found to have been worn down by 0.01 mm and the diameter of the channel by 0.02 mm. With the aid of this result and that of two reoperated replacements (after 3 and 4.5 years respectively) Walldius calculated the wear in the vertical direction in the channel of the inner axle journal as being 1 mm in 10 years.

In the following years Walldius modified his knee replacement using metal only (Vitallium). In 1969 Freeman et al. (14) reported on operational tests with this prosthesis and indicated a wear rate of approximately 0.1 g/100 000 cycles. In 1973 the same authors published a detailed report on newly taken up friction and wear test in the simulator regarding Walldius' and Shiers' knee replacements. A summary of the results is given in Tables 1 and 2. Recent tests carried out by Thull, whose simulator, including the test conditions, was mentioned in a previous paragraph, show interesting results in a comparison of the Walldius and GSB knees. In the Walldius knee, tibial and femoral parts are connected by a fixed axis whose bearing components are made exclusively of Vitallium. The GSB joint in contrast, shows a variable axis with the gliding combination HDPE on cast CoCrMo-alloy.

At the joint axis in the Walldius knee a material loss of maximal 40 μm was observed, on the other hand no significant influence of the valgus angle was established. The GSB joint provided totally different results. A metal loss within the range of up to 300 μm

Table 1 Results from a simulator test after Swanson, Freeman, and Heath. Constant load of 890 Newton, Ringer's solution

Prosthesis	Number of cycles	Frictional moment (Newton · meters) flexion	extension
Walldius knee	0	5.0	4.5
	2600	8.9	11.6
	9700	9.9	9.9
	1,836,000	17.6	17.6

Table 2 Frictional moments measured in the simulator after Swanson, Freeman, and Heath. Constant load of 890 Newton, Ringer's solution

Prosthesis	Number of cycles before removal of fluid	Amounts of metal in sediment (mg) Co	Cr	Mo
Shiers knee	0 – 1,080,100	28.6	15.8	2.35
	1,080,100 – 1,236,400	16.6	0.3	3.2
Walldius knee	0 – 110,200	7.1	5.0	0.16
	110,200 – 301,400	27.0	19.1	0.87
	301,400 – 1,275,100	total 640		
	1,275,100 – 1,836,100	total 550		

(after 10^6 load cycles, load 300 Kp) develops through direct metal-to-metal contact at the femoral side part. The plastic bearings of the tibial part show wear and distortion up to a maximum of 600 /um, the right bearing shell being much more stressed than the left. Thull attributes this to the influence of the valgus angle as well as the clearance between tibial and femoral parts, what effects an unsymetrically distribution of forces (Fig. 16).

Mazas et al. (21) report on the resistance to wear of the Guepar prosthesis. The combination of bearing materials in this joint is CoCrMo-alloy/CoCrMo-alloy. The test conditions in the machine included: flexion motion to 120 ^{o} at 70 cycles per minute; varying load of 0–100 Kp; duration of test 4,200,000 cycles. The maximum material loss between axis and element was 0.237 mm for an initial slack of 0.044 mm. The authors conclude from this that this wear rate seems quite acceptable.

In our hospital we observed high abrasive wear in the axle bolt in the case of reoperated Guepar replacements. In Fig. 17 one can see deep grooves in the plane flexion-extension.

A further hinge knee joint is the prosthesis type "LL". In this artificial joint we find a gliding combination of HDPE/CoCrMo-alloy. Letournel and Lagrange (19) report on experiments to determine the wear of the HDPE components in the walking simulator. A wear of about 0.1 mm after 1 million cycles was found, corresponding to approximately two years of walking.

NEW DEVELOPMENTS

What new materials are presently being tested and evaluated for their qualifications as implant material with specially favourable tribological behaviour?

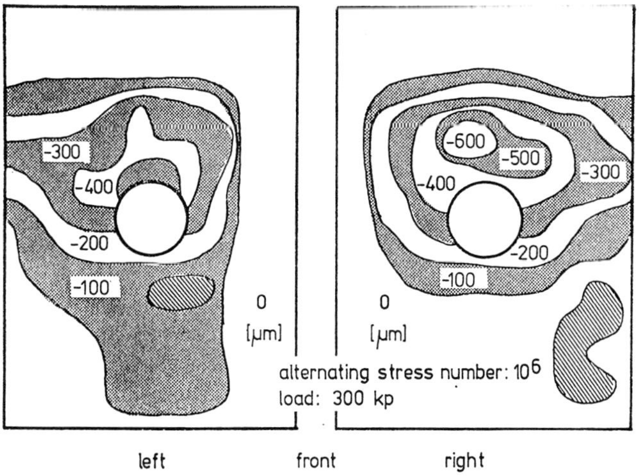

Fig. 16 Abrasion and deformation of the GSB plastic bearings (after Thull)

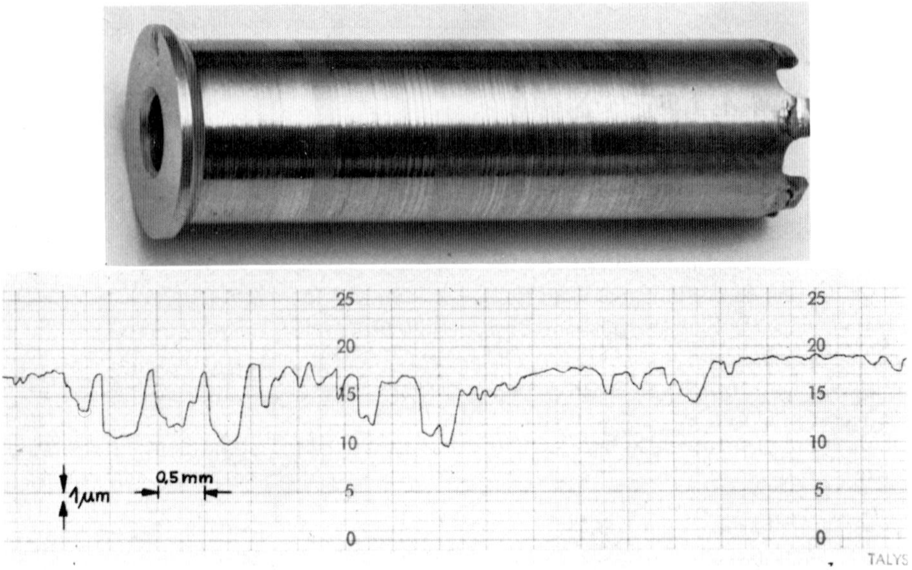

Fig. 17 Above: axle bolt of a Guepar-knee replacement after 1.5 years implantation – high abrasive wear
Below: roughness profile diagram of this bolt – the deep grooves are clearly visible

The question as to what possibilities exist for the improvement of the wear behaviour of HDPE is repeatedly posed in the literature.

In a thrust-washer type testing machine Dumbleton et al. (11,12) found that the wear resistance of polyethylene may be improved by gamma irradiation. At a radiation dose of 200 Mrad he found a decrease in the wear factor k of about two-and-a-half-fold.

In the biomechanical laboratory of our hospital we also tested the influence of the radiation dose. Of special interest to us was, above all, the change in the mechanical properties of HDPE under a second sterilization by γ-rays, as is often carried out. In pin-on-disc studies we observed an increase in wear and indentation hardness with a higher radiation dose (these results correspond to doses up to 15 Mrad). On the basis of these results it seems advisable to avoid second sterilizations by γ-rays (Fig. 18).

Seedhom et al. (31) propose a solid phase forming of HDPE, because the resulting material, under favourable conditions of moulding, has a wear rate that is nearly one half to one order of magnitude lower than that of the unmoulded material.

Experiments by Miller et al. (23) showed that the Ti 6Al 4V is satisfactory for total joint replacements when used in combination with HDPE. As a comparative material CoCrMo-alloy and 316 stainless steel were used. The TiO_2 layer showed sufficient adhesion and mechanical strength so as not to be damaged by the opposite HDPE surface. As already observed by Amstutz (1), the authors noticed a transferring of a polyethylene film on all metal counterfaces. Dowson et al. (8,9) are of the opinion, that all these transfer films can effect an increase as well as a decrease in the wear rate, depending on the initial condition of the surface roughness of the counterface.

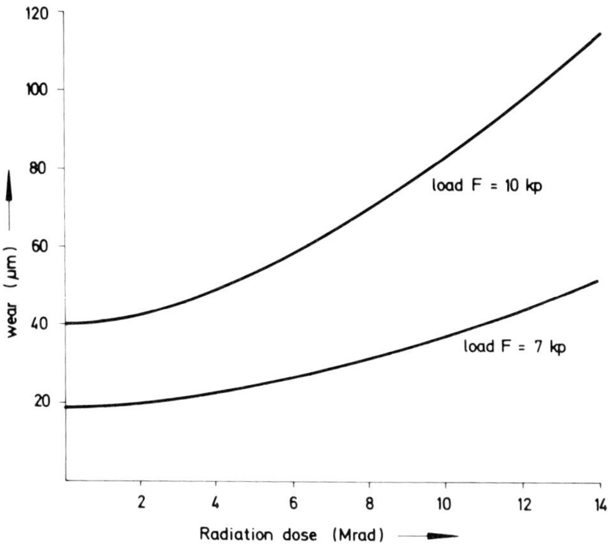

Fig. 18 Dependence of the wear rate on radiation dose in HDPE (results from the pin-on-disc study)

In contrast with the results of Miller et al. (23), Galante and Rostoker (15) noticed a high rate of wear in Ti 6Al 4V in their laboratory tests with a disc-on-plate wear testing machine. For this reason it must be urged that this alloy should not be used in artificial joints.

With the intention of developing a material of superior wear resistance Galante and Rostoker tested a graphite-filled HDPF composite against Vitallium alloy. "Wear rates of this material were well below those of the other combinations tested and were shown to be only 1/7–1/30 of that found for HDPE" (37). We, however, have not been able to confirm these results in our own test series. We established that a graphite-filled HDPE manifested higher wear rates than the pure one.

On the way to ideal bearing components for artificial hip joints, Mathys and Mathys (20) tested a series of thermoplastic and metal materials in a model testing machine. From these experiments it was seen that in a combination of two different polymers a more favourable wear behaviour can be created than in a polymer-metal-combination. Especially favourable is the combination of polyester with acetal-copolymer.

A completely new material for use in endoprosthetics are the oxide-ceramics. In 1973, Galante and Rostoker (15) in the USA eliminated aluminium oxide from usage in total joint replacements because of high wear. Boutin (4) in France implanted hundreds of artificial hip joints of pure, high-density Al_2O_3. In this model, cup and head consisted of ceramic, while the stem was made from resin-covered metal. Al_2O_3 is absolutely biocompatible, inert, and chemically consistent. It resists extremly high compression forces. According to reports from Boutin, laboratory experiments have shown that wear drops to zero after an initial walking phase between 300 and 600 hours.

Beutler et al. (2) have come to the conclusion, after carrying out their own test series, that without doubt also in a material combination of Al_2O_3/Al_2O_3 a constant yet extremely low loss of material takes place (the limit of identification of the loss was at 0.1 mg).

In Germany several teams have also been working for years on the application of dense Al_2O_3-ceramic for joint replacements (7,16,29). Heimke et al. (17) carried out tribological experiments with this material after the pin-on-disc method applying synovial fluid. After the first 1000 gliding meters, a minor initial wear turned up.

In our own experiments we were able to demonstrate the change in surface roughness after 1 million load-motion cycles in the hip simulator (Figs. 19,20). The gliding surfaces of an Al_2O_3/Al_2O_3 prosthesis showed an initial roughness of CLA = 0.55 μm. After the test a

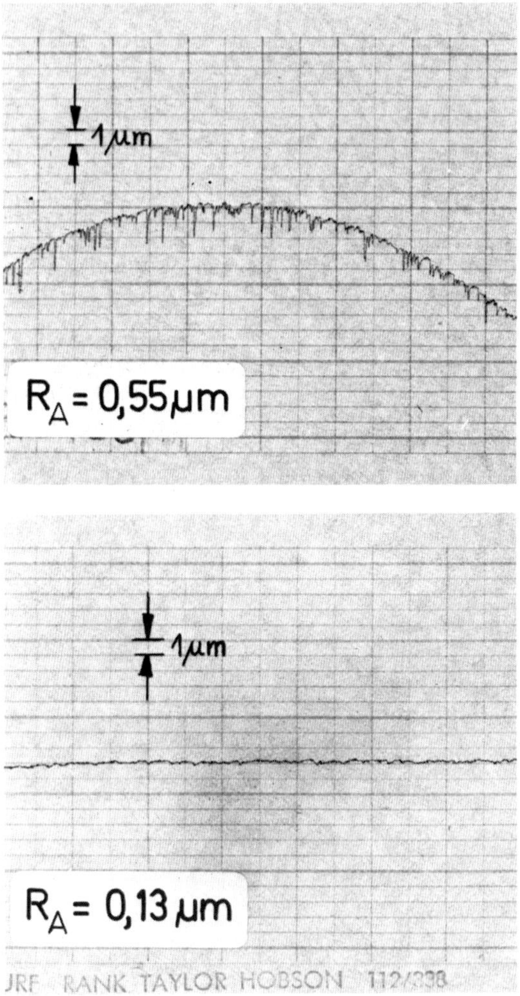

Fig. 19
Surface roughness of an Al_2O_3-head (cup same material) before (above) and after (below) the simulator test

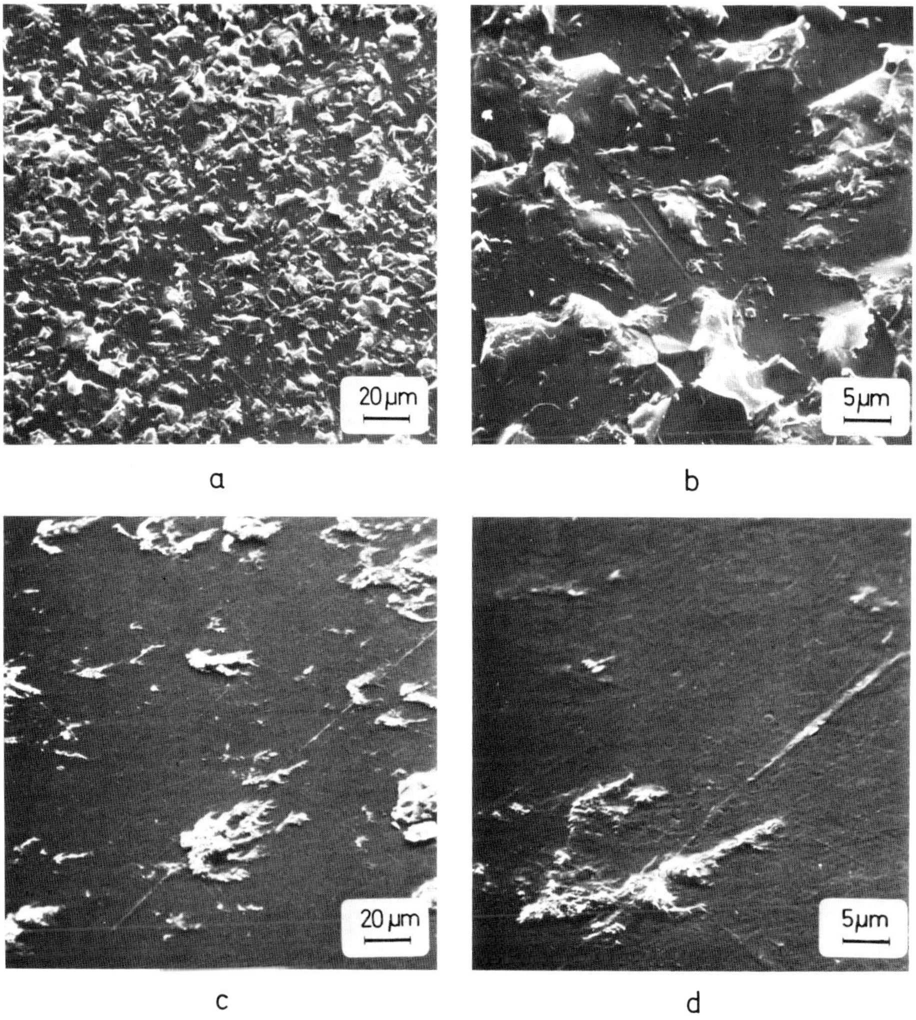

Fig. 20 The same results as in Fig. 19 presented in scanning electron microscope pictures.
a,b: before the test
c,d: after the test

CLA-rate of 0.13 µm was observed. The smoothing of the bearing surfaces was also demonstrated exactly in different scanning electron microscopic pictures. Meanwhile some producers of ceramic protheses have found a way of largely abolishing an initial polishing process during the manufacturing period. In the biomechanical laboratory of our hospital various new developments in the field of ceramic hip replacements are submitted to a detailed comparative examination in the joint simulator.

Latest tribological tests with a material combination HDPE/Al_2O_3-ceramic showed a lower wear rate in the HDPE-cup compared with the HDPE/metal-combinations now in use (32). As an explanation for this it is indicated, above all, that in contrast to metal in the gliding movement between HDPE and Al_2O_3-ceramic no transferance of a polyethylene film to the ceramic ball develops. Moreover it is mentioned that ceramic has a better wettability by fluid than metal.

CONCLUSION

From all these details it may be concluded that many test results cannot be compared with one another, on account of the different testing parameters. Due to the varying testing conditions it can be explained that positive and negative results exist for one single material with regard to its tribological behaviour. Therefore it is certainly in the interest of manufacturer and surgeon, but also in the interest of the patient, to demand an international standardization in the field of a mechanical and biological testing of implants.

REFERENCES

1. Amstutz, H.C.: Polymers as bearing materials for total hip replacement: a friction and wear analysis. Journal of Biomedical Materials Research 3, 547 (1968)
2. Beutler, H., Lehmann, M., Staehli, G.: Wear behaviour of medical engineering materials. Wear 33, 337 (1975)
3. Bousquet, G., Grammont, P.: Etude experimentale de la longevite des protheses de hanche du point de vue mecanique. Acta Orthopaedica Belgica 38, suppl. I, 123 (1972)
4. Boutin, P.: Arthroplastie totale de la hanche par prothese en alumine frittee. Revue d'orthopedie 58, 229 (1972)
5. Charnley, J.: The long-term result of low friction arthroplasty of the hip performed as a primary intervention. Journal of Bone and Joint Surgery 54-B, 61 (1972)
6. Charnley, J., Kamangar, A., Longfield, M.D.: The optimum size of prosthetic heads in relation to the wear of plastic sockets in total replacement of the hip. Medical and Biological Engineering 7, 31 (1969)
7. Dörre, E., Geduldig, D., Happel, M., Lade, R., Prüssner, P., Willert, H.-G., Zichner, L.: Welche Aussicht hat die Biokeramik als Implantatmaterial in der Orthopädie? 23. Annual meeting of the Vereinigung Süddeutscher Orthopäden e.V., Baden-Baden 1975
8. Dowson, D., Atkinson, R., Brown, K.: The wear of high molecular weight polyethylene with particular reference to its use in artificial human joints. Amer. Chem. Soc. Div. Org. Coat., Plast. Chem. Pap. 34, 35 (1974)
9. Dowson, D., Walker, P.S., Longfield, M.D., Wright, V.: A joint simulating machine for load-bearing joints. Medical and Biological Engineering 8, 37 (1970)
10. Duff-Barclay, I., Spillman, D.T.: Lubrication and wear in living and artificial human joints. Proc. Instn. Mech. Engrs. 181, (1966/67) 3J
11. Dumbleton, J.H., Miller, D.A., Miller, E.H.: A simulator for load-bearing joints. Wear 20, 165 (1972)

12. Dumbleton, J.H., Shen, C., Miller, E.H.: A study of the wear of some materials in connection with total hip replacement. Wear 29, 163 (1974)

13. Erhard, G., Strickle, E.: Gleitelemente aus thermoplastischen Kunststoffen. Kunststoffe 62, 282 (1972)

14. Freeman, M.A.R., Swanson, S.A.V., Heath, J.C.: Study of the wear particles produced from cobalt-chromium-molybdenum-manganese total joint replacement prostheses. Annals of the Rheumatic Diseases 28 Suppl., 29 (1969)

15. Galante, J.O., Rostoker, W.: Wear in total hip prostheses. Acta Orthopaedica Scandinavica Suppl., 145 (1973)

16. Griss, P., v.Andrian-Werbug, H., Heimke, G., Krempien, B., Silber, R., Jaissle, R., Merkle, B.: Erste Erfahrungen mit der Keramik-Metall-Verbund-Endoprothese. 23. Annual meeting of the Vereinigung Süddeutscher Orthopäden e.V., Baden-Baden 1975

17. Heimke, G., Beisler, W., v.Andrian-Werbug, H., Griss, P., Krempien, B.: Untersuchungen an Implantaten aus Al_2O_3-Keramik. Berichte der Deutschen Keramischen Gesellschaft 50, 4 (1973)

18. Hoffmann-Daimler, S.: Zur Entwicklung neuer Hüftgelenkprothesen. Medizinisch-Orthopädische Technik 93, 31 (1973)

19. Letournel, E., Lagrange, J.: Total knee replacement with the LL type prosthesis. Clinical Orthopaedics and Related Research 94, 249 (1973)

20. Mathys, R. sen., Mathys, R. jun.: Die Grenzflächen Metall-Metall, Metall-Kunststoff, Kunststoff-Kunststoff. In: Biopolymere und Biomechanik von Bindegewebssystemen, Berlin-Heidelberg-New York: Springer-Verlag 1974

21. Mazas, F.B. and Guepar: Guepar total knee prosthesis. Clinical Orthopaedics and Related Research 94, 211 (1973)

22. Miller, D.A.: Reducing wear in total hip prosthesis. University of Cincinnati, College of Engineering (1971)

23. Miller, D.A., Ainsworth, R.D., Dumbleton, J.H., Page, D., Miller, E.H., Chi Shen: A comparative evaluation of the wear of ultra-high molecular weight polyethylene abraded by Ti-6Al-4V. Wear 28, 207 (1974)

24. Paul, J.P.: Forces transmitted by joints in the human body. Proc. Instn. Mech. Engrs. 181 (1966/67) 3J

25. Pauwels, F.: Der Schenkelhalsbruch. Stuttgart: Enke-Verlag 1935

26. Rabinowicz, E.: Friction and wear of materials. New York: J. Wiley 1965

27. Rydell, N.: Forces in the hip joint. In: R.M. Kenedi, edit., Biomechanics and related bioengineering topics, Oxford: Pergamon Press 1965

28. Ruckelshausen, M.C.: Haltbarkeitserwartungen von Hüfttotalprothesen in Abhängigkeit von Verschleiß, Reibungskoeffizient und Kopfdurchmesser. In: Cotta u. Schulitz, edit., Der totale Hüftgelenkersatz, Stuttgart: Thieme 1973

29. Salzer, M., Zweymüller, K., Locke, H., Plenk jr. H.: Erste Erfahrungen mit einer Hüfttotalendoprothese aus Biokeramik. 23. Annual meeting of the Vereinigung Süddeutscher Orthopäden e.V., Baden-Baden 1975

30. Scales, J.T., Lowe, S.A.: Some factors influencing bone and joint replacements. In: M. Jayson, edit., Total hip replacement, London: Sector Publishing 1971

31. Seedhom, B.B., Dowson, D., Wright, V.: Wear of solid phase formed high-density polyethylene in relation to the life of artificial hips and knees. Wear 24, 35 (1973)

32. Semlitsch, M., Willert, H.G., Dörre, E.: Discussion remark. 62. DGOT-Tagung, Tübingen 1975

33. Shaw, J.A., Murray, D.G.: Knee joint simulator. Clinical Orthopaedics and Related Research 94, 15 (1973)

34. Shikita, T., Oonishi, H.: Abnutzung und Schmierung der Totalendoprothesen des Hüftgelenks. In: Cotta u. Schulitz, edit., Der totale Hüftgelenkersatz, Stuttgart: Thieme 1973

35. Simon, S.R., Paul, I.L., Rose, R.M., Radin, E.L.: Stiction-friction of total prostheses and its relationship to loosening. Journal of Bone and Joint Surgery 57-A, 226 (1975)

36. Swanson, S.A.V., Freeman, M.A.R., Heath, J.C.: Laboratory tests on total joint replacement prostheses. Journal of Bone and Joint Surgery 55-B, 759 (1973)

37. Tetik, R.D., Galante, J.O., Rostoker, W.: A wear resistant material — tissue biocompatibility of an ultra-high molecular weight (UHMW) polyethylene-graphite composite. Journal of Biomedical Materials Research 8, 231 (1974)

38. Thomas, G., Uhr, H.E.: Experimentelle Untersuchungen zur Leistungsfähigkeit der totalen Hüftgelenksprothese. Zeitschrift für Orthopädie 106, 694 (1969)

39. Thull, R., Schaldach, M.: Funktionssimulation an Kniegelenkprothesen. Biomedizinische Technik 20, Ergänzungsband, 111 (1975)

40. Thull, R.: Investigations of artificial knee joints — testing and biomechanical aspects. Proceedings of the fifth International Congress of Biomechanics, Iyväskylä (Finland) 1975

41. Ungethüm, M.: Tribologische Aspekte beim totalen Gelenkersatz. Zeitschrift für Orthopädie 112, 168 (1974)

42. Ungethüm, M., Jäger, M., Witt, A.N., Hildebrandt, J.: Sphericity examinations of arthroplastic total hip prostheses. Acta Orthopaedica Scandinavica 45, 421 (1974)

43. Ungethüm, M., Zenker, H.: Abrieb- und Oberflächenuntersuchung bei einer Totalendoprothese nach McKee-Farrar. Archiv für orthopädische und Unfall-Chirurgie 76, 212 (1973)

44. Ungethüm, M., Hildebrandt, J., Jäger, M., Mosle, H.G.: Ein neuer Simulator zur Testung von Totalendoprothesen für das Hüftgelenk. Archiv für orthopädische und Unfall-Chirurgie 77, 304 (1973)

45. Walker, P., Dowson, D., Longfield, M., Wright, V.: A joint simulator. In: Wright, V., edit., Lubrication and wear in joints, London: Sector Publishing 1969

46. Walker, P.S. Bullough, P.G.: The effects of friction and wear in artificial joints. Orthop. clin. North America 4, 275 (1973)

47. Walker, P.S., Gold, B.L.: Comparison of the bearing performance of normal and artificial human joints. J. Lubr. Techn. 95, 333 (1973)

48. Walker, P.S., Gold, B.L.: The tribology (friction, lubrication and wear) of all-metal artificial hip joints. Wear 17, 285 (1971)

49. Walldius, B.: Arthroplasty of the knee using an endoprosthesis. Acta Orthopaedica Scandinavica Suppl. 24, 22 (1957)

50. Weightman, B.O., Paul, I.L., Rose, R.M., Simon, S.R., Radin, E.L.: A comparative study of total hip replacement prostheses. Journal of Biomechanics 6, 299 (1973)

51. Weightman, B., Simon, S., Paul, I., Rose, R., Radin, E.: Lubrication mechanism of hip joint replacement prostheses. J. Lubr. Techn., Transactions of the ASME 1972, pp. 131-135

52. Wilson, J.N., Scales, J.T.: Loosening of total hip replacements with cement fixation. Clinical Orthopaedics 72, 145 (1970)

SUMMARY OF THE BIOENGINEERING ASPECTS OF ARTIFICIAL JOINT REPLACEMENT

M. Schaldach, R. Thull, and F. Hein

The advances in artificial hip and knee joint technology of the last few years show that, with the implants presently available, the patient can already largely be re-habilitated. The success of the treatment depends not only on the indication and on the implantation technique, but, in addition, also on the nature of the implant used. Questions of design with respect to function and fixation, the mechanical properties of the materials employed, and a knowledge of the interactions of the material with the biological environment, however, continue to present problems. These occasionally involve considerable set-backs and their solution can be achieved only by close co-operation between clinician, engineer and scientist.

The difficulties of application and development of a total artificial joint, can be eliminated only by the use of experimental technologies, which represent the most advanced state of the art. Physical chemistry, chemistry and the science of materials must be utilized to the full extent of their possibilities in order to develop mechanically stable and abrasion-resistant materials which do not react with the electrolytes in the body. Since, at the present time, it is impossible to say what materials will finally turn out to be optimal for the artificial joint, their development must be on as broad a basis as possible. Metals and their alloys, ceramics, glass ceramics and plastics re-inforced with additional materials must all be improved simultaneously, in order, by making use of the results of investigations into biomechanical forces in the bone and in the prosthesis, to be able to design the optimal artificial joint. Here, inventiveness with respect to the form of the joint, should not be exhausted in a mere simulation of the natural models, but, rather, efforts must be made to tailor the design to the materials to be used, while ensuring conformity of function to the anatomical and physiological conditions pertaining. With respect both to the development and testing of new materials, and to the design of new prosthesis, a number of advances have been made in recent times. In Germany, at least, these advances have been initiated and supported by financial aid from the state. A comprehensive promotion program drawn up by the Federal Ministry for Research and Technology has made it possible for the results of engineering and scientific efforts from almost all fields of technology to be concentrated on the solution of the problems associated with artificial joints. The results available to date indicate how important communication between the various scientific disciplines is for the promotion of individual medico-technical developmental projects. But here, too, the rule of all applied sciences should be taken into account, namely, that basic research should be limited to what is really necessary and technical advances realized in a form expedient for effecting practical therapy in the patient.

An examination of the development of the artificial joint from the end of the 19th century onwards and a consideration of the joints available today show that considerable advances have been made. At the same time, however, fundamental shortcomings are clearly recognizable. Since the advantages of the designs have largely been dealt with, attention might now profitably be turned to the three most important weaknesses, which may be described by the headings:

A. Matching of the stress distribution to the natural situation, after implantation of the prosthesis
B. Materials for prostheses
C. Fixation of the prostheses

A serious problem with prostheses fixed with the aid of bone cement has proved to be the loosening of the fixation. Not infrequently, fractures of the implanted material, usually in the region of the stem, are the result.

The clarification of the causal factors of this type of therapeutic failure is, with the present state of our knowledge, only inadequately possible. This also applies to the forces acting upon the hip joint during stressing and movement, in particular the calculation of the stress distribution in bony structures, in the region of the acetabulum, in the proximal femur and in the prosthesis itself. Our ideas as to the forces acting upon the hip are mainly based on the work of Pauwels. For the evaluation of the static and dynamic processes in the hip joint after total hip replacement, our knowledge would seem to be inadequate. For example, we simply know too little about the forces acting within the prosthesis, at the interfaces implant/bone cement and cement/bone. Only a greater knowledge of these, to date largely unknown, factors will make possible a decisive improvement in the operation and help avoid the type of failure mentioned.

The materials presently available for implants do not meet the requirements with respect to mechanical properties and inert behaviour within the body. For example skeletal prostheses must, at one and the same time, be able to tolerate the specific bending, buckling and torsional forces, possess a considerable ability to damp mechanical vibrations and meet stringent requirements with respect to surface hardness and resistance to abrasion. In addition, any electrochemical reactions occurring must not give rise to unphysiological concentrations of ions.

No spectacular developments have been seen in the metals most frequently used in orthopaedics. The development of new cobalt-chromium alloys is characterized by only slight changes in composition; by the addition of nickel and tungsten, the facecentered cubic phase is stabilized and, at the same time, ductility and workability are improved. Of considerable interest are the porous implants, produced by powder-metallurgics, which allow both hard and soft tissue to grow into the pores, thus improving the fixation of the prosthesis. With a pore diameter of less than 100 μm, penetration is predominantly by soft tissue. In experimental studies, a satisfactory fixation through hard tissue was observed at a pore diameter of between 100 and 250 μm.

Sintered aluminium oxide is one of the chemically and mechanically stable oxide ceramic materials, and, for this reason is being used in the field of orthopaedics in the form of dense-sintered prosthetic parts, both experimentally and, in some cases, also clinically.

Hulbert has reviewed the state of the art of this technology in this book. The same working group has also described experience obtained with calcium aluminate, which has also been tested as a prosthetic material.

A possible alternative to porous metallic or ceramic prostheses are the biocompatible forms of glass proposed by Hench. They are characterized by the fact that the fixation of the prosthesis is effected by chemical bonds that form between the tissue and the surface of the glass.

That plastics are widely used in the field of medicine must not close our eyes to the fact that, in particular in the case of materials used in orthopaedic tasks, not inconsiderable problems still have to be resolved. In particular their stability leaves much to be desired. At the present time, the only plastic material widely used is high-density polyethylene.

Generally speaking, progress in biomaterials research should be most profitable when dealing with fundamentals rather than individual materials. It is by work on the fundamentals of tissue ingrowth into porous implants and of the nature of in vivo degradation that stability and implant incorporation will be achieved. This does not mean that individual materials are not important, for their properties must be relevant to the biological situation. However, it is the principles that are important and apart from a few mechanical properties and the questions of local tissue reaction and systemic toxicity effects, it is likely that, under optimal circumstances, many materials could perform the same tasks with equal suitability.

It must be clear that the most urgent problems associated with the use of materials in the body are concerned with reactions at interfaces.

The problem of fixation of the endoprosthesis has been given a new impetus with the trials of ceramic prostheses, which can be implanted without the use of cement. However, until long-term results are available, the development of improved cements should be hurried along.

Cold polymerizing polymethylmethacrylate (PMMA) has gained an important place in operative orthopaedics and surgery as a bone cement for the fixing of joint endoprostheses and in combination with metallic implants for combined osteosyntheses. The conditions at the cement/bone interface must, however, be described as less than ideal since, as already established, there is no bonding of the cement and bone. It is possible that the addition of powdered glass ceramic will bring an improvement. The favourable interface properties of the physiologically matched glass ceramic as proposed by Deutscher might well improve the fixation properties of the bone cement. The expectation behind this hope is that the glass ceramic particles in the secondarily polymerized PMMA matrix adhering to the free surface adjacent to the bone will form a firm bond with the newly formed bone tissue. The desirable solution to the fixation problem can only be a cement-free bonding of the prosthesis with the bone. This will, however, be realizable only through physiological fusion with the bone.

Future improvements can take account of the requirements and the criticisms set out here only if we can achieve a situation, in which scientists, engineers and doctors tackle the outstanding problems in close cooperation with one another. As a first step it will be necessary to set up a research and development program, using a language common to all three groups, that can serve as a working basis. We must here distinguish between tasks that can be dealt with in the short, middle and long term.

There are many pointers which suggest that in the short term, improvements can be achieved by employing the available prostheses optimally with respect to their specific design, and by actually taking into consideration the physical and polymer-chemical properties of bone cements. Model-specific indications for the multitude of available prostheses and the willingness on the part of the surgeon, in each and every case, first to analyze the joint problem presenting and then to implant the most suitable prosthesis, should bring a therapeutic advance.

Material developments specifically for applications in the field of highly-stressed joints are conceivable as an objective that may be attained in the middle-term. The investigations presently being carried out in many places, on the biological compatibility of various materials hold out the hope that we shall soon see a standardized test program for the testing of new developments. If known procedures and techniques are resolutely and systematically employed, the determination of mechanical and chemical properties of materials certainly represents no particular problem. Nevertheless, the interpretation of the results with respect to the clinical situation often presents difficulties.

In the long term, the development of new fixing mechanisms for the coupling of the implant to the bone, can be expected. Now that the biomechanical problems have been thoroughly examined, we still lack a materials-scientific and biological basis that would enable us to match the mechanical properties of the implant material to the biological structure of the bone. How successfully we shall meet this typically biomedical engineering requirement depends to no small extent, on how the communication between clinician, scientist and engineer develops in the future.

INDEX